ACS SYMPOSIUM SERIES **1115**

Galectins and Disease Implications for Targeted Therapeutics

Anatole A. Klyosov, Editor
Galectin Therapeutics, Inc.
Norcross, Georgia

Peter G. Traber, Editor
Galectin Therapeutics, Inc.
Norcross, Georgia

American Chemical Society, Washington, DC

Distributed in print by Oxford University Press

Library of Congress Cataloging-in-Publication Data

Galectins and disease implications for targeted therapeutics / Anatole A. Klyosov, editor, Galectin Therapeutics, Inc., Newton, Massachusetts, Peter G. Traber, editor, Galectin Therapeutics, Inc., Newton, Massachusetts.
pages cm. -- (ACS symposium series ; 1115)
Includes bibliographical references and index.
ISBN 978-0-8412-2880-1
1. Lectins--Therapeutic use. I. Klesov, A. A. (Anatolii Alekseevich) II. Traber, Peter G.
QP552.L42G354 2012
572′.69--dc23
2012042318

The paper used in this publication meets the minimum requirements of American National Standard for Information Sciences—Permanence of Paper for Printed Library Materials, ANSI Z39.48n1984.

Distributed in print by Oxford University Press

PRINTED IN THE UNITED STATES OF AMERICA

Foreword

The ACS Symposium Series was first published in 1974 to provide a mechanism for publishing symposia quickly in book form. The purpose of the series is to publish timely, comprehensive books developed from the ACS sponsored symposia based on current scientific research. Occasionally, books are developed from symposia sponsored by other organizations when the topic is of keen interest to the chemistry audience.

Before agreeing to publish a book, the proposed table of contents is reviewed for appropriate and comprehensive coverage and for interest to the audience. Some papers may be excluded to better focus the book; others may be added to provide comprehensiveness. When appropriate, overview or introductory chapters are added. Drafts of chapters are peer-reviewed prior to final acceptance or rejection, and manuscripts are prepared in camera-ready format.

As a rule, only original research papers and original review papers are included in the volumes. Verbatim reproductions of previous published papers are not accepted.

ACS Books Department

Contents

Galectin Mechanisms and Therapeutic Approaches in Cancer

Galectin Mechanisms and Therapeutic Approaches in Inflammation and Fibrosis

Indexes

Preface

Symposium ‘Galectin Function and Therapeutics’, which took place from September 17-19, 2012 in Boston, has had an important mission: to show the participants and the world where we stand with understanding galectins and their functions and the direct applications of galectin management in practical medicine.

This is a very complex and challenging issue. As is shown in Chapter 1, there are more than 3900 articles on galectins; on their structure and functions, published in academic literature since the middle of the 1990’s. Most of these papers came from academia. As a result, we have a very advanced science on galectins, 15 of which were identified; on their chemical structure, interactions of galectins with their ligands of both carbohydrate and peptide nature, (alleged) mechanisms of their intracellular and intercellular operations, interception of various biochemical processes, their expression and regulatory effects of the expression, etc. Significant amounts of work have been done with experimental animals, including knockout gal(-/-) mice, as well on effects of galectins and their inhibitors on experimental pathologies in mice, rats, dogs, monkeys. In a few instances galectin inhibitors (galectin blockers) are being tested in human clinical trials, or will be tested soon.

It all sounds very encouraging. However, a bird’s eye view at these vast research areas reveals a somewhat troubling, though not an unusual pattern. An observant eye will notice that the galectin-related field of science, which is essentially biomedical science, consists of four largely disconnected areas. They are connected by only one feature – galectins themselves, which is the main object of attention for the researchers. However, methodologically, by experimental design, by aims set, and by essence of conclusions advanced, these four areas are practically disconnected, and the translation of data and conclusions from one area to another is still in its infancy.

One area of research aims at studying isolated and purified galectins and their (desirably) specific inhibitors, that is galectin blockers. It has resulted in wonderful science. Great synthetic chemistry has been accomplished. Some very potent galectin blockers were designed, tested, and their (apparent) binding constants (actually, dissociation constants) have been measured; the best of which occur in the low nanomolar range (10-40 nM). However, those great numbers stay, as a rule, within that *in vitro* area. Commonly, they are not translated to the next (disconnected) area, which is essentially the cell biology of galectins.

The second area is comprised of studies into model cell systems, such as those focused on (alleged) galectin ligands and galectin interactions inside the cells, protein-carbohydrate and protein-protein interactions and recognitions. This is a highly sophisticated and advanced scientific endeavor, which brings about remarkable fundamental knowledge, particularly when produced by skillful hands and minds. However, the same galectin blockers, when tested in cell cultures, show much less impressive (apparent) binding constants, often some 10,000-100,000 times less efficient, that is in the high micromolar range (100-600 μM). In other words, something is not right with the translation from the purified galectins to the intra- and/or extracellular galectins. Could it be that in the "chemical" system we study the effects of direct galectin blockers, and in the cellular system we study the effect of the same galectin blockers but at the output of the "rate-limiting" signaling system? Or maybe *in vitro* we study the "wrong binding", with a "wrong binding site", albeit very tight, while *in vivo* we see only those types of binding which produce specific biological effects which we actually observe and measure? This effect is well known in enzyme kinetics, for example, where it is called "non-productive binding". Probably it could be, however, it is seemingly beyond the current research interest. Maybe because of that the areas are sufficiently disconnected.

The thoughts described above do not appear to be some groundless suggestions. In 2009 the Glycobiology journal published a paper "The α-galactomannan Davanat binds galectin-1 at a site different from the conventional galectin carbohydrate binding domain". Then, another paper was published in the same 2009, now in Biochemical Journal, entitled "The carbohydrate-binding domain on galectin-1 is more extensive for a complex glycan than for simple saccharides…". It is hard to tell how significant those findings might be for other galectins and for their *in vivo* effects. However, it should be noticed here, that for the polymer α-galactomannan the translation between *in vitro* and *in vivo* effects, including those in human clinical trials, is appear to be more direct. For said polymer-based galactomannan its apparent K_d *in vitro* (with purified galectin-1 and -3) is 0.9 and 0.2 mg/mL, respectively, while in humans the galactomannan dose in the clinical trials was 0.5 mg/mL (280 mg/m^2, that is 7 mg/kg, or 0.5 mg/mL of blood, taking 7% for the amount of blood in humans, which is about the same 7% in the rats). With mice, the employed dose of the galactomannan was 120 mg/kg (Preclinica, 2003), that is 2.5 mg/mouse, or about the same 0.5 mg/mL of blood.

It seems that a careful consideration of data obtained with low-molecular and high-molecular galectin blockers as drug candidates might shed more light on translational regularities for *in vitro* - *in vivo* systems.

The third area is associated with animal experiments and attempts to handle the respective galectin management *in vivo*. Terms such as "intracellular signaling", "cross-linking by galectins of the cell surface receptors", "segregated membrane microdomains", "galectins in pre-mRNA splicing" are "left behind", in the preceding area of cell studies. They are not used in work with experimental animals and in the respective data interpretations. A galectin blocker is administered by one or other means, and a readout such is commonly tumor shrinkage, reduction of a pathological manifestation, such as liver fibrosis stage and grade, portal blood pressure, biomarker levels, etc., is recorded. Translation of the cellular data from the "preceding" area to experimental animals is commonly absent. A mode of administration of a galectin blocker, such as IV, IP, sub-Q, oral, often (or always) rules a significant part of the outcome of the animal experiments.

The "highest" in that hierarchy, the fourth area, concerns human clinical trials. Some translation from the preceding level is obvious, such as with respect to toxicity of the galectin blocker. If it is toxic in experimental animals, it is automatically assumed to be toxic in humans, and it is commonly so. Efficacy of the galectin blocker is hard to translate from animal to man, and these data are practically absent. Hence, the disconnection again. Even the dosages are hard to translate from the animals to humans, and mg/kg in animals is now often mg/m2 (typically in cancer patients) in humans, being recalculated using some standard coefficients. Again, the mode of administration (IV, IP, sub-Q, oral) and bioavailability of the drug (if not administered IV) can completely change the pattern of the drug behavior in the human body.

Without telling examples, what is said above can appear to be just some theorization (except the example with the galactomannan polysaccharide *in vitro* and *in vivo*, on mice and humans, presented above). However, it is not a unique situation related only to galectins and galectin blockers. It is a rather common situation in biomedicine and drug design, when translation is often difficult to achieve.

At this point I would recall when – a long time ago - I was working with alcoholdehydrogenase (ADH) in a laboratory at Harvard Medical School, using ethanol as the principal substrate for the enzyme. It seemed strange that the highest amount of ADH was found in the horse liver, since horses were not known as heavy drinkers of alcohol. Soon, however, I learned that ethanol was not the "right" substrate for ADH in most of mammals; though a very standard one in biochemical studies. Some steroids were right substrates for ADH. Therefore, ethanol would not have been a good choice for translational studies, unless we specifically consider ethanol for the translation. By the way, octanol (with eight carbon atoms in the molecule), which is thousands of times better substrate of ADH compared to ethanol, would not have been a right substrate either for translational studies. So, being good is not necessarily being right in that area.

Following are some specific examples with respect to galectins:

Thiodigalactoside diesters TD131 and TD139 are very potent inhibitors of galectin-3 with an estimated K_d of 30-50 nM (Nilsson, Leffler et al, see Chapter 2 in this book), that is approximately 0.00002-0.00003 mg/mL. This value has been determined employing competitive fluorescence polarization assays, apparently via competition with lactose and/or other standard low-molecular weight ligands, that is the binding was to the "conventional binding site" in the galectin. An attempt to translate this binding constant to mice via IP (intraperitoneal) injection led to injection of 0.3 mg of the inhibitor to mouse (Hepatology, 2012), that was approximately 10,000-15,000 times higher concentration compared to the above K_d value. In cell culture experiments the biological effect was reached at the amount of the inhibitor 100-600 μM, that is 0.06-0.40 mg/mL, or 3,000-15,000 times higher concentration compared to the above K_d value. The apparent K_d in the cell culture, which was measured as IC_{50}, that is a concentration of the compound which results in the 50% inhibitory (or other biological) effect, was 300 μM, or 5,000-10,000 higher compared with the K_d in vitro. Taking into account what was said above about two binding sites at some (or all?) galectins, it might be suggested that small molecular weight galectin inhibitors first saturate the tightly binding "non-productive" site (which binds with the K_d in a sub-μM and even low nM range), and only then, at concentrations of the inhibitor of ~ 10,000 times higher, they begin to occupy the second, "right" binding site of the galectin. Galectin-based polysaccharides, however, bind to the "right" substrate in the first place, and, being not so tight inhibitors, match the low-molecular weight inhibitors with their efficacy *in vivo*. This apparent match in efficacy might turn out for the low-molecular weight galectin blockers to be an impressive mismatch in the price of the drug candidate and its toxicity. This, of course, has to be studied in detail.

These considerations are given here, in the preface of the book, to tune the reader to the complexity of the therapy-related issues described in various chapters of this book. The most important mission of the Symposium was in realizing this complexity not only from the fundamental standpoint, but also – and foremost – in terms of the potential therapeutic applications of galectin-related therapy.

The above were just quick examples showing that the translation from *in vitro* to *in vivo* data needs to be addressed more attentively. Right now a choice of galectin blockers for studies in galectin therapy is highly empirical, on strictly a "trial and error" basis. The overall aim of the Symposium was to consider the situation and offer some directions to make the search for the right galectin blockers more justified and stemming from *in vitro* experimental data, if possible. To show that it is not possible, if it turned out that way, would also be a step in the right direction, meaning that we cannot rely on data obtained with purified galectins. This will save the biomedicinal industry time and money. To forego many *in vitro* data on galectins would not be the best outcome, at least for the time being. However, it would spare us from hopes based on wrong experimental systems. We are not there yet, and that is why we need translational data as described above.

Leo Tolstoy wrote in the first line of his "Anna Karenina" – "Happy families are all alike in their happiness; every unhappy family is unhappy in its own way". I would dare to say that happy drugs are all alike in their happiness, while every unhappy drug is unhappy in its own way.

Anatole A. Klyosov
Galectin Therapeutics, Inc.
4960 Peachtree Industrial Blvd., Suite 240
Norcross, Georgia 30071

Overview

Chapter 1

Galectins in Disease and Potential Therapeutic Approaches

Anatole A. Klyosov* and Peter G. Traber*

Galectin Therapeutics, Inc., 4960 Peachtree Industrial Blvd., Suite 240, Norcross, Georgia 30071
***E-mail: klyosov@galectintherapeutics.com (A.A.K); Traber@galectintherapeutics.com (P.G.T.)**

The Galectin protein family includes 15 members that are characterized by galactose binding domains and are widely expressed in diverse cell types. Galectins are found in multiple intracellular compartments and are secreted into the extracelluar space. There has been an explosion in information on these fascinating proteins in pathological states, particularly inflammation, fibrosis, and cancer. This book, in conjunction with an international conference, attempts to cover the key areas of galectin-dependent disease and review the approaches to developing pharmaceutical approaches to treatment. The time is right for major efforts to advance galectin-based therapies into multiple human diseases.

Introduction

The term "galectins" was coined only 18 years ago (*1*), and for the preceding 15 years (see Figure 1) scientists had been reporting on what they called "galactose-binding proteins". Over the last decade there has been a near exponential increase in the yearly publication rate of research papers on galectins (Figure 1). By August 2012, the number of publications on galectins reached 3776.

The number of pubications and the important findings for biology and disease has led to a general recognition that galectins are an important class of molecules for multiple pathological processes and potential targets for therapy.

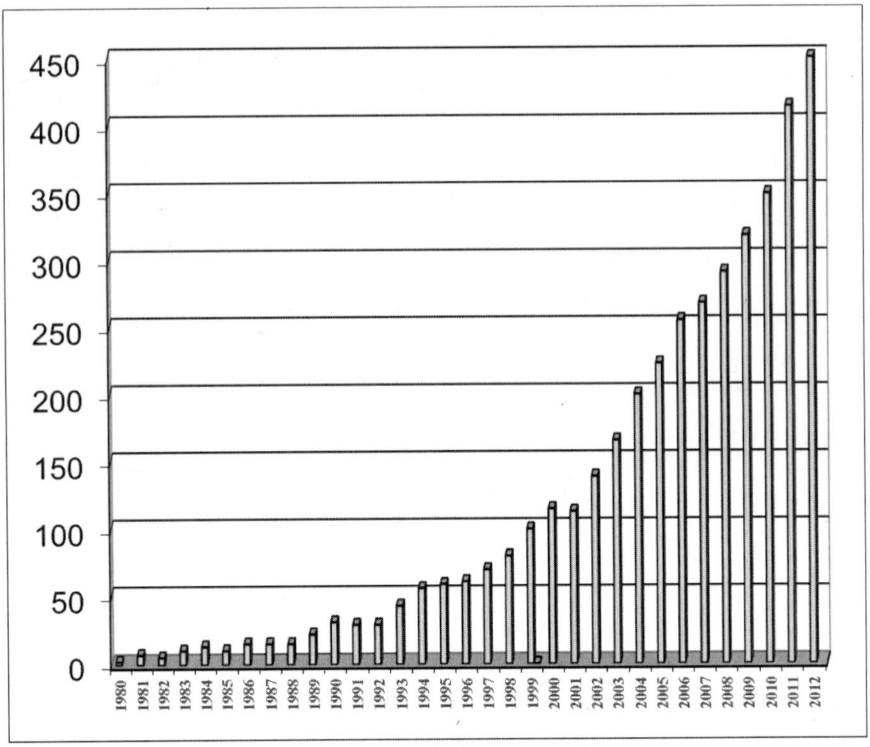

Figure 1. PubMed (U.S. National Library of Medicine, Medical Institutes of Health) records on academic publications on galectins, total 3776 by August 1, 2012. Data for 2012 are projected.

Galectins as a group are characterized by a galactose-specific carbohydrate binding domain which interacts with galactose moieties located on glycoproteins. Nature has created as many as 15 different galectins, known today, which have already been identified, isolated, and in some cases characterized – structurally and functionally (*2*). In addition to cellular glycoproteins, all galectins show an affinity for galactose residues attached to other organic compounds, such as in lactose [(β-D-Galactosido)-D-glucose], N-acetyl-lactosamine, poly-N-acetyllactosamine, galactomannans, fragments of pectins, as well as others. Galactose by itself does not bind to galectins, or binds so weakly that the binding can hardly be detected. Galectins also have domains which promote homodimerization. Thus, they are capable of acting as a "molecular glue" of sorts between glycoproteins. Galectins are found in multiple cellular compartments, including the nucleus and cytoplasm, and are secreted into the extracellular space where they interact with cell surface and extracellular matrix glycoproteins. The mechanism of molecular interactions depends on the localization. While galectins interact with glycoproteins in the extracellular space, in the intracellular space the interactions with other proteins occurs via protein domains (Chapter 4). In the extracellular space the association of cell surface receptors may increase or decrease receptor signaling or the ability to interact with ligands. Additionally, galectins may promote cell-cell and cell-matrix interactions. Because of the critical importance of the interaction of glycoproteins and cells for tissue function, it is no wonder that galectins have been ascribed a plethora of functions in cellular and animal models.

The collective literature shows that galectins are instrumental to many crucial biological and pathobiological functions, such as inflammation, angiogenesis (blood supply, including that to cancer tumor cells), immune response (they were shown to turn off the "friend or foe" immune recognition system), cancer cell migration (leading to metastasis), and many others.

With respect to targeting galectins for therapy of disease, we believe that the understanding of biology and pathology associated with galectins is coming of age. In several disease areas there is sufficient evidence to suggest that targeting galectins may have an efficacious effect on disease processes. One of the primary reasons for this is that galectins are normally expressed in relatively low levels but are markedly increased in disease states such as cancer, inflammation and fibrosis. Therefore, a strategy to knock down expression or function may be effective while not interferring with normal basal function. If the past decade can be described as the decade of galectin function discovery, the coming decade may be the decade of the realization of galectin targeting therapeutics.

While there are a number of biotechnology companies in the early phases of developing galectin targeted therapeutics, programs in large pharmaceutical companies are either early and not yet visible to the public or non-existent. While we believe this will change over the next few years, there are a number of reasons for this situation:

- Galectin targeting therapeutics is in the very early stages and there is as yet no convincing evidence of efficacy in a human disease. The pharmaceutical industry likes proven targets and once there is evidence of an effect in human disease, acivity will increase.
- Galectins, as with many other lectins, present a challenge to researchers in terms of quantitative description of ligand-receptor interactions, which is density-dependent when glycan epitopes are located on the surface of cells. In other words, a quantitative description for galectin-cell interactions should include the density and number of glycan epitopes on the surface of cells, as well as the dissociation constant (K_d) that is not a single, well-defined (at least in theory) value as with respect to monovalent glycans in solution, but a relative $K_{d\,(eff)}$ value that includes density and number of epitopes on the cell surface (*3*).
- A number of the current galectin targeting approaches utilize complex carbohydrate drugs which are not common in the industry and do not have tried and true regulatory pathways.

Galectins in Human Diseases

The majority of the 3776 papers on galectins are academic studies that invsestigate various aspects of galectin structure and function without a focus on a particular disease. Very few address pharmacological approaches to galectin targeting therapies. In order to analyze the published papers with respect to human diseases and pathologies, we have considered the most recent thousand articles, from July 2012 back through August 2007, and broke them into categories according to diseases and pathologies. In more than one-third of those articles certain diseases and pathologies have been mentioned. Table 1 lists the number of publications according to PubMed in which a specific disease was identified and galectins were mentioned in association with the disease (in the order of that number). Some diseases might be combined under more general names, however, we prefer to be more specific at the expense of extending the list. The many diseases that have been linked to galectins underlies the pleotropic function of these proteins. There are a number of groupings that fall out of examining this list, with cancer, inflammation, fibrosis, and immune function being prominent.

Table 1. Number of publications according to PubMed in which a specific disease was identified and galectins were mentioned in association with the disease[a]

1. Thyroid carcinoma	63	14. Follicular thyroid adenomas/carcinomas	10
2. Colorectal/gastric cancer/adenoma	54	15. Ovarian cancer	10
3. Heart failure/myocardial dysfunction/injury	42	16. Cancer, carcinoma (non-specified)	10
4. Breast cancer	37	17. Hepatocellular carcinoma	9
5. Papillary thyroid carcinoma	31	18. Asthma/lung inflammation	9
6. Pancreatic cancer/ adenocarcinoma	25	19. Pituitary tumors/ adenocarcinoma/blastoma	9
7. Melanoma	22	20. Spinal cord injury	9
8. Rheumatoid arthritis/ osteoarthritis	21	21. Bladder cancer	7
9. Oral/laryngeal squamous cell carcinoma	20	22. Liver fibrosis	7
10. Prostate cancer/ adenocarcinoma	16	23. Lung cancer/non-small cell lung cancer	7
11. Diabetes	13	24. Renal carcinoma	7
12. Glioma-associated cancer/glioblastoma	12	25. Myelogeneous leukemia	5
13. Preeclampsia	11	26. Ischemia (non-specified)	5

Continued on next page.

Table 1. (Continued). Number of publications according to PubMed in which a specific disease was identified and galectins were mentioned in association with the disease[a]

27. HIV-1	5	51. Gynecological cancer	2
28. Lymphoid malignancies/ lymphomas	4	52. Lymphocytic leukemia	2
29. Human cervical (epithelial) adenocarcinoma	4	53. Nasal polyposis	2
30. Multiple sclerosis	4	54. Cartilage tumor	2
31. Ophthalmology	4	55. Lymphoblastic leukemias	2
32. Nasopharyngeal carcinoma	4	56. Adenoid cystic carcinoma	2
33. Renal fibrosis	4	57. Servical squamous cell carcinoma	2
34. NASH	4	58. Celiac disease	2
35. Lung diseases/pneumonia	3	59. Amyotrophic lateral sclerosis	2
36. Neuroblastoma	3	60. Hodgkin lymphoma	2
37. Myeloma, multiple myeloma	3	61. Chronic lymphocytic leukemia	2
38. Lupus erythematosus	3	62. Malignant pheochromocytoma	2
39. Brain cancer	3	63. Cystic fibrosis	2
40. Cholangiocarcinoma	3	64. Parathyroid carcinoma	2
41. Hypoxic-ischemic brain injury	3	65. Glaucoma	2
42. Malignant mesothelioma	3	66. Tongue carcinoma	2
43. Head and neck cancer	2	67. Invasive globular carcinoma	2
44. Ulcer/ulcerative colitis	2	68. Cardiomyopathy	2
45. T-cell leukemia/lymphoma	2	69. Renal ischemia	2
46. Venous thrombosis	2	70. Carcinomas of the endometrium	2
47. Cancer vaccines	2	71. Liver ischemia	2
48. Malaria	2	72. Diabetic nephropathy	2
49. Chondrosarcoma	2	73. Cutaneous melanoma	2
50. Trypanoso	2	74. Forebrain ischemia	1

Continued on next page.

Table 1. (Continued). Number of publications according to PubMed in which a specific disease was identified and galectins were mentioned in association with the disease[a]

75. Nasal papillomamiasis	101. Eosinophilic pneumonia
76. Intestinal inflammation	102. Cell carcinoma
77. Proliferative vitreoretinopathy	103. Leiomyosarcoma
78. Hepatitis C	104. Endometrioid adenocarcinoma
79. Invasive trophoblasts	105. Large cell lymphoma
80. Liver cancer	106. Testicular cancer
81. Kaposi's sarcoma	107. Thyroiditis
82. Invasive pathogens	108. Ductal adenocarcinoma
83. Pilocytic astrocytomas	109. Myeloid leukemia
84. Peripheral nerve injury	110. Leukemia (non-specified)
85. Psoriasis/skin inflammation	111. Ischemic stroke
86. Atopic dermatitis	112. Salivary gland tumor
87. Encephalomyelitis	113. Ulcerative colitis
88. Cystic tumors of the pancreas	114. Crohn's disease
89. Nephritis	115. Acute kidney injury
90. Renal injury	116. Liver cirrhosis
91. Venereal diseases	117. Encephalitis
92. Intestinal fibrosis	118. Cardiac toxicity (non-specified)
93. Digestive diseases	119. Behcet's disease
94. Parkinson's disease	120. GVH disease
95. Malignant endothelia	121. Serous carcinomas
96. Corticotroph adenomas	122. Cerebral ischemia
97. Pneumococcal meningitis	123. Choriocarcinoma
98. Esophageal cancer	124. Fibrosis (non-specified)
99. Connective tissue disease	125. Insulin allergy
100. Histocytic sarcoma	126. Spindle cell oncocytoma

[a] (Diseases from number 75 through 126 have been found to be described in one paper each).

Galectins in Cancer

It is clear from the literature that galectin proteins are increased in expression in the majority of cancers and they serve a variety of functions in cancer cell biology ((*4–6*) and references therein). When considering functions in cancer, a critical issue is whether the functional locations of the galectin proteins are intracellular or extracellular. This has important implications related to fundamental function, but also the ability to target galectin function with therapeutic agents. Intracelluar functions in cancer related to apoptosis and signaling have been described ((*7*) and references therein). The Figure 2 shows the major areas in cancer biology where galectins may function in the extracellular environment.

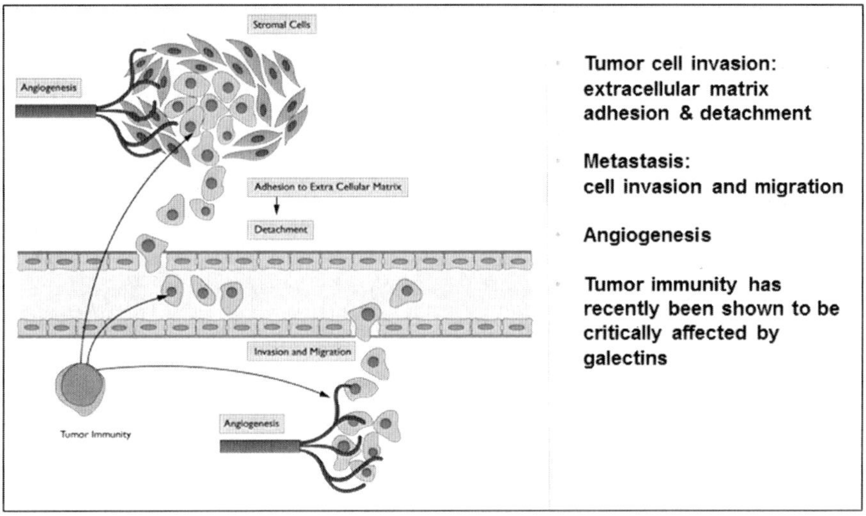

Figure 2. The major areas in cancer biology where galectins may function in the extracellular environment. (see color insert)

The importance of galectins for tumor cell invasion and metastasis has been reviewed extensively ((*8–10*) and references therein). Additionally, it has been well documented that galectin proteins, in particular galectin 1 and galectin 3, are markedly increased in expression in cancer cells and contribute to the pathogenesis of tumor progression ((*4–10*) and references therein).

This volume has a number of chapters which review and extend our knowledge on how galectins function in cancer. Chapters 9, 10, 11, 14, and 17 review the role of galectins in melanoma, glioma, breast cancer, leukemia, and myeloma, respectively. Analysis of these cancers hightlight the variety of functions of galectins in cancers. Chapter 12 reviews the potential use of a truncated galectin-3 protein, Galectin-3C, as a treatment for cancers, which also reveals potential functions of galectins in cancer. Chapter 18 reviews approaches for using galectin targeting for prevention of cancer metastases.

Tumor Angiogenesis

Tumor growth depends on a continuous blood supply to deliver oxygen, nutrients, and other biologically important factors to the tumor. The growth of new capillaries from preexisting blood vessels is called neovascularization or angiogenesis, which is a complex process involving endothelial cell activation, disruption of vascular basement membranes, proliferation of endothelial cells and their migration. This multistep cellular process, the molecular machinery, leading to growth of new vessels into the tumor, hence, tumor angiogenesis, is dependent on a number of galectins, among them galectin-1, -2, -3, -4, -8, which presumably play important roles in mediating cell-cell and cell-matrix interactions. Chapter 13 reviews the role of galectins in tumor angiogenesis and the potential of targeting galectins for therapy.

For example, galectin-1-null mice showed much slower tumor growth because of reduced tumor angiogenesis. Galectin-3 stimulates capillary tube formation *in vitro* and angiogenesis *in vivo*. It has been shown that vessel walls of normal lymphoid tissues do not express galectin-1, while blood vessel walls of lymphomas express it in relation to their vascular density. These and other relevant data are reviewed in (*11*, *12*), as well as in other recent articles. A study (*13*) notes: "Recent studies have shown that a carbohydrate-binding protein, galectin-3, is a novel pro-angiogenic molecule. The mechanism by which galectin-3 promotes angiogenesis remains unknown". In the follow-up study (*14*) the authors confirmed that angiogenesis is heavily influenced by VEGF-A and by VEGF receptor 2 (VEGF-R2), which is glycosylated like most cell surface proteins, although, as the authors mentioned, the function of VEGF-R2 with respect to its glycosylation pattern is poorly characterized. The authors have shown that galectin-3 interacts with the EGF and TGFβ receptors, retaining them on the plasma membrane and altering their signal transduction via phosphorylation of VEGF-R2 in endothelial cells. The authors concluded that galectin-3 contributes to the plasma membrane retention and proangiogenic function of VEGF-R2.

Another review (*10*) has noted that "galectin-3 is an important regulator of a broad range of cancer cell activities and plays important roles in cancer cell growth, transformation, apoptosis, angiogenesis, adhesion, invasion and metastasis. Such a divergent influence of galectin-3 on cancer cell activities derives from its multiple inter- and sub-cellular localizations where it interacts with a range of different binding partners".

It was also shown that galectin-3 promotes adhesion of disseminating tumor cells to vascular endothelium *in vitro* and experimental metastasis *in vivo*. Furthermore, the presence of galectin-2, -3, -4, and -8 enhances cancer-endothelial adhesion by interaction with the TF epitope (Gal-β-1,3GalNAc α-) disaccharide on cancer-associated MUC1 glycan and promote cancer-endothelial adhesion (*15*).

Nearly this same group of galectins (galectins-1, -3, -4, and -8) are expressed in human colon and rectal cancer, and upregulated during colorectal cancer development and metastasis. Their upregulation has been correlated with cancer cell growth, apoptosis, and angiogenesis (*16*).

Galectin-8 is a rather common target when deciphering the angiogenesis-related process, and it was suggested to be one of the "pro-angiogenic" lectins. Galectin-8 is a bivalent "tandem-repeat"-type galectin, whose two carbohydrate-recognition domains are connected covalently by a linker peptide. This galectin is expressed both in the cytoplasm and nucleus in endothelial cells of normal and tumor vessels; hence, it might play an essential role in the regulation of angiogenesis in general and tumor angiogenesis in particular (*17*).

Recently, it was shown that tumor cells can stimulate tumor angiogenesis by secretion of galectin-1 in wild-type mice; however, this effect is hampered in galectin-1-null mice (*18*). The authors concluded that galectin-1 is a pro-angiogenic factor.

A significant study describing the role of galectin-1 in angiogenesis and immune dysregulation in murine cancer was recently published (*19*). It was shown that galectin-1 is a tumor promoting protein produced by cancer cells, and that the low-molecular weight galectin blocker, thiodigalactoside (TDG), a non-metabolized drug candidate, suppressed tumor growth, angiogenesis, immune cell dysregulation. Furthermore, intra-tumoral (B16F10 melanoma and breast cancer model) injection of TDG significantly increased the level of tumor-infiltrating CD8+ lymphocytes, and TDG treatment of tumors in nude mice, defective in T cell immunity, reduced angiogenesis and slowed tumor growth by ~ 30% less than in immunocompetent mice. At the same time, Dings et al. (*20*) showed that anti-angiogenic compounds could also enhance T-cell mediated anti-tumor responses and function as angiostatic adjuvants to immunotherapy against cancer. These are apparently the first cases demonstrating that low-molecular weight galectin-1 blockers are potential immune system modulating anti-cancer agents.

Tumor Immunology

A growing literature shows that the recognition and killing of tumor cells by the cellular immune system is modulated by galectins. In a seminal paper for the field, Pierre Van der Bruggen and his colleagues have shown that galectin-3 has a critical effect on tumor specific CD8+ cells (*21*). They showed that in the presence of galectin-3, cytotoxic T cells lose the colocalization of the T-cell receptor and CD8, which results in relative anergy of the T cells when confronted with tumor antigen. The function of CD8+ cells and the TCR-CD8 colocalization was restored when galectin ligands were added. This has led to the hypothesis that tumor secreted galectin-3 binds to cytotoxic T cells and renders them anergic, unable to kill tumor cells. A summary of this "galectin effect" as described by the van der Bruggen group is illustrated in the Figure 3 and reviewed in Chapter 16.

Galectin-1 has also been shown to be important in modulating cellular immunity to tumor cells. In an elegant set of experiments using knockout mice and syngeneic tumors with variable galectin-1 expression, it was shown that tumor associated expression of galectin-1 was involved in mediating tumor progression through intratumoral immunomodulation (*22*). It is possible that other galectins are involved in modulating the cellular immune response to tumors and it appears that inhibition of galectins may be an approach to enhance tumor killing by cytotoxic T cells.

Another example of this immunomodulatory effect is in malignant glioma. Malignant gliomas are the most common primary brain tumors. A clinical prognosis in those pathologies is rather bleak, making an average survival time around one year in unselected series ((*23*), and references therein). The immune response of the patients typically is not effective, due to high migratory capacity of the brain tumor and its aggressive growth. It was suggested that a number of galectins, such as galectin-1, -3, -4, and -8 contribute to malignant gliomas growth and resistance against antineoplastic therapy (ibid.). In an earlier work the authors have provided evidence of a role of galectin-1 in the regulation of glioma cell proliferation and migration (*24*). The authors concluded that targeting galectin-1 (and possibly other galectins) may have therapeutic benefits in the treatment of malignant glioma. Robert Kiss and his Laboratory of Experimental Immunology in Leuven, Belgium, continue to uncover the role of galectin-1 in immunotherapy for brain cancer as an important player in glioma-mediated immune escape (*25–27*). It was shown that galectin-1 is abundantly expressed in high-grade glioma, and active specific immunotherapy by dendritic cell vaccination apparently generates an anti-tumoral immune response, when accompanied by down-regulation of counteracting tolerogenic signals (*27*), see also (*28–32*).

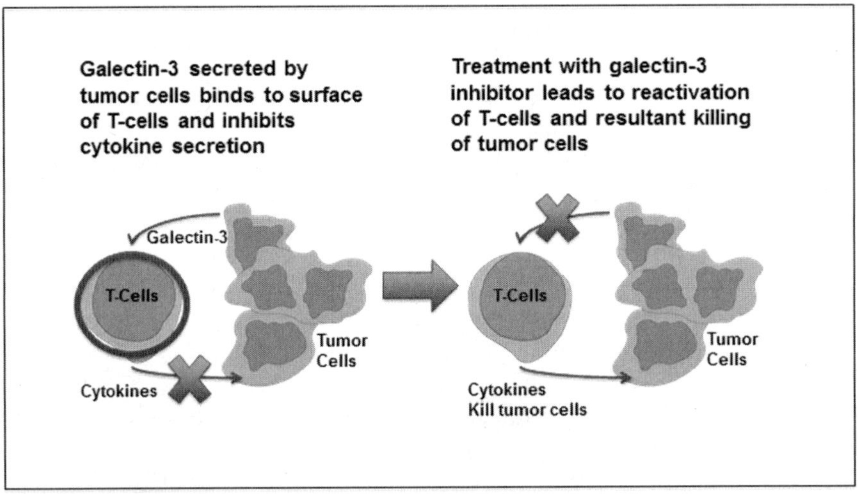

Figure 3. The "galectin effect", illustrating the hypothesis that tumor-secreted galectin-3 binds to cytotoxic T cells and renders them anergic, unable to kill tumor cells. (see color insert)

We believe there is the potential for galectin inhibition to play a key role in the burgeoning area of cancer immunotherapy. For example, there have been two recent approvals of drugs for using the patient's immune system to fight cancer, Provenge (Dendreon; a dendritic cell tumor vaccine) and Yervoy (BMC; a monoclonal inhibitor of CTLA4 which activates cytotoxic T-cells). There are many additional vaccines and immune stimulatory agents in development. An effective galectin targeting agent that enhances the immune system's ability to fight cancer would be a complementary approach to these tumor immunotherapies. Chapter 16 describes an ongoing clinical trial that aims to evaluate an anti-galectin thereapy, GM-CT-01, in combination with a peptide vaccine in metastatic melanoma.

Galectins in Inflammation, Immune Cell Function, and Fibrosis

The process of inflammation and repair involves multiple cell types including cells of the immune system and many inflammatory mediators in a complex and interconnected cascade of events. Acute inflammation can be terminated or progress to a chronic phase which may lead to fibrosis. The enormous complexity of this process cannot be summarized in this review, but we evaluate some of the data related to the components of inflammation, immune cell function, and fibrosis. It should be stated up front that separating these three only facilitates discussion because the processes in tissues are all intertwined.

Inflammation

Acute inflammation is a critical defense mechanism against invading pathogens and tissue damage. When inflammation becomes chronic, systemically or locally, multiple pathologies ensue with negative consequences. Most of the information on galectins involvement in inflammation results from studies of chronic inflammatory models. However, as discussed in Chapter 19 (A therapeutic role for galectins in acute inflammation?), galectins also play a role in acute inflammation, particularly galectin-1, 3, and 9.

Multiple studies show that galectins are important in regulating chronic inflammatory responses; however, the current data do not provide a clear picture. Some galectins appear to suppress responses of inflammatory cells, while some galectins stimulate and promote them. It seems that the specific effect of a galectin depends on the targeted cell, its microenvironment (such as a pattern of the specific glycosylation of target cells), and the inflammatory stimulus. It has been suggested that differing results may be related to the fact that studies are performed *in vitro* which employ recombinant galectins, typically lacking certain portions of the protein (*33*). Where more relevant studies were conducted, for instance, with galectin-3-null mice, it was found that galectin-3 promotes inflammatory responses (reviewed by Liu et al, in (*34*)). Much of the confusion in the field is likely related to the relevancy of *in vitro* models and non-physiological proteins and concentrations. Chapter 21 reviews relevant data in intack animal models of multiple inflammatory diseases. This analysis begins to unwind the stories of galectin involvement in chronic inflammatory disorders.

In a number of cases, galectins can accompany inflammatory responses, and often it is hard to determine whether the appearance of galectins (as an elevated expression) post-injury is causal or a biomarker. For example, spinal cord injury in rats induces secondary tissue damage that is associated with inflammation, and up to six months post-injury a cluster of genes (including galectin-3) has been reported to show elevated expression in macrophages. The authors (*35*) concluded that "inflammation-related genes are chronically up-regulated after spinal cord injury".

In another interesting line of work, it appears that polymorphisms in galectin molecules may be important in chronic inflammatory processes. It was shown that it is not just galectin-3 that contributes to development of rheumatoid arthritis (RA), but it may be related to its polymorphic forms (*36*). Indeed in synovium of RA, an elevated expression of galectin-3 has been found; however, the allelic carriage of LGALS3 +292C was increased in RA patients (151 RA patients and 182 healthy subjects as control) from 66.9% in RA vs. 52.7% in control. The two polymorphic forms (SNP) of galectin-3 gene were located at rs4644 and rs4652 sites in the DNA. Another study (*37*) showed that galectin-3 is present in the inflamed synovium in patients with rheumatoid arthritis, and plays a pathogenic role in the development and progression of antigen-induced arthritis. The authors showed that the joint inflammation and bone erosion in mice were markedly suppressed in galectin-3 null mice as compared with wild-type mice. The reduced arthritis in galectin-3 null mice was accompanied by decreased levels of proinflammatory cytokines.

Henderson and Sethi (*38*) noted that galectin-3 is a specific regulator of many biological systems, including inflammation. For example, in acute tissue damage, galectin-3 is a key component in the host defense against microbes, such as *Streptococcus pneumoniae*. However, if tissue injury becomes repetitive, galectin-3 also appears to be involved in the transition to chronic inflammation, facilitating the walling off of tissue injury with fibrogenesis and organ scarring. Therefore galectin-3 can be viewed as a regulatory molecule acting at various stages along the continuum from acute inflammation to chronic inflammation and tissue fibrogenesis.

According to Norling et al (*39*), evidence is accruing that indicates that galectins fall into a category of immunoregulatory mediators, signifying their potential as prospective novel anti-inflammatory agents. In their review, they describe the immunoregulatory bioactivities of three members of the galectin superfamily, galectin-1, -3 and -9. As the authors emphasize, these galectins are emerging as pertinent players in the modulation of acute and chronic inflammatory diseases, autoimmunity and cancer, and thus are being increasingly recognized as molecular targets for innovative drug discovery. These findings arc further explored in Chapters 19 and 20.

Wound healing is the critical end process of the inflammatory cascade. The role of galectins in wound healing is reviewed in Chapter 26.

Immune Cells

While immune cells are critcally involved in the inflammatory process, it is useful to look directly at the effects of galectins on individual effector and regulatory cells of the immune system. The function of galectins with respect to immune cells is complex and, at times appears contradictory. It appears that the function varies depending on the source and stage of immune activation. Some galectins can disable T cells by inducing apoptosis. For example, galectin-1 induces apoptosis in activated human T cells, apparently through the binding to T cell surface glycoproteins, such as CD7, CD43, and CD45. This mechanism may be concentration dependent and has not been observed by all investigators.

A recent study (*40*) identified galectin-1 as an intracellular binding partner of Bam32, the B lymphocyte adaptor molecule which is strongly induced during human dendritic cell maturation. These authors noted that galectin-1 demonstrates many immunological activities, among them regulating immune responses via regulatory T cells modulation. Galectin-1 is also an important element along with its immunoregulatory activity in controlling immune cell trafficking, dendritic cell physiology, and T-cell fate (*41*).

Galectin-9 plays a role in a murine acute lung injury by preferentially suppressing macrophage function to release pro-inflammatory cytokines through down-regulation of Toll-like receptors. In those experiments, mice were pretreated with galectin-9 by subcutaneous injection prior to intranasal LPS inoculation, and the authors found that galectin-9 suppresses pathological changes in acute lung-injured mice by reducing levels of pro-inflammatory cytokines and chemokines, such as tumor necrosis factor (TNF)-α, IL-1b, IL-6, decreased neutrophils, and increased IL-10 (*42*).

Galectin-9 has also been shown to bind T cell Ig mucin-3 (Tim-3) expressed on different cells which triggers T cell death and activates innate immune cells. The authors found some evidence that two carbohydrate recognition domains of galectin-9 (N- and C-terminal regions) have different activities in promoting T-cell death (*43*).

Chapters 6 and 7 present intriguing approaches to modulating T cells. Chapter 6 describes the role of a cross-linking GM1 ganglioside in the suppression of autoimmune disorders. Chapter 7 describes the use of fluiorinated glucosamine analogs to enhance the activity of anti-tumor T cells.

Fibrosis

Chronic inflammation in organs often leads to an accumulation of fibrotic tissue. In fact, the end result of inflammation from multiple underlying etiologies is fibrosis and resultant organ dysfunction. This is evident in lung, heart, kidney, pancreas, and liver. Multiple lines of evidence point to galectin proteins, and galectin-3 in particular, as critical in the pathogenesis of organ fibrosis. The best evidence in this regard comes from experiments in knockout mice. Galectin-3 null mice are resistant to fibrosis of the liver in response to hepatotoxins, lung fibrosis in response to intrathecal bleomycin , kidney and heart fibrosis, and chronic pancreatitis (for review see (*38*)). This important area of pathology is reviewed in Chapter 22 (Galectin-3: A central regulator of chronic inflammation and tissue fibrosis). In addition, a novel mechanism for the activation of stellate cells in the liver, the primary fibrogenic cell in the liver, is discussed in Chapter 23 (The role of galectin-3 in stellate cell activation and liver fibrosis).

An important liver diease that results in fibrosis is non-alcoholic steatohepatitis (NASH). Fatty liver and NASH with liver fibrosis, which was invariably detected in galectin-3 (+/+) mice on a high fat diet, was much less pronounced and was found in only 38% of these galectin-3 null mice (*44*). Taken together, these data suggest that galectin-3 is an attractive therapeutic target for liver fibrosis that occurs as a result of multiple liver diseases as well as fibrotic conditions in multiple organs.

Cardiovascular Disease

Atherosclerosis is and inflammatory lipid accumulation in arterial vessels which is the cause of a huge burden of morbidity and mortality world wide. Chapters 5, 22 and 24 review the roles of galectins in atherosclerosis, representing a potentially new approach to this disease.

Heart failure is generally defined as a failure of the heart to supply sufficient blood volume to meet the requirements of the body. Heart failure is the result of myocardial injury or hemodynamic overload, which goes beyond mechanical dysfunction; heart failure is associated with a number of pathophysiologic mechanisms, including inflammation, tissue remodeling, endocrine signaling, and interactions with the renal and nervous systems; it is the result of interplay of a number of biochemical factors, collectively referred to a biomarkers.

A series of studies (*45–54*) have convincingly showed an importance of galectin-3 in heart failure and mortality. Chapter 24 reviews data that shows galectin-3 is important in heart fibrosis and failure and may be an important target for therapy.

Asthma

Asthma is a chronic disease characterized by airway inflammation, airway hyperresponsiveness, reversible airway obstruction, predominance of Th2 cells and eosinophilic inflammation. A number of studies point at an important role of galectins in these outcomes and mechanisms leading to them. Chapter 22 reviews some data in galectin-3 knockout mice on the role of this galectin in allergic disease and airway inflammation. Below we discuss studies which show the involvement of galectin-3, -7, -9 and -10 in the allergic disorder.

Ge et al (*55*) investigated a murine model of chronic allergic airway inflammation aiming at the role played by galectin-3 in airway remodeling, a characteristic feature of asthma that leads to airway dysfunction and poor clinical outcome in humans. They found that the higher degree of airway remodeling in wild-type mice was associated with higher Gal-3 expression. Furthermore, using galectin-3-null mice they found diminished remodeling of the airways with significantly reduced mucus secretion, subepithelial fibrosis, smooth muscle thickness, and peribronchial angiogenesis. The authors concluded that Gal-3 promotes airway remodeling via airway recruitment of inflammatory cells, specifically eosinophils, and the development of a Th2 phenotype, as well as increased expression of eosinophil-specific chemokines and profibrogenic and angiogenic mediators (*55*).

In another study, a gene therapy approach, which employed plasmid encoding galectin-3 in chronic asthmatic mice, was shown to improve Th2 allergic inflammation. A correlation was found between galectin-3 treatment and inhibition of cytokine signaling proteins in lungs which act as negative regulators of cytokine signaling, and play an important role in immune response by controlling the balance between Th1 and Th2 cells. The authors concluded that Gal-3 treatment could be a valuable therapeutic approach in allergic disease (*56*).

Galectin-9 was found to play a potential role in the pathogenesis of asthma (*57*). Galectin-9 is an eosinophil chemoattractant and inducer of Th1 cell apoptosis. The authors used a group of BALB/c mice sensitized and challenged with ovalbumin, which develop airway inflammation and mucus hypersecretion, and found that galectin-9 protein levels were elevated in lungs of those mice compared to controls. The authors concluded that galectin-9 contributes to the development of allergic airway inflammation (*57*). Galectin-9 was also found to inhibit allergic inflammation of the airway and airway hyperresponsiveness (AHR) by modulating CD44-dependent leukocyte recognition of the extracellular matrix (*58*).

Another study (*59*) reported that galectin-9 and Tim-3 mRNA levels in lungs increased in mice with asthma and significantly correlated with the levels of blood Th1/Th2 cytokines. Rosiglitazone treatment apparently decreased the expression of galectin-9 and Tim-3. This was shown in a group of 45 BALB/c SPF female mice which were randomized into control group and asthma groups with and without rosiglitazone intervention. Also, it has been shown that the expression of galectin-9 and Tim-3 mRNA was positively correlated with blood IL-4 level, but negatively correlated with blood IFN-γ level (*59*).

A recent review (*60*) considers an important role of galectin-9 in health and disease, including asthma. In normal physiology, galectin-9 appears to be a pivotal modulator of T-cell immunity by inducing apoptosis in specific T-cell subpopulations. However, since these T-cell populations are associated with autoimmunity, inflammatory disease, and graft rejection, it was found that application of exogenous (such as recombinant) galectin-9 may limit pathogenic T-cell activity in various preclinical models of autoimmunity and allograft graft rejection. In many solid cancers, the loss of galectin-9 expression is closely associated with metastatic progression, and treatment with recombinant galectin-9 prevents metastatic spread in various preclinical cancer models. The review discusses the therapeutic potential of galectin-9 in various diseases, including autoimmunity, asthma, infection, and cancer.

Galectin-10 mRNA was found to be over-expressed in aspirin-induced asthma (AIA), suggesting a novel candidate gene and a potentially innovative pathway for mucosal inflammation in aspirin intolerance (*61*). The choice of the model was made following the observation that in sensitive patients, aspirin is associated with nasal and bronchial inflammation, eliciting local symptoms.

Rogerio et al (*62*) do not mention galectins specifically; however, they identify a "D-galactose-binding lectin" from *Synadenium carinatum* latex. The lectin, which is very likely a galectin, increased interferon-gamma and IL-10 in an asthma inflammatory model, suggesting that it might induce a TH2 to TH1 shift in the adaptive immune response. Extracts from this latex are widely used in popular medicine to treat a great number of inflammatory disorders.

Galectin-7 was found to be involved in asthma development in children (*63*). Asthmatic and non-asthmatic children were compared, and galectin-7 was found to be 8-fold greater in bronchial epithelial cells from asthmatic children.

Arthritis

Arthritis is an inflammatory disease of one or more joints in the body. Rheumatoid arthritis (RA), a common autoimmune form of arthritis, is a chronic, systemic inflammatory disorder that may affect many tissues and organs, and destroys cartilages or bones at the joints. RA is initiated by self-attack using own immune system, but the detail of pathological mechanism is unclear. Galectins appear to be involved in the pathogenesis of RA and autoimmune disccorders, particularly galectin-3 and galectin-9. We report below a number of studies suggesting involvement of galectins in autoimmune arthritis.

In a recent study of Wang et al (*64*) lentiviral vectors encoding galectin-3 small hairpin RNA (shRNA) and galectin-1, as well as two control vectors expressing luciferase shRNA and green fluorescent protein, were individually injected intra-articularly into the ankle joints of rats with collagen-induced arthritis. The authors showed that both knockdown of galectin-3 and overexpression of galectin-1 induced higher percentages of antigen-induced T-cell death in the lymph node cells from arthritic rats. Based on the data obtained the authors suggest a hypothetical model of a cross talk between galectin-1 and galectin-3 in the circumstance of rheumatoid joints, and implicate galectin-3 and galectin-1 as potential therapeutic targets for the treatment of rheumatoid arthritis.

Li et al. (*65*) investigated an involvement of galectin-3 in the regulatory process of inflammatory bone resorption in rats with adjuvant-induced arthritis (AA rats) accompanying severe bone destruction in the ankle joints. The level of galectin-3 in the ankle-joint extracts was markedly augmented at week 3 after adjuvant injection, at the time when severe bone destruction was observed. Immunohistochemical analysis revealed an extremely high expression of galectin-3 in macrophages and granulocytes infiltrated in the area of severe bone destruction. Recombinant galectin-3 was added to *in vitro* culture systems, and found to markedly inhibit the formation of osteoclasts in cultures of murine osteoclast precursor cell line as well as in rat bone marrow culture systems. This inhibition was not observed by heat-inactivated galectin-3 or by galectin-7. Furthermore, *in vivo* studies clearly showed a significant suppression of bone destruction and osteoclast recruitment accompanying arthritis, when galectin-3 was injected into the cavity of ankle joint of AA rats. The authors concluded that abundant galectin-3 observed in the area of severe bone destruction may act as a negative regulator for the upregulated osteoclastogenesis accompanying inflammation to prevent excess bone destruction.

In a murine model of arthritis, it was shown that the joint inflammation and bone erosion of AIA were markedly suppressed in galectin 3(-/-) mice as compared with WT mice, and the reduced arthritis in galectin 3(-/-) mice was accompanied by decreased levels of antigen-specific IgG and proinflammatory cytokines (*37*). The frequency of IL-17-producing cells in the spleen was reduced in galectin 3(-/-)

mice as compared with WT mice. Exogenously added recombinant galectin 3 could partially restore the reduced arthritis and cytokines in galectin 3(-/-) mice. The authors concluded that galectin 3 plays a pathogenic role in the development and progression of AIA and that the disease severity is accompanied by alterations of antigen-specific IgG levels, systemic levels of TNFα and IL-6, and frequency of IL-17-producing T cells.

The importance of galectin-9 in rheumatoid arthritis was discussed in the study (*66*), in which galectin-9 is considered as a ligand of TIM-3, a novel transmembrane protein that is involved in the regulation of T-helper 1 (Th1)-cell-mediated immunity, and containing T-cell immunoglobulin- and mucin-domain. The goal of the study was to investigate the expression of TIM-3 along with galectin 9 with respect to disease activity in rheumatoid arthritis (RA). Blood was collected from 39 RA patients and 31 healthy controls, and blood leucocyte TIM-3 and Gal-9 mRNA levels and RA disease activity were determined. It was found that TIM-3 mRNA expression was significantly higher in the synovial tissue (ST) of RA patients than in the ST of osteoarthritis (OA) patients. The authors concluded that TIM-3 and its interaction with Gal-9 are closely associated with RA disease activity and may play an important role in the pathogenesis of RA. Besides, in addition to the negative regulatory effect of Gal-9 mediated through the TIM-3-Gal-9 pathway, Gal-9 may exert its suppressive effect on RA disease activity by modulation of regulatory T (Treg) cells.

The study described above was part of a more general work by the authors (*67*) aimed at the role of expression of TIM-3 from CD4+ T cells from rheumatoid arthritis (RA) patients and healthy controls, and a contribution of galectin-9 to apoptosis of CD4+ T cells in these patients. It was shown that TIM-3 mRNA expression was significantly lower in CD4+ T cells from RA patients compared with those in healthy controls. CD4+ T cell survival was significantly higher in RA patients than in healthy controls.

Galectin-9 was found to suppress collagen-induced arthritis (CIA) in a mouse model in a dose-dependent manner (*68*). Such suppression was observed even when treatment was started on 7 days after the booster, indicating its preventive and therapeutic effects. The authors have suggested that galectin-9 ameliorates CIA by suppressing the generation of Th17, promoting the induction of regulatory T cells.

In was found that the synovial fluid (SF) cells from rheumatoid arthritis (RA) patients express and secrete galectin-8, to a concentration of 25-65 nM, well within the concentration of Gal-8 required to induce apoptosis of SF cells (*69*). Besides, Gal-8 was found to be a novel high-affinity ligand of CD44vRA, a specific CD44 variant, with an apparent binding constant of 6 nM (*69*). Besides, it was found that galectin-1 was found to be overexpressed in rheumatoid arthritis (RA) synovium (*70*).

It was found that galectin-3 was over expressed in the synovial tissue of patients with rheumatoid arthritis (RA), particularly at sites of joint destruction (*71*). The same authors showed that galectin 3 is not only involved in inflammation, but also contribute to the activation of synovial fibroblasts. In contrast, the authors found that expression of galectin-1 was not uniform in different RA specimens, and was never found at sites of invasion. The authors

(Neidhart, Gay et al.) concluded that galectin 3 represents novel markers of disease activity in rheumatoid arthritis (*71*, *72*).

Other Diseases

Because of the ubiquitous nature of inflammatory processes in disease, it is not surprising that galectins have been implicated as potentially important in a diverse number of disorders. Here we provide information on a number of other diseases that have been evaluated.

Galectin-3 has been evaluated in Behçet's disease (BD), a rare immune-mediated systemic vasculitis, often manifested by mucous membrane ulceration and ocular involvements. In a 2-year study, 131 subjects, 39 of which were BD active, 31 inactive, 22 disease controls with leucocytoclastic vasculitis confirmed with a skin biopsy, and 39 healthy control subjects were evaluated. It was found that serum galectin-3 levels were significantly higher in active BD patients compared to inactive BD patients and healthy control subjects. There was no significant difference between the leucocytoclastic vasculitis and active BD patients. Serum galectin-3 levels were positively correlated with clinical activity scores of active BD patients. In addition, galectin-3 levels were significantly higher during the active disease period when compared with the inactive period during follow-ups. It was also reported that patients with vascular involvement had significantly higher galectin-3 levels than other active BD patients (*73*).

Galectins have been evaluated in multiple sclerosis lesions (*74*). Among 11 different galectins tested, those which were present at detectable levels in control white matter were galectins-1, -3, -8 and -9, and their expression was significantly enhanced in active multiple sclerosis lesions. Galectin-9 showed a distinctly different intracellular localization in microglia/macrophages when comparing active and inactive MS lesions. In active lesions, it was mainly found in nuclei, while in inactive lesions, it was primarily located in the cytoplasm. The authors concluded that some galectins are associated with multiple sclerosis pathology.

In a series of papers (*75–78*), St-Pierre, Sato et al. have suggested a role for galectin-1 as a host factor that influences HIV-1 pathogenesis by increasing its drug resistance. In brief, galectin-1 increases HIV-1 infectivity by accelerating its binding to susceptible cells. By comparison, it seems that galcctin-1 directly binds to HIV-1 through recognition of clusters of N-linked glycans on the viral envelope gp120, by binding to CD_4, the host receptor for gp120. In turn, it results in promoting of virus attachment and infection events, since viral adhesion is a rate-limiting step for HIV-1 entry. The authors have tested some glycosides, such as mercaptododecyl glycosides with a terminal β-galactosyl group, and for some derivatives found "high binding responses" with galectin-3, -4, and 8. This opens possibilities in developing new drugs to prevent and treat HIV-1 infection.

Galectin-3 was suggested as a biomarker for amyotrophic lateral sclerosis (ALS), a neurodegenerative disease (*79*), after studying the appropriate mouse model and then validating the finding in human tissues. 14 of 1299 proteins evaluated were found to be dramatically altered in the ALS mice compared with the two control groups. Galectin-3 emerged as a lead biomarker candidate on the basis of its differential expression. Spinal cord tissue from ALS patients also exhibited 2-fold increased levels of galectin-3 when compared to controls.

Galectin-Based Diagnostics and Clinical Survival Prognosis in Patients

Increased expression of galectins is associated with multiple disease states, making measurement of the protein in serum or tissues an attractive surrogate biomarker. Since there are no specific chapters in this book on diagnostics, here we review a number of examples of that use of galectins as disease markers.

Heart Failure

The most advanced example of using galectin as a marker of disease comes from the work of BG Medicine of Waltham, MA. This company has commercialized an FDA approved assay for galectin-3 and evaluated in a variety of cardiovascular situations. Among biomarkers in heart failure, which includes brain natriuretic peptides, inflammatory markers, neurohormones (such as aldosterone), cardiorenal markers, galectin-3 has shown great promise in a number of studies (*46*, *47*).

A recent study (*49*) showed that an elevated galectin-3 level was associated with advanced age, poor renal function and predicted all-cause mortality (hazard ratio 1.86, 95% confidence interval 1.36 to 2.54). These data were based on measured plasma galectin-3 levels in 133 subjects with chronic heart failure (HF) and 45 with advanced decompensated HF using echocardiographic and hemodynamic evaluations. In the chronic HF cohort, median plasma galectin-3 level was 13.9 ng/ml (interquartile range 12.1 to 16.9). In multivariate analysis, galectin-3 remained an independent predictor of all-cause mortality after adjusting for age and other myocardial indications. The authors reported that galectin-3 level, however, did not predict the combined end point of all-cause mortality, cardiac transplantation, or HF hospitalization. In the advanced decompensated HF cohort, there was no relationship between galectin-3 levels and echocardiographic or hemodynamic indexes. The authors concluded that high plasma galectin-3 levels were associated with renal insufficiency and poorer survival in patients with chronic systolic HF.

It was found recently that the level of galectin-3 in plasma (determined using a novel ELISA kit, Galectin-3 Assay™, BG Medicine, Waltham, MA) is a prognostic marker in patients with chronic heart failure (HF), and a significant predictor of mortality risk. In the study (*50*) 232 patients with chronic HF were studied, 98 of whom died in the 6.5 year follow-up period. The 98 patients who died during the follow-up period had galectin-3 levels that were significantly higher compared the survivors.

In another study (*51*), galectin-3 was measured in 599 patients with acute dyspnea who presented to the emergency room, of whom 209 were diagnosed as "acute heart failure". Galectin-3 levels were higher in those with acute heart failure (9.2 ng/mL) than in those who did not (6.9 ng/mL). The same study was described by de Boer et al (*45*) who reported that galectin-3 was the most powerful predictor in a short-term prognosis (60 days, primary end-point rehospitalization caused by heart failure or all-cause mortality, n = 17). The study was later extended to 592 heart failure patients (*52*) with preserved and reduced left ventricular ejection fraction (LVEF), and results were compared this to other biomarkers. The primary end-point of the study was a composite of all-cause mortality and HF hospitalization. The observed doubling of galectin-3 levels was associated with a hazard ratio (HR) of 1.97 (1.62-2.42) for the primary outcome. After correction for age, gender, and other factors, such as diabetes, the HR was 1.38 (1.07-1.78). The authors concluded that galectin-3 is an independent marker for outcome in HF and appears to be particularly useful in HF patients with preserved LVEF.

Galectin-3 levels in 55 patients with end-stage HF were compared with those in 40 healthy controls, and again galectin-3 levels were higher in HF patients (11 ng/mL) than in control (4.1 mg/mL) (*53*). Furthermore, patients who died or developed multi-organ failure had significantly higher galectin-3 levels compared to those who successfully bridged to transplantation.

Another recent study (*54*) evaluated 115 patients presenting to the emergency room with acute dysphonea and diagnosed with heart failure (ADHF) have their galectin-3 level measured. Those patients who had galectin-3 levels above the median value had a 63% mortality in the following four years; patients with less that the median value had a 37% mortality. Therefore, as the authors noted, a single admission galectin-3 level predicts mortality to four years, independent of echocardiographic markers of disease severity.

Thus, galectin-3 appears to be a useful biomarker for prognosis in heart failure. Rather than just a marker of disease, it may be that galectin-3 plays a critical role in the progression of heart failure through its role in fibrogenesis (discussed in Chapter 24).

Cancer

Expression of galectin-3 in patients with colorectal cancer following surgery and/or under chemotherapy treatment and the relationship of galectin-3 expression and clinical aspects or tumor evolution have been studied in 75 samples of colorectal tissues (*80*). The highest percentage of staining cells (an immunohistochemical test for galectin-3 expression) appeared in the most advanced cancer. The immunoexpression of galectin-3 was strong or moderate in 42% of the colorectal tumors. Patients with strong or moderate immunoexpression of galectin-3 died or had recurrence more frequently. The authors noted that galectin-3 cytoplasmatic immunoexpression seems to be a prognostic factor in colorectal cancer, because a higher risk of recurrence had been observed in tumors with a high score of galectin-3.

A high level of expression of galectin-3 was found in malignant lesions of breast (n = 60) compared with that in benign breast lesions (n = 30) (*81*). Besides, the 5-year survival rate and mean survival period were significantly lower in the gal-3 expression positive cases than those in the negative cases of breast cancer. The authors concluded that the expressive level of gal-3 might have important effect on the carcinogenesis, progression and biologic behaviors of breast cancer, and that the positive cases of gal-3 expression might have poor prognosis.

Canesin et al. provide an example of galectin-3 expression in bladder cancer (*82*). Galectin-3 expression was assessed by transcript profiling (U133A arrays) in a series or frozen bladder tumors (n = 105). Immunohistochemistry was performed on tissue arrays containing bladder tumors (n = 389) to evaluate associations of protein expression patterns of galectin-3 with proliferation, apoptosis, and clinical pathologic variables. Galectin-3 protein levels were then quantified in 160 urinary specimens of bladder cancer patients and controls by ELISA test. It was found that galectin-3 gene expression levels increased in invasive tumors as compared with non-muscle invasive lesions and were associated with poor survival in patients with advanced disease. Protein expression patterns also correlated galectin-3 with tumor stage, grade, and apoptosis, and overall survival in patients with tumors. Furthermore, galectin-3 urinary levels segregated bladder cancer patients from controls with high diagnostic accuracy. The authors (*82*) concluded that galectin-3 can be considered as a biomarker for bladder cancer diagnostics, staging, and outcome prognosis.

Galectin-3 is considered to be the most-well-studied molecular candidate for thyroid cancer diagnosis. Despite great variance in methodology, the majority of immunohistochemical studies found that galectin-3 was differentially expressed in thyroid carcinoma compared with benign and normal thyroid specimens. This suggests that galectin-3 is a good diagnostic marker for thyroid cancer. The authors (*83*) noted that, on the other hand, galectin-3 genomic expression studies have shown inconsistent results for diagnostic utility and are not recommended. They emphasized that consideration of galectin-3 as a diagnostic marker for thyroid cancer represents a promising avenue for future study, and its clinical application could significantly reduce the number of diagnostic thyroid operations and thus positively impact the current management of thyroid nodular disease. A separate study (*84*) has also shown that galectin-3 demonstrated highest specificity and sensitivity in the diagnosis of thyroid cancer. A recent study (*85*) notes – "galectin-3 is strongly expressed in thyroid carcinomas but not in benign tumors or normal glands". Anaplastic thyroid carcinomas are deadly tumors that are highly invasive, particularly into bone (there are two more types of malignant thyroid tumors – papillary and follicular). The authors of the study concluded that galectin-3 contributes to thyroid carcinoma malignancy. In another study, expression of galectin-3 in papillary thyroid carcinoma (PTC) [40 cases of papillary microcarcinoma, 74 cases of classic PTC, and several rare variants in 155 PTC cases have been considered] occurred in 92% (142/155) of all cases, and was found to be at much higher levels than that in the control group (*86*).

Prostate cancer, which is the second most common cancer and the second leading cause of cancer death in men, can be effectively treated if it is diagnosed at an early stage when the tumor is confined to the prostate. The PSA test and screening method, which has been widely used for detection of prostate cancer, is unreliable due to the high prevalence of false positive and false negative results. A recent study (*87*) points out that epigenetic alterations, including hyper-methylation of gene promoters, are believed to be early events in neoplastic progression, and thus these methylated genes can serve as biomarkers for the detection of cancer from clinical specimens. This study considers methylated galectin-3 DNA sequence during prostate carcinogenesis and evaluates its usefulness for early detection of prostate cancer in tissue biopsies, serum, and urine.

Galectin-3 expression as a prognostic marker or therapeutic target has been immunohistochemically studied in epithelial ovarian carcinoma (EOC), in which levels of galectin-3, mainly cytoplasmic in location, were evaluated in 71 patients with 54 serous, 13 endometrioid, and 4 mucinous ovarian carcinomas. In vitro, Gal-3 was inhibited using siRNA to evaluate its role in cell growth and sensitivity to chemotherapeutic agents in ovarian carcinoma cell lines. High Gal-3 expression was observed in a majority (88.7%) of the EOCs but not in normal ovarian tissues, and it was correlated with shorter progression-free survival of patients, 43.1 and 49.5 months, respectively (*88*).

Galectin-3 has also been suggested to be a marker of disease progression in primary cutaneous melanoma (PCM) in patients due to its over-expression in the pathology. To examine this point, galectin-3 expression was evaluated using immunohistochemistry in 104 PCM samples, two-thirds of those were superficial spreading (SSM) and one-third was nodular melanomas (NM). Significant differences in galectin-3 expression between SSM and NM was observed, and increased galectin-3 expression was positively correlated with tumor thickness, Clark and Breslow stage, mitotic rate, presence of tumor ulceration, lymphatic invasion, positive sentinel lymph node and distant metastases. The data showed an association between increased galectin-3 expression and reduced recurrence-free survival, as well as with reduced disease-specific survival. The authors concluded that galectin-3 could serve as an additional prognostic marker of disease progression and metastasis in patients with PMC (*89*).

All of the above examples are related to galectin-3. However, this simply reflects the attention that researchers have paid to galectin-3 and the availability of test kits for galectin-3. Recently, galectin-8 was shown to be a robust biomarker for recurrence of bladder cancer (*90*), as demonstrated by galectin-8 staining patterns from 162 samples of non-muscle-invasive transitional cell carcinoma, 25 samples of muscle-invasive transitional cell carcinoma, and 10 samples of normal urothelium. Loss of galectin-8 was associated with the likelihood of tumor recurrence, with no significance for tumor progression. Patients whose specimens showed weak galectin-8 expression had a shorter recurrence-free interval (42 vs. 12 months). All of the 10 normal urothelium samples showed high galectin-8 expression. Decreased staining was found to be associated with higher tumor stages and grades. The authors concluded that loss of galectin-8 might be an early step in the development of malignant lesions of the bladder and a significant independent predictor of recurrence.

Aside from galectin-3 and -8, galectin-1 and -4 have been reported to be clinically significant as colorectal cancer markers (*91*). These authors showed early on that galectin-1 is over-expressed in colorectal carcinoma (CRC) tissues. In this paper (*91*), they showed in 105 CRC patients and 100 healthy volunteers (control) that levels of circulating galectin-1 and -4 reflect the presence of CRC and/or its state of progression. Circulating levels of galectin-1/-3/-4 in plasma of CRC patients were significantly higher compared to those in controls. Galectin-1 and -4 levels significantly decreased post surgery, and the level of galectin-4 in most patients fell below the threshold value. The levels of circulating galectin-4 significantly increased as tumor stage progressed, whereas those for galectin-1 were relatively high at an early stage. These data suggested that galectin-4 may be a tumor biomarker for use in patient follow-ups, while galectin-1 could be used potentially for tumor screening.

In terms of galectin-1-based diagnostic screening, the Nicolay group in Eindhoven, The Netherlands, have employed molecular MRI and a novel galectin-1-targeting peptide, Anginex, with liposome-based nanoparticles to assess and combat tumor growth *in vivo* (*92*, *93*).

The expression pattern of galectin-1 was determined in 73 vulvar tissues by a standard immunohistochemical method: 12 benign vulvar specimen, 41 vulvar intraepithelial lesions (VIN), according to their differentiation were subdivided into VIN I, II and III and 20 invasive squamous cell carcinomas (ISCC). The immunohistochemical analyses showed that the intensity of galectin-1 expression on stromal cells next to the neoplastic cells steadily increased according to the pathological grade: benign vulvar tissue <VIN I<VIN II<VIN II<VIN III<ISCC ($p<0.0001$). In epithelial cells, negative or weak reactivity for galectin-1 was observed. These findings indicate that the galectin-1 expression on stromal cells increases with the histopathological grade of vulvar tissues, and it can be suggested that these changes might be associated with the progression of vulvar neoplasia (*94*).

Liver Diseases

A recent study of 33 patients with alcoholic liver cirrhosis and 11 patients with normal liver function has shown higher galectin-3 in portal venous serum compared to hepatic venous serum (HVS) in patients with normal liver function, which suggested hepatic removal of galectin-3 (*95*). However, galectin-3 was cleared by healthy livers, but not from cirrhotic livers, and subsequently HVS and SVS (systemic venous blood) galectin-3 levels were significantly increased in patients with liver cirrhosis compared to controls. In summary, systemic, portal and hepatic levels of galectin-3 were found to be negatively associated with liver function in patients with alcoholic liver cirrhosis.

Another study questioning the importance of galectin-3 in liver disease to non-alcoholic fatty liver disease (*96*) concluded that galectin-3 may not be a biomarker. In this study, serum levels of galectin-3 in 71 patients with NAFLD and 39 controls were assayed, and it was shown that they did not differ in patients with NAFLD (median 4.1 ng/mL; interquartile range: 1.5-5.5 ng/mL) compared with healthy controls (median 3.1 ng/mL; interquartile range: 0.8-7.5 ng/mL).

Galectin Targeting Agents and Approaches

Clearly, one of the obvious approaches to galectin therapy would be to design galectin blockers that specifically inhibit galectins, and examine those inhibitors against certain pathologies, first, of course, in experimental animal models. This, however, is not so easy. First of all, "classical" ligands of galectins are rather weak binders, and are not really applicable as drugs. For example, lactose (4-O-β-D-Galactopyranosyl-D-glucose) binds to galectin-3 with K_d between 0.2 and 1 mM, to galectin-4 with K_d of 0.9-2.0 mM, and quite poorly binds to galectin-7, -10, 13 ((*33*) and references therein). N-acetyllactosamine binds better, however, still not good enough to become a drug: 50 μM with galectin-1, 30-200 μM with galectin-3, 1-2 mM with galectin-4 (ibid).

A number of approaches have been taken to developing molecules that target galectin proteins for therapeutic purposes. These include small organic molecules that target primarily the carbohydrate binding domain (*97*, *98*), peptidomiemetics that target other areas on the protein, and natural plant derived complex carbohydrates that have exposed galactose residues. There are two primary groups of plant-derived compounds that have been explored, pectin-based compounds exemplified by modified citrus pectin, and 1,4-β-D-galactomannan-based compounds exemplified by GM-CT-01 (DAVANAT®). While there are other potential approaches, these are the primary ones that have been reported and are in various stages of development.

Small Galectin Ligands Molecules as Potential Galectin Blockers

As detailed in Chapter 2, a group of researchers at Lund University, Sweden, has synthesized small organic compounds, derivatives of galactose, and tested them with respect to binding to the carbohydrate binding domain of different galectins. Inhibitors of galectin-3 were the most potent, with K_d values as low as 29 nM (3,3′-ditriazolyl thiodigalactoside), 50 nM (3,3′-diamido thiodigalactoside), 320 nM (3′-amido lacNAC derivative), and 660 nM (3′-triazolyl lacNac derivative). Their strategy so far has been less successful for inhibiting galectin-1, since apparent K_d values indicated rather weak binding, varying from 40 μM (digalactosyl sulfone) and 313 μM (C-galactoside derivative) to 1.25 mM (3-O-triazolylmethyl galactose derivative). Inhibitors of galectin-4, -7, and -9 were also relatively weak, with K_d values as high as 160 μM (2,3-dibenzoyl taloside, galectin-4), and 23 μM; 140 μM (3′-thiourea lacNac and phenyl thio-galactoside derivatives, respectively, galectin-7), and 540 μM (3′-triazolyl mannoside, galectin-9).

The galectin-3 inhibitors are promising therapeutic agents, but little is known about critical drug characteristics such as *in vivo* potency, absorption, metabolism, pharmacokinetics, and toxicology. While they have been shown to be active in certain disease models, more work is needed on the mechanism of action and to determine if they are active in a therapeutically acceptable delivery and dosing model. For example, the thiodigalactoside diester galectin-3 inhibitor (K_d = 660 nM; named Td131_1), when tested against papillary thyroid cancer (PTC) cell lines and human *ex vivo* PTC, actually increased the percentage of apoptotic cells in a dose-dependent manner (with 100-600 μM of the inhibitor, that is in the 150-1000 higher concentrations compared with the K_d value). However, this treatment was found to be largely ineffective in terms of the chemosensitivity of PTC cell lines to doxorubicin, which is normally enhanced upon suppression of galectin-3. Administration of as much as 0.6 mM of the thiodigalactoside compound actually decreased the IC_{50} of doxorubicin by 43-46%, or showed no detectable change in caspase-3 or PAEP cleavage (*99*).

Peptidomeimetics

As detailed in Chapter 3, an alternative approach has been used to design compounds that target galectin-1 at a site different from the canonical β-galactoside binding site. Initially, they designed a peptide 33mer, called Anginex, based on structural and compositional features common to many anti-angiogenic proteins (e.g. endostatin, angiostatin, PF4, thrombospondin, gamma interferon-inducible protein-10 (IP-10), tumor necrosis factor, BPI, thrombospondin type 1 repeat peptides, Flt-1 peptide) (*100*, *101*). Anginex was shown to effectively inhibit tumor angiogenesis and tumor growth in mouse models (*102*) by targeting galectin-1 (*103*). Subsequently, these researchers were able to design peptidomimetics of Anginex (6DBF7 and PTX008) that were reduced in size and peptidic character from the peptide 33mer. 6DBF7 has only 13 amino acid residues, 20 less than parent Anginex, and maintains a requisite anti-parallel β-sheet fold via a dibenzofuran β-turn mimetic scaffold (*104*). PTX008 is a fully non-peptidic calixarene-scaffolded compound (a.k.a. compound 0118 in (*97*)) that displays chemical substituents to approximate the molecular dimensions and amphipathic features of Anginex and 6DBF7. All three compounds (Anginex, 6DBF7 and PTX008) target galectin-1 and function similarly *in vitro* and *in vivo* in terms of e.g. inhibiting endothelial cell proliferation, angiogenesis, and tumor growth (*97*, *102*, *104*). Moreover, in targeting galectin-1, they are quite different from traditional sugar-based compounds, because they act as allosteric inhibitors of galectin-1 carbohydrate ligand binding (*105*). A Swiss-based company, OncoEthix Inc. is currently engaged in a Phase I clinical trial in cancer patients with PTX-008, also reviewed in Chapter 15.

Pectin-Based Compounds

Modified citrus pectin (MCP) is a product of partial degradation of highly branched citrus pectin. Despite numerous studies published since 1992 (*106*), none of them showed a structure of a MCP, except for some vague wording about "linear" and "hairy" parts of the polymer. "Average" molecular weights of various MCPs range from about 10,000 to 120,000 Da; however, these are only crude estimates. Each MCP variant likely represents a wide range of molecules of various molecular weights.

In initial studies in the 1990's and the first half of the 2000's, it was assumed that MCPs bind to galectin-3, although this was more conjecture than experimentally-based fact (*107*, *108*). The first studies showed that intravenous injection of B16-F1 murine melanoma cells with MCP into mice resulted in a significant decrease of lung colonization, unlike injection of non-modified pectin solution, which led to the opposite effect, i.e. an increase of lung colonization (*106*). In addition, MCP inhibited B16-F1 melanoma cells adhesion to laminin and asialofetuin-induced homotypic aggregation (*107*). MCP was also found to be active by oral intake in mice (as a 1 and 2.5 mg/mL in drinking water solutions), reducing tumor growth, angiogenesis, and spontaneous metastasis *in vivo* (*109*). One particular MCP, called GCS-100, was shown to induce apoptosis in various multiple myeloma cell lines, the growth of which was induced by adhesion to bone marrow stromal cells (*108*). It should be noted that GCS-100 by itself did not alter galectin-3 expression, but was active in that regard in a mixture with dexamethasone (ibid.). The effects of pectin-derived GCS-100 on tumor infiltrating lymphocytes is detailed in Chapter 16 (see also (*21*, *110*)). GCS-100 has been advanced into clinical trials, which are discussed below.

MCP was found to be active in the suppression of liver metastasis of colon cancer in mice (*111*). Mice fed with a drinking water solution of MCP in concentrations of 0 (control), 10, 25, and 50 mg/mL showed rates of liver metastasis of 100%, 80%, 73%, and 60%, respectively, and median volumes from primary lesions in the spleen of 1.51, 0.93, 0.77 and 0.70 cm^3, respectively.

Commercially available fractionated pectin powder (FPP) (molecular weight of pectin fragments and their distribution in FPP were not available, and the meaning of the term "fractionated" was unclear, whether the "native", pH-untreated pectin was fractionated or fractionation was performed with its partially degraded form) was shown to be capable of inducing apoptosis in human prostate cancer cells, and the level of apoptosis was reported to be 40 times above that in untreated cells. Interestingly, PectaSol (pH-treated citrus pectin) had little or no apoptotic activity, even though there were no detectable (or significant) differences found among the pectins (*112*). The pattern is complicated by the fact that chemical removal of ester linkages in FPP (by mild alkaline treatment) which yield homogalacturonan oligosaccharides, completely destroyed the apoptotic activity. Conversely, removing galacturonosyl carboxymethylesters and/or breaking the nonmethylesterified homopolygalacturonan chains in FPP by enzymatic treatment (with pectinmethylesterase and/or emdopolygalacturonase) did not significantly reduce the apoptotic activity of FPP. Furthermore, heat treatment (by autoclaving) of citrus pectin solutions led to the induction of significant levels of apoptosis comparable to that of FPP (ibid.). In other words, the biological activity of citrus pectin can be modulated by chemical and physical means, which makes the picture not easily manageable in order to obtain a reproducible drug formulation.

Apparently, the first time the interaction of pectin fragments, galactans (from potato pectin) with galectin-3 was demonstrated in 2009 (*113*). The galactans contain 88% galactose residues (6% galacturonic acid, 3% arabinose, and 3% rhamnose). For a comparison, rhamnogalacturonan 1 (containing 12% galactose, 62% galacturonic acid, 20% rhamnose, 3% arabinose) and polygalacturonic acid from MCP (96% galacturonic acid, 1% galactose, 1.2% rhamnose, 1% xylose, 0.2% arabinose) were also tested for their interaction with galectin-3. It was found that all three compounds, fluorescently labeled, bind to galectin-3 at pH 7.2 (at which pH galectin-3 is positively changed), but not at pH 12, at which only galactans retained a high level of binding to Gal-3.

A more recent article supporting this last conclusion reported an effect of a galactan from an almost pure pectic rhamnogalacturonan 1 (from okra pods) on the proliferation and apoptosis of highly metastatic B16-F10 melanoma cells *in vitro*

(*114*). The study suggests that the pectic galactan induced apoptosis in melanoma cells by interacting with galectin-3.

The inhibitory effect of citrus pectin on the proliferative capacity of several malignant carcinoma and erythroleukemia cell lines was studied at various doses of the pectin, and it was suggested that the observed antiproliferative effect may be due to this pectin's ability to inhibit galectin expression (*115*).

Another study was based on the known ability of galectin-3 to be upregulated in acute kidney injury, and was aimed at suppressing galectin-3 with MCP. Indeed, MCP-treated mice demonstrated reduced levels of galectin-3 in association with decreased renal fibrosis, macrophages, proinflammatory cytokine expression and apoptosis. However, levels of other renal galectins, galectin-1 and -9, were unchanged (*116*).

A recent review article summarizes the various biological effects of MCP possibly due to its binding galectin-3 (*117*). Pectin-dervied complex carbohydrates are promising therapeutic agents, but for this therapy to come to fruition it will necessary to have a pharmaceutical compound that is reproducible in scale up manufacture and is both chemically and biologically well characterized.

Galactomannan-Derived Compounds: GM-CT-01

Pro-Pharmaceuticals Inc., now Galectin Therapeutics, Inc., has pursued a strategy to produce galactose-containing polysaccharides that serve as galectin ligands and interfere with their function. To this end, the company manufactured GM-CT-0l (also called DAVANAT® in the literature), a modified galactomannan, through a patented method of controlled chemical degradation of natural galactomannans (*118*). Since galactomannans are present in nearly all plants, an industrial-level source that is readily available for processing, reducing the cost of goods which will make the drug more affordable. Galactomannan from the seeds of *Cyamopsis tetragonoloba* was chosen as a readily available product which is produced in ton quantities for use as a gel food industry. From this raw material, which is approximately 50% high molecular weight galactomannan and water insoluble, we produced a pharmaceutical grade, low-molecular weight, pure galactomannan product suitable for human parenteral administration. The process and compound GM-CT-01 is patented, a Drug Master File is on record with the FDA, there is an open IND with the FDA, and an open IMPD with the EMA. Clinical trial results (*118–120*) are described below.

The backbone of GM-CT-01 is made of mannose, and approximately every second mannose residue carries a galactose substituent, Figure 4 (*118*, *120*). The average repeating unit of GM-CT-01 is made up of seventeen β-D-Man residues and ten α-D-Gal residues, and an average polymeric molecule contains approximately 12 of such repeating units, at an average molecular weight of about 55 kDa. GM-CT-01 compound for clinical trials has a specified molecular weight in the range of 42,000 to 60,000 Da. The molecular structure of GM-CT-01 was analyzed using chemical analysis and ^{1}H- and ^{13}C-NMR spectroscopy (*120*), its absolute molecular weight was determined using HPLC/RI-MALLS and a ZIMM plot analysis (ibid.), and the weight-averaged molecular weight was also measured by pulsed field gradient NMR diffusion spectroscopy (*121*).

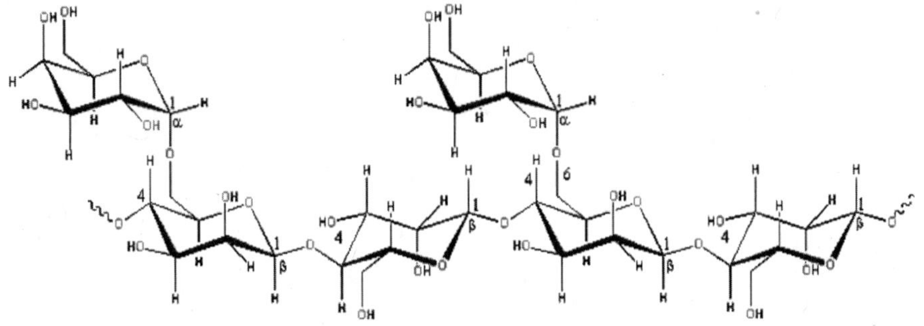

Figure 4. Structure of the basic repeating building block of DAVANAT. Each DAVANAT® molecule consists of 54 such units (119). (see color insert)

The binding of GM-CT-01 to galectin-1 was recently characterized by in terms of its specificity, dissociation constant and stoichiometry of binding (*122*, *123*). As far as we know, GM-CT-01 is the first polymeric carbohydrate-based drug candidate proven to be an effective ligand for galectin-1 (*122*). In addition, analysis has shown that GM-CT-01 binds to galectin-3 with approximately three times the avidity as it does to galectin-1 using the same assay system (unpublished data, Mayo, Klyosov, 2012). There is some recent data in a bioassay system (CD4+ and CD8+ tumor infiltrating lymphocytes, with interferon-γ secreted as a readout of the assay) that suggests that GM-CT-01 has an effect on inhibiting galectin-3 with an an apparent binding avidity of 60-70 nM (*110*).

Other Galectin Targeting Approaches

The truncated galectin-3 protein, galectin-3C, has been used to inhibit the galectin-3 protein with promising pre-clinical results, as described in Chapter 12. Chapter 7 describes a fascinating new approach whereby fluorinated analogs of glucosamine may reduce synthesis of galactosamines and reduce the ability of galectin-1 to affect lymphocyte function. This takes the opposite approach to galectin inhibitors by reducing molecules binding to galectin.

Summary Comments on Galectin Inhibitors

In general, more characterization of the various approaches would be helpful in sorting out the mechanimsm of action. One should be cautioned to assume that all compounds that bind to galectins will act similarly in biological systems and in disease. For example, the small organic molecules are designed to target a single galectin molecule at the carbohydrate binding domain. In contrast, GM-CT-01 binds up to three galectin molecules per drug molecule and occupies a larger potion of the galectin molecule that includes the dimerization domain. These differences in binding characteristics could have important implications for function.

Another important, and largely unexplored issue, is what happens following binding of these agents to galectins. Is the effect simply a result of competitive inhibition, or are there changes in degradation, trafficking, or synthesis as a result of binding? Additionally, the downstream effects after binding of galectins are largely unknown for these agents.

Development of Galectin Targeting Therapy in Human Disease

Current Human Data

Three are currently limited data using galectin inhibitors in human disease. What data are available has all been obtained in cancer patients. Two galectin targeting agents have been tested in previously completed or terminated clinical trials for the treatment of cancer, including GM-CT-01, a galactomannan derivative (described above), and GCS-100, a citrus pectin derivative. OTX-008, a peptidomeimetic compound, is reported in Chapter 15 to be a phase 1 clinical trial at the time of this writing.

GM-CT-01

GM-CT-01 was evaluated in colorectal cancer based on pre-clinical studies that demonstrated efficacy when combined with 5-FU against cancer and seemed to additionally mitigate 5-FU toxicity. (*118–120*). Four clinical trials were performed by Pro-Pharmaceuticals (now Galectin Therapeutics), as indicated on ClinicalTrials.gov:

1. http://clinicaltrials.gov/ct2/show/NCT00054977?term=GM-CT-01&rank=3
2. http://clinicaltrials.gov/ct2/show/NCT00110721?term=GM-CT-01&rank=2
3. http://clinicaltrials.gov/ct2/show/NCT00388700?term=GM-CT-01&rank=4
4. http://clinicaltrials.gov/ct2/show/NCT00386516?term=GM-CT-01&rank=1

A Phase I dose-escalating safety clinical trial enrolled patients with different types of solid tumors and had failed (as indicated in the history of the disease) standard, approved treatments. This study evaluated the tolerability of six rising doses of GM-CT-01 alone ranging from 30 to 280 mg/m2 and in combination with 5-FU (500 mg/m2) over 2 cycles of therapy. Treatment of a total of 40 patients enrolled in the study demonstrated that GM-CT-01 was well tolerated without dose limiting toxicity identified.

Three phase 2, open label clinical trials were partially completed, two in patients with metastatic colorectal cancer, and one in patients with cholangiocarcinoma. While the three trials were not completed, there was evidence of efficacy in metastatic colorectal cancer and a reduction in 5-FU related side effects. Trial number 2 listed above, which enrolled 20 patients, had 1 patient with a partial response and 6 patients with stable disease. Additionally, there was a 46% increase in Median Overall Survival of 5-FU plus GM-CT-01 when compared to a contemporaious colorectal cancer trial which reported best standard of care [data submitted to the FDA].

The reduction in side effects occurred despite the fact that 5-FU serum levels were not reduced, and were possibly increased when compared to historical pharmacokinetic data, widely known by the clinicians. Adverse events related to 5-FU were evaluated by combining the 57 patients from all four clinical trials and comparing them to the results of adverse events reported in the literature. The table below shows the comparison. There was a markedly lower incidence of grade 3-4 adverse events associated with 5-FU when GM-CT-01 was combined with 5-FU. While the data are not compared to direct control patients in the studies, this analysis suggests that, in addition to potentially having an effect on treatment of the cancer, there may be an amelioration of 5-FU adverse events. Since gut epithelial damage and inflammation are important components of 5-FU side effects, it is possible that galectins are involved in this pathology. This hypothesis requires additional research, but raises the possibility that galectin inhibition may have a role in cancer supportive care in combination with chemotherapy.

Event in percent of patients (%)	Kabbinavar 5-FU/LV	Cunningham 5-FU/LV	Bolus 5-FU/LV	5-FU/LV (Mayo)	5-FU+GM-CT-01
	N=104	N=212	N=219	N=593	N=57
Adverse Events	Grade 3-4 (%)	Grade 3-4 (%)	Grade 3-4 (%)	Grade 3-4 (%)	Grade 3-4(%)
Diarrhea	40	14	13	12	0
Nausea/Vomiting	NR	9	4	7	<2
Mucositis	NR	22	17	NR	<2
Neutropenia/ Leukopenia	7	7	67	21	<2

*Studies included in table compilation (Bolus 5-FU/LV and 5-FU (Mayo)

1. Rothenberg ML, Meropol NJ, Poplin EA, et al.: Mortality associated with irinotecan plus bolus fluorouracil/leucovorin: summary findings of an independent panel. J Clin Oncol 19(18):3801-7, 2001.
2. Chiara S, Nobile MT, Vincenti M, et al.: Advanced colorectal cancer in the elderly: results of consecutive trials with 5-fluorouracil-based chemotherapy. Cancer Chemother Pharmacol 42 (4): 336-40, 1998.
3. Goldberg RM, Hatfield AK, Kahn M, et al.: Prospectively randomized North Central Cancer Treatment Group trial of intensive-course fluorouracil combined with the l-isomer of intravenous leucovorin, oral leucovorin, or intravenous leucovorin for the treatment of advanced colorectal cancer. J Clin Oncol 15 (11): 3320-9, 1997.
4. Sloan JA, Goldberg RM, Sargent DJ, et al.: Women experience greater toxicity with fluorouracil-based chemotherapy for colorectal cancer. J Clin Oncol 20(6):1491-8, 2002.
5. Tsalic M, Bar-Sela G, Beny A, et al.: Severe toxicity related to the 5-fluorouracil/leucovorin comibination (the Mayo Clinic regimen): a prospective study in colorectal cancer patients. Am J Clin Oncol 26(1): 103-6, 2003.

**Study Summaries

1. Kabbinavar, FF, et al *Journal of Clinical Oncology* 23:3697-370, 2005. The study was a randomized, phase II trial comparing bevacizumab plus fluorouracil and leucovorin (FU/LV) versus placebo plus FU/LV as first-line therapy in patients with metastatic colorectal cancer. Regimen: LV 500 mg/m^2 over 2 hours and FU 500 mg/m^2 as a bolus midway through the LV infusion was administered weekly for the first 6 weeks of each 8-week cycle.
2. Cunningham, D, et. al. Annals of Oncology 7:961-965, 1996. This reports the results of a randomized trial comparing Tomudex (raltritrexed) with 5-fluorouracil plus leucovorin in advanced colorectal cancer. Regimen: The control group was treated with LV 20 mg/m2 and 5-FU 425 mg/m2 once daily for 5 days every 4 weeks.

In addition to these four previous clinical trials, there is a clinical trial that is currently enrolling patients. As described in Chapter 16, GM-CT-01 is being used in combination with a peptide vaccine in patients with metastatic melanoma.

GCS-100

GCS-100, a modified citrus pectin compound, was evaluated in three clinical trials performed by GlycoGenesys/Prospect Therapeutics, all suspended for lack of funding, as found on ClinicalTrials.gov:

1. http://clinicaltrials.gov/ct2/show/NCT00776802?term=gcs-100&rank=1
2. http://clinicaltrials.gov/ct2/show/NCT00514696?term=gcs-100&rank=2
3. http://clinicaltrials.gov/ct2/show/NCT00609817?term=gcs-100&rank=3

Preliminary data from two of these trials was reported in abstract form. In a phase 1 dose escalating trial, GCS-100 was administered to patients with refractory solid tumors to determine dose-limiting toxicity (DLT), maximum tolerated dose (MTD), and pharmacokinetics (PK) and efficacy. The DLT was a Grade 3 erythematous, maculopapular rash, resolving with systemic steroid treatment. Skin biopsy revealed a vasculitis similar to findings seen in dog models. Other adverse events included nausea, vomiting, diarrhea, fatigue, fever and hyperglycemia. Sustained periods of stable disease were achieved in a number of patients with previously treated advanced solid tumors (*124*). A phase 2 clinical trial was conducted in elderly patients with CLL, in which it was reported that 6 of 24 patients had partial responses and two patients had to discontinue treatment because of rash (*125*).

Considerations for Development of Human Therapeutics

This overview and the excellent set of associated chapters reveal that there are multiple galectin dependent diseases that may be amenable to therapies targeted at galectins. It is now time for efforts to shift from academic descriptions and experiments into pharmaceutical development. As part of this effort, as stated above, the current set of therapeutic agents need to be characterized in relation to binding and mechanism of action. The diseases to target need to be carefully chosen based on the relevance to human disese. While there is some data in human cancer, careful thought needs to be given to the right cancers and approach to therapy, including combinations with existing therapy. We believe that the next decade will be an exciting and formative one that will see successes of galectin-targeted therapy in human disease. It may be the start of a new class of agents for a target that could have widespread use.

References

1. Barondes, S. H.; Castronovo, V.; Cooper, D. N. W.; Cummings, R. D.; Drickamer, K.; Feizi, T.; Gitt, M. A.; Hirabayashi, J.; Hughes, C.; Ken-ichi, K.; Leffler, H.; Liu, F. T.; Lotan, R.; Mercurio, A. M.; Monsigny, M.; Pillai, S.; Poirer, F.; Raz, A.; Rigby, P. W. J.; Rini, J. M.; Wang, J. L. Galectins: A family of animal β-galactoside-binding lectins. *Cell* **1994**, *76*, 597–598.

2. *Galectins*; Klyosov, A. A., Witzhak, Z. A., Platt, D., Eds.; John Wiley & Sons: Hoboken, NJ, 2008.
3. Dam, T. K.; Brewer, C. F. Lectins as pattern recognition molecules: The effects of epitope density in innate immunity. *Glycobiology* **2010**, *20*, 270–279.
4. Ito, K.; Stannard, K.; Gabutero, E.; Clark, A. M.; Neo, S. Y.; Onturk, S.; Blanchard, H.; Ralph, S. J. Galectin-1 as a potent target for cancer therapy: Role in the tumor microenvironment. *Cancer Metastasis Rev.* **2012**; Epub ahead of print, June 17, 2012; PMID: 22706847.
5. Nangia-Makker, P.; Balan, V.; Raz, A. Galectin-3 binding and metastasis. *Methods Mol. Biol.* **2012**, *878*, 251–266.
6. Toussaint, I. L. G.; Nilson, A. E.; Goble, J. M.; Ballman, K. V.; James, C. D.; Lefranc, F.; Kiss, R.; Uhm, J. H. Galectin-1, a gene preferentially expressed at the tumor margin, promotes glioblastoma cell invasion. *Mol. Cancer* **2012**, *11*, 32; Epub ahead of print, May 14, 2012; PMID: 22583806.
7. Liu, F. T.; Yang, R. Y.; Hsu, D. K. Galectins in acute and chronic inflammation. *Ann. N. Y. Acad. Sci.* **2012**, *1253*, 80–91.
8. Ito, K.; Ralph, S. J. Inhibiting galectin-1 reduces murine lung metastasis with increased CD4(+) and CD8(+) T cells and reduced cancer cell adherence. *Clin. Exp. Metastasis* **2012**, *29*, 561–572.
9. Yang, L. P.; Jiang, S.; Liu, J. Q.; Miao, X. Y.; Yang, Z. L. Association of immunostaining of Galectin-3 and *Sambucus nigra* agglutinin with invasion, metastasis and poor progression of gallbladder adenocarcinoma. *Hepatogastroenterology* **2012**, *12* (119), 59; Epub ahead of print, April 12, 2012; DOI: 10.5754/hge12129.
10. Newlaczyl, A. U.; Yu, L. G. Galectin-3: A jack-of-all-trades in cancer. *Cancer Lett.* **2011**, *313*, 123–128.
11. Camby, I.; Le Mercier, M.; Lefranc, F.; Kiss, R. Galectin-1: A small protein with major functions. *Glycobiology* **2006**, *16*, 137R–157R.
12. Lefranc, F.; Le Mercier, M.; Mathieu, V.; Kiss, R. Galectin-1: Cancer cell migration, angiogenesis, and chemoresistance. In *Galectins*; Klyosov, A. A., Witzhak, Z. A., Platt, D., Eds.; John Wiley & Sons: Hoboken, NJ, 2008; pp 157−191.
13. Markowska, AI; Liu, F. T.; Panjwani, N. Galectin-3 is an important mediator of VEGF- and bFGF-mediated angiogenic response. *J. Exp. Med.* **2010**, *207* (9), 1981–1993; Epub ahead of print, August 16, 2010.
14. Markowska, A. I.; Jefferies, K. C.; Panjwani, N Galectin-3 protein modulates cell surface expression and activation of vascular endothelial growth factor receptor 2 in human endothelial cells. *J. Biol. Chem.* **2011**, *286* (34), 29913–29921.
15. Barrow, H.; Guo, X.; Wandall, H. H.; Pedersen, J. W.; Fu, B.; Zhao, Q.; Chen, C.; Rhodes, J. M.; Yu, L. G. Serum galectins -2, -4 and -8 are greatly increased in colon and breast cancer patients and promote cancer cell adhesion to blood vascular endothelium. *Clin. Cancer Res.* **2011**, *17* (22), 7035–7046; Epub ahead of print, September 20, 2011.
16. Barrow, H.; Rhodes, J. M.; Yu, L. G. The role of galectins in colorectal cancer progression. *Int. J. Cancer* **2011b**, *129*, 1–8.

17. Delgado, V. M.; Nugnes, L. G.; Colombo, L. L.; Troncoso, M. F.; Fernandez, M. M.; Malchiodi, E. L.; Frahm, I.; Croci, D. O.; Compagno, D.; Rabinovich, G. A.; Wolfenstein-Todel, C.; Elola, M. T. *FASEB J.* **2011**, *25*, 242–254.
18. Thijssen, V. L.; Barkan, B.; Shoji, H.; Aries, I. M.; Mathieu, V.; Deltour, L.; Hackeng, T. M.; Kiss, R.; Kloog, Y.; Poirier, F.; Griffioen, A. W. Tumor cells secrete galectin-1 to enhance endothelial cell activity. *Cancer Res.* **2010**, *70*, 6216–6224.
19. Ito, K.; Scott, S. A.; Cutler, S.; Dong, L. F.; Neuzil, J.; Blanchard, H.; Ralph, S. J. Thiodigalactoside inhibits murine cancer by concurrently blocking effects of galectin-1 on immune dysregulation, angiogenesis and protection against oxidative stress. *Angiogenesis* **2011**, *14*, 293–307.
20. Dings, R. P. M.; Vang, K. B.; Castermans, K.; Popescu, F. E.; Zhang, Y.; Noesser, E.; Oude Egbrink, M. G. A.; Mescher, M. F.; Farrar, M. A.; Griffioen, A. W.; Mayo, K. H. *Enhancement Clin. Cancer Res.* **2011**, *17*, 3134–3145.
21. Demotte, N.; Wieërs, G.; Van Der Smissen, P.; Moser, M.; Schmidt, C.; Thielemans, K.; Squifflet, J. L.; Weynand, B.; Carrasco, J.; Lurquin, C.; Courtoy, P. J.; van der Bruggen, P. A galectin-3 ligand corrects the impaired function of human CD4 and CD8 tumor-infiltrating lymphocytes and favors tumor rejection in mice. *Cancer Res.* **2010**, *70*, 7476–7488.
22. Banh, A; Zhang, J; Cao, H; Bouley, DM; Kwok, S; Kong, C; Giaccia, AJ; Koong, AC; Le, QT Tumor galectin-1 mediates tumor growth and metastasis through regulation of T-cell apoptosis. *Cancer Res.* **2011**, *71*, 4423–4431.
23. Strik, H. M.; Kolodziej, M.; Oertel, W.; Bäsecke, J. Glycobiology in malignant gliomas: Expression and functions of galectins and possible therapeutic options. *Curr. Pharm. Biotechnol.* **2011**, *13* (11), 2299–2307; PMID: 21605067.
24. Strik, H. M.; Schmidt, K.; Lingor, P.; Tönges, L.; Kugler, W.; Nitsche, M.; Rabinovich, G. A.; Bähr, M. Galectin-1 expression in human glioma cells: Modulation by ionizing radiation and effects on tumor cell proliferation and migration. *Oncol. Rep.* **2007**, *18*, 483–488.
25. Lefranc, F.; Sadeghi, N.; Camby, I.; Metens, T.; Dewitte, O.; Kiss, R. Present and potential future issues in glionlastoma treatment. *Expert Rev. Anticancer Therapy* **2006**, *6*, 719–732.
26. Lefranc, F.; Marhieu, V.; Kiss, R. Galectin-1 mediated biochemical controls of melanoma and glioma aggressive behavior. *World J. Biol. Chem.* **2011**, *2*, 193–201.
27. Verschuere, T.; De Vleeschouwer, S.; Lefranc, F.; Kiss, R.; Van Gool, S. W. Galectin-1 and immunotherapy for brain cancer. *Expert Rev. Neurother.* **2011**, *11*, 533–543.
28. Bruyère, C.; Madonna, S.; Van Goietsenoven, G.; Mathieu, V.; Dessolin, J.; Kraus, J. L.; Lefranc, F.; Kiss, R. JLK1486, a bis 8-hydroxyquinoline-substituted benzylamine, displays cytostatic effects in experimental gliomas through MyT1 and STAT1 activation and, to a lesser extent, PPARγ activation. *Transl. Oncol.* **2011**, *4* (3), 126–137.

29. Bruyère, C.; Abeloos, L.; Lamoral-Theys, D.; Senetta, R.; Mathieu, V.; Le Mercier, M.; Kast, R. E.; Cassoni, P.; Vandenbussche, G.; Kiss, R.; Lefranc, F. Temozolomide modifies caveolin-1 expression in experimental malignant gliomas *in vitro* and *in vivo*. *Transl. Oncol.* **2011**, *4*, 92–100.
30. Bruyère, C.; Mijatovic, T.; Lonez, C.; Spiegl-Kreinecker, S.; Berger, W.; Kast, R. E.; Ruysschaert, J. M.; Kiss, R.; Lefranc, F. Temozolomide-induced modification of the CXC chemokine network in experimental gliomas. *Int. J. Oncol.* **2011**, *38*, 1453–1464.
31. Suñol, M.; Cusi, V.; Cruz, O.; Kiss, R.; Lefranc, F. Immunohistochemical analyses of alpha1 and alpha3 Na+/K+-ATPase subunit expression in medulloblastomas. *Anticancer Res.* **2011**, *31*, 953–958.
32. Le Calvé, B.; Rynkowski, M.; Le Mercier, M.; Bruyère, C.; Lonez, C.; Gras, T.; Haibe-Kains, B.; Bontempi, G.; Decaestecker, C.; Ruysschaert, J. M.; Kiss, R.; Lefranc, F. Long-term in vitro treatment of human glioblastoma cells with temozolomide increases resistance in vivo through up-regulation of GLUT transporter and aldo-keto reductase enzyme AKR1C expression. *Neoplasia* **2011**, *12*, 727−739. Erratum in *Neoplasia* **2011**, *13* (9), following p 886.
33. Klyosov, A. A. Galectins and Their Functions in Plain Language. In *Galectins*; Klyosov, A. A., Witzhak, Z. A., Platt, D., Eds.; John Wiley & Sons: Hoboken, NJ, 2008; pp 9–31.
34. Liu, F.-T.; Hsu, D. K.; Yang, R.-Y.; Chen, H.-Y.; Saesuga, J. Galectins in Regulation of Inflammation and Immunity. In *Galectins*; Klyosov, A. A., Witzhak, Z. A., Platt, D., Eds.; John Wiley & Sons: Hoboken, NJ, 2008; pp 97−113.
35. Byrnes, K. R.; Washington, P. M.; Knoblach, S. M.; Hoffman, E.; Faden, A. I. Delayed inflammatory mRNA and protein expression after spinal cord injury. *J. Neuroinflammation* **2011**, *8*, 130.
36. Hu, C. Y.; Chang, S. K.; Wu, C. S.; Tsai, W. I.; Hsu, P. N. Galectin-3 gene (LGALS3) +292C allele is a genetic predisposition factor for rheumatoid arthritis in Taiwan. *Clin. Rheumatol.* **2011**, *30*, 1227–1233.
37. Forsman, H.; Islander, U.; Andreasson, E.; Andersson, A.; Onnheim, K.; Karlstrom, A.; Savman, K.; Magnusson, M.; Brown, K. L.; Karlsson, A. Galectin 3 aggravates joint inflammation and destruction in antigen-induced arthritis. *Arthritis Rheum.* **2011**, *63*, 445–454.
38. Henderson, N. C.; Sethi, T. The regulation of inflammation by galectin-3. *Immunol. Rev.* **2009**, *230*, 160–171.
39. Norling, L. V.; Perretti, M.; Cooper, D. Endogenous galectins and the control of the host inflammatory response. *J. Endocrinol.* **2009**, *201*, 169–184.
40. Ortner, D.; Grabher, D.; Hermann, M.; Kremmer, E.; Hofer, S.; Heufler, C. The adaptor protein Bam32 in Human dendritic cells participates in the regulation of MHC Class I-induced CD8+ T cell activation. *J. Immunol.* **2011**, *187*, 3972–3978.
41. Cooper, D.; Llarregui, J. M.; Pesoa, S. AQ.; Croci, D. O.; Perretti, M.; Rabinovich, G. A. Multiple functional targets of the immunoregulatory activity of galectin-1: Control of immune cell trafficking , dendritic cell physiology, and T-cell fate. *Methods Enzymol.* **2010**, *480*, 199–244.

42. Kojima, K.; Arikawa, T.; Saita, N.; Goto, E.; Tsumura, S.; Tanaka, R.; Masunaga, A.; Niki, T.; Oomizu, S.; Hirashima, M.; Kohrogi, H. Galectin-9 attenuates acute lung injury by expanding CD14- plasmacytoid dendritic cell-like macrophages. *Am. J. Respir. Crit. Care Med.* **2011**, *84* (3), 328–329; Epub ahead of print, May 11, 2011.
43. Li, Y.; Feng, J.; Geng, S.; Wei, H.; Chen, G.; Li, X.; Wang, L.; Wand, R.; Peng, H.; Han, G.; Shen, B.; Li, Y. The N- and C-terminal carbohydrate recognition domains of galectin-9 contribute differently to its multiple functions in innate immunity and adaptive immunity. *Mol. Immunol.* **2011**, *48*, 670–677.
44. Iacobini, C.; Menini, S.; Ricci, C.; Fantauzzi, C. B.; Scipioni, A.; Salvi, L.; Gordone, S.; Delucchi, F.; Serino, M.; Federici, M.; Pricci, F.; Pugliese, G. Galectin-3 ablation protects mice from diet-induced NASH: A major scavenging role for galectin-3 in liver. *J. Hepatol.* **2011**, *54*, 975–983.
45. de Boer, R. A.; Yu, L.; van Veldhuisen, D. J. Galectin-3 in cardiac remodeling and heart failure. *Curr. Heart Fail. Rep.* **2010**, *7*, 1–8.
46. Bohm, M.; Voors, A. A.; Ketelslegers, J. M.; Schirmer, S. H.; Turgonyl, E.; Bramlage, P.; Zannad, F. Biomarkers: Optimizing treatment guidance in heart failure. *Clin. Res. Cardiol.* **2011**, *100* (11), 973–981; Epub ahead of print, July 16, 2011.
47. Ueland, T.; Aukrust, P.; Broch, K.; Aakhus, S.; Skårdal, R.; Muntendam, P.; Gullestad, L. Galectin-3 in heart failure: High levels are associated with all-cause mortality. *Int. J. Cardiol.* **2011**, *150*, 361–364.
48. Yanavitski, M.; Givertz, M. M. Novel biomarkers in acute heart failure. *Curr. Heart Fail. Rep.* **2011**, *8*, 206–221.
49. Tang, W. H.; Shrestha, K.; Shao, Z.; Borowski, A. G.; Troughton, R. W.; Thomas, J. D.; Klein, A. L. Usefulness of plasma galectin-3 levels in systolic heart failure to predict renal insufficiency and survival. *Am. J. Cardiol.* **2011**, *108*, 385–390.
50. Lok, D. J.; Van Der Meer, P.; de la Porte, P. W.; Lipsic, E.; Van Wijngaarden, J.; Hillege, H. L.; van Veldhuisen, D. J. Prognostic value of galectin-3, a novel marker of fibrosis, in patients with chronic heart failure: Data from the DEAL-HF study. *Clin. Res. Cardiol.* **2010**, *99*, 323–328.
51. van Kimmenade, R. R.; Januzzi, J. L., Jr; Ellinor, P. T.; Sharma, U. C.; Bakker, J. A.; Low, A. F.; Martinez, A.; Crijns, H. J.; MacRae, C. A.; Menheere, P. P.; Pinto, Y. M. Utility of amino-terminal pro-brain natriuretic peptide, galectin-3, and apelin for the evaluation of patients with acute heart failure. *J. Am. Coll. Cardiol.* **2006**, *48*, 1217–1224.
52. de Boer, R. A.; Lok, D. J.; Jaarsma, T.; van der Meer, P.; Voors, A. A.; Hillege, H. L.; van Veldhuisen, D. J. Predictive value of plasma galectin-3 levels in heart failure with reduced and preserved ejection fraction. *Ann. Med.* **2011**, *43*, 60–68.
53. Milting, H.; Ellinghaus, P.; Seewald, M.; Cakar, H.; Bohms, B.; Kassner, A.; Körfer, R.; Klein, M.; Krahn, T.; Kruska, L.; El Banayosy, A.; Kramer, F. Plasma biomarkers of myocardial fibrosis and remodeling in terminal heart failure patients supported by mechanical circulatory support devices. *J. Heart Lung Transplant* **2008**, *27*, 589–596.

54. Shah, R. V.; Chen-Tournoux, A. A.; Picard, M. H.; van Kimmenade, R. R.; Januzzi, J. L. Galectin-3, cardiac structure and function, and long-term mortality in patients with acutely decompensated heart failure. *Eur. J. Heart Fail.* **2010**, *12*, 826–832.
55. Ge, X. N.; Bahaie, N. S.; Kang, B. N.; Hosseinkhani, M. R.; Ha, S. G.; Frenzel, E. M.; Liu, F. T.; Rao, S. P.; Sriramarao, P. Allergen-induced airway remodeling is impaired in galectin-3-deficient mice. *J. Immunol.* **2010**, *185*, 1205–1214.
56. López, E.; Zafra, M. P.; Sastre, B.; Gámez, C.; Lahoz, C.; del Pozo, V. Gene expression profiling in lungs of chronic asthmatic mice treated with galectin-3: Downregulation of inflammatory and regulatory genes. *Mediators Inflamm.* **2011**, 823279; Epub ahead of print, March 20, 2011.
57. Sziksz, E.; Kozma, G. T.; Pállinger, E.; Komlósi, Z. I.; Adori, C.; Kovács, L.; Szebeni, B.; Rusai, K.; Losonczy, G.; Szabó, A.; Vannay, A. Galectin-9 in allergic airway inflammation and hyper-responsiveness in mice. *Int. Arch. Allergy Immunol.* **2010**, *151*, 308–317.
58. Katoh, S.; Ishii, N.; Nobumoto, A.; Takeshita, K.; Dai, S. Y.; Shinonaga, R.; Niki, T.; Nishi, N.; Tominaga, A.; Yamauchi, A.; Hirashima, M. Galectin-9 inhibits CD44-hyaluronan interaction and suppresses a murine model of allergic asthma. *Am. J. Respir. Crit. Care Med.* **2007**, *176*, 27–35.
59. Zhang, Z. Y.; Luan, B.; Feng, X. X. To study the expression of galectin-9 and tim-3 in lungs of mice with asthma and the effect of rosiglitazone (PPAR-γ agonist) on their expression. *Zhongguo Dang Dai Er Ke Za Zhi* **2011**, *13*, 406–410 (in Chinese).
60. Wiersma, V. R.; de Bruyn, M.; Helfrich, W.; Bremer, E. Therapeutic potential of galectin-9 in human disease. *Med. Res. Rev.* **2011**, 20249; Epub ahead of print, July 26, 2011; DOI: 10.1002/med.20249.
61. Devouassoux, G.; Pachot, A.; Laforest, L.; Diasparra, J.; Freymond, N.; Van Ganse, E.; Mougin, B.; Pacheco, Y. Galectin-10 mRNA is overexpressed in peripheral blood of aspirin-induced asthma. *Allergy* **2008**, *63*, 125–131.
62. Rogerio, A. P.; Cardoso, C. R.; Fontanari, C.; Souza, M. A.; Afonso-Cardoso, S. R.; Silva, E. V.; Koyama, N. S.; Basei, F. L.; Soares, E. G.; Calixto, J. B.; Stowell, S. R.; Dias-Baruffi, M.; Faccioli, L. H. Anti-asthmatic potential of a D-galactose-binding lectin from Synadenium carinatum latex. *Glycobiology* **2007**, *17*, 795–804.
63. Yin, G. Q.; Zhao, S. Y.; Guo, S. P.; Zhao, Y. H.; Liu, X. C.; Jiang, Z. F. Galectin-7 is associated with bronchial epithelial cell apoptosis in asthmatic children. *Zhonghua Er Ke Za Zhi* **2006**, *44*, 523–526 (in Chinese).
64. Wang, C. R.; Shiau, A. L.; Chen, S. Y.; Cheng, Z. S.; Li, Y. T.; Lee, C. H.; Yo, Y. T.; Lo, C. W.; Lin, Y. S.; Juan, H. Y.; Chen, Y. L.; Wu, C. L. Intra-articular lentivirus-mediated delivery of galectin-3 shRNA and galectin-1 gene ameliorates collagen-induced arthritis. *Gene Ther.* **2010**, *17* (10), 1225–1233; Epub ahead of print, June 3, 2010.
65. Li, Y. J.; Kukita, A.; Teramachi, J.; Nagata, K.; Wu, Z.; Akamine, A.; Kukita, T. A possible suppressive role of galectin-3 in upregulated osteoclastogenesis accompanying adjuvant-induced arthritis in rats. *Lab. Invest.* **2009**, *89*, 26–37.

66. Lee, J.; Oh, J. M.; Hwang, J.; Ahn, J.; Bae, E. K.; Won, J.; Koh, E. M.; Cha, H. S. Expression of human TIM-3 and its correlation with disease activity in rheumatoid arthritis. *Scand. J. Rheumatol.* **2011**, *40*, 334–440.
67. Lee, J.; Park, E. J.; Noh, J. W.; Hwang, J. W.; Bae, E. K.; Ahn, J. K.; Koh, E. M.; Cha, H. S. Underexpression of TIM-3 and blunted galectin-9-induced apoptosis of CD4+ T cells in rheumatoid arthritis. *Inflammation* **2012**, *35* (2), 633–637; Epub ahead of print, June 30, 2011.
68. Seki, M.; Oomizu, S.; Sakata, K. M.; Sakata, A.; Arikawa, T.; Watanabe, K.; Ito, K.; Takeshita, K.; Niki, T.; Saita, N.; Nishi, N.; Yamauchi, A.; Katoh, S.; Matsukawa, A.; Kuchroo, V.; Hirashima, M. Galectin-9 suppresses the generation of Th17, promotes the induction of regulatory T cells, and regulates experimental autoimmune arthritis. *Clin. Immunol.* **2008**, *127*, 78–88.
69. Eshkar, S. L.; Ronen, D.; Levartovsky, D.; Elkayam, O.; Caspi, D.; Aamar, S.; Amital, H.; Rubinow, A.; Golan, I.; Naor, D.; Zick, Y.; Golan, I. The involvement of CD44 and its novel ligand galectin-8 in apoptotic regulation of autoimmune inflammation. *J Immunol.* **2007**, *179*, 1225–1235.
70. Kim, C. W.; Cho, E. H.; Lee, Y. J.; Kim, Y. H.; Hah, Y. S.; Kim, D. R. Disease-specific proteins from rheumatoid arthritis patients. *J. Korean Med. Sci.* **2006**, *21*, 478–484.
71. Neidhart, M.; Zaucke, F.; von Knoch, R.; Jüngel, A.; Michel, B. A.; Gay, R. E.; Gay, S. Galectin-3 is induced in rheumatoid arthritis synovial fibroblasts after adhesion to cartilage oligomeric matrix protein. *Ann. Rheum. Dis.* **2005**, *64*, 419–424.
72. Ohshima, S.; Kuchen, S.; Seemayer, C. A.; Kyburz, D.; Hirt, A.; Klinzing, S.; Michel, B. A.; Gay, R. E.; Liu, F. T.; Gay, S.; Neidhart, M. Galectin 3 and its binding protein in rheumatoid arthritis. *Arthritis Rheum.* **2003**, *48*, 2788–2795.
73. Ozden, M. G.; Caycı, Y. T.; Tekin, H.; Coban, A. Y.; Aydın, F.; Sentürk, N.; Bek, Y.; Cantürk, T.; Turanlı, A. Y. Serum galectin-3 levels in patients with Behçet's disease: Association with disease activity over a long-term follow-up. *J. Eur. Acad. Dermatol. Venereol.* **2011**, *25*, 1168–1173.
74. Stancic, M.; van Horssen, J.; Thijssen, V. L.; Gabius, H. J.; van der Valk, P.; Hoekstra, D.; Baron, W. Increased expression of distinct galectins in multiple sclerosis lesions. *Neuropathol. Appl. Neurobiol.* **2011**, *37*, 654–671.
75. St-Pierre, C.; Ouellet, M.; Tremblay, M. J.; Sato, S. Galectin-1 and HIV-1 infection. *Methods Enzymol.* **2010**, *480*, 267–294.
76. St-Pierre, C.; Ouellet, M.; Giguère, D.; Ohtake, R.; Roy, R.; Sato, S.; Tremblay, M. J. Galectin-1 specific inhibitors as a new class of compounds to treat HIV-1 infection. *Antimicrob. Agents Chemother.* **2011**, *56* (1), 154–162; Epub ahead of print, November 7, 2011; PMID: 22064534.
77. St-Pierre, C.; Manya, H.; Ouellet, M.; Clark, G. F.; Endo, T.; Tremblay, M. J.; Sato, S. Host-soluble galectin-1 promotes HIV-1 replication through a direct interaction with glycans of viral gp120 and host CD4. *J. Virol.* **2011**, *85*, 11742–11751.
78. Murakami, T.; Yoshioka, K.; Sato, Y.; Tanaka, M.; Niwa, O.; Yabuki, S. Synthesis and galectin-binding activities of mercaptododecyl glycosides

containing a terminal β-galactosyl group. *Bioorg. Med. Chem. Lett.* **2011**, *21*, 1265–1269.

79. Zhou, J. Y.; Afjehi-Sadat, L.; Asress, S.; Duong, D. M.; Cudkowicz, M.; Glass, J. D.; Peng, J. Galectin-3 Is a candidate biomarker for amyotrophic lateral sclerosis: Discovery by a proteomics approach. *J. Proteome Res.* **2010**, *9* (10), 5133–5141.
80. Povegliano, Z. L.; Oshima, C. T.; de Oliveira Lima, F.; Andrade Scherholz, P. L.; Manoukian, F. N. Immunoexpression of galectin-3 in colorectal cancer and its relationship with survival. *J. Gastrointest. Cancer* **2010**, *42* (4), 217–221.
81. Chen, G.; Zou, Q.; Yang, Z. Expression of galectin-3 and *Sambucus nigra* agglutinin and its clinicopathological significance in benign and malignant lesions of breast. *Zhong Nan Da Xue Xue Bao Yi Xue Ban* **2010**, *35*, 584–589 (in Chinese).
82. Canesin, G.; Gonzalez-Peramato, P.; Palou, J.; Urrutia, M.; Cordón-Cardo, C.; Sánchez-Carbayo, M. Galectin-3 expression is associated with bladder cancer progression and clinical outcome. *Tumour Biol.* **2010**, *31*, 277–285.
83. Chiu, C. G.; Strugnell, S. S.; Griffith, O. L.; Jones, S. J.; Gown, A. M.; Walker, B.; Nabi, I. R.; Wiseman, S. M. Diagnostic utility of galectin-3 in thyroid cancer. *Am. J. Pathol.* **2010**, *176*, 2067–2081.
84. Sethi, K.; Sarkar, S.; Das, S.; Mohanty, B.; Mandal, M. Biomarkers for the diagnosis of thyroid cancer. *J. Exp. Ther. Oncol.* **2010**, *8*, 341–352.
85. Levy, R; Grafi-Cohen, M; Kraiem, Z.; Kloog, Y. Galectin-3 promotes chronic activation of K-Ras and differentiation block in malignant thyroid carcinomas. *Mol. Cancer Ther.* **2010**, *9*, 2208–2219.
86. Zhu, X.; Sun, T.; Lu, H.; Zhou, X.; Lu, Y.; Cai, X.; Zhu, X. Diagnostic significance of CK19, RET, galectin-3 and HBME-1 expression for papillary thyroid carcinoma. *J. Clin. Pathol.* **2010**, *63* (9), 786–789; Epub ahead of print, July 19, 2010 .
87. Ahmed, H. Promoter methylation in prostate cancer and its application for the early detection of prostate cancer using serum and urine samples. *Biomark. Cancer* **2010**, *2*, 17–33.
88. Kim, M. K.; Sung, C. O.; Do, I. G.; Jeon, H. K.; Song, T. J.; Park, H. S.; Lee, Y. Y.; Kim, B. G.; Lee, J. W.; Bae, D. S. Overexpression of galectin-3 and its clinical significance in ovarian carcinoma. *Int. J. Clin. Oncol.* **2011**, *16*, 352–358.
89. Buljan, M.; Situm, M.; Tomas, D.; Milošević, M.; Krušlin, B. Prognostic value of galectin-3 in primary cutaneous melanoma. *J. Eur. Acad. Dermatol. Venereol.* **2011**, *25*, 1174–1181.
90. Kramer, M. W.; Waalkes, S.; Serth, J.; Hennenlotter, J.; Tezval, H.; Stenzl, A.; Kuczyk, M. A.; Merseburger, A. S. Decreased galectin-8 is a strong marker for recurrence in urothelial carcinoma of the bladder. *Urol. Int.* **2011**, *87*, 143–150; Epub ahead of print, July 14, 2011.
91. Watanabe, M.; Takemasa, I.; Kaneko, N.; Yokoyama, Y.; Matsuo, E.; Iwasa, S.; Mori, M.; Matsuura, N.; Monden, M.; Nishimura, O. Clinical

significance of circulating galectins as colorectal cancer markers. *Oncol. Rep.* **2011**, *25*, 1217–1226.
92. Mulder, W. J. M.; van der Schaft, D. W. J.; Hautvast, P. A. I.; Strijkers, G. J.; Koning, G. A.; Storm, G.; Mayo, K. H.; Griffioen, A. W.; Nicolay, K. Early in vivo assessment of angiostatic therapy efficacy by molecular MRI. *FASEB J.* **2007**, *21*, 378–383.
93. Kluza, E.; van der Schaft, D. W. J.; Hautvast, P. A. I.; Mulder, W. J. M.; Mayo, K. H.; Griffioen, A. W.; Strijkers, G. J.; Nicolay, K. Synergistic targeting of aVb3 integrin and galectin-1 with heteromultivalent paramagnetic liposomes for combined MR imaging and treatment of angiogenesis. *Nano Lett.* **2010**, *10*, 52–58.
94. Kohrenhagen, N.; Voelker, H. U.; Kapp, M.; Dietl, J.; Kämmerer, U. The expression of galectin-1 in vulvar neoplasia. *Anticancer Res.* **2010**, *30*, 1547–1552.
95. Wanninger, J.; Weigert, J.; Wiest, R.; Bauer, S.; Karrasch, T.; Farkas, S.; Scherer, M. N.; Walter, R.; Weiss, T. S.; Hellerbrand, C.; Neumeier, M.; Schäffler, A.; Buechler, C. Systemic and hepatic vein galectin-3 are increased in patients with alcoholic liver cirrhosis and negatively correlate with liver function. *Cytokine* **2011**, *55*, 435–440.
96. Yilmaz, Y.; Eren, F.; Kurt, R.; Yonal, O.; Polat, Z.; Senates, E.; Bacha, M.; Imeryuz, N. Serum galectin-3 levels in patients with nonalcoholic fatty liver disease. *Clin. Biochem.* **2011**, *44*, 955–958.
97. Dings, R. P. M.; Chen, X.; Hellebrekers, D. M. E. I.; van Eijk, L. I.; Hoye, T. R.; Griffioen, A. W.; Mayo, K. H. Design of non-peptidic topomimetics of anti-angiogenic proteins with anti-tumor activities. *J. Natl. Cancer Inst.* **2006**, *98*, 932–936.
98. Oberg, C. T.; Leffler, H.; Nilsson, U. J. Inhibition of galectins with small molecules. *Chimia* **2011**, *65*, 18–23.
99. Lin, C.-L.; Whang, E. E.; Donner, D. B.; Jiang, X.; Price, B. D.; Carothers, A. M.; Delaine, T.; Leffler, H.; Nilsson, U. J.; Nose, V.; Moore, F. D.; Ruan, D. T. Activates apoptosis and enhances both chemosensitivity galectin-3 targeted therapy with a small molecule inhibitor. *Mol. Cancer Res.* **2009**, *7*, 1655–1662.
100. Griffioen, A. W.; van der Schaft, D.; Barandsz-Janson, A.; Cox, A.; Struijker-Boudier, H. A.; Hillen, H. F. P.; Mayo, K. H. Anginex, a designed Peptide that inhibits angiogenesis. *Biochem. J.* **2001**, *354*, 233–242.
101. Dings, R. P. M.; Mayo, K. H. A journey in structure-based discovery: From designed peptides to protein-surface topomimetics as antibiotic and antiangiogenic agents. *Acc. Chem Res.* **2007**, *40*, 1057–1065.
102. Dings, R. P. M.; Hargittai, B.; Haseman, J.; Griffioen, A. W.; Mayo, K. H. Anti-tumor activity of the novel angiogenesis inhibitor anginex. *Cancer Lett.* **2003**, *194*, 55–66.
103. Thijssen, V. L.; Postel, R.; Brandwijk, R. J. M. G. E.; Dings, R. P. M.; Nesmelova, I.; Satijn, S.; Verhofstad; Nakabeppu, Y.; Baum, L. G.; Bakkers, J.; Mayo, K. H.; Poirier, F.; Griffioen, A. W. Galectin-1 is essential in tumor angiogenesis and is a target for anti-angiogenesis therapy. *Proc. Natl. Acad. Sci. USA* **2006**, *103*, 15975–15980.

104. Mayo, K. H.; Dings, R. P. M.; Flader, C.; Nesmelova, I.; Hargittai, B.; van der Schaft; van Eijk, L. I.; Walek, D.; Haseman, J.; Hoye, T. R.; Griffioen, A. W. Design of a partial-peptide mimetic of anginex with antiangiogenic and anticancer activity. *J. Biol. Chem.* **2003**, *278*, 45746–45752.
105. Dings, R. P. M.; Miller, M. C.; Raymond, E.; Nesmelova, I.; Astorgues-Xerri, L.; Kumar, N.; Serova, M.; Mayo, K. H. Anti-tumor agent calixarene 0118 targets human galectin-1 as an allosteric inhibitor of carbohydrate binding. *J. Med. Chem.* **2012**, *55* (11), 5121–5129.
106. Platt, D.; Raz, A. Modulation of the lung colonization of B16-F1 melanoma cells by citrus pectin. *J. Natl. Cancer Inst.* **1992**, *84*, 438–442.
107. Inohara, H.; Raz, A. Effects of natural complex carbohydrate (citrus pectin) on murine melanoma cell properties related to galectin-3 functions. *Glycoconjugate J.* **1994**, *11*, 527–532.
108. Chauhan, D.; Li, G.; Podar, K.; Hideshima, T.; Neri, P.; He, D.; Mitsiades, N.; Richardson, P.; Chang, Y.; Schindler, J.; Carver, B.; Anderson, K. C. A novel carbohydrate-based therapeutic GCS-100 overcomes bortezomib resistance and enhances dexamethasone-induced apoptosis in multiple myeloma cells. *Cancer Res.* **2005**, *65*, 8350–8358.
109. Nangia-Makker, P.; Hogan, V.; Honjo, Y.; Baccarini, S.; Tait, L.; Bresalier, R.; Raz, A. Inhibition of human cancer cell growth and metastasis in nude mice by oral intake of modified citrus pectin. *J. Natl. Cancer Inst.* **2002**, *94*, 1854–1862.
110. Demotte, N.; Wieers, G.; Klyosov, A.; van der Bruggen, P. Is It Possible To Correct the Impaired Function of Human Tumor-Infiltrating Lymphocytes? *Keystone Symposium on Molecular and Cellular Biology. New Frontiers at the Interface of Immunity and Glycobiology*, Lake Louise, AB, Canada, March 6−11, 2011; Abstract 23F11.
111. Liu, H.-Y.; Huang, Z.-L.; Yang, G.-H.; Lu, W.-Q.; Yu, N.-R. Inhibitory effect of modified citrus pectin on liver metastases in a mouse colon cancer model. *World J Gastroenterol* **2008**, *14*, 7386–7391.
112. Jackson, C. L.; Dreaden, T. M.; Theobald, L. K.; Tran, N. M.; Beal, T. L.; Eid, M.; Gao, M. Y.; Shirley, R. B.; Stoffel, M. T.; Kimar, M. V.; Mohnen, D. M. Pectin induces apoptosis in human prostate cancer cells: Correlation of apoptotic function with pectin structure. *Glycobiology* **2007**, *17*, 805–819.
113. Gunning, A. P.; Bongaerts, R. J.; Morris, V. J. Recognition of galactan components of pectin by galectin-3. *FASEB J.* **2009**, *23*, 415–424.
114. Vayssade, M.; Sengkhamparn, N.; Verhoef, R.; Delaigue, C.; Goundiam, O.; Vigneron, P.; Voragen, A. G.; Schols, H. A.; Nagel, M. D. Antiproliferative and proapoptotic actions of okra pectin on B16F10 melanoma cells. *Phytother. Res.* **2010**, *24*, 982–989.
115. Bergman, M.; Djaldetti, M.; Salman, H.; Bessler, H. Effect of citrus pectin on malignant cell proliferation. *Biomed. Pharmacother.* **2010**, *64*, 44–47.
116. Kolatsi-Joannou, M.; Price, K. L.; Winyard, P. J.; Long, D. A. Modified citrus pectin reduces galectin-3 expression and disease severity in experimental acute kidney injury. *PLoS One* **2011**, *6*, e18683; DOI: 10.1371/journal.pone.0018683.

117. Glinsky, VV; Raz, A. Modified citrus pectin anti-metastatic properties: One bullet, multiple targets. *Carbohydr. Res.* **2009**, *344* (14), 1788–1791Epub ahead of print, September 26, 2008.
118. Klyosov, A. A.; Platt, D.; Zomer, E. Preclinical studies of anticancer efficacy of 5-fluorouracil when co-administered with the 1,4-beta-d-galactomannan. *PRECLINICA* **2003**, *1*, 175–186.
119. Klyosov, A. A.; Zomer, E.; Platt, D. Davanat® and Colon Cancer: Preclinical and Clinical (Phase I) Studies. In *Carbohydrate Drug Design*; Klyosov, A. A., Witczak, Z. J., Platt, D., Eds.; ACS Symposium Series 932; American Chemical Society: Washington, DC, 2006; pp 67−104.
120. Platt, D.; Klyosov, A. A.; Zomer, E. Development of a Polysaccharide as a Vehicle To Improve the Efficacy of Chemotherapeutics. In *Carbohydrate Drug Design*; Klyosov, A. A., Witczak, Z. J., Platt, D., Eds.; ACS Symposium Series 932; American Chemical Society: Washington, DC, 2006; pp 49−66.
121. Miller, M.; Klyosov, A. A.; Platt, D.; Mayo, K. Using pulse field gradient NMR diffusion measurements to define molecular size distributions in glycan preparations. *Carbohydr. Res.* **2009**, *344*, 1205–1212.
122. Miller, M. C.; Klyosov, A. A.; Mayo, K. H. The α-galactomannan davanat binds galectin-1 at a site different from the conventional galectin carbohydrate binding domain. *Glycobiology* **2009b**, *19*, 1034–1045.
123. Miller, M. C.; Nesmelova, I. V.; Platt, D.; Klyosov, A. A.; Mayo, K. H. The carbohydrate-binding domain on galectin-1 is more extensive for a complex glycan than for simple saccharides: Implications for galectin-glycan interactions at the cell surface. *Biochem. J.* **2009**, *421*, 211–221.
124. Grous, J. J.; Redfern, C. H.; Mahadevan, D.; Schindler, J. GCS-100, a Galectin-3 Antagonist, in Refractory Solid Tumors: A Phase I Study. *Journal of Clinical Oncology*, 2006, ASCO Annual Meeting Proceedings, 24, No. 18S, June 20 Supplement, 13023.
125. Cotter, F.; Smith, D. A.; Boyd, T. E.; Richards, D. A.; Alemany, D.; Loesch, D.; Salogub, G.; Tidmarsh, G. F., Gammon, G. M.; Gribben, J. Single-Agent Activity of GCS-100, A First-in-Class Galectin-3 Antagonist, in Elderly Patients with Relapsed Chronic Lymphocytic Leukemia. *Journal of Clinical Oncology Advertisement, Journal of Clinical Oncology*, 2009, ASCO Annual Meeting Proceedings Post-Meeting Edition, 27, No. 15S, May 20 Supplement.

Galectin and Galectin Inhibitors: Structural Aspects

Chapter 2

Low-Molecular Weight Inhibitors of Galectins

Hakon Leffler[1] and Ulf J. Nilsson[*,2]

[1]Section MIG, Department of Laboratory Medicine, Lund University, Sölvegatan 23, SE-223 62, Lund, Sweden
[2]Center for Analysis and Synthesis, Lund University, POB 124, SE-221 00 Lund, Sweden
[*]E-mail: ulf.nilsson@organic.lu.se

The galectins are known to be able to recognize and cross-link ß-D-galactopyranoside-containing glycoconjugates as a result of presenting multiple binding sites. This review summarizes efforts in our group for the last ten years towards low-molecular weight chemically modified carbohydrate derivatives. In addition to providing an avenue for improved affinity and galectin-selectivity, we have focused on the chemical synthesis of low-molecular weight inhibitors, since synthetic derivatives offer opportunities to design more "drug-like" in order to circumvent drawbacks typically associated with natural oligosaccharides and fragments, such as low affinity (high μM to mM for galectins), limited chemical and metabolic stability, and high polarity leading to low bioavailability and rapid clearance. The examples described in the review provide evidence that it is possible to improve both affinity and selectivity of low-molecular weight compounds for galectins by chemically modifying galactose (and other monosaccharides) with non-carbohydrate structural elements targeting ligand sub-sites flanking the core galactose-binding sub-site C. Indeed, inhibitors have been made that possess both low-nM affinities for galectins and that show potent *in vivo* efficacy. Hence, promising low-molecular weight galectin-targeting lead structures have been identified, although it remains to investigate and optimize ADME and toxicology aspects of these compounds in order to fully reach the status of identifying clinical candidates.

Introduction

The galectins are proteins that display a multitude of biological functions. Several of these are related to their ability to recognize and cross-link ß-D-galactopyranoside-containing glycoconjugates as a result of presenting multiple binding sites in the form of dimers, multimers, or tandem-repeat of binding sites (*1*). The functional outcome in specific situation depends on the particular subtype of galectin(s) expressed and the bound glycoconjugate fine structure flanking the bound core galactoside. Most functional effects on cellular and organismal level are related to inflammation and cancer (*2–4*), which are detailed elsewhere in this book. Due key rate-limiting roles in *e.g.* inflammation and cancer, efforts towards selective and efficient galectin inhibitors are today considered being of great importance. Several chemical strategies for galectin inhibition have been reported and used in experimental situations, including the use of natural saccharide fragments, multivalent structures and glycodendrimers, peptides, antibodies, anti-sense nucleotides, dominant-negative galectin-3 fragments, and low-molecular weight synthetic inhibitors. This mini-review will summarize efforts in our group for the last ten years towards low-molecular weight chemically modified carbohydrate derivatives (*5*, *6*). In addition to providing an avenue for improved affinity and galectin-selectivity, we have focused on the chemical synthesis of low-molecular weight inhibitors because synthetic derivatives offer opportunities to design more "drug-like" in order to circumvent drawbacks typically associated with natural oligosaccharides and fragments, such as low affinity (high µM to mM for galectins), limited chemical and metabolic stability, and high polarity leading to low bioavailability and rapid clearance.

Low-Molecular Weight Inhibitors

The galectins are stable, soluble, and readily expressed which is why structural studies are relatively frequent and more than 100 structures deposited in the Protein Data Bank. Hence, a substantial body of structural data on galectin carbohydrate recognition domains (CRD) available for inhibitor design has aided in the development of low-molecular weight inhibitors over the last decade. The galectin CRD is a slightly bent β-sandwich with the carbohydrate–binding site as a groove on the concave side. This may be divided in five sub-sites (*7–9*), where the central C sub-site harbors the key ß-D-galactoside and mono-saccharide residues (or other moieties) flanking the ß-D-galactoside are positioned in sub-sites A-B and D-E (Figure 1).

Synthetic low-molecular weight inhibitors can be categorized as being targeting one or more of the sub-sites A-B and D-E, as well as sub-sites not known to bind natural ligands. These latter sub-sites are in many cases unique to only one or a few galectins, which opens up possibilities for creating inhibitors with improved selectivities. The low-molecular weight galectin inhibitors presented herein are classified according which sub-sites are targeted by their synthetic modifications.

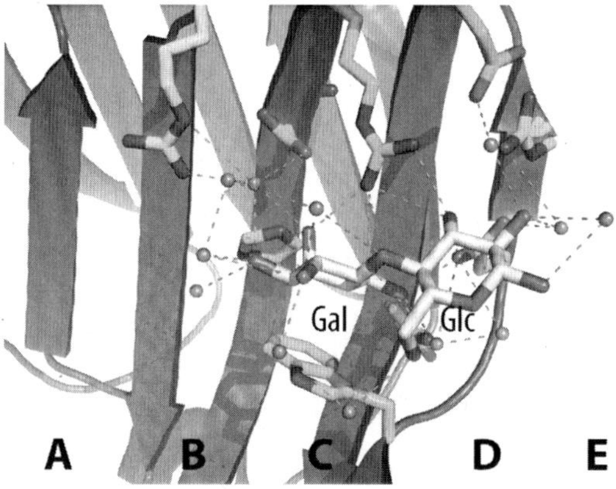

Figure 1. An ultra-high resolution (0.86Å) X-ray structure of galectin-3 in complex with lactose (10) showing the core ß-D-galactoside situated in sub-site C and the D-glucose in sub-site D. Sub-sites A-B and E protrudes beyond gal-HO3 and glc-HO1, respectively, and are unoccupied. (see color insert)

Sub-Site A-B

X-ray structures of galectins in complex with natural ligands early on revealed binding grooves or valleys extending beyond the key galactose O1 and O3 positions (sub-sites A-B and D-E in Figure 2). Hence, an attractive strategy emerging in the late '90s was to create synthetic low-molecular weight inhibitors occupying these sub-sites by derivatizing galactose at O1/C1 or O3/C3. Targeting sub-sites A-B was accomplished through synthesis of several series of O3/C3-modified lacNAc derivatives; 3-*O*-benzyl ethers (*14*), C3-amides (*13*, *15*), C3-thioureas (*16*), and 1,2,3-triazoles (*17*, *18*). In particular, the aromatic nature of these lacNAc-modifications proved to enhance affinities for galectin-1 (4-phenyl-1,2,3-triazole), galectin-3 (benzyl ethers, benzamides, and 4-phenyl-1,2,3-triazoles), and galectin-7 (aryl thioureas). In addition, 4-carbamoyl-1,2,3-triazol-1-yl substitution at C3 of lacNAc resulted in an affinity enhancement for galectin-3 in the same range as the corresponding 4-phenyl-1,2,3-triazol-1-yl derivatives. The role of the aromatic group in the C3-benzamides was discovered to reside in stacking interactions with galectin-3 arg144 (*13*, *19*), suggesting that cation-π interactions together with desolvation effects may contribute the affinity enhancement. Interestingly, the aromatic substitution pattern of the C3-benzamide has a profound effect on the interaction mode, while as an unsubstituted benzamide simply stacked onto the galectin-3 arg144 side chain (Figure 2b) (*19*), a less well solvated 2,3,5,6-tetrafluoro-4-methoxy-benzamide minimized water contact by inducing a 3Å move of the entire arg144 side chain to create and insert into a novel cavity (Figure 2c) (*13*). This observation hints towards possibilities to control galectin conformations via properly designed inhibitor groups and thus create novel inhibitor interaction sites.

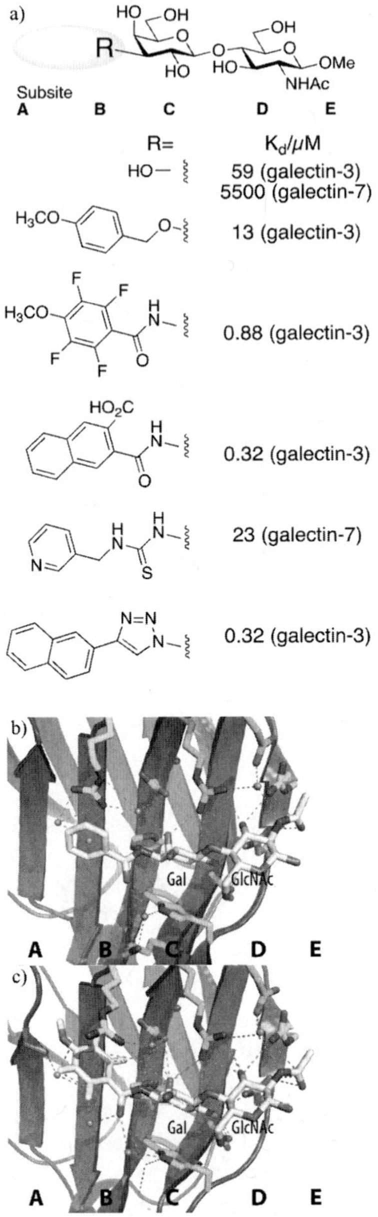

Figure 2. a) Derivatives of N-acetyllactosamine carrying aromatic moieties at O3' or C3' interacting favorably in galectin sub-sites A-B. K_d values are determined by a competitive fluorescence polarization assay (11, 12). X-ray structure of galectin-3 co-crystallized with a b) 3'-benzamido-LacNAc derivative (10) and a c) 3'-(2,3,5,6-tetrafluoro-4-methoxy)-benzamido-LacNAc derivative (13). (see color insert)

More recently, we demonstrated that association of galectin-3 with the C3-benzamido lacNAc derivatives discussed above and with lactose induces large increases in protein conformational entropy (*19*). The increases in conformational entropy were in the range of the enthalpic contributions to the free energy of binding. This somewhat unexpected observation suggests that design of galectin inhibitors should not only take into account enthalpic interactions, but also the under-exploited and often neglected, or at best, under-estimated inhibitor effects on protein conformational entropy changes. Although several of these O3/C3-modified lacNAc derivatives often possess improved affinities and selectivities compared to natural ligands, all compounds still contain an (almost) intact lacNAc disaccharide and thus the associated disadvantages such as high polarity/low bioavailability and chemical/enzymatic lability *in vivo*. Hence, further optimization is desirable to improve affinity, selectivity, and ADMET properties.

Sub-Site E

The discovery that C3-substitution of lacNAc with aromatic moieties could provide a significant affinity enhancement and improved galectin sub-type selectivity through aromatic-arginine stacking interactions stimulated efforts to design inhibitors that presented on aromatic group to interact with the galectin-conserved arginine residue, *e.g.* arg74, 186, 75, and 87 in galectin-1, 3, 7, 9 N-terminal (9N), respectively, that are located near bound lactose O2 (Figure 1). Along this hypothesis, we designed and synthesized structurally simple lactosides carrying at O2 benzoate derivatives, which provided inhibitor orders of magnitude more potent (K_d low μM) than the parent lac or lacNAc disaccharides for galectin-1, 3, and 9N (Figure 3) (*20*). However, as for the sub-site A-B-binding compounds discussed above, the low-μM affinity of the lactose *O*2-esters would still need to be improved, together with ADMET properties, in order to reach the status of promising candidates for therapeutic interventions.

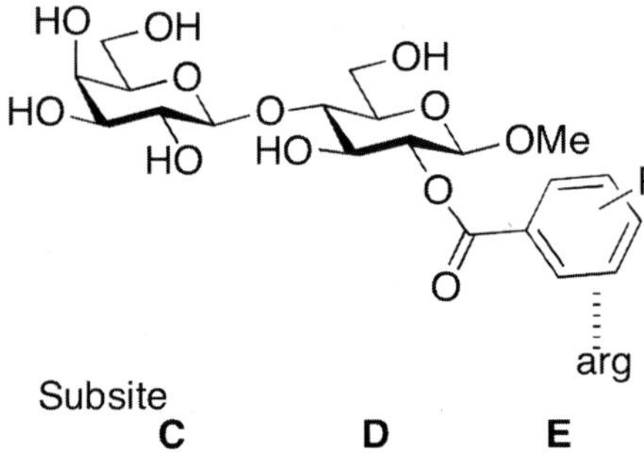

K_d

R= H: 4.4 μM (galectin-1)

R= 3,5-di-OMe: 2.2 μM (galectin-3)

R= 1-naphthoate: 1.6 μM (galectin-9N)

Figure 3. 2-O-Aryloyl lactose derivative targeting galectin sub-site E.

Sub-Site A-B and E

Taking cue from our successful studies of sub-site A-B and E interactions with aromatic ligand appendices, we subsequently embarked on combining these interactions into one single inhibitor by attaching two aromatic structural elements onto a disaccharide scaffold. Symmetrically 3,3′-substituted thiodigalactoside derivatives appeared particularly attractive in this respect as the two 3,3′-substituents would end up in sub-sites A-B and E, respectively, and in these potentially also interact favorably with arginine side chains discussed above, *e.g.* arg144 and arg186 in galectin-3. Indeed, such thiodigalactosides carrying aromatic esters (*21*) or amides (*22*, *23*) or at both C3-positions proved to be exceptionally potent inhibitors of galectin-3 and 9N with association constants in sub-μM and double-digit nM range, respectively (Figure 4). Other galectins investigated were generally less well inhibited. Subsequently, we continued with an investigation into the possibility of 3,3′-triazolyl-thiodigalactosides being able of forming similar affinity-enhancing double arginine interactions with galectins (Figure 4). Indeed, the 3,3′-triazolyl-thiodigalactosides proved to be about as efficient galectin-3 and 9N inhibitors as the corresponding aromatic amides (*17*).

The 3,3′-disubstituted thiodigalactosides are the most potent low-molecular weight galectin inhibitors reported to date and they have been demonstrated to be promising lead structures in cancer and inflammation relevant *in vitro* and *in vivo* experiments including anti-motility effects on (*21*) and enhancing sensitivity towards pro-apoptotic drugs in tumor cells (*24*), fibrosis (*25*, *26*), and hepatitis (*27*). Hence, these classes of compound constitute the most promising low-molecular weight lead structures to date with high affinity and good solubility-polarity balance (clogP 0 to 2), although further optimization is needed with respect to size, galectin selectivity, polar surface area, number of hydrogen bonding sites, and ADMET properties etc.

Sub-Site D

As reasonable affinity (low μM) is achieved by occupying sub-site C-D with saccharides, most inhibitors have been developed based on disaccharide scaffolds such as lactose, N-acetyllactosamine, or thiodigalactoside. However, this often leaves the inhibitors with a varying risk of acidic or enzymatic cleavage of the disaccharide glycoside bond. Hence, we have also investigated the possibility of replacing the sub-site D-binding saccharide moiety with non-carbohydrate structural elements and galactosyl oximes and phenyl thioglycosides. Aromatic *O*-galactosyloximes were thus discovered to be very selective inhibitors of galectin-3 (*28*) and substituted phenyl thio-galactosides to be selective inhibitors of galectin-7 (*29*), both with affinities in the range of natural disaccharide fragments (Figure 5). The inhibitory efficiency of the *O*-galactosyl oximes could be significantly improved by adding the affinity-enhancing sub-site B-binding aromatic amides or triazoles (*30*) described above (Figure 5).

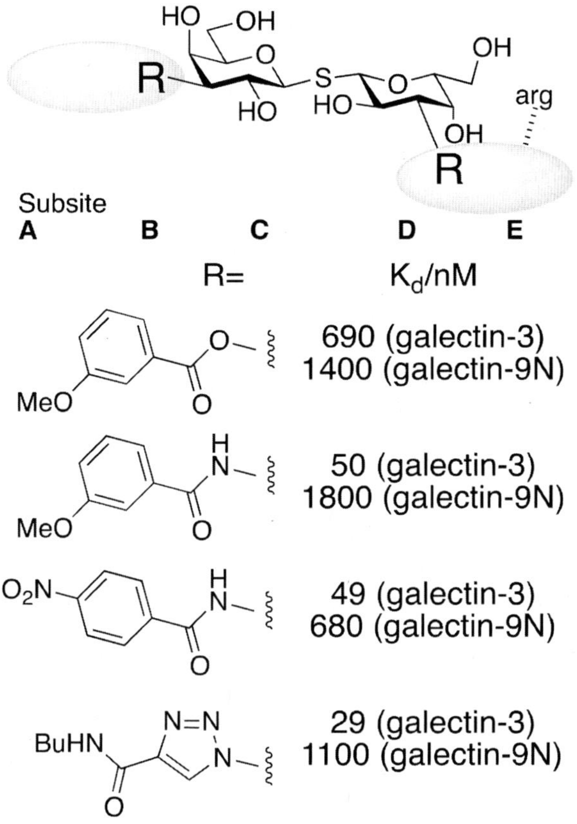

Figure 4. 3,3'-Di-benzoyl, -benzamido, and -triazolyl-thiodigalactosides. Other galectins showed a lower binding capacity. The 3,3'-di-(3-methoxybenzoyl) derivative was named TD131 in an investigation of its effects of enhancing thyroid tumor cell apoptosis (24), the 3,3'-di-3-(3-methoxybenzamido derivative was evidenced to block alternative macrophage activation (25), and an analog of the 3,3'-di-triazole was named TD139 in investigations of anti-fibrotic (26) and anti-inflammatory (27) effects in vivo.

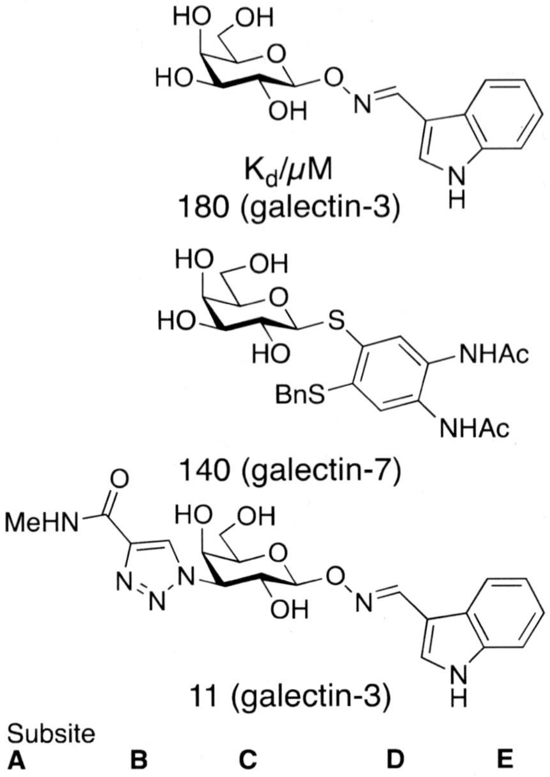

Figure 5. Sub-site D-binding O-galactosyl oximes and phenyl thio-galactosides.

Sub-Site C

The core ß-D-galactopyranose bound in sub-site C interacts primarily with galectins by it's α-face stacking onto a trp side chain and HO4 and HO6 forming hydrogen bonds to other conserved amino acids. Presumably, any monosaccharide or other molecule that can mimic these interactions would potentially bind sub-site C. In accordance with this hypothesis, ß-mannosyl triazoles were demonstrated to inhibit galectin-3 and 9N (Figure 6) (*31*). The triazole moiety presumably interacts with sub-site (A-)B, as discussed for other inhibitors above, while the mannose HO2 mimics the hydrogen bonding pattern of galactose HO4. Furthermore, galactose HO2 does not form any interactions within sub-site C, suggesting that the structural and/or stereochemical variations at this position may very well be tolerated by galectins. Indeed, inversion at galactose C2 resulted in taloside derivatives that inhibit galectin-3, 4C and 8N well. In fact, galectin-4C and 8N bound talose derivatives stronger than the parent galactose derivatives (*32*). Taking these structures one step further by introducing novel functionalities at talose O2 resulted in inhibitors engaging in previously un-exploited interactions with sub-sites perpendicular to the natural ligand-binding sub-sites A-E; see below.

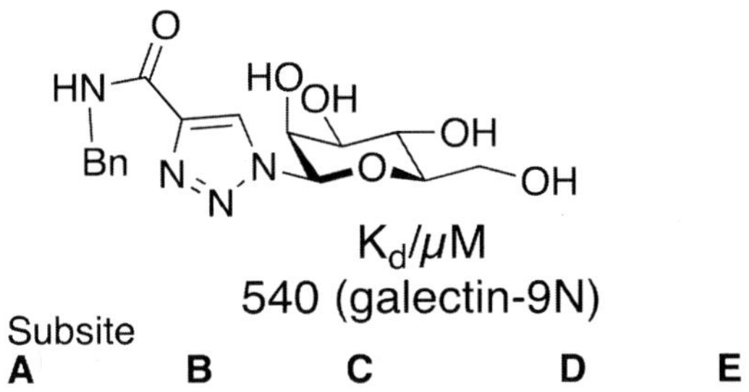

Figure 6. Triazol-1-yl ß-mannosyl amides hypothesized to mimic the binding of 3-(triazol-1-yl)-galactosides in sub-site B-C.

Other Sub-Sites

The cases above all describe galectin inhibitors that interact with sub-sites A-E, *i.e.* sub-sites typically occupied by natural oligosaccharide ligands. However, most galetins have more or less pronounced sub-sites perpendicular to the 5 ß-sheet-traversing A-E sub-sites. In particular, a sub-site stretching out from the ß-side of a galactoside bound in sub-site C varies significantly between galectins, which renders this site an attractive target for developing selective inhibitors. Our first series of compounds intended to exploit such a sub-site were galactosides derivatized at O2 (Figure 7). Among these compounds, anionic substituents, a 2-*O*-sulfates in particular, resulted in enhanced affinity for galectin-3 (*33, 34*), while 2-*O*-alkylphosphates were improved inhibitors of galectin-7 (*34*). The 2-*O*-anionic substituents may enhance the affinity for galectin-3 by interacting with *e.g.* arg 144, while a 2-*O*-benzyl-phosphate was evidenced by X-ray crystallography to favorably interact with arg31 in galectin-7 (*35*). Although the anionic 2-*O*-substituents proved to be potent inhibitors of galectin-3 and 7 in a protein affinity assay, their polar and ionic nature presumably limits the use in *in vivo* and as drug leads.

Extending the 2-*O*-substitution strategy to the sub-site C-binding galactose-mimicking talosides, described above, and combining it with sub-site B-binding aromatic esters or amides was productive and resulted in promising inhibitors of galectin-4C (*32, 36*) and 8N (*32*). Importantly, any doubts to whether the talosides actually mimic galactosides in binding sub-site C was recently put aside by X-ray structural studies with the substituted talosides in complex with galectin-1 and 3 (*37*). In this study, the talosides indeed bound sub-site C by stacking onto the conserved trp side chain and by forming hydrogens bond via HO4 and HO6 in a manner identical to that of natural galactoside-containing ligands (Figure 8).

The examples described above evidence that it is possible to improve both affinity and selectivity of low-molecular weight compounds for galectins by chemically modifying galactose (and other monosaccharides) with non-carbohydrate structural elements targeting ligand sub-sites flanking the core galactose-binding sub-site C. Indeed, inhibitors have been made that possess both low-nM affinities for galectins (*in vitro*) and they show potent *in vivo* efficacy. Hence, promising low-molecular weight galectin-targeting lead structures have been identified, although it remains to investigate and optimize ADME and toxicology aspects of these compounds in order to fully reach the status of identifying clinical candidates.

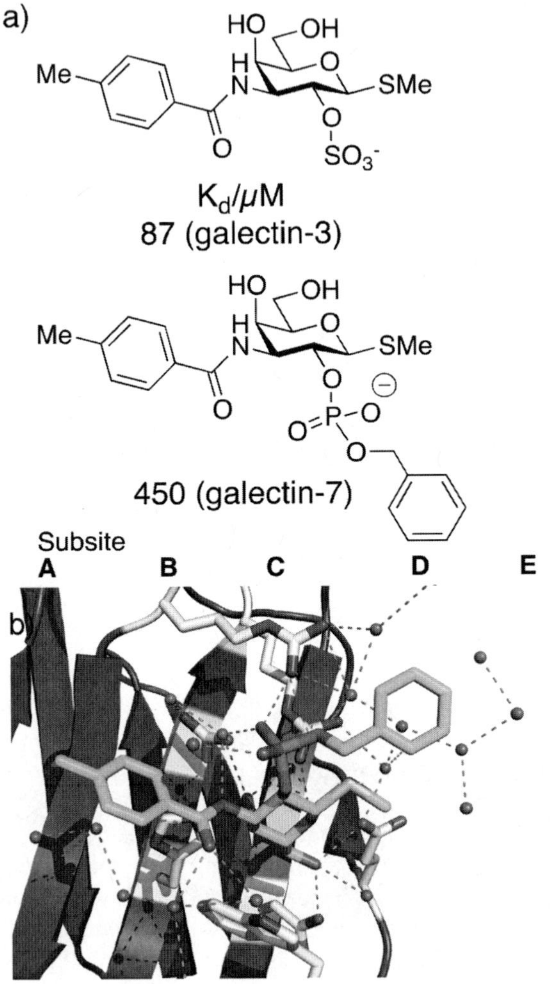

Figure 7. a) 2,3-Disubstituted galactosides interacting with sub-sites perpendicular to the A-E sub-sites. b) A 2-O-benzylphosphate in complex with galectin-7. (see color insert)

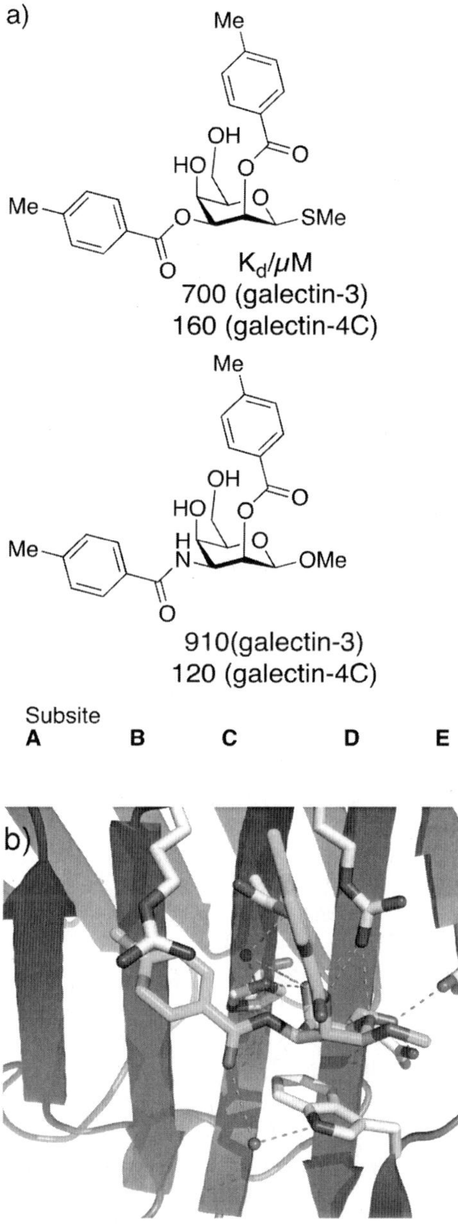

Figure 8. a) 2,3-Disubstituted talosides interacting with sub-sites perpendicular to the A-E sub-sites. b) A 2,3-disubstituted taloside in complex with galectin-3. (see color insert)

Acknowledgments

This work was supported by the Swedish Research Council (Grant No. 621-2003-4265), the foundation "Olle Engkvist Byggmästare", and the Royal Fysiographic Society, Lund.

References

1. Leffler, H. *Glycoconjugate J.* **2004**, *19*, 433.
2. Liu, F.-T.; Rabinovich, G. A. *Nat. Rev. Cancer* **2005**, *5*, 29.
3. Liu, F. T.; Rabinovich, G. A. *Ann. N. Y. Acad. Sci.* **2010**, *1183*, 158.
4. Rabinovich, G. A.; Croci, D. O. *Immunity* **2012**, *36*, 322.
5. Ingrassia, L.; Camby, I.; Lefranc, F.; Mathieu, V.; Nshimyumukiza, P.; Darro, F.; Kiss, R. *Curr. Med. Chem.* **2006**, *13*, 3513.
6. Oberg, C.; Leffler, H.; Nilsson, U. J. *Chimia* **2011**, *65*, 1.
7. Leffler, H.; Carlsson, S.; Hedlund, M.; Qian, Y.; Poirier, F. *Glycoconjugate J.* **2004**, *19*, 433.
8. Hirabayashi, J.; Hashidate, T.; Arata, Y.; Nishi, N.; Nakamura, T.; Hirashima, M.; Urashima, T.; Oka, T.; Futai, M.; Muller, W. E. G.; Yagi, F.; Kasai, K.-i. *Biochem. Biophys. Acta* **2002**, *1572*, 232.
9. Knibbs, R.; Agrwal, N.; Wang, J. L.; Goldstein, I. J. *J. Biol. Chem.* **1993**, *268*, 14940.
10. Saraboji, K.; Håkansson, M.; Genheden, S.; Diehl, C.; Qvist, J.; Weininger, U.; Nilsson, U.; Leffler, H.; Ryde, U.; Akke, M.; Logan, D. *Biochemistry* **2011**, *51*, 296.
11. Sörme, P.; Kahl-Knutsson, B.; Huflejt, M.; Nilsson, U. J.; Leffler, H. *Anal. Biochem.* **2004**, *334*, 36.
12. Sörme, P.; Kahl-Knutsson, B.; Wellmar, U.; Nilsson, U. J.; Leffler, H. *Meth. Enzymol.* **2003**, *362*, 504.
13. Sörme, P.; Arnoux, P.; Kahl-Knutsson, B.; Leffler, H.; Rini, J. M.; Nilsson, U. J. *J. Am. Chem. Soc.* **2005**, *127*, 1737.
14. Sörme, P.; Kahl-Knutsson, B.; Wellmar, U.; Magnusson, B.-G.; Leffler, H.; Nilsson, U. J. *Methods Enzymol.* **2003**, *363*, 157.
15. Sörme, P.; Qian, Y.; Nyholm, P.-G.; Leffler, H.; Nilsson, U. J. *ChemBioChem* **2002**, *3*, 183.
16. Salameh, B. A.; Sundin, A.; Leffler, H.; Nilsson, U. J. *Bioorg. Med. Chem.* **2006**, *14*, 1215.
17. Salameh, B. A.; Cumpstey, I.; Sundin, A.; Leffler, H.; Nilsson, U. J. *Bioorg. Med. Chem.* **2010**, *18*, 5367.
18. Salameh, B. A.; Leffler, H.; Nilsson, U. J. *Bioorg. Med. Chem. Lett.* **2005**, *15*, 3344.
19. Diehl, C.; Engström, O.; Delaine, T.; Håkansson, M.; Genheden, S.; Modig, K.; Leffler, H.; Ryde, U.; Nilsson, U. J.; Akke, M. *J. Am. Chem. Soc.* **2010**, *132*, 14577.
20. Cumpstey, I.; Salomonsson, E.; Sundin, A.; Leffler, H.; Nilsson, U. J. *ChemBioChem* **2007**, *8*, 1389.

21. Delaine, T.; Cumpstey, I.; Ingrassia, L.; Le Mercier, M.; Okechukwu, P.; Leffler, H.; Kiss, R.; Nilsson, U. J. *J. Med. Chem.* **2008**, *51*, 8109.
22. Cumpstey, I.; Salomonsson, E.; Sundin, A.; Leffler, H.; Nilsson, U. J. *Chem. Eur. J.* **2008**, *14*, 4233.
23. Cumpstey, I.; Sundin, A.; Leffler, H.; Nilsson, U. J. *Angew. Chem., Int. Ed.* **2005**, *44*, 5110.
24. Lin, C.-I.; Whang, E. E.; Donner, D. B.; Jiang, X.; Price, B. D.; Carothers, A. M.; Delaine, T.; Leffler, H.; Nilsson, U. J.; Nose, V.; Moore, F. D.; Ruan, D. T. *Mol. Cancer Res.* **2009**, *7*, 1655.
25. MacKinnon, A. C.; Farnworth, S. L.; Hodkinson, P. S.; Henderson, N. C.; Atkinson, K. M.; Leffler, H.; Nilsson, U. J.; Haslett, C.; Forbes, S. J.; Sethi, T. *J. Immunol.* **2008**, *180*, 2650.
26. Mackinnon, A. C.; Gibbons, M. A.; Farnworth, S. L.; Leffler, H.; Nilsson, U. J.; Delaine, T.; Simpson, A. J.; Forbes, S. J.; Hirani, N.; Gauldie, J.; Sethi, T. *Am. J. Resp. Crit. Care Med.* **2012**, *185*, 537.
27. Volarevic, V.; Milovanovic, M.; Ljujic, B.; Pejnovic, N.; Arsenijevic, N.; Nilsson, U.; Leffler, H.; Lukic, M. L. *Hepatology* **2012**; DOI: 10.1002/hep.25542.
28. Tejler, J.; Leffler, H.; Nilsson, U. J. *Bioorg. Med. Chem. Lett.* **2005**, *15*, 2343.
29. Cumpstey, I.; Carlsson, S.; Leffler, H.; Nilsson, U. J. *Org. Biomol. Chem.* **2005**, *3*, 1922.
30. Tejler, J.; Salameh, B.; Leffler, H.; Nilsson, U. J. *Org. Biomol. Chem.* **2009**, *7*, 3982.
31. Tejler, J.; Skogman, F.; Leffler, H.; J., N. U. *Carbohydr. Res.* **2007**, *342*, 1869.
32. Öberg, C. T.; Blanchard, H.; Leffler, H.; Nilsson, U. J. *Bioorg. Med. Chem. Lett.* **2008**, *18*, 3691.
33. Öberg, C. T.; Leffler, H.; Nilsson, U. J. *J. Med. Chem.* **2008**, *51*, 2297.
34. Öberg, C. T.; Noresson, A.-L.; Leffler, H.; Nilsson, U. J. *Chem. Eur. J.* **2011**, *17*, 8139.
35. Masuyer, G.; Jabeen, T.; Oberg, C. T.; Leffler, H.; Nilsson, U. J.; Acharya, K. R. *FEBS J.* **2011**, *279*, 193.
36. Öberg, C. T.; Noresson, A.-L.; Leffler, H.; Nilsson, U. J. *Tetrahedron* **2011**, *67*, 9164.
37. Collins, P. M.; Oberg, C. T.; Leffler, H.; Nilsson, U. J.; Blanchard, H. *Chem. Biol. Drug Des.* **2012**, *79*, 339.

Chapter 3

From Carbohydrate to Peptidomimetic Inhibitors of Galectins

Kevin H. Mayo*

Department of Biochemistry, Molecular Biology & Biophysics, 6-155 Jackson Hall, University of Minnesota, 321 Church Street, Minneapolis, Minnesota 55455
***E-mail: mayox001@umn.edu**

Although the roles that galectins play in controlling and mediating various biological processes is ever growing, only recently have galectins been accepted as valid therapeutic targets for clinical intervention. Because galectin inhibitors have therapeutic potential in many areas, e.g. as anti-inflammatory, anti-cancer, and even anti-HIV-1 agents, considerable efforts are being made by many laboratories to discover or design galectin antagonists. However, none are presently available for standard-of-care use in the clinic. To date, most galectin antagonists target the carbohydrate binding site, and as such are generally ß-galactoside-analogs and glycomimetics. Several peptide-based galectin inhibitors have also been reported, and one of these, calixarene-based peptidomimetic PTX008 that targets galectin-1, is presently in a phase I clinical trial. This review provides an overview of various galectin inhibitors reported to date.

Keywords: NMR, nuclear magnetic resonance spectroscopy; CRD, carbohydrate binding domain; RMSD, root mean square deviation

Galectin Structure: The Starting Point for Inhibitor Design

High resolution structures have been reported for many galectins (*1*). In all instances, the galectin CRD folded structure is composed of two antiparallel β-sheets of five (β1 to β5) and six (β6-β11) β-strands, arranged in a β-sheet sandwich motif, that has an overall "jelly roll" topology (e.g. galectin-1, PDB 1gzw (*2*) in Figure 1a). Most importantly is the fact that monomer folds of all CRDs are highly homologous, not only between the same galectin from different species, but also between/among all galectins, with RMSD values for β-strand backbone atoms of < ~1 Å. In these structures, loops are more variable due in part to increased flexibility and differences in amino acid type and number of residues.

Galectins are also known to self-associate, mostly forming dimers, especially those from the prototype group, and despite homology of their monomer structures, these galectins can form different types of dimers. The so-called "terminal" dimer is formed through hydrophobic interactions between N- and C-terminal residues of the two monomer subunits, with the subunits being related by a 2-fold rotation axis that runs approximately perpendicular to the plane of the β-sheets (e.g. galectin-1 in Figure 1a). This dimer interface involves β-strands β1 and β11 from each subunit (*1*). Another prototype dimer is exemplified with galectin-7 (Figure 1b) whose interface is formed by electrostatic interactions among charged residues on the convex surfaces of two monomers.

Oligomerization increases the number of CRDs in the galectin complex, and this allows galectins in general to function by cross-linking glycans on the surfaces of cells (*1*).

The carbohydrate binding site of galectin CRDs, which is highly conserved (e.g. arginine, histidine, asparagine, glutamine, and a totally conserved tryptophan that interacts with the hydrophobic surface of the galactose ring) among all galectins, is located at the top of the six-stranded β-sheet (*1*), as illustrated in Figures 1a,b, with bound lactose molecules shown in green. Lactose is essentially "grabbed" by the peptide loop above the lactose molecule and the relatively large and flat tryptophan side chain at the bottom of the disaccharide. NMR structural studies indicate that this loop is relatively flexible when the disaccharide is absent, and is more firmly positioned when the disaccharide is bound (*3*). However, conformational flexibility, at least in galectin-1 (*3*) and galectin-3 (*4*), is actually increased upon ligand binding which contributes favorably to thermodynamic stability of the ligand-bound complex. Lactose is the simpliest disaccharide to which galectins bind, with affinities usually in the micromolar range, i.e. 64×10^{-6} M to 80×10^{-6} M (*3*). Carbohydrate binding affinity can be increased by modifying the lactose disaccharide, e.g. to *N*-acetyllactosamine (*1*). Although galectins were originally identified as β-galactoside binding lectins, they can also bind to carbohydrates with various other linkages, e.g. α-galactosides (*5–7*). Moreover, actual carbohydrate moieties of glycoconjugates on the cell surface are far more complicated than simple β-galactosides like lactose or *N*-acetyllactosamine, and it is likely that other saccharide units in those glycans interact to some extent with galectins to determine and/or differentiate the function of various galectins. In fact, the carbohydrate binding site on galectin-1 has been reported to be larger than that covered by simple disaccharides (*8*).

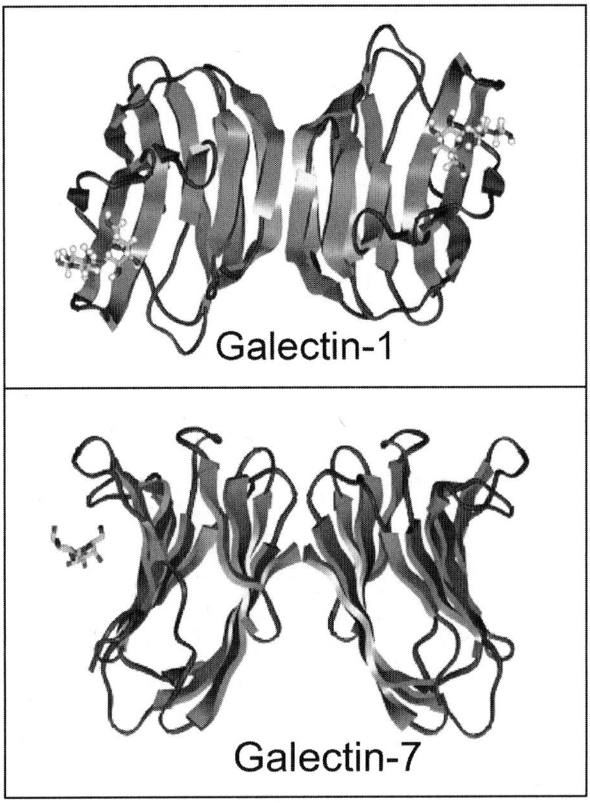

Figure 1. The structure of prototype galectin-1 dimer (PDB access code 1gzw) (upper panel) and prototype galectin-7 dimer (PDB access code 1bkz) (lower panel). The carbohydrate binding site in each monomer subunit (upper panel) or in one of the monomer subunits in the dimer (lower panel) is indicated by a lactose molecule shown as a ball-and-stick structure in green. (see color insert)

Because specific interactions with different β-galactosides like lactose are generally quite similar for all galectin CRDs (*1*), these have usually been at the heart of designing galectin inhibitors. Three hydroxy groups of lactose (or N-acetyl-lactosamine), i.e., the C4-OH and C6-OH of Gal and the C3-OH of GlcNAc (or Glc), are required to form hydrogen bonds with side chains of hydrophilic residues from galectins. The galactose ring in particular forms several H-bonds between its oxygen atoms O4, O5 and O6, and H44, E71, and N61 of galectin-1. The O3 of the glucose ring forms H-bonds with residues R48 and E71. H52 and W68 are proposed to have van der Waals interactions with both the glucose and galactose rings, respectively. The non-polar side of the galactose ring (composed primarily of its C1, C3, and C5 hydrogen atoms and distinguished by its axial C4-OH on the more polar side) interacts primarily with the tryptophan residue. This hydrophobically mediated interaction contributes favorably to the binding free energy, and plays a role in the binding site discrimination between the galactose and glucose rings. In contrast to galactose, glucose has its C4-OH group in an equatorial position, which decreases the apolar nature of the corresponding surface and attenuates hydrophobic interactions with the conserved tryptophan (*1*). Aside from lactose, galectin structures in complex with *N*-acetyllactosamine, linear trisaccharde, and *N*-acetyllactosamine octasaccharide have also been reported (*1*). In all cases, a carbohydrate disaccharide moiety binds the galectin in a similar fashion.

In addition, the number of ligand contacts is correlated with the binding affinities. For example, substitution of the hydroxyl group by deoxy-acetamido in position 2 of the reducing sugar (glucose vs. N-acetyl-glucose) increases binding affinity by about 5-fold (*1*). This increase may be due to interaction with the acetyl group. Furthermore, derivatization of the β-galactoside in N-acetyllactosamine at the 3′ position with the charged substituent sialic acid increases binding affinity by 2-fold compared to that from LacNAc, and addition of the α1-2fucoside further consolidates binding by reducing the K_d by 4-fold over that of LacNAc. Perhaps the largest effect is observed with the linear B2 trisaccharide or Galili pentasaccharide, where the K_d value (1×10^{-6} M) is about 10-fold lower (i.e. better) than with LacNAc. Working with more complex N-acetyllactosamine-based carbohydrates, Leppanen *et al.* (*9*) reported that human galectin-1 binds to immobilized extended glycans (i.e. poly- N-acetyllactosamine, $(\text{-3Gal}\beta\text{1-4GlcNAc}\beta\text{1-})_n$ sequences, complex-type biantennary N-glycans, modified chitin-derived glycans, and even to native and desialylated human pro-myelocytic HL-60 cells) with similar K_d values of 2 to 4 $\times 10^{-6}$ M. Interestingly, galectin-1 binding affinity fell when these glycans were free in solution (i.e. not immobilized), suggesting that the N-acetyllactosamine recognition element on surface-bound glycans is more optimally conformed for favorable interactions with galectin-1. Working with even more complex carbohydrates, Hirabayashi *et al.* (*10*) demonstrated that some galectins, like galectin-1 and galectin-7, showed increased binding affinity with an increase in branching number up to triantennary *N*-glycans. In general, binding affinity to branched *N*-glycans could be increased by up to about a factor of 5 to 10 compared to monovalent analogs. However, for other galectins like galectin-8, *N*-glycan branching lead to decreased affinity. Of further note, galectin-9 showed the greatest affinity for both repeated oligolactosamines and branched type *N*-glycans, with K_d values e.g. of 0.7×10^{-6} M for bianntenary *N*-glycans, and 0.16×10^{-6} M for both trianntenary and tetraanntenary *N*-glycans. These K_d values indicate about 100 times greater affinity for these branched glycans compared to analogous monovalent *N*-glycans. Overall, these data suggest that binding of some galectins to glycans *in situ* will be much stronger than anticipated from results of routine galectin binding assays that employ standard disaccharides like lactose. Moreover, this galectin-dependent variance of *N*-glycan binding (e.g. branched vs. non-branched) may be one way in which galectins could differentially modulate biological activity. This angle, along with maximizing the number of ligand contacts with the lectin, has been exploited in designing selective galectin inhibitors.

Targeting the Carbohydrate Binding Site

Given the structural and functional significance of the galectin CRD carbohydrate binding site, the obvious site in galectins to target is its carbohydrate binding site, and therefore, most investigators have focused their efforts on designing low molecular weight saccharide-based inhibitors that target the CRD carbohydrate binding site. The general approach has been to design competitive inhibitors where binding affinities are greater than that of e.g. lactose or N-acetyllactosamine. Moreover, the multivalent way in which galectins can cross-link glycans has also been exploited in the design of some galectin antagonists.

Galectin antagonists reported to date are mostly ß-galactoside-analogs and glycomimetics that target the obvious, canonical carbohydrate binding site. Most of these compounds were designed to antagonize galectins 1, 3, 7, 8, and 9 (primarily gal-3) and include aryl *O*- and *S*-galactosides and lactosides (*11*, *12*), carbohydrate-based triazoles and isoxazoles (*12*), 3-(1,2,3-triazol-1-yl)-1-thio-galactosides (*13*), anomeric oxime ether derivatives of ß-galactose (*O*-galactosyl aldoximes) (*14*), phenyl thio-ß-**D**-galactopyranoside analogs (*15*), thioureido *N*-acetyllactosamine derivatives (*16*), and multi-valent arene thiodigalactoside bis-benzamido analogs with groups on each end of the carbohydrate moiety to interact with arginine residues within the carbohydrate binding domain (*17*). Other multivalent inhibitors include functionalized unnatural amino acids (phenyl-bis-alanine and phenyl-tris-alanine) with 2-azidoethyl ß-**D**-galactopyranosyl-(1-4)-ß-**D**-glucopyranoside (*18*), a bi-lactosylated steroid-based compound (*19*), and polymethylene-spaced di-lactoseamine derivatives (*20*). The play on attaching hydrophobic groups to a lactose-based compound took a different slant when Fort *et al.* (*21*) attached linear alkyl chains of varying length to the anomeric carbon of the glucose or *N*-acetyl glucose ring of lactose. By screening their synthetic "lacto-*N*-biose" libraries for binding to galectin-3 using microscale affinity chromatography and mass spectrometry, they identified compounds with K_d values ranging from 11 x 10^{-6} M to 73 x 10^{-6} M. These and other related compounds are discussed more thoroughly in Chapter 2.

There are several problems with designing galectin inhibitors for use in the clinic, e.g. weak ligand binding affinity, galectin selectivity, low *in vivo* exposure. Although some of the carbohydrate-based compounds mentioned above bind various galectins *in vitro* with single digit micromolar K_d values, most bind galectins rather weakly with K_d's >100 μM. Galectin selectivity is another significant issue, due primarily to the conserved structural homology of ß-galactoside binding sites among galectins, as discussed above. This issue is being addressed. For example, Collins et al. (*22*) has replaced galactose with talose (C2 epimer of galactose), because O2 substituents are more solvent exposed and should enhance the potential for designing more selective galectin inhibitors. These authors established proof-of-concept by demonstrating differential effects between galectin-1 and galectin-3.

Galectin-3 may in fact be the easiest galectin to target selectively, because its binding site is somewhat different in footprint and composition vis-à-vis other galectins (*1*). This may be important because galectin-3 is crucial to many pathologies. Galectin-3 is anti-apoptotic, and plays a role in tumor development, as well as in cardiac inflammation, fibrosis, hypertrophy, and dysfunction. A number of galectin-3 selective inhibitors have been reported. Glinsky et al. (*23*) found that lactulosyl-L-leucine (Lac-L-Leu) targets galectin-3 to promote apoptosis in human cancer cells, and augments paclitaxel activity by increasing its efficacy against established metastases. Liu et al. (*24*) reported that the naturally-occuring tetrapeptide N-acetyl-seryl-aspartyl-lysyl-proline (Ac-SDKP) prevents Gal-3-induced cardiac inflammation and collagen deposition in the heart in hypertension and heart failure post-myocardial infarction. Lin et al. (*25*) reported that a galectin-3 targeting thio-lactose-based compound, Td131_1, promoted apoptosis, improved radiosensitivity, and synergistically enhanced chemosensitivity to doxorubicin in papillary thyroid cancer (PTC) cell lines (8505-C and TPC-1). However, the *in vitro* inhibitory concentration of Td131_1 was found to be in the 200 μM to 600 μM range for about 50% effect, indicating that it is a relatively weak inhibitor of Gal-3. Nevertheless, as an adjuvant, Td131_1 did enhance effects from doxorubicin and increased radiosensitivity in clonogenic assays.

Although few of these galectin inhibitors has been tested *in vivo*, bioavailabilty of simple carbohydrate-based compounds will also likely be problematic in *in vivo* settings, primarily due to hydrolysis, metabolism, and short half-lives. Unless these issues can be overcome, it appears that targeting galectins with carbohydrate-based inhibitors will remain an academic exercise. One solution to this issue may be to use larger glycans that would be less subject to clearance and metabolism.

Galectin Therapeutics, Inc. already has a plant-derived α-galactomannan, GM-CT-01(Davanat), in the clinic (see http://clinicaltrials.gov/ct2/show/NCT00110721). This glycan has a weight average molecular weight of 59 kDa (*26*), allowing it to cleared more slowly from circulation vis-à-vis simple carbohydrates. Its larger size also should make it less susceptible to rapid metabolism *in vivo*. In addition, GM-CT-01 has a larger footprint for binding to galectin-1 (*5*). GCS-100 (La Jolla Pharmaceuticals; Prospect Therapeutics) is a large modified glycan (~1000 kDa) derived from citrus pectin that targets galectin-3. In the clinic, GCS-100 has an acceptable human safety profile, as well as an anti-myeloma effect in the context of bortezomib resistance (*27*). It is active in several animal tumor models and in phase 1 studies with solid tumors and CLL32 with minimal toxicity to normal lymphocytes or myelopoiesis.

Non-Carbohydrate-Based Inhibitors

For reasons discussed above, low molecular weight carbohydrates may not be the best galectin inhibitors for use in the clinic. An alternative approach is to target galectins at sites other than their carbohydrate binding site with peptides or peptidomimetics. These sites on galectins are likely to be less conserved and may allow for better galectin-specific targeting. Complex glycans found on the surface of cells may in fact interact with galectins at surface patches that are not within, or are more distant from, the canonical carbohydrate binding site. In fact, such a site has been observed for the binding of GM-CT-01 to galectin-1 (*5*). This is one site that may be targeted with non-carbohydrate inhibitors. Although an obvious site to target is at galectin oligomer interfaces (*28*), no inhibitors that target this site have been reported.

Rotblat *et al.* (*29*) identified a hydrophobic patch on galectin-1 that is analogous to the Cdc42 geranylgeranyl binding site on RhoGDI from the X-ray structure of the RhoGDI/Cdc42 complex (*30*). By comparing the Cdc42 geranylgeranyl- binding cavity on RhoGDI with the surface of homologously folded galectin-1, Rotblat *et al.* (*29*) identified a homologous hydrophobic isoprenoid-binding site on galectin-1. This proposed farnesyl-like binding site incorporates galectin-1 residues L9, L11, L17, F30, F32, and I128, which lie within the β-sheet sandwich fold. Because a binding analysis suggested that L11 was most crucial for interactions with a farnesyl-like group, Rotblat *et al.* (*29*) used site-directed mutagenesis to generate a L11A mutant of galectin-1 and provide proof for their model. Their work demonstrated that the L11A mutant destabilized Ras-GTP and its association with the membrane, and subsequently inhibited Ras function (fibroblast transformation and PC12-cell neurite outgrowth). Moreover, the L11A mutant possessed normal galectin-1 carbohydrate binding and dimerization properties, allowing them to conclude that intracellular galectin-1/Ras interactions are not dependent on galectin-1 β-galactoside (lactose) binding (*29*). Whether H-Ras/galectin-1 interactions indeed involve insertion of the farnesyl moiety of Ras into the described hydrophobic pocket in galectin-1 will need to be validated structurally.

In a related study, Ashery *et al.* (*31*) confirmed that hydrophobic prenyl-binding surfaces on galectin-1 and galectin-3 interact with the farnesyl group on the C-terminus of Ras, thereby contributing to the prolongation of Ras signals in the plasma membrane. More recently, Gorfe *et al.* (*32*) modeled the structure of farnesyl-modified H-Ras protein in a DMPC bilayer, and showed that part of the farnesyl group (the farnesyl cysteine carboxymethylester) in fact lies over a hydrophobic domain on the β-sheet surface of Ras, which in many respects resembles a part of the β-sheet domain in galectins, reminiscent of the Rotblat *et al.* study discussed above. It may be that one face of the β-sheet sandwich of galectin-1 interacts with the β-sheet surface of Ras, as well as with the farnesyl moiety, in a sort of hydrophobic ternary complex.

Competitive inhibitors of glycan binding have also been explored. Moise et al. (*33*) combined proteolytic fragmentation without/with ligand and mass spectrometry to identify two peptides from the carbohydrate recognition domains of galectin-1 (64-73 DGGAWGTEQR and 37-48 DSNNLCLHFNPR) and galectin-3 (152-162 GNDVAFHFNPR and 177-183 LDNNWGR). These peptides harbor key residues in contact with the ligand and therefore represent bioactive sequences in these two galectins. These peptides work by competing with galectins for binding to glycans. For example, the galectin-3-derived hexapeptide FHFNPR (residues 157-162) was able to reduce galectin-3 binding to lactose presented by a surface-adsorbed neoglycoprotein and even interfered with the binding of galectin-3 to the surfaces of cells. However, the peptide concentrations needed are rather high, i.e. 0.5 mM to 2 mM, and this generation of peptide inhibitor will not be a useful therapeutic. Nevertheless, the potential for optimization of this competitive inhibitor is evident.

In a different peptide-based approach, Zou *et al.* (*34*) used combinatorial bacteriophage display and identified 13 peptides, two of which (G3-A9 and G3-C12, with amino acid sequences PQNSKIPGPTFLDPH and ANTPCGPYTHDCPVKR, respectively) bound specifically to galectin-3 (at its carbohydrate binding site) (and not to any other galectins or plant lectins) and with relatively high affinity (K_d of 80 x 10^{-9} M) and inhibited metastasis-associated cancer cell adhesion *in vitro*. Both peptides recognized cell surface galectin-3 on cultured carcinoma cells and monocytes; blocked interaction between galectin-3 and TFAg (Thomsen-Friedenreich glycoantigen), and inhibited adhesion of human breast carcinoma cells to endothelial cells under flow conditions. However, the *in vivo* effectivity of these peptides is not known, as animal model studies have not been performed. Moreover, although these peptides bind galectin-3 and inhibit its biological function *in vitro*, it remains unclear where they bind on the surface of galectin-3, or if they actually block the binding of carbohydrate ligand to galectin-3. Nevertheless, it seems likely that the peptides bind somewhere on the surface of the galectin, and not directly at the carbohydrate binding site, especially because both peptides carry a net positive charge like the actual carbohydrate binding site.

A Galectin-1-Targeting Peptidomimetic in the Clinic

Early on, we designed a series peptide 33mers that formed well-folded β-sheets and remained soluble in aqueous solution under physiological conditions, the βpep series (*35*, *36*). Using NMR spectroscopy, we elucidated the solution structure of βpep-4 and found that this designed peptide folded as an anti-parallel ß-sheet (*37*). Other βpep peptides also formed relatively stable β-sheet structures in aqueous solution (*36*, *38*, *39*). Because most antiangiogenic proteins and peptides (e.g. endostatin, angiostatin, PF4, thrombospondin, gamma interferon-inducible protein-10 (IP-10), tumor necrosis factor, BPI, thrombospondin type 1 repeat peptides, Flt-1 peptide) are structurally and compositionally homologous to βpep peptides (anti-parallel ß-sheet structure and a preponderance of positively charged and hydrophobic residues) (*40*), we screened our βpep library for the ability to inhibit endothelial cell (EC) proliferation, an *in vitro* indicator of angiogenic potential (*41*), and identified ßpep-25 (anginex) as a potent angiogenesis inhibitor. Anginex inhibits tumor growth by attenuating angiogenesis within the tumors in mice (*42–47*), and was most effective against slower growing tumors.

Using yeast 2-hybrid screening and other approaches, galectin-1 has been identified as the molecular target of anginex (*48*). Most importantly, we used NMR spectroscopic HSQC chemical shift mapping using uniformly ^{15}N-enriched galectin-1 to identify the anginex binding site on galectin-1, which lies on the surface of galectin-1 near to the carbohydrate binding site, as illustrated in Figure 2. A molecule of lactose is shown in blue for visual orientation. Since anginex does block adhesion of endothelial cells to the extracellular matrix, it is likely that anginex functions to interfere somehow with molecular interactions between complementary components of the matrix and the endothelial cell surface (*48*).

An SAR study of anginex identified residues responsible for its angiostatic activity (*49*, *50*). This region on anginex includes several hydrophobic residues within the first two ß-strands that were most important to promote the activity of anginex and interact with galectin-1 (Figure 2).

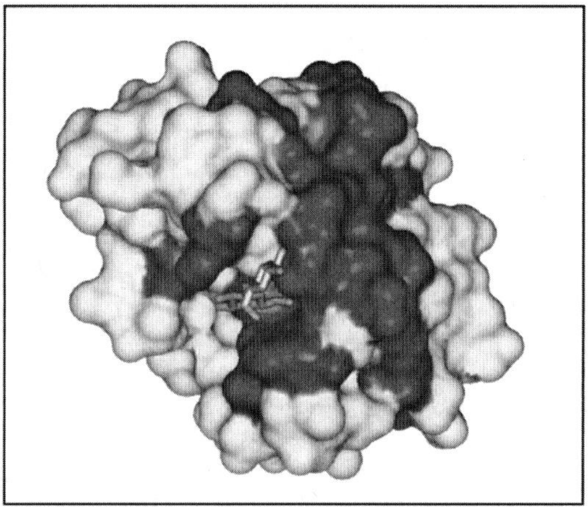

Figure 2. A space filling model of the surface of galectin-1 (PDB access code 1gzw) is shown in yellow, with the anginex interaction site in red, and a molecule of lactose at its binding site in blue (Nesmelova et al, unpublished results). (see color insert)

Moreover, these hydrophobic residues in anginex occur at alternating positions (*i*, *i*+2), consistent with a β-strand motif, as well as at cross-strand positions that comprise the hydrophobic face of the amphipathic ß-sheet structure. We also found that positive charge character was important to angiostatic activity (*51*). Cysteine-substituted, disulfide-linked analogs of anginex firmly established that antiparallel ß-sheet defines the bioactive conformation (*52*).

This SAR information indicated which peptide segments were non-essential (C-terminal residues G27–D33 and the loop (R12-W19) between β-strands 1 and 2) and allowed us to design a partial peptide mimetic of Anginex, called 6DBF7 (*49*), wherein the mimetic has remnants of β-strands 1 and 2 from anginex and a ß-turn mimetic scaffold (dibenzofuran, DBF) (*53*, *54*) to induce ß-sheet formation. The anti-parallel β-sheet structure of 6DBF7 was confirmed by NMR spectroscopy (*49*), with the general topology having an alternating sequence of non-polar vs. polar amino acid residues, as in anginex, which results in one face of the sheet being adorned largely with hydrophobic substituents and the other face with largely positively charged, neutral and hydrophilic negatively charged, respectively, as illustrated in Figure 3.

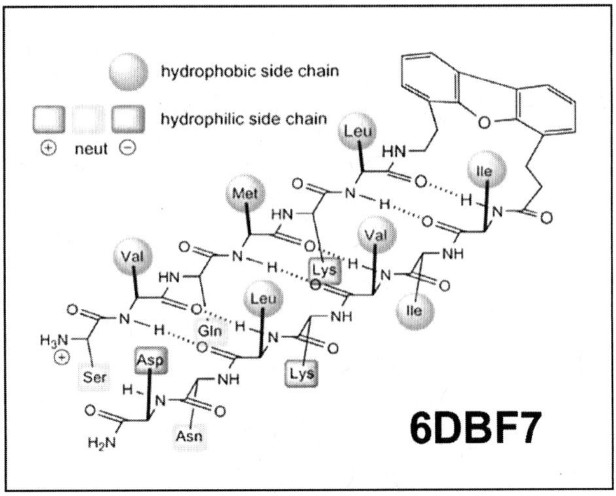

Figure 3. A cartoon structure of 6DBF7. The dibenzofuran moiety is shown head-on at the top right, and polar residues on the hydrophilic side of the amphipathic β-sheet are highlighted with squares and non-polar residues on the hydrophobic side of the amphipathic β-sheet are highlighted with circles. (see color insert)

Using EC proliferation, migration, and sprouting assays, we found that 6DBF7 displayed antiangiogenic activity with an IC_{50} of 15 μM in the EC proliferation assay compared to 4 βM for parent anginex. However, in mice, 6DBF7 was about 2-fold better at inhibiting tumor growth compared to anginex, likely due to better *in vivo* exposure of 6DBF7 (*49*). In these *in vivo* experiments, there was no apparent sign of toxicity from 6DBF7 or anginex, as assessed by unaltered behavior and normal weight gain of the animals, and no change in hematocrit and creatinine levels in the blood. Moreover, macro- and micro-scopic morphology of internal organs were observed to be normal within all experimental groups of animals.

The final step was to re-design the peptidomimetic to eliminate all peptide components and further reduce the size of the inhibitor. With proteins, any interaction surface is defined by the spatial arrangement of amino acid side chains (i.e. chemical groups) that are scaffolded in place by the peptide backbone, which by itself is often irrelevant to the interaction surface. Because of this, we found that we could use an organic scaffold with appropriate chemical appendages to mimic the molecular dimensions, surface topology, and chemical composition of the biofunctional structural unit in anginex and 6DBF7.

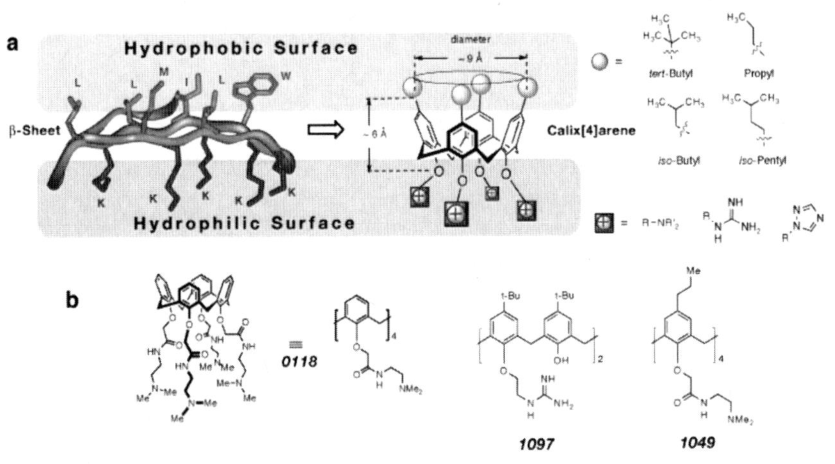

Figure 4. (A) The design concept for β-sheet topomimetics of anginex is shown, with topological features influencing the choice of the calix[4]arene scaffold for arraying hydrophobic and hydrophilic substituents to mimic the structural and compositional characteristics of anginex. In the folded structure of anginex, hydrophobic and hydrophilic surfaces, as well as specific amino acid residues in one letter code, are indicated. The calix[4]arene scaffold is shown to scale, and hydrophobic (t-Bu = tert-butyl; Me = methyl) and basic group chemical substituents that were used on the two faces of the calix[4]arene scaffold are indicated. (B) Two structural representations of the tetra-amine compound 0118 and two related analogs, diguanidine 1097 and inactive tetraamine 1049 are shown. (see color insert)

Figure 4a illustrates the design concept with the calix[4]arene scaffold. The structural unit encompassing key residues in anginex covers approximately the dimensions of a 2-stranded ß-sheet only about four amino acid residues in length on each strand. The overall backbone dimensions are similar to those of a calix[4]arene scaffold. Adding hydrophobic and basic chemical groups to the calix[4]arene scaffold can increase the molecular surface span on each side of the scaffold up to about 15 Å, which approximates maximal distances between proximal side chains in the ß-sheet. From structural biology and synthetic chemistry perspectives, calixarene provides a good scaffold from which to position chemical groups that mimic the character and surface topology of key amino acid side chains in anginex. Based on this rationale, we synthesized a relatively small library of 23 calixarene-based compounds, with each analog displaying chemical substituents (Figure 4b) to mimic the approximate molecular dimensions and amphipathic features of folded anginex (*46, 55*). Nearly all could be prepared rather easily via a four to six step long synthetic route, with a yield of multi-ten mg quantities.

This "small molecule" library of calixarene compounds is unique because calixarene-based protein surface topomimetics maintain volume like that found in small segments of β-sheet (or helix for that matter). Moreover, calixarenes are not "traditional" therapeutics, because they are structurally unlike most, if not all, compounds found in "small molecule" libraries. In drug discovery, a chemical library is only as good as the breadth and variety of the compounds in it. We screened the topomimetic library using an EC proliferation assay and identified two members 0118 and 1097 (see chemical structures in Figure 4) as potent inhibitors of EC growth (*46*), with topomimetic 0118 (IC_{50} = 2 μM) being more active than 1097 (IC_{50} = 8 μM) or anginex (IC_{50} = 4 μM). Both topomimetics were subsequently found to be angiostatic *in vivo* and inhibited tumor growth (60% to 80%) in mouse models at daily doses of 10 mg/Kg (*42–44*, *46*, *47*, *56*). In all *in vivo* experiments, there were no signs of general toxicity from 0118 or 1097, as assessed in the animals by unaltered behavior, normal weight gain, and hematocrit and creatinine levels in the blood. Moreover, macro- and microscopic morphology of internal organs were also observed to be normal within all experimental groups of animals.Calixarene compound 0118 is also known as PTX008 (from PepTx Inc.) and OTX008 (from OncoEthix Inc).

NMR spectroscopy demonstrated that 0118 indeed interacts with galectin-1 and on the surface of the lectin near to, but not at, its carbohydrate binding site (*57*), as observed for anginex and 6DBF7. Topomimetic 0118 functions as a non-competitive, allosteric inhibitor of carbohydrate binding to galectin-1, as demonstrated by several approaches (*57*). Flow cytometry shows that FITC-labeled gal-1 binding to natural glycans on splenocytes (leukocytes ($CD4^+$ and $CD8^+$ cells) and endothelial cells ($CD31^+$)) is inhibited in a dose dependent manner as the concentration of 0118 is increased. This finding is supported by results from agglutination assays where addition of 0118 significantly attenuates RBC and leukocyte agglutination. The concentration responsiveness from 0118 in flow cytometry and agglutination experiments with galectin-1 parallels that observed in cell proliferation inhibition studies using a series of human cell lines that express varying amounts of gal-1.

As an antagonist of galectin-1, calixarene 0118 is unique, primarily because it binds at a site on the lectin that is located on the side to back face of the lectin away from its ß-galactoside-binding site. Since galectin-1 is crucial to several processes required for tumor growth, this may explain why 0118, like anginex and 6DBF7, displays multimodal activities (inhibition of EC proliferation and promotion of leukocyte infiltration into tumors). For instance, interfering with gal-1 function could (i) prevent tumor angiogenesis (*48*), (ii) abrogate tumor escape from immunity through blockade of gal-1-induced apoptosis in activated T lymphocytes (*58*), and (iii) prevent metastasis formation through inhibition of gal-1 facilitated tumor cell-EC interactions.

Preclinical work with 0118 has been promoted by PepTx Inc. and further developed by OncoEthix Inc. who brought the galectin-1 inhibitor into the clinic in a Phase I trial with terminal cancer patients starting in February 2012. At this point, it appears that 0118 is well tolerated in patients, as discussed in Chapter 15.

Acknowledgments

We would like to acknowledge the generous research support of the National Institutes of Health (National Cancer Institute grant CA-096090) that made possible work described in this chapter.

References

1. Nesmelova, I. V.; Dings, R. P. M.; Mayo, K. H. Understanding Galectin Structure-Function Relationships To Design Effective Antagonists. In *Galectins*; Klyosov, A. A., Witczak, Z. J., Platt, D., Eds.; John Wiley & Sons: Hoboken, NJ, 2008; pp 33–69.
2. Lopez-Lucendo, M. F.; Solis, D.; Andre, S.; Hirabayashi, J.; Kasai, K.; Kaltner, H.; Gabius, H. J.; Romero, A. Growth-regulatory human galectin-1: Crystallographic characterisation of the structural changes induced by single-site mutations and their impact on the thermodynamics of ligand binding. *J. Mol. Biol.* **2004**, *343*, 957–970.
3. Nesmelova, I. V.; Ermakova, E.; Daragan, V. A.; Pang, M.; Menéndez, M.; Lagartera, L.; Solís, D.; Baum, L. G.; Mayo, K. H. Lactose binding to galectin-1 modulates structural dynamics, increases conformational entropy, and occurs with apparent negative cooperativity. *J. Mol. Biol.* **2010**, *397*, 1209–1230.
4. Zhuang, T.; Leffler, H.; Prestegard, J. H. Enhancement of bound-state residual dipolar couplings: Conformational analysis of lactose bound to Galectin-3. *Protein Sci.* **2006**, *15*, 1780–1790.
5. Miller, M. C.; Klyosov, A.; Mayo, K. H. The α-galactomannan Davanat binds galectin-1 at a site different from the conventional galectin carbohydrate binding domain. *Glycobiology* **2009**, *19*, 1034–1045.
6. Miller, M. C.; Ribeiro, J. P.; Roldós, V.; Martín-Santamaría, S.; Cañada, F. J.; Nesmelova, I. A.; André, S.; Pang, M.; Klyosov, A. A.; Baum, L. G.; Jiménez-Barbero, J.; Gabius, H. J.; Mayo, K. H. Structural aspects of binding of α-linked digalactosides to human galectin-1. *Glycobiology* **2011**, *21*, 1627–1641.
7. Miller, M. C.; Klyosov, A. A.; Mayo, K. H. Structural features for α-galactomannan binding to galectin-1. *Glycobiology* **2012**, *22*, 543–551.
8. Miller, M. C.; Nesmelova, I. V.; Platt, D.; Klyosov, A.; Mayo, K. H. The carbohydrate-binding domain on galectin-1 is more extensive for a complex glycan than for simple saccharides: Implications for galectin-glycan interactions at the cell surface. *Biochem. J.* **2009**, *421*, 211–221.
9. Leppanen, A.; Stowell, S; Blixt, O.; Cummings, R. D. Dimeric galectin-1 binds with high affinity to alpha2,3-sialylated and non-sialylated terminal *N*-acetyllactosamine units on surface-bound extended glycans. *J. Biol. Chem.* **2005**, *280*, 5549–5562.
10. Hirabayashi, J.; Hashidate, T.; Arata, Y.; Nishi, N.; Nakamura, T.; Hirashima, M.; Urashima, T.; Oka, T.; Futai, M.; Muller, W. E.; Yagi, F.; Kasai, K. Oligosaccharide specificity of galectins: a search by frontal affinity chromatography. *Biochim. Biophys. Acta* **2002**, *1572*, 232–254.

11. Sirois, S.; Giguere, D.; Roy, R. A first QSAR model for galectin-3 glycomimetic inhibitors based on 3D docked structures. *Med. Chem.* **2006**, *2*, 481–489.
12. Giguere, D.; Patnam, R.; Bellefleur, M. A.; St-Pierre, C.; Sato, S.; Roy, R. Carbohydrate triazoles and isoxazoles as inhibitors of galectins-1 and -3. *Chem. Commun.* **2006**, *22*, 2379–2381.
13. Salameh, B. A.; Leffler, H.; Nilsson, U. J. 3-(1,2,3-Triazol-1-yl)-1-thio-galactosides as small, efficient, and hydrolytically stable inhibitors of galectin-3. *Bioorg. Med. Chem. Lett.* **2005**, *15*, 3344–3346.
14. Tejler, J.; Leffler, H.; Nilsson, U. J. Synthesis of O-galactosyl aldoximes as potent LacNAc-mimetic galectin-3 inhibitors. *Bioorg. Med. Chem. Lett.* **2005**, *15*, 2343–2345.
15. Cumpstey, I.; Carlsson, S.; Leffler, H.; Nilsson, U. J. Synthesis of a phenyl thio-beta-D-galactopyranoside library from 1,5-difluoro-2,4-dinitrobenzene: Discovery of efficient and selective monosaccharide inhibitors of galectin-7. *Org. Biomol. Chem.* **2005**, *3*, 1922–1932.
16. Salameh, B. A.; Sundin, A.; Leffler, H.; Nilsson, U. J. Thioureido N-acetyllactosamine derivatives as potent galectin-7 and 9N inhibitors. *Bioorg. Med. Chem.* **2006**, *14*, 1215–1220.
17. Cumpstey, I.; Sundin, A.; Leffler, H.; Nilsson, U. J. C2-symmetrical thiodigalactoside bis-benzamido derivatives as high-affinity inhibitors of galectin-3: efficient lectin inhibition through double arginine-arene interactions. *Angew. Chem., Int. Ed. Engl.* **2005**, *44*, 5110–5112.
18. Tejler, J.; Tullberg, E.; Frejd, T.; Leffler, H.; Nilsson, U. J. Synthesis of multivalent lactose derivatives by 1,3-dipolar cycloadditions: selective galectin-1 inhibition. *Carbohydr. Res.* **2006**, *341*, 1353–1362.
19. Ingrassia, L.; Nshimyumukiza, P.; Dewelle, J.; Lefranc, F.; Wlodarczak, L.; Thomas, S.; Dielie, G.; Chiron, C.; Zedde, C.; Tisnes, P.; van Soest, R.; Braekman, J. C.; Darro, F.; Kiss, R. A lactosylated steroid contributes in vivo therapeutic benefits in experimental models of mouse lymphoma and human glioblastoma. *J. Med. Chem.* **2006**, *49*, 1800–1807.
20. Rabinovich, G. A.; Cumashi, A.; Bianco, G. A.; Ciavardelli, D.; Iurisci, I.; D'Egidio, M.; Piccolo, E.; Tinari, N.; Nifantiev, N.; Iacobelli, S. Synthetic lactulose amines: Novel class of anticancer agents that induce tumor-cell apoptosis and inhibit galectin-mediated homotypic cell aggregation and endothelial cell morphogenesis. *Glycobiology* **2006**, *16*, 210–220.
21. Fort, S.; Kim, H. S.; Hindsgaul, O. Screening for galectin-3 inhibitors from synthetic lacto-N-biose libraries using microscale affinity chromatography coupled to mass spectrometry. *J. Org. Chem.* **2006**, *71*, 7146–7154.
22. Collins, P. M.; Oberg, C. T.; Leffler, H.; Nilsson, U. J.; Blanchard, H. Taloside Inhibitors of galectin-1 and galectin-3. *Chem. Biol. Drug Des.* **2012**, *79*, 339–346.
23. Glinsky, V. V.; Kiriakova, G.; Glinskii, O. V.; Mossine, V. V.; Mawhinney, T. P.; Turk, J. R.; Glinskii, A. B.; Huxley, V. H.; Price, J. E.; Glinsky, G. V. Synthetic galectin-3 inhibitor increases metastatic cancer cell sensitivity to taxol-induced apoptosis *in vitro* and *in vivo*. *Neoplasia* **2009**, *11*, 901–909.

24. Liu, H.; D'Ambrosio, M.; Liao, T.; Peng, H.; Rhaleb, N. E.; Sharma, U.; Andre, S.; Gabius, H. J.; Carretero, O. A. N-acetyl-seryl-aspartyl-lysyl-proline prevents cardiac remodeling and dysfunction induced by galectin-3, a mammalian adhesion/growth-regulatory lectin. *Am. J. Physiol. Heart Circ. Physiol.* **2009**, *296*, 404–412.
25. Lin, C. I.; Whang, E. E.; Donner, D. B.; Jiang, X.; Price, B. D.; Carothers, A. M.; Delaine, T.; Leffler, H.; Nilsson, U. J.; Nose, V.; Moore, F. D.; Ruan, D. T. Galectin-3 targeted therapy with a small molecule inhibitor activates apoptosis and enhances both chemosensitivity and radiosensitivity in papillary thyroid cancer. *Mol. Cancer Res.* **2009**, *7*, 1655–1662.
26. Miller, M. C.; Klyosov, A.; Platt, D.; Mayo, K. H. Using pulse field gradient NMR diffusion measurements to define molecular size distributions in glycan preparations. *Carbohydr. Res.* **2009**, *344*, 1205–1212.
27. Streetly, M. J.; Maharaj, L.; Joel, S.; Schey, S. A.; Gribben, J. G.; Cotter, F. E. GCS-100, a novel galectin-3 antagonist, modulates MCL-1, NOXA, and cell cycle to induce myeloma cell death. *Blood* **2010**, *115*, 3939–3948.
28. Miyanishi, N.; Nishi, N.; Abe, H.; Kashio, Y.; Shinonaga, R.; Nakakita, S.; Sumiyoshi, W.; Yamauchi, A.; Nakamura, T.; Hirashima, M.; Hirabayashi, J. Carbohydrate-recognition domains of galectin-9 are involved in intermolecular interaction with galectin-9 itself and other members of the galectin family. *Glycobiology* **2007**, *17*, 423–432.
29. Rotblat, B.; Niv, H.; Andre, S.; Kaltner, H.; Gabius, H. J.; Kloog, Y. Galectin-1(L11A) predicted from a computed galectin-1 farnesyl-binding pocket selectively inhibits Ras-GTP. *Cancer Res.* **2004**, *64*, 3112–3118.
30. Hoffman, G. R.; Nassar, N.; Cerione, R. A. Structure of the Rho family GTP-binding protein Cdc42 in complex with the multifunctional regulator RhoGDI. *Cell* **2000**, *100*, 345–356.
31. Ashery, U.; Yizhar, O.; Rotblat, B.; Elad-Sfadia, G.; Barkan, B.; Haklai, R.; Kloog, Y. Spatiotemporal organization of Ras signaling: rasosomes and the galectin switch. *Cell. Mol. Neurobiol.* **2006**, *26*, 471–495.
32. Gorfe, A. A.; Hanzal-Bayer, M.; Abankwa, D.; Hancock, J. F.; McCammon, J. A. Structure and dynamics of the full-length lipid-modified H-Ras protein in a 1,2-dimyristoylglycero-3-phosphocholine bilayer. *J. Med. Chem.* **2007**, *50*, 674–684.
33. Moise, A.; André, S.; Eggers, F.; Krzeminski, M.; Przybylski, M.; Gabius, H. J. Toward bioinspired galectin mimetics: identification of ligand-contacting peptides by proteolytic-excision mass spectrometry. *J. Am. Chem. Soc.* **2011**, *133*, 14844–14847.
34. Zou, J.; Glinsky, V. V.; Landon, L. A.; Matthews, L.; Deutscher, S. L. Peptides specific to the galectin-3 carbohydrate recognition domain inhibit metastasis-associated cancer cell adhesion. *Carcinogenesis* **2005**, *26*, 309–318.
35. Ilyina, E.; Mayo, K. H. Multiple native-like conformations trapped via self-association-induced hydrophobic collapse of the 33-residue β-sheet domain from platelet factor 4. *Biochem. J.* **1995**, *306*, 407–419.
36. Mayo, K. H.; Ilyina, E.; Park, H. A recipe for designing water-soluble, beta-sheet-forming peptides. *Protein Sci.* **1996**, *5*, 1301–1315.

37. Ilyina, E.; Roongta, V.; Mayo, K. H. NMR structure of a de novo designed, peptide 33mer with two distinct, compact beta-sheet folds. *Biochemistry* **1997**, *36*, 5245–5250.
38. Cox, A.; Arroyo, M. M.; Mayo, K. H. Folding of βpep-4 beta-sheet sandwich dimers and tetramers is influenced by aliphatic hydrophobic residues at the intersubunit interface. *Biochem J* **2001**, *357*, 739–747.
39. Arroyo, M. M.; Mayo, K. H. NMR solution structure of the angiostatic peptide anginex. *Biochem. Biophys. Acta* **2007**, *1774*, 645–651.
40. Dings, R. P. M.; Nesmelova, I; Griffioen, A. W.; Mayo, K. H. Discovery and development of anti-angiogenic peptides: A structural link. *Angiogenesis* **2003**, *6*, 83–91.
41. Griffioen, A. W.; van der Schaft, D. W.; Barendsz-Janson, A. F.; Cox, A.; Struijker Boudier, H. A.; Hillen, H. F.; Mayo, K. H. Anginex, a designed peptide that inhibits angiogenesis. *Biochem. J.* **2001**, *354*, 233–242.
42. van der Schaft, D. W.; Dings, R. P. M.; de Lussanet, Q. G.; van Eijk, L. I.; Nap, A. W.; Beets-Tan, R. G.; Bouma-Ter Steege, J. C.; Wagstaff, J.; Mayo, K. H.; Griffioen, A. W. The designer anti-angiogenic peptide anginex targets tumor endothelial cells and inhibits tumor growth in animal models. *FASEB J.* **2002**, *16*, 1991–1993.
43. Dings, R. P. M.; van der Schaft, D. W.; Hargittai, B.; Haseman, J.; Griffioen, A. W.; Mayo, K. H. Anti-tumor activity of the novel angiogenesis inhibitor anginex. *Cancer Lett.* **2003**, *194*, 55–66.
44. Dings, R. P. M.; Yokoyama, Y.; Ramakrishnan, S.; Griffioen, A. W.; Mayo, K. H. The designed angiostatic peptide anginex synergistically improves chemotherapy and antiangiogenesis therapy with angiostatin. *Cancer Res.* **2003**, *63*, 382–385.
45. Dings, R. P. M.; Williams, B. W.; Song, C. W.; Griffioen, A. W.; Mayo, K. H.; Griffin, R. J. Anginex synergizes with radiation therapy to inhibit tumor growth by radiosensitizing endothelial cells. *Int. J. Cancer* **2005**, *115*, 312–319.
46. Dings, R. P. M.; Chen, X.; Hellebrekers, D. M.; van Eijk, L. I.; Zhang, Y.; Hoye, T. R.; Griffioen, A. W.; Mayo, K. H. Design of non-peptidic topomimetics of antiangiogenic proteins with antitumor activities. *J. Natl. Cancer Inst.* **2006**, *98*, 932–936.
47. Dings, R. P. M.; Mayo, K. H. A journey in structure-based drug discovery: From designed peptides to protein surface topomimetics as antibiotic and antiangiogenic agents. *Acc. Chem. Res.* **2007**, *40*, 1057–1065.
48. Thijssen, V. L.; Postel, R.; Brandwijk, R. J.; Dings, R. P. M.; Nesmelova, I.; Satijn, S.; Verhofstad, N.; Nakabeppu, Y.; Baum, L. G.; Bakkers, J.; Mayo, K. H.; Poirier, F.; Griffioen, A. W. Galectin-1 is essential in tumor angiogenesis and is a target for antiangiogenesis therapy. *Proc. Natl. Acad. Sci. U.S.A.* **2006**, *103*, 15975–15980.
49. Mayo, K. H.; Dings, R. P. M.; Flader, C.; Nesmelova, I.; Hargittai, B.; van der Schaft, D. W.; van Eijk, L. I.; Walek, D.; Haseman, J.; Hoye, T. R.; Griffioen, A. W. Design of a partial peptide mimetic of anginex with antiangiogenic and anticancer activity. *J. Biol. Chem.* **2003**, *278*, 45746–45752.

50. Mayo, K. H. Galectins: From Theory to therapy. *IDrugs* **2008**, *11*, 97–100.
51. Mayo, K. H.; Griffioen, A. W. Designing betapep peptides: A rational approach to discovery of novel pharmaceutical agents and small molecules. *Drugs Fut.* **2003**, *28*, 337–346.
52. Dings, R. P. M.; Arroyo, M. M.; Lockwood, N. A.; Van Eijk, . LI.; Haseman, J. R.; Griffioen, A. W.; Mayo, K. H. β-sheet is the bioactive conformation of the anti-angiogenic anginex peptide. *Biochem. J.* **2003c**, *23*, 281–288.
53. Kim, H. O.; Kahn, M. A merger of rational drug design and combinatorial chemistry: Development and application of peptide secondary structure mimetics. *Comb. Chem. High Throughput Screening* **2000**, *3*, 167–183.
54. Tsang, K. Y.; Diaz, H.; Graciani, N.; Kelly, J. W. Hydrophobic cluster formation is necessary for dibezofuran-based amino acids to function as ß-sheet nucleators. *J. Am. Chem. Soc.* **1994**, *116*, 3988–4005.
55. Chen, X.; Dings, R. P.; Nesmelova, I.; Debbert, S.; Haseman, J. R.; Maxwell, J.; Hoye, T. R.; Mayo, K. H. Topomimetics of amphipathic b-sheet and helix-forming bactericidal peptides neutralize lipopolysaccharide endotoxins. *J. Med. Chem.* **2006**, *49*, 7754–7765.
56. Dings, R. P. M.; Loren, M.; Heun, H.; McNiel, E.; Griffioen, A. W.; Mayo, K. H.; Griffin, R. J. Scheduling of radiation with angiogenesis inhibitors Anginex and Avastin improves therapeutic outcome via vessel normalization. *Clin. Cancer Res.* **2007**, *13*, 3395–3402.
57. Dings, R. P. M.; Miller, M. C.; Nesmelova, I.; Astorgues-Xerri, L.; Kumar, N.; Serova, M.; Chen, X.; Raymond, E.; Hoye, T.; Mayo, K. H. Anti-tumor agent calixarene 0118 targets human galectin-1 as an allosteric inhibitor of carbohydrate binding. *J. Med. Chem.* **2012**, *55*, 5121–5129.
58. Dings, R. P. M.; Vang, K. B.; Castermans, K.; Popescu, F.; Zhang, Y.; Oude Egbrink, M. G.; Mescher, M. F.; Farrar, M. A.; Griffioen, A. W.; Mayo, K. H. Enhancement of T-cell-mediated antitumor response: angiostatic adjuvant to immunotherapy against cancer. *Clin. Cancer Res.* **2011**, *17*, 3134–3145.

Galectin Extra- and Intra-Cellular Functions and Their Therapeutic Implications

Chapter 4

Intracellular Galectins: Platforms for Assembly of Macromolecular Complexes

John L. Wang,[*,1] Kevin C. Haudek,[1] Patricia G. Voss,[1] Ronald J. Patterson,[2] and Eric J. Arnoys[3]

[1]Department of Biochemistry and Molecular Biology, Michigan State University, East Lansing, Michigan 48824
[2]Department of Microbiology and Molecular Genetics, Michigan State University, East Lansing, Michigan 48824
[3]Department of Chemistry and Biochemistry, Calvin College, Grand Rapids, Michigan 49546
[*]E-mail: wangj@cns.msu.edu

Although members of the galectin family were initially isolated on the basis of their saccharide-binding activity and cell surface localization, at least 11 of the 15 galectins identified in mammalian systems have been reported to be in the nucleus, as well as in the cytoplasm of cells. More interestingly, the precise intracellular localization and activity of the various galectins also cover a wide range. In most instances, distinct galectins give rise to the same or similar cellular responses. At the inner surface of plasma membranes, for example, galectin-1 (Gal1) and galectin-3 (Gal3) exhibit similar activities by binding to the Ras oncogene product to direct effector usage and signaling pathway. Gal1 and Gal3 also interact with Gemin4 and TFII-I as a part of ribonucleoprotein complexes and the two galectins have been documented to be required, but redundant, factors in pre-mRNA splicing. On the other hand, however, it appears that, although Gal3 and galectin-7 (Gal7) both bind to the apoptosis repressor protein Bcl-2, the ultimate cellular response is opposite: Gal3 is anti-apoptotic while Gal7 is pro-apoptotic. In all of these interactions, the ligands bind to the galectins through protein-protein interactions rather than via protein-carbohydrate recognition. The emergent general theme is that the galectins can serve to organize macromolecular platforms for a variety of activities.

Introduction

The galectins are a family of carbohydrate-binding proteins that share two key properties: (a) binding affinity for β-galactoside; and (b) conserved sequence elements in the saccharide-binding site (*1*). In mammalian systems studied to date, this family contains at least 15 members. Galectins have also been identified in many non-mammalian species, including birds, amphibians, fish, worms, sponges, and fungi. Screening the databases of genomic DNA sequences and expressed sequence tags has revealed putative galectins in plants and viruses (*2*). In addition to binding to galactose-containing glycoconjugates, many members of the galectin family share another property in terms of their cell biology --- they exhibit the phenomenon of dual localization (*3*), being found in both the intracellular (cytoplasm and nucleus) and the extracellular (cell surface and medium) compartments.

Of the 15 galectins identified, at least 11 have been reported to be in the nucleus, as well as in the cytoplasm, of cells. Surprisingly, many of these same galectins are also found outside of the cell. The present essay will focus on the association of galectins with distinct subcellular structures at different locations within the cytoplasm and the nucleus. These two compartments are connected by an aqueous channel of the nuclear pore complex and thus, are topological equivalent to each other but are separated from the lumen of intracellular vesicles and the outside of the cell by a lipid membrane barrier.

Galectin-1 and Galectin-3 Serve as Escorts of Ras Proteins

In the cytoplasm of H-Ras(12V)-transformed Rat-1 (EJ) cells, galectin-1 (Gal1) binds to and mediates the membrane anchorage of the H-Ras oncogene product, thereby allowing cell transformation (*4*). A similar direct interaction has been documented between galectin-3 (Gal3) and K-Ras (*5*). Ras signaling and oncogenesis depend on its dynamic localization between raft and non-raft plasma membrane microdomains, dictated in part by a farnesyl isoprenoid modification. Indeed, the galectins bind to Ras in a farnesyl-dependent manner and the binding is inhibited by S-farnesylthiosalicylic acid. Computational modeling studies have identified a hydrophobic pocket in Gal1, analogous to the geranylgeranyl-binding pocket of RhoGDI (*6*). A similar hydrophobic pocket can be found in the CRD of Gal3 as well (*7*).

Interaction of the farnesyl group in H-RasGTP with Gal1 strengthens their co-localization in non-raft microdomains (*7*, *8*). Immuno-gold labeling and electron microscopy revealed the localization of both Gal1 and H-Ras(G12V) in clusters on the inner surface of the plasma membrane. Downregulation of Gal1 by antisense reagents resulted in the disappearance of the Gal1-H-Ras(G12V) clusters. Similarly, Gal3 is an integral component of K-RasGTP, but not K-RasGDP, nanoclusters (*9*). Gal3 binding confers on Ras a conformation that reduces the efficiency of GTP hydrolysis by RasGAP (*5*), thereby prolonging Ras signals and determination of Ras effector usage. Gal3 promotes K-Ras signaling to both Raf and phosphoinositide 3-kinase (*5*) while Gal1 promotes H-Ras signaling to Raf at the expense of phosphoinositide 3-kinase and Ral guanine nucleotide exchange factor (*7, 10*). All of these results suggest that Gal1 and Gal3 can serve as escorts of Ras proteins into membrane microdomains, which in turn operate as robust platforms for signaling.

Galectin-3 at the Centrosome

Because none of the galectin polypeptides appears to carry a typical signal sequence for sequestration into the endomembrane pathway for secretion, several non-classical mechanisms of externalization have been proposed: for specific galectins, in specific cell types and, in some cases, restricted to specific developmental/differentiation stages (*11–13*). A common requirement of these mechanisms is that the galectin polypeptide must traverse across one lipid bilayer into the lumen of vesicular compartments, which is topologically equivalent to the outside of the cell. Nevertheless, studies on the activities of galectins within various secretory or endosomal vesicles have pointed to a novel intracellular interaction and function in polarized epithelial cells. Within transport vesicles of intestinal enterocytes, for example, galectin-4 (Gal4) associates with lipid microdomains to stabilize "superraft" platforms for sorting and delivery of components destined for the apical membrane of polarized epithelial cells (*14–16*). On the other hand, Gal3 appears to be responsible for clustering raft-independent glycoproteins (e.g. lactase phlorizine hydrolase and neurotrophin receptor p75NTR) in the same apical sorting and delivery process, as was observed in Madin-Darby canine kidney (MDCK) cells and in the adult mouse intestine (*17, 18*).

In the course of these studies, it was noted that, in small intestines of mice in which the Gal3 gene has been inactivated (*Lgals3-/-*), there were indeed defects in the apical trafficking of glycoproteins. However, the role of Gal3 in glycoprotein trafficking could not account for all of the other observed alterations in cytoarchitecture of the normally polarized epithelial cells. This raised the possibility that Gal3 may be involved in some more fundamental aspect in the establishment of cell polarity (*18*). Indeed, depletion of Gal3 (by siRNA treatment of renal epithelial MDCK cells that form domes in three-dimensional cultures or by gene inactivation in kidneys of *Lgals3-/-* mice) resulted in: (a) perturbations of the microtubular network, which normally arrays from the apical domain and runs along the apical-basolateral axis; (b) alterations in the morphology of the primary cilium, which appeared longer and abnormally shaped in the Gal3 deficient cells; and (c) appearance of abnormal centrosome-like structures (*19*). Immunofluorescence experiments showed that Gal3 could be co-localized with centrosomal proteins: centrin-2, pericentrin and γ-tubulin. Interestingly, Gal3 could be co-immunoprecipitated with centrin-2 but only over a limited period (day 3 - day 5) when confluent MDCK cells undergo polarization. The data clearly implicate that Gal3 plays a role in epithelial morphogenesis, most likely through its interactions at the centrosome.

Intracellular Galectin-3, Galectin-7, and Galectin-12 and Their Effects on Apoptosis

Human T lymphoma Jurkat cells ectopically expressing Gal3 survive longer than control cells when subjected to a variety of apoptosis-inducing agents (*20*). It has also been shown that Gal3 inhibits apoptosis caused by the loss of cell anchorage (anoikis) (*21*). Therefore, Gal3 exhibits anti-apoptotic activity. Several lines of studies have provided hints regarding the pathways by which Gal3 antagonizes apoptosis. First, Gal3 binds to the apoptosis repressor Bcl-2, mimicking the ability of Bcl-2 family members to form heterodimers (*20*). Second, in human breast epithelial cells, Gal3 inhibits anoikis by down-regulating cyclins E and A while up-regulating their inhibitory proteins $p21^{WAF/Cip1}$ and $p27^{KIP1}$ (*22*). Third, in cisplatin-induced apoptosis of the breast carcinoma cells, Gal3 is translocated to mitochondrial membranes, where it prevents mitochondrial damage, cytochrome c release, and the consequent apoptosome activity (*23*). This translocation is dependent on synexin, a Ca^{2+}- and phospholipid-binding protein. Down-regulation of synexin by antisense oligonucleotides inhibited Gal3 translocation and abolished its anti-apoptotic activity. Finally, Gal3 may also negatively regulate apoptosis by directly interacting with nucling, which is involved with cytochromc c/Apaf-1/caspase 9 apoptosome induction following pro-apoptotic stress (*24*). Thus, Bcl-2, nucling, and synexin are three ligands of Gal3 related to the latter's anti-apoptosis activity from within the cell.

Galectin-7 (Gal7) is expressed in various stratified epithelia and its overexpression is correlated with the induction of apoptosis in UVB-induced sunburn keratinocytes (*25*). Similarly, Gal7 transfection of the human cervical carcinoma cell line HeLa and the colon carcinoma cell line DLD-1 rendered the cells more sensitive to apoptosis induced by a variety of distinct stimuli (*26*, *27*). The Gal7 transfectants displayed up-regulated Jun N-terminal kinase (JNK) activity, enhanced caspase-3 activity, as well as accelerated mitochondrial release of cytochrome c. More recently, Villeneuve *et al.* (*28*) documented that a fraction of intracellular Gal7 was constitutively localized at mitochondria in a Bcl-2-dependent manner and sensitizes the mitochondria to apoptotic signals. Using highly purified mitochondrial fractions isolated from human HCT16 colon carcinoma cells, a proteomic analysis following Bcl-2 immunocapture revealed Gal7 as an interacting partner. Gal7 binds directly to Bcl-2, suggesting a mechanism for its enhancement of the apoptotic pathway. In this connection, it might be important to note that: (a) Gal3 was not amongst the 127 potential Bcl-2 interacting proteins identified through the proteomic analysis, despite the fact that *in vitro* binding studies had shown a direct interaction between Gal3 and Bcl-2 (*20*); and (b) inside cells, Gal3 is anti-apoptotic (*20*, *21*) while Gal7 is pro-apoptotic (*25*, *26*), possibly reflecting the fact that, while the polypeptides of the two galectins share a homologous CRD, Gal3 contains an unusual amino-terminal domain rich in Pro- and Gly-residues fused onto a carboxyl-terminal CRD while Gal7 contains only the CRD.

Galectin-12 (Gal12) contains two CRDs arranged as a tandem repeat (*29*) and is expressed predominantly in adipose tissue and in differentiated 3T3-L1 adipocytes (*30*). In the mouse, the Gal12 gene is one of the few genes that are expressed specifically in adipose tissue (*31*). Caloric restriction and treatment of obese animals with troglitazone (a synthetic ligand of peroxisome proliferator activated receptor γ) increased Gal12 expression. The increase in Gal12 mRNA in troglitazone-treated animals is accompanied by an increase in the number of apoptotic cells in adipose tissue. Moreover, transfection of COS-1 cells with Gal12 cDNA induced apoptosis in the recipient cells. On the basis of these results, it was suggested that Gal12 may participate in the apoptosis of adipocytes (*30*). In these studies, Gal12 was localized in the nucleus of adipocytes (*30*). More recently, however, Yang *et al.* (*32*) reported that the protein is primarily localized on lipid droplets and regulates lipolytic protein kinase A signaling through cAMP levels. Mice in which the Gal12 gene has been inactivated (*Lgals12-/-*) were found to have increased adipocyte mitochondrial respiration, reduced adiposity, and less severe insulin resistance. The results suggest that Gal12 functions as an intracellular regulator of lipolysis.

Ribonucleoprotein Complexes of Galectin-1 and Galectin-3

The nuclear localization of Gal3, coupled with its co-sedimentation with hnRNPs and snRNPs, provided the initial hint that it might play a role in pre-mRNA splicing (*33*, *34*). Using a cell-free system, several key findings indicate that Gal1 and Gal3 are two of the many proteins involved in splicing: (a) nuclear extracts (NE) derived from HeLa cells, capable of carrying out splicing of pre-mRNA, contained both Gal1 and Gal3 (*35*); (b) depletion of both galectins from NE, either by lactose affinity chromatography or by antibody adsorption, resulted in the concomitant loss of splicing activity (*35*, *36*); (c) either recombinant Gal1 or recombinant Gal3 was able to reconstitute the splicing activity in the galectin-depleted extract, suggesting that their activities were redundant (*35*); (d) saccharides which bind to Gal1 and Gal3 with high affinity, such as lactose and thiodigalactoside, inhibited the splicing reaction when added to a complete NE whereas non-binding saccharides such as cellobiose failed to have any effect (*36*); and (e) when a splicing reaction containing ^{32}P-labeled pre-mRNA was subjected to immunoprecipitation with either anti-Gal1 or anti-Gal3, radiolabeled RNA species corresponding to the starting substrate, intermediates of the splicing reaction, and mature mRNA products of active spliceosomes were all co-precipitated with the specific galectin (*37*).

More recently, glycerol gradient fractionation of NE resulted in the identification of a complex (~10S) in which Gal3 is associated with U1 snRNP (*38*). This complex was sufficient to load Gal3 onto the pre-mRNA substrate during spliceosome assembly. Of particular significance was the observation that splicing activity in a NE depleted of U1 snRNP can be reconstituted by the Gal3 – U1 snRNP particle, isolated by immunoprecipitation of the 10S region of the glycerol gradient with anti-Gal3 antibodies. In contrast, parallel anti-Gal3 immunoprecipitation of free Gal3 molecules not in a complex with U1 snRNP (fraction 1 of the same gradient), failed to restore splicing activity. These results indicate that the Gal3 - U1 snRNP-pre-mRNA ternary complex is a productive complex and that U1 snRNP is required to assemble Gal3 onto an active spliceosome.

This Gal3-U1 snRNP particle also contains the general transcription factor TFII-I. When NE of HeLa cells was subjected to adsorption on a fusion protein containing glutathione S-transferase (GST) and Gal3, TFII-I was identified by mass spectrometry as one of the polypeptides specifically bound (*39*). Lactose and other saccharide ligands of the galectins inhibited GST-Gal3 pull-down of TFII-I, while non-binding carbohydrates failed to yield the same effect. Similar results were also obtained using GST-Gal1. The association of TFII-I with Gal3 (and Gal1) was of interest because a prior proteomic analysis of the spliceosome had found TFII-I as one of its proteins (*40*). Site-directed mutants of Gal1, expressed and purified as GST fusion proteins, were compared with the wild-type (WT) in three assays: (a) binding to asialofetuin-Sepharose as a measure of the carbohydrate-binding activity; (b) pull-down of TFII-I from NE; and (c) reconstitution of splicing in NE depleted of galectins as a test of the *in vitro* splicing activity. The binding of GST-Gal1(N46D) to asialofetuin-Sepharose was less than 10% of that observed for GST-Gal1(WT), indicating that the mutant was deficient in carbohydrate-binding activity. In contrast, both GST-Gal1(WT) and GST-Gal1(N46D) were equally efficient in pull-down of TFII-I and in reconstitution of splicing activity in the galectin-depleted NE. Moreover, while the splicing activity of the wild-type protein can be inhibited by saccharide ligands, the carbohydrate-binding deficient mutant was insensitive to such inhibition. These results suggest that the carbohydrate-binding and the splicing activities of Gal1 can be dissociated and thus, saccharide-binding, *per se*, is not required for the splicing activity (*39*).

Gal1 and Gal3 associate with other complexes containing splicing factors in the absence of pre-mRNA. Gal3 was identified through mass spectrometry as a member of a large complex (~60S) termed the PCC (PSF-containing complex) (*41*). In addition to containing PSF (pyrimidine track binding protein (PTB)-associated splicing factor), this PCC contained many other proteins identified in complexes with Gal3 such as Gemin4, SMN, and TFII-I. Both Gal1 and Gal3 interact with the carboxyl-terminal 50 amino acids of Gemin4 (*42*), a member of the SMN (survival of motor neuron) complex that assembles the Sm proteins onto snRNAs in the normal biogenesis of these ribonucleoprotein complexes (*43*). Finally, there is also a report that Gal3 stabilizes heterogeneous nuclear ribonucleoprotein (hnRNP) Q (*44*).

Other Complexes and Interactions

Shimura *et al.* (*45*) reported that in the human breast cancer cell line BT-549, Gal3 binds β-catenin/Tcf and co-localizes with the complex to the nucleus to induce trancriptional activity in the Wnt signaling pathway. Using purified proteins and GST pull-down assays, direct binding between Gal3 and β-catenin was documented; the CRD of Gal3 and the NH2-terminal portion of β-catenin were required for this interaction (*45*). More recent studies have supported a role for Gal3 in stabilizing β-catenin and its nuclear accumulation in Wnt signaling in human colorectal cancer cells (*46*, *47*). However, the direct interaction between Gal3 and β-catenin has been called into question (*47*). It was proposed that Gal3 mediates AKT phosphorylation of glycogen synthase kinase-3β, decreasing the latter's activity on β-catenin. This, in turn, stabilizes β-catenin in the cytoplasm, allowing for nuclear accumulation and transcriptional activity.

In a survey of different human cancer cell lines, Gal3 was found maximally expressed in nuclei of thyroid cancer cells. Gal3 interacts directly with the thyroid-specific transcription factor TTF-1, up-regulating its transcriptional activity and thus contributing to the proliferation of the thyroid cells. Concomitant expression of nuclear Gal3 and TTF-1 was associated with a worse clinical outcome (*48*). It has also been reported that OCA-B, a B-cell specific coactivator for the OCT transcription factors, interacts with Gal1 and Gal3, with a possible role in regulating B-cell receptor mediated cell proliferation (*49*). Through interactions with the Gli family of transcription factors, Sufu serves as a negative regulator of the Hedgehog signal transduction pathway. A yeast two-hybrid screen using Sufu as bait identified Gal3 as a potential interacting protein (*50*). This direct interaction was confirmed by GST pull-down assays using GST-Sufu fusion protein and radiolabled Gal3. Like Gal3, Sufu shuttles between the cytoplasm and nucleus. The possibility is raised, then, that Gal3 may play a role in the nuclear versus cytoplasmic distribution of Sufu, thereby affecting transcriptional activity.

The shuttling of Gal3 between the nucleus and cytoplasm (*51*) is dependent on both a nuclear localization signal (NLS) (*52*, *53*) as well as a nuclear export signal (NES) (*54*), both of which have been identified on the Gal3 polypeptide. Thus, another set of important interactions is the association of the nucleo-cytoplasmic transport receptors with Gal3 as their cargo. Although active transport of Gal3 into the nucleus requires both importin-α and importin-β, Gal3 only binds directly to importin-α (*52*). The NES of Gal3 fits the spacing of hydrophobic leucine/isoleucine residues in the canonical nuclear export sequence recognized by the nuclear export transporter exportin-1 (CRM1), which is inactivated by the antibiotic leptomycin B (*54*). Indeed, incubation of cells in the presence of leptomycin B results in the accumulation of Gal3 in the nucleus.

Concluding Remarks

The present essay has focused on the ligands and interactions of galectins inside cells (Table I). Although this family of proteins was initially identified as galactose-specific carbohydrate-binding proteins, all the ligands discussed here bind to galectins via protein-protein interactions rather than protein-carbohydrate recognition. Despite this fact, however, it should be noted that the domain responsible for interacting with the majority of the partners is the CRD and, in many cases, saccharide ligands such as lactose can perturb the interaction (e.g. Bcl-2 binding to Gal3 (*20*)). In addition, some of the ligands appear to be location specific (e.g. Ras proteins bind to Gal1 and Gal3 at the inner face of the plasma membrane) while still other interactions are location and temporally specific (e.g. centrin-2 binding to Gal3 at the centrosome only at specific stage of differentiation). Despite these variations, however, it seems clear that a general theme has become apparent: the galectins can serve to organize macromolecular complexes at different locations within the cell.

Table I. Polypeptides interacting with galectins inside cells

Ligand	*Galectin*	*Location*	*Feature and Activity*	*Ref*
Bcl-2	3	cytoplasm	anti-apoptosis activity via the apoptosis repressor Bcl-2	(*20*, *21*)
	7	mitochondria	pro-apotosis activity by counteracting apoptosis repressor Bcl-2	(*25*, *26*)
β-catenin	3	cytoplasm	translocation of β-catenin/Tcf complex from cytoplasm to nucleus to induce transcriptional activity in the Wnt signaling pathway	(*45*)
centrin-2	3	centrosome	transient direct interaction dependent on stage of epithelial morphogenesis	(*19*)
exportin-1 (CRM1)	3	nucleus to cytoplasm	nuclear export signal-dependent transport of Gal3 from nucleus to cytoplasm	(*53*)
Gemin4	1 3	nucleus	component of Survival of Motor Neuron (SMN) complex in the biogenesis of small nuclear ribonucleoprotein complexes (snRNPs)	(*42*)
hnRNP Q	3	nucleus	stablizes the heterogeneous nuclear ribonucleoprotein complex	(*44*)
importin-α	3	cytoplasm to nucleus	nuclear localization signal-dependent localization of Gal3	(*51*)
nucling	3	cytoplasm	inhibits nucling in cytochrome c/Apaf-1/caspase 9 apoptosome induction	(*24*)
OCA-B	1 3	cytoplasm and nucleus	transcriptional coactivation and B cell proliferation	(*49*)

Continued on next page.

Table I. (Continued). Polypeptides interacting with galectins inside cells

Ligand	Galectin	Location	Feature and Activity	Ref
H-Ras K-Ras	1 3	inner surface of plasma membrane	dependent on hydrophobic interactions with farnesyl modification on Ras, prolonging RasGTP signaling	(*4*)
synexin	3	cytoplasm to mitochondria	translocation to mitochondrial membrane and prevention of cytochrome c release	(*23*)
Sufu	3	cytoplasm	regulation of nuclear versus cytoplasmic distribution of Sufu, which negatively regulates Gli family of transcription factors in the Hedgehog signaling pathway	(*49*)
TFII-I	1 3	nucleus	component of spliceosome in pre-mRNA processing; associated with U1 snRNP	(*39*) (*38*)
TTF-1	3	nucleus	up-regulate thyroid-specific transcription factor activity, contributing to the proliferation of thyroid cells	(*48*)

Acknowledgments

The work carried out in the authors' laboratories has been supported by grants GM-38740 from the National Institutes of Health (JLW), MCB-0092919 from the National Science Foundation (RJP), 09-CDFP-2001 from the Michigan State University Intramural Research Program (RJP), and a Calvin Research Fellowship from Calvin College (EJA).

References

1. Barondes, S. H.; Castronovo, V.; Cooper, D. N. W.; et al. Galectins: A family of animal β-galactoside-binding lectins. *Cell* **1994**, *76*, 597–598.
2. Cooper, D. N. W. Galectinomics: Finding themes in complexity. *Biochim. Biophys. Acta* **2002**, *1572*, 209–231.
3. Arnoys, E. J.; Wang, J. L. Dual localization: Proteins in extracellular and intracellular compartments. *Acta Histochem.* **2007**, *109*, 89–110.
4. Paz, A.; Haklai, R.; Elad-Sfadia, G.; Ballan, E.; Kloog, Y. Galectin-1 binds oncogenic H-Ras to mediate Ras membrane anchorage and cell transformation. *Oncogene* **2001**, *20*, 7486–7493.
5. Elad-Sfadia, G.; Haklai, R.; Ballan, E.; Kloog, Y. Galectin-3 augments K-Ras activation and triggers a Ras signal that attenuates ERK but not phosphoinositide 3-kinase activity. *J. Biol. Chem.* **2004**, *279*, 34922–34930.

6. Rotblat, B.; Niv, H.; Andre, S.; Kaltner, H.; Gabius, H.-J.; Kloog, Y. Galectin-1(L11A) predicted from a computed galectin-1 farnesyl-binding pocket selectively inhibits Ras-GTP. *Cancer Res.* **2004**, *64*, 3112–3118.
7. Ashery, U.; Yizhar, O.; Rotblat, B.; Elad-Sfadia, G.; Barkan, B.; Haklai, R.; Kloog, Y. Spatiotemporal organization of Ras signaling: Rasosomes and the galectin switch. *Cell. Mol. Neurobiol.* **2006**, *26*, 471–495.
8. Hancock, J. F.; Parton, R. G. Ras plasma membrane signaling platforms. *Biochem. J.* **2005**, *389*, 1–11.
9. Shalom-Feuerstein, R.; Plowman, S. J.; Rotblat, B.; Ariotti, N.; Tian, T.; Hancock, J. F.; Kloog, Y. K-Ras nanoclustering is subverted by overexpression of the scaffold protein galectin-3. *Cancer Res.* **2008**, *68*, 6608–6616.
10. Elad-Sfadia, G.; Haklai, R.; Ballan, E.; Gabius, H.-J.; Kloog, Y. Galectin-1 augments Ras activation and diverts Ras signals to Raf-1 at the expense of phosphoinositide 3-kinase. *J. Biol. Chem.* **2002**, *277*, 37169–37175.
11. Hughes, R. C. Secretion of the galectin family of mammalian carbohydrate-binding proteins. *Biochim. Biophys. Acta* **1999**, *1473*, 172–185.
12. Nickel, W.; Rabouille, C. Mechanisms of regulated unconventional protein secretion. *Nature Rev. Mol. Cell Biol.* **2009**, *10*, 148–155.
13. Delacour, D.; Koch, A.; Jacob, R. The role of galectins in protein trafficking. *Traffic* **2009**, *10*, 1405–1413.
14. Delacour, D.; Gouyer, V.; Zanetta, J. P.; et al. Galectin 4 and sulfatides in apical membrane trafficking in enterocyte-like cells. *J. Cell Biol.* **2005**, *169*, 491–501.
15. Braccia, A.; Villani, M.; Immerdal, L.; Niels-Christiansen, L. L.; Nystrom, B. T.; Hansen, G. H.; Danielsen, E. M. Microvillar membrane microdomains exist at physiological temperature. Role of galectin-4 as lipid raft stabilizer revealed by "superrafts". *J. Biol. Chem.* **2003**, *278*, 15679–15684.
16. Stechly, L.; Morelle, W.; Dessein, A. F.; et al. Galectin-4 regulated delivery of glycoproteins to the brush border membrane of enterocyte-like cells. *Traffic* **2008**, *9*, 2206–2220.
17. Delacour, D.; Cramm-Behrens, C. I.; Drobecq, H.; Le Bevic, A.; Naim, H. Y.; Jacob, R. Requirement for galectin-3 in apical protein sorting. *Curr. Biol.* **2006**, *16*, 408–414.
18. Delacour, D.; Koch, A.; Ackermann, W.; et al. Loss of galectin-3 impairs membrane polarization of mouse enterocytes *in vivo*. *J. Cell Sci.* **2008**, *121*, 458–465.
19. Koch, A.; Poirier, F.; Jacob, R.; Delacour, D. Galectin-3, a novel centrosome-associated protein required for epithelial morphogenesis. *Mol. Biol. Cell* **2010**, *21*, 219–231.
20. Yang, R. Y.; Hsu, D. K.; Liu, F.-T. Expression of galectin-3 modulates T-cell growth and apoptosis. *Proc. Natl. Acad. Sci. U.S.A.* **1996**, *93*, 6737–6742.
21. Akahani, S.; Nangia-Makker, P.; Inohara, H.; Kim, H.-R.; Raz, A. Galectin-3: A novel anti-apoptotic molecule with a functional BH1 (NWGR) domain of Bcl-2 family. *Cancer Res.* **1997**, *57*, 5272–5276.

22. Kim, H.-R.; Lin, H.-M.; Biliran, H.; Raz, A. Cell cycle arrest and inhibition of anoikis by galectin-3 in human breast epithelial cells. *Cancer Res.* **1999**, *59*, 4148–4154.
23. Yu, F.; Finley, R. L.; Raz, A.; Kim, H.-R. Galectin-3 translocates to the perinuclear membrane and inhibits cytochrome c release from the mitochondria. A role for synexin in galectin-3 translocation. *J. Biol. Chem.* **2002**, *277*, 15819–15827.
24. Liu, L.; Sadi, T.; Sano, N.; Fukui, K. Nucling mediates apoptosis by inhibiting expression of galectin-3 through interference with nuclear factor κB signaling. *Biochem. J.* **2004**, *380*, 31–41.
25. Bernerd, F.; Sarasin, A.; Magnaldo, T. Galectin-7 overexpression is associated with the apoptotic process in UVB-induced sunburn keratinocytes. *Proc. Natl. Acad. Sci. U.S.A.* **1999**, *96*, 11329–11334.
26. Kuwabara, I.; Kuwabara, Y.; Yang, R. Y.; et al. Galectin-7 (PIG1) exhibits pro-apoptotic function through JNK activation and mitochondrial cytochrome c release. *J. Biol. Chem.* **2002**, *277*, 3487–3497.
27. Ueda, S.; Kuwabara, I.; Liu, F.-T. Suppression of tumor growth by galectin-7 gene transfer. *Cancer Res.* **2004**, *64*, 5672–5676.
28. Villeneuve, C.; Baricault, L.; Canelle, L.; et al. Mitochondrial proteomic approach reveals galectin-7 as a novel Bcl-2 binding protein in human cells. *Mol. Biol. Cell* **2011**, *22*, 999–1013.
29. Yang, R. Y.; Hsu, D. K.; Yu, L.; Ni, J.; Liu, F.-T. Cell cycle regulation by galectin-12, a new member of the galectin superfamily. *J. Biol. Chem.* **2001**, *276*, 20252–20260.
30. Hotta, K.; Funahashi, T.; Matsukawa, Y.; et al. Galectin-12, an adipose-expressed galectin-like molecule possessing apoptosis-inducing activity. *J. Biol. Chem.* **2001**, *276*, 34089–34097.
31. Kouadjo, K. E.; Nishida, Y.; Cadrin-Girard, J. F.; Yoshioka, M.; St-Amand, J. House-keeping and tissue-specific genes in mouse tissues. *BMC Genomics* **2007**, *8*, 127.
32. Yang, R. Y.; Yu, L.; Graham, J. L.; Hsu, D. K.; Lloyd, K. C. K.; Havel, P. J.; Liu, F.-T. Ablation of a galectin preferentially expressed in adipocytes increases lipolysis, reduces adiposity, and improves insulin sensitivity in mice. *Proc. Natl. Acad. Sci. U.S.A.* **2011**, *108*, 18696–18701.
33. Laing, J. G.; Wang, J. L. Identification of carbohydrate binding protein 35 in heterogeneous nuclear ribonucleoprotein complex. *Biochemistry* **1988**, *27*, 5329–5334.
34. Hubert, M.; Wang, S.-Y.; Wang, J. L.; Seve, A.-P.; Hubert, J. Intranuclear distribution of galectin-3 in mouse 3T3 fibroblasts: Comparative analyses by immunofluorescence and immunoelectron microscopy. *Exp. Cell Res.* **1995**, *220*, 397–406.
35. Vyakarnam, A.; Dagher, S. F.; Wang, J. L.; Patterson, R. J. Evidence for a role for galectin-1 in pre-mRNA splicing. *Mol. Cell. Biol.* **1997**, *17*, 4730–4737.
36. Dagher, S. F.; Wang, J. L.; Patterson, R. J. Identification of galectin-3 as a factor in pre-mRNA splicing. *Proc. Natl. Acad. Sci. U.S.A.* **1995**, *92*, 1213–1217.

37. Wang, W.; Park, J. W.; Wang, J. L.; Patterson, R. J. Immunoprecipitation of spliceosomal RNAs by antisera to galectin-1 and galectin-3. *Nucleic Acids Res.* **2006**, *34*, 5166–5174.
38. Haudek, K. C.; Voss, P. G.; Locascio, L. E.; Wang, J. L.; Patterson, R. J. A mechanism for incorporation of galectin-3 into the spliceosome through its association with U1 snRNP. *Biochemistry* **2009**, *48*, 7705–7712.
39. Voss, P. G.; Gray, R. M.; Dickey, S. W.; et al. Dissociation of the carbohydrate-binding and splicing activities of galectin-1. *Arch. Biochem. Biophys.* **2008**, *478*, 18–25.
40. Rappsilber, J.; Ryder, U.; Lamond, A. I.; Mann, M. Large-scale proteomic analysis of the human spliceosome. *Genome Res.* **2002**, *12*, 1231–1245.
41. Peng, R.; Hawkins, I.; Link, A. J.; Patton, J. G. The splicing factor PSF is part of a large complex that assembles in the absence of pre-mRNA and contains all 5 snRNPs. *RNA Biol.* **2006**, *3*, 69–76.
42. Park, J. W.; Voss, P. G.; Grabski, S.; Wang, J. L.; Patterson, R. J. Association of galectin-1 and galectin-3 with Gemin4 in complexes containing the SMN protein. *Nucleic Acids. Res.* **2001**, *29*, 3595–3602.
43. Neuenkirchen, N.; Chari, A.; Fischer, U. Deciphering the assembly pathway of Sm-class U snRNPs. *FEBS Lett.* **2008**, *582*, 1997–2003.
44. Yoo, B. C.; Hong, S. H.; Ku, J. L.; et al. Galectin-3 stabilizes heterogeneous nuclear ribonucleoprotein Q to maintain proliferation of human colon cancer cells. *Cell Mol. Life Sci.* **2009**, *66*, 350–364.
45. Shimura, T.; Takenaka, Y.; Tsutsumi, S.; Hogan, V.; Kikuchi, A.; Raz, A. Galectin-3, a novel binding partner of β-catenin. *Cancer Res.* **2004**, *64*, 6363–6367.
46. Shi, Y.; He, B.; Kuchenbecker, K. M.; et al. Inhibition of Wnt-2 and galectin-3 synergistically destabilizes β-catenin and induces apoptosis in human colorectal cancer cells. *Int. J. Cancer* **2007**, *121*, 1175–1181.
47. Song, S.; Mazurek, N.; Liu, C.; et al. Galectin-3 mediates nuclear β-catenin accumulation and Wnt signaling in human colon cancer cells by regulation of glycogen synthase kinase-3β activity. *Cancer Res.* **2009**, *69*, 1343–1349.
48. Paron, I.; Scaloni, A.; Pines, A.; et al. Nuclear localization of Galectin-3 in transformed thyroid cells: A role in transcriptional regulation. *Biochem. Biophys. Res. Commun.* **2003**, *302*, 545–553.
49. Yu, X.; Siegel, R.; Roeder, R. G. Interaction of the B cell-specific transcriptional coactivator OCA-B and galectin-1 and a possible role in regulating BCR-mediated B cell proliferation. *J. Biol. Chem.* **2006**, *281*, 15505–15516.
50. Paces-Fessy, M.; Boucher, D.; Petit, E.; Paute-Briand, S.; Blanchet-Tournier, M. F. The negative regulator of Gli, Suppressor of fused (Sufu), interacts with SAP18, galectin-3 and other nuclear proteins. *Biochem. J.* **2004**, *378*, 353–362.
51. Davidson, P. J.; Davis, M. J.; Patterson, R. J.; Ripoche, M. A.; Poirier, F.; Wang, J. L. Shuttling of galectin-3 between the nucleus and cytoplasm. *Glycobiology* **2002**, *12*, 329–337.
52. Nakahara, S.; Hogan, V.; Inohara, H.; Raz, A. Importin-mediated nuclear translocation of galectin-3. *J. Biol. Chem.* **2006**, *281*, 39649–39659.

53. Davidson, P. J.; Li, S.-Y.; Lohse, A. G.; et al. Transport of galectin-3 between the nucleus and cytoplasm. I. conditions and signals for nuclear import. *Glycobiology* **2006**, *16*, 602–611.
54. Li, S.-Y.; Davidson, P. J.; Lin, N. Y.; Patterson, R. J.; Wang, J. L.; Arnoys, E. J. Transport of galectin-3 between the nucleus and cytoplasm. II. Identification of the signal for nuclear export. *Glycobiology* **2006**, *16*, 612–622.

Chapter 5

Galectins as Novel Regulators of Platelet Signaling and Function: Therapeutic Implications

Gabriel A. Rabinovich[1] and Mirta Schattner[*,2]

[1]Laboratory of Immunopathology, Institute of Experimental Medicine (IMEX), and National Academy of Medicine, Argentina
[2]Laboratory of Experimental Thrombosis, Institute of Biology and Experimental Medicine (IBYME), CONICET, National Academy of Medicine, Argentina
[*]E-mail: mschattner@hematologia.anm.edu.ar

Platelet activation at sites of vascular injury leads to the formation of a hemostatic plug. Activation of platelets is therefore crucial for normal hemostasis. However, uncontrolled platelet activation may also lead to the formation of occlusive thrombi that can cause ischemic events. Platelets can be activated by soluble molecules including thrombin, TXA_2, ADP, serotonin or by adhesive extracellular matrix proteins such as von Willebrand factor and collagen. By acting either in soluble or immobilized form, Galectin-1 and 8 trigger platelet activation through modulation of discrete signaling pathways. These novel findings offer new hypotheses and some speculations about the role of platelet-galectin interactions not only in hemostasis and thrombosis but also in inflammation and related diseases such as atherosclerosis and cancer.

Platelets are enucleated blood cells derived from megakaryocytes that are essential for proper hemostasis and thrombosis and also play critical roles in inflammatory processes, atherosclerosis, tumor metastasis and host defense. When platelets perceive activating signals through their cell surface receptors, they undergo dramatic structural and chemical changes, involving a complex interplay of cell adhesion and signaling molecules. Activated platelets rapidly bind circulating platelets via membrane integrin αIIbβ3 (GPIIb/IIIa) and fibrinogen, to form a thrombus for preventing bleeding at sites of vascular injury. However, platelet aggregation can also occlude atherosclerotic arteries causing cardiac and cerebrovascular diseases (*1*).

Galectins are structurally related carbohydrate-binding proteins, which are defined by their affinity for poly-N-acetyllactosamine-enriched glycoconjugates and sequence similarities in the carbohydrate recognition domain (CRD) (*2*). Although experimental and clinical studies have extensively implicated galectins in the regulation of immune cell homeostasis and host-pathogens interactions, there is increasing evidence that these proteins are also involved in the pathogenesis of cardiovascular diseases, in particular development of atherosclerosis (*3*, *4*). Moreover, recent work from our laboratory has shown that galectin (Gal)-1 and Gal-8 can trigger platelet activation by interacting with different platelet receptors and promote the formation of platelet-leukocyte aggregates suggesting a novel mechanism of thrombus formation mediated by galectin-glycan interactions (*5*, *6*).

Galectins and Platelet Aggregation

The capacity of platelets to form a thrombus depends on their ability to aggregate. At a molecular level, platelet aggregation is mediated by a specific receptor on the platelet surface: the $\alpha_{IIb}\beta_3$ integrin (*7*). Like most traditional platelet agonists, both soluble Gal-1 and Gal-8 promote the transition of this integrin from a low-affinity state (resting state) to a high-affinity state (active state), which results in the unmasking of neoepitopes in the $\alpha_{IIb}\beta_3$ complex, and allows fibrinogen binding which acts as a bridging molecule between platelets to form aggregates. This conformational change of $\alpha_{IIb}\beta_3$ integrin triggered by galectins is accompanied by a raise in intracellular calcium levels as well as morphological changes of platelets involving the rearrangement of the cytoskeleton including extension of filopodia and lamellipodia (spreading) and F-actin polymerization.

Both Gal-1 and Gal-8 induce aggregation of platelets suspended either in plasma or buffer which indicates a relevant role of these lectins in physiological media (*5*, *6*). Although cell agglutination was one of the first biological activities described for these lectins, this effect on platelets was only observed at high Gal-1 and Gal-8 concentrations. Platelet aggregation at lower concentrations is absent in fixed platelets, in the presence of calcium chelating agents, or eptifibatide (an αIIbβ3 antagonist), implying that platelet responses mediated by galectins could be related either to cell activation or to a clustering effect of platelet surface receptors depending on their concentration. Although both galectins were capable of promoting aggregation, Gal-8 was found to be ten times more potent than Gal-1 in this stimulatory effect. Although the dimeric structure of Gal-8 would anticipate a more robust effect of this galectin compared to Gal-1, the observation that only the N-terminal domain was also able to trigger platelet activation indicates that lectin bivalency is not essential to promote activating effects on platelets. The differences in the concentration required to achieve a similar effect, could therefore reflect different downstream molecular signals triggered by each galectin.

The initial formation of platelet thrombus is rapidly reinforced by the generation and release of platelet TXA_2 and ADP (the main metabolite of arachidonic acid by the cyclooxigenase pathway, and a component of platelet dense granules respectively) which acting in a paracrine and autocrine manner promote further platelet activation (*1*). Both molecules are generated on platelet stimulation by Gal-1 and Gal-8. Moreover, although the aggregation response triggered by low Gal-8 concentrations was inhibited in the presence of aspirin (cyclooxigenase inhibitor) and/or an ADP-scavenger, a full response was obtained at higher concentrations indicating that Gal-8 is a strong agonist that activate platelets independently from TXA_2 formation or ADP release (*6*).

Galectins Trigger Proinflammatory and Procoagulant Platelet-Mediated Responses

The role of platelets in inflammation and vascular repair is mainly associated to the release of α granule content which includes among others cell adhesion molecules that favor platelet/endothelial and leukocyte interaction (P-selectin, CD40L) prothrombotic substances (vWF) and pro- and anti-angiogenic molecules (vascular endothelial growth factor (VEGF) or endostatin respectively) (*8*).

Gal-1 and Gal-8 are strong inducers of P-selectin expression. The major role of P-selectin on the platelet surface is the interaction with PSGL-1, its major counterreceptor on leukocytes, to form platelet-leukocyte aggregates (*9*). In fact, activation of platelets by Gal-1 in the presence of polymorphonuclear leukocytes results in a significant formation of heterotypic cell aggregates (*5*). This interaction promotes activation of both cell types, which is a crucial condition for triggering inflammation, vascular remodelling and thrombosis. Platelet-leukocyte aggregates represent an established link between inflammation and thrombosis in acute syndromes including coronary diseases and related disorders (*10*, *11*). Furthermore, the interaction of P-selectin with PSGL-1 induces the up-regulation of tissue factor in the leukocyte membrane and the production of procoagulant microparticles, thereby contributing to a pro-thrombotic state. In addition, a role for P-selectin in platelet aggregation and the formation of arterial thrombi, has also been described (*12*).

vWF is a large multimeric glycoprotein that allows platelet-endothelium, platelet-subendothelium and platelet-platelet interaction and is therefore important for platelet adhesion and thrombus formation. Similarly to P-selectin, vWF is stored in platelet α granules and in Weibel-Palade bodies of endothelial cells from which is released during injury or inflammation. vWF is a biomarker for endothelial dysfunction and cardiovascular risk and high levels of vWF are found in both chronic and acute inflammation (*13*). The release of alpha granule stored vWF occurs after activation of platelets by Gal-1 (unpublished data) or Gal-8 (*6*).Thus, P-selectin expression and vWF release mediated by galectins might play an important role in the pathogenesis of thrombus formation and the modulation of inflammatory responses.

Vesiculation of the platelet membrane and formation of platelet microparticles (PMPs) is a characteristic effect of certain agonists such as collagen, thrombin or C5b-9 complement fragment (*14*). PMPs are released not only during platelet activation *in vitro* but are also detected *in vivo* (*15*, *16*). They are thought to provide catalytic surface for several enzyme complexes of the coagulation system and to underlie the pro-coagulant responses elicited by platelet activation. Moreover, PMPs may themselves evoke cellular responses in the immediate microenvironment including platelet adhesion to the site of endothelial injury and angiogenesis (*17*). The ability of Gal-1 (*5*) to induce phosphatidylserine-expressing PMPs suggests that this lectin not only promotes platelet activation, but could also indirectly activate the coagulation cascade.

Galectins and Platelet Adhesion

Platelet adhesion to the extracellular matrix (ECM) at sites of vascular injury represents a key step for limiting bleeding but, if uncontrolled, can lead to occlusion. Under low shear rate, such as that found in veins and larger arteries, platelet adhesion to the vessel wall primarily involves binding to fibrilar collagen, fibronectin and laminin. However at conditions of elevated shear stress, the initial tethering and firm adhesion of platelets to the exposed subendothelium is mediated by the interaction of the platelet GP Ib/IX/V complex and the subendothelial bound vWF (*1*). However, as vWF-deficient mice have delayed but not absent arterial thrombus formation it was suggested that under these conditions GPIb may bind other ligands that can mediate platelet adhesion (*18*). Interestingly, *in vitro* studies have shown that Gal-8 (*6*) and Gal-1 (*19*) promote platelet adhesion and spreading. $\alpha_{IIb}\beta_3$ integrin was identified as a functional receptor for Gal-1 (*19*) and GPIbα was identified for Gal-8 (*6*). Thus, it could be conceivable that galectins may act directly as a substrate or may either behave as matricellular proteins that bind to platelet GPIb-V-IX complex thus contributing to the platelet adhesion to the ECM. Of note, GPIb-V-IX complex plays a wide role in vascular biology since it not only binds to vWF but also recognizes several ligands on leukocytes and endothelium allowing the interaction of platelets with other vascular and blood cells (*18*). These data identify Gals as unique platelet agonists that have the ability to activate platelets in both soluble and immobilized conformations.

Platelet Receptors for Galectins

Most of the extracellular functions mediated by galectins involve the interaction of these proteins with cell surface glycoconjugates containing repeating units of N-acetyllactosamine [Galβ1,4GlcNAc]. Platelet activation mediated by Gal-1 or Gal-8 is prevented by lactose but not sucrose (*5*, *6*) indicating that these effects involve the interaction of these lectins with specific carbohydrate ligands on the platelet surface. Among the different receptors, integrins are known to be involved in Gal-1 mediated biological responses. Given the relevance of different integrins in platelet function, these molecules may represent potential binding partners for Gal-1.

We identified α_{IIb} integrin as a Gal-1 binding partner by mass spectrometry. Studies using blocking antibodies and platelets derived from patients who are deficient in $\alpha_{IIb}\beta_3$ established that this integrin acts as a functional receptor for Gal-1 in platelets. Because galectins in general, have the ability to form lattices, we hypothesized that Gal-1 binding to platelet surface results in the clustering of $\alpha_{IIb}\beta_3$ molecules, a phenomenon known to trigger outside-in signaling. In fact, stimulation of platelets by Gal-1 resulted in the activation of the major signaling pathways involved in the outside-in signaling including phosphorylation of the β_3 cytoplasmic tail and activation of the tyrosine kinases Syk and Akt and the enzyme phospholipase C γ 2 (PLCγ2) (*19*).

MALDI/TOF mass spectrometry analyses determined that Gal-8 binds platelet surface GPs, subunit α_{IIb} from the $\alpha_{IIb}\beta_3$ integrin and GPIb and V from GPIb-IX-V complex (*6*). However, the use of platelets derived from patients who are deficient in $\alpha_{IIb}\beta_3$ or in GPIb, revealed that only GPIb is essential for Gal-8-dependent signal transduction and therefore represents a functional Gal-8 counter-receptor (*6*). Moreover, Src, PI3K/Akt and PLCγ2 (well known downstream signaling molecules related to GPIb-IX-V complex) (*20*), are involved in platelet activation induced by Gal-8, giving additional support to the notion that GPIb is an essential receptor for transducing Gal-8 signaling (*6*).

Thus, extracellular Gal-1 and Gal-8 induce platelet activation by engaging distinct cell surface receptors. Whether this phenomenon implies a synergism between different members of the galectin family to trigger platelet activation requires further investigation.

Platelets Express Galectins

In addition to almost all of the vascular cells, human platelets express substantial levels of Gal-1 and Gal-8 (*5*, *6*). Although both galectins are secreted proteins, they are mainly found in the cytosol of different cell types. Human platelets express the two splice variants of Gal-8. Moreover, whereas Gal-8, like P-selectin, is absent on the surface of resting platelets, it is exposed on the membrane of thrombin-stimulated platelets. In contrast, Gal-1 is not expressed on platelet surface upon activation (unpublished observation). The differences between both galectins are still not clear. Interestingly, addition of lactose and thiodigalactoside moderately inhibits the aggregation induced by classical agonists suggesting that platelet-derived galectins might contribute to platelet activation.

Role of Endogenous Gal-1 in Hemostasis

We investigated the role of Gal-1 in platelet function using wild-type mice and Gal-1 deficient mice. In vivo evaluation of hemostasis by tail bleeding revealed increased bleeding time in KO animals, which was not associated to a lower platelet count. Using ex vivo techniques, we showed that Gal-1-deficient platelets exhibited impaired kinetics of clot retraction and platelet spreading on fibrinogen in the presence of normal integrin $\alpha_{IIb}\beta_3$ expression. Gal-1-deficient platelets showed normal alpha granule secretion and normal platelet aggregation. Therefore, Gal-1 appears to regulate integrin $\alpha_{IIb}\beta_3$ "outside-in" signaling events in platelets and is necessary for normal primary hemostasis in vivo (*19*).

Pathophysiologic Implications of Galectin-Platelet Interactions

Hemostasis, Thrombosis, and Inflammation

Given the described effects of Gal-1 and Gal-8 in platelet physiology, exposure of these endogenous lectins in the subendothelium or in activated endothelial cells (*21*) is expected to trigger platelet adhesion, spreading and thrombus formation (Figure 1A). Moreover, in the vascular system, platelets are another source of Gal-8 that would be accessible upon platelet activation to eventually promote further thrombus growth. Studies in galectin-null mutant mice reveal the relevance of these lectins in physiological hemostasis.

The expression of P-selectin on the platelet surface, the formation of leukocyte-platelets aggregates and leukocyte activation are relevant events in deep vein thrombosis (DVT). Given that galectins promote all these responses, binding of these lectins to platelets might represent potentially novel mechanism involved in DVT. Interestingly, Gal-3 binding protein has been found to be up-regulated in proteomics analysis of microparticles during DVT (*22*). While Gal-8 has been linked to proinflammatory processes (*23*, *24*), both, anti- and pro-inflammatory activities have been ascribed to Gal-1 (*25*). Whether anti-inflammatory effects occur at low concentrations of Gal-1, while pro-inflammatory effects prevail at high concentrations, still remains to be established. The fact that Gal-1 promotes platelet activation support to the notion that under certain circumstances, Gal-1 could also act as a pro-inflammatory factor.

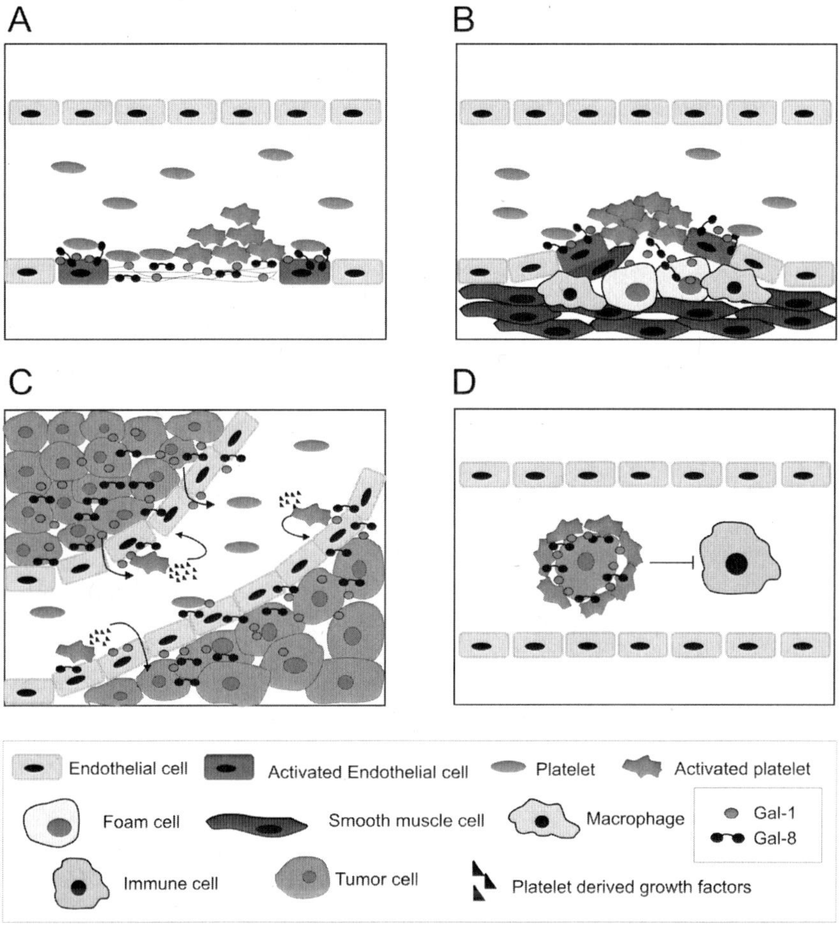

Figure 1. Potential Galectins roles in physiopathological platelet responses. A- When endothelial injury occurs, platelets could recognize Gal-1 and Gal-8 present in the surface of activated endothelial cells and in the exposed subendothelial extracellular matrix. Galectins would be able to trigger platelet adhesion, spreading and thrombus formation. B- Galectins might be involved in atheroma plaque formation and progression. When plaque rupture occurs platelets may bind to galectins present in the plaque and in the activated endothelium thus enhancing thrombus formation. C- Tumor cells overexpress Gal-1 and Gal-8. The lectins are released or exposed in the tumor cell surface and this might activate platelets which release the content of their granules that is rich in growth factors that can promote tumor development and angiogenesis. D- A circulating tumor cell that express Gal-1 and Gal-8 on its surface can bind platelets, thus forming heterotypic aggregates which may possibly protect tumor cells against immune attack, favouring metastasis. (see color insert)

Atherosclerosis

Although the expression and role of Gal-8 in human atherosclerotic lesions has not yet been explored, several groups demonstrated that galectins including Gal-1 participate in the initiation, progression and rupture of an atheroma plaque. Gal-1, -3 and -8 are not only expressed by the different cellular components of the atheroma lesions (*26–28*) but they also promote smooth muscle cell proliferation and transformation of macrophages into foam cells through the uptake of modified lipoproteins or AGEs (*29*, *30*).

Platelets are essential mediators in atherothrombosis. Platelet adhesion and mural thrombosis are ubiquitous in the initiation and generation of the lesions of atherosclerosis in animals and humans. Platelets can adhere to dysfunctional endothelium, exposed collagen, and macrophages. When activated, platelets release their granules, which contain cytokines and growth factors that contribute to the migration, activation and proliferation of smooth-muscle cells, monocytes and T-leukocytes (*31*).

The expression of galectins in the inner of atheroma plaque may not only represent strong amplifiers of platelet activation but may also be key components of the extremely thrombogenic core exposed after plaque rupture, the main trigger for acute thrombus formation and cause of unstable angina, myocardial infarction, transient ischemic attack, and stroke. Evidence for a role of galectins in atherosclerosis has also emerged from whole-genome association studies for myocardial infarction in Asian populations (*26*) although these findings were not reproduced in studies of populations with other ancestries (*32*).

Tumor Progression

It has been extensively shown that depletion or functional inactivation of platelets through a variety of genetic and pharmacological manipulations markedly reduces tumor progression and metastasis. Platelets may influence the metastatic potential of tumor cells via several mechanisms: a) through the release of a variety of inflammatory mediators which may influence tumor growth and stroma formation, b) through the expression of P-selectin, platelets may contribute to the stable adhesion to endothelium and/or transmigration of tumor cells outside of the vasculature, c) through the formation of heterotypic aggregates between mucins in circulating cancer and P-selectin in activated platelets which may protect tumor cells against immune attack (*33*).

The overexpression of galectins in tumor cells might also be a trigger for platelet activation allowing the release of alpha granules content that include growth factors which can promote tumor development and angiogenesis (Figure 1C). Furthermore, the formation of mixed-cell aggregates between tumor cells expressing high levels of galectins and platelets might also represent a complementary molecular mechanism to mucins and P-selectin interaction by which platelets contribute to tumor progression and metastasis (Figure 1D).

Cancer-Associated Thrombosis

Thrombosis and disseminated intravascular coagulation are common complications in cancer patients. A hypercoagulable or pro-thrombotic state of malignancy occurs due to the ability of tumor cells to activate platelets and the coagulation system. Pro-thrombotic factors in cancer include the ability of tumor cells to produce and secrete pro-coagulant/fibrinolitic substances and inflammatory cytokines and the physical interaction between tumor cell and platelets (*34*). However, the mechanisms allowing the occurrence of prothrombotic states in cancer patients are not completely understood.

The observed increased levels of Gal-1 and Gal-8 in tumoral endothelial cells as well as in other malignant cells could represent a pathogenic mechanism involved in thrombosis and disseminated intravascular coagulation complications, commonly present in cancer patients. Given the pivotal role of Gal-1 and Gal-8 in tumor progression, it could be conceivable that galectin-induced platelet activation might contribute to the pathogenesis of thrombosis in cancer patients.

Perspectives

Over the last decade we have witnessed impressive advances regarding the biology of galectins and their role in cell homeostasis, in particular as regulators of the immune response. The information currently available indicates that galectins are expressed and secreted by several cell types in normal and pathological conditions.

The emerging evidence showing that galectins are also capable of triggering platelet activation opens a completely new field of research where so far there are more questions than answers. The study of platelet activation mediated by galectins will certainly provide further insight into the mechanisms linking inflammatory mediators to thrombus formation and could expand our view of the role of platelets much beyond homeostasis to their pathophysiologic role during inflammation and cancer.

References

1. Rivera, J.; Lozano, M. L.; Navarro-Nunez, L.; Vicente, V. *Haematologia* **2009**, *94*, 700–711.
2. Rabinovich, G. A.; Baum, L. G.; Tinari, N.; Paganelli, R.; Natoli, C.; Liu, F. T.; Iacobelli, S. *Trends Immunol.* **2002**, *23*, 313–320.
3. Papaspyridonos, M.; McNeill, E.; de Bono, J. P.; Smith, A.; Burnand, K. G.; Channon, K. M.; Greaves, D. R. *Arterioscler. Thromb. Vasc. Biol.* **2008**, *28*, 433–440.
4. Al-Ansari, S.; Zeebregts, C. J.; Slart, R. H.; Peppelenbosch, M.; Tio, R. A. *Trends Cardiovasc. Med.* **2009**, *19*, 164–169.
5. Pacienza, N.; Pozner, R. G.; Bianco, G. A.; D'Atri, L. P.; Croci, D. O.; Negrotto, S.; Malaver, E.; Gomez, R. M.; Rabinovich, G. A.; Schattner, M. *FASEB J.* **2008**, *22*, 1113–1123.

6. Romaniuk, M. A.; Tribulatti, M. V.; Cattaneo, V.; Lapponi, M. J.; Molinas, F. C.; Campetella, O.; Schattner, M. *Biochem. J.*, *432*, 535–547.
7. Shattil, S. J.; Kim, C.; Ginsberg, M. H. *Nat. Rev. Mol. Cell Biol.*, *11*, 288–300.
8. Dole, V. S.; Bergmeier, W.; Mitchell, H. A.; Eichenberger, S. C.; Wagner, D. D. *Blood* **2005**, *106*, 2334–2339.
9. Furie, B.; Furie, B. C. *Trends Mol. Med.* **2004**, *10*, 171–178.
10. Michelson, A. D.; Barnard, M. R.; Krueger, L. A.; Valeri, C. R.; Furman, M. I. *Circulation* **2001**, *104*, 1533–1537.
11. Dotsenko, O.; Chaturvedi, N.; Thom, S. A.; Wright, A. R.; Mayet, J.; Shore, A.; Schalkwijk, C.; Hughes, A. D. *J. Thromb. Haemostasis* **2007**, *5*, 2036–2042.
12. Celi, A.; Lorenzet, R.; Furie, B. C.; Furie, B. *Dis. Markers* **2004**, *20*, 347–352.
13. Vischer, U. M. *J. Thromb. Haemostasis* **2006**, *4*, 1186–1193.
14. Bode, A. P.; Sandberg, H.; Dombrose, F. A.; Lentz, B. R. *Thromb. Res.* **1985**, *39*, 49–61.
15. Pereira, J.; Alfaro, G.; Goycoolea, M.; Quiroga, T.; Ocqueteau, M.; Massardo, L.; Perez, C.; Saez, C.; Panes, O.; Matus, V.; Mezzano, D. *Thromb. Haemostasis* **2006**, *95*, 94–99.
16. van den Goor, J. M.; van den Brink, A.; Nieuwland, R.; van Oeveren, W.; Rutten, P. M.; Tepaske, R.; Tijssen, J. G.; Sturk, A.; de Mol, B. A.; Eijsman, L. *J. Thorac. Cardiovasc. Surg.* **2003**, *126*, 1101–1106.
17. Brill, A.; Dashevsky, O.; Rivo, J.; Gozal, Y.; Varon, D. *Cardiovasc. Res.* **2005**, *67*, 30–38.
18. Bergmeier, W.; Piffath, C. L.; Goerge, T.; Cifuni, S. M.; Ruggeri, Z. M.; Ware, J.; Wagner, D. D. *Proc. Natl. Acad. Sci. U.S.A.* **2006**, *103*, 16900–16905.
19. Romaniuk, M. A.; Croci, D. O.; Lapponi, M. J.; Tribulatti, M. V.; Negrotto, S.; Poirier, F.; Campetella, O.; Rabinovich, G. A.; Schattner, M. *FASEB J.* **2012**.
20. Ozaki, Y.; Asazuma, N.; Suzuki-Inoue, K.; Berndt, M. C. *J. Thromb. Haemostasis* **2005**, *3*, 1745–1751.
21. Thijssen, V. L.; Hulsmans, S.; Griffioen, A. W. *Am. J. Pathol.* **2008**, *172*, 545–553.
22. Diaz, J. A.; Ramacciotti, E.; Wakefield, T. W. *Thromb. Res.* **2009**.
23. Tribulatti, M. V.; Cattaneo, V.; Hellman, U.; Mucci, J.; Campetella, O. *J. Leukoc. Biol.* **2009**.
24. Cattaneo, V.; Tribulatti, M. V.; Campetella, O. *Biochem. J.*, *434*, 153–160.
25. Yang, R. Y.; Rabinovich, G. A.; Liu, F. T. *Expert Rev. Mol. Med.* **2008**, *10*, e17.
26. Ozaki, K.; Inoue, K.; Sato, H.; Iida, A.; Ohnishi, Y.; Sekine, A.; Sato, H.; Odashiro, K.; Nobuyoshi, M.; Hori, M.; Nakamura, Y.; Tanaka, T. *Nature* **2004**, *429*, 72–75.
27. Nachtigal, M.; Al-Assaad, Z.; Mayer, E. P.; Kim, K.; Monsigny, M. *Am. J. Pathol.* **1998**, *152*, 1199–1208.

28. Chellan, B.; Narayani, J.; Appukuttan, P. S. *Exp. Mol. Pathol.* **2007**, *83*, 399–404.
29. Papaspyridonos, M.; Smith, A.; Burnand, K. G.; Taylor, P.; Padayachee, S.; Suckling, K. E.; James, C. H.; Greaves, D. R.; Patel, L. *Arterioscler. Thromb. Vasc. Biol.* **2006**, *26*, 1837–1844.
30. Moiseeva, E. P.; Javed, Q.; Spring, E. L.; de Bono, D. P. *Cardiovasc. Res.* **2000**, *45*, 493–502.
31. Ross, R. *N. Engl. J. Med.* **1999**, *340*, 115–126.
32. Kimura, A.; Takahashi, M.; Choi, B. Y.; Bae, S. W.; Hohta, S.; Sasaoka, T.; Nakahara, K. I.; Chida, K.; Sawabe, M.; Yasunami, M.; Naruse, T.; Izumi, T.; Park, J. E. *Tissue Antigens* **2007**, *69*, 265–269.
33. Borsig, L. *Expert Rev.Anticancer Ther.* **2008**, *8*, 1247–1255.
34. Noble, S.; Pasi, J. *Br. J. Cancer* **2010**, *102* (Supplement 1), S2–S9.

Chapter 6

Galectin-1 Cross-Linking of GM1 Ganglioside in Autoimmune Suppression

Robert W. Ledeen,[*,1] Gusheng Wu,[1] David Bleich,[2] Zi-Hua Lu,[1] and Hans-Joachim Gabius[3]

[1]Department of Neurology and Neurosciences and New Jersey Medical School, University of Medicine and Dentistry of New Jersey, Newark, New Jersey 07101
[2]Department of Medicine, New Jersey Medical School, University of Medicine and Dentistry of New Jersey, Newark, New Jersey 17101
[3]Institute of Physiological Chemistry, Faculty of Veterinary Medicine, Ludwig-Maximilians-University Munich, Munich, Germany
[*]E-mail: ledeenro@umdnj.edu

Galectins are a crucial element in the adaptive immune system that maintains immune tolerance through suppression of autoreactive T cells. The homodimeric (proto-type) galectin-1 (Gal-1) is recognized as having a prominent role in this regulatory process based on its presence in regulatory T cells (Tregs) and ability to induce anergy and/or apoptosis in effector T cells (Teffs). While Gal-1 is known to interact with distinct glycoproteins in a variety of cell types, its primary counter-receptor in Teffs was shown to be the GM1 ganglioside, a glycosphingolipid which experiences significant elevation upon Teff activation. Complementary activation upregulates Gal-1 in Tregs, which upon release then reacts with GM1 in the Teff cell membrane. The resulting lattice formation causes cross-linking of integrin heterodimer (e.g. $\alpha_5\beta_1$) with which GM1 is associated, thereby triggering a signaling cascade that culminates in TRPC5 Ca^{2+} channel activation. The resultant Ca^{2+} influx, when achieved beyond a threshold level, initiates further downstream signaling that suppresses proliferation of autoreactive Teffs. Failure to achieve this threshold in Teffs from non-obese diabetic (NOD) mice was shown to result from marked deficiency of GM1, which could be remedied both *in vitro* and *in vivo* by GM1 supplementation. Alleviation of type 1 diabetes in the NOD mouse by Gal-1 supplementation is thought to result from pushing cross-linking of deficient GM1 in the Teff membrane to higher levels, sufficient to elevate Ca^{2+} influx to the required threshold level. There is potential therapeutic advantage in examining autoimmune conditions in general for possible points of failure in this galectin-based regulatory mechanism.

Introduction

The pivotal role of regulatory T cells (Tregs) in controlling the expansion of pathogenic effector T cells (Teffs) is now well recognized (*1*) and has led to efforts to increase the number or potency of Tregs as a means of controlling autoimmune disorders. This approach has registered some success with animal models, as in type 1 diabetes (T1D) which was prevented or consigned to delayed onset by this strategy (*2–4*). However, detailed investigations of Tregs have revealed a diversity of cell types, especially in humans where FoxP3 has proved less reliable as marker of suppressor activity than was the case with mouse Tregs (*5–7*). A novel aspect of Treg function now in view is the occurrence in these cells of galectin-1 (Gal-1), a homodimeric (proto-type) member of a family of endogenous lectins that promotes self tolerance through suppression of autoreactive Teffs (*8–10*). Galectins, by selectively binding to cell surface glycans, are potent adhesion/growth-regulatory effectors (*11*). In fact, Gal-1 amelioration of a number of animal models has been described, this work having started with *in vivo* application in 1983 on autoimmune myasthenia gravis and rabbits (*12*) and continued with TID (*13*), collagen-induced arthritis (*14*), experimental colitis (*15*), concanavalin A-induced hepatitis (*16*), and experimental autoimmune encephalitis (EAE) (*9*, *10*, *17*) The particular glycan(s) targeted by Gal-1 in promoting immune tolerance and details of the underlying mechanisms have not been clearly identified. In this review we summarize evidence pointing to GM1 ganglioside as the key counter-receptor for Gal-1 in autoreactive Teffs and provide evidence for increased Ca^{2+}-influx as effector signaling.

Galectin-1 Interaction with GM1 Promotes Immunosuppression: *In Vitro Evidence*

Galectin-1 is strongly upregulated in activated Tregs (*8*, *10*) and released by a non-classical secretory mechanism (*18*) following which it can bind to glycoconjugates on its own cell surface for further (cell-cell) interaction or function in *trans* as effector. The target in either case is a functionally interactive glycoconjugate(s) on the membrane of another cell. Consideration has been accorded glycoproteins as binding sites, well delineated examples being the fibronectin receptor or CD7 as functional counter-receptor in Gal-1-dependent growth regulation, even at the clinical level [for review, see ref. (*19*); for case studies on mentioned glycoproteins, see refs. (*20*, *21*)]. Also indicating glycoprotein involvement was correlation of α2,6-sialylation of cell surface protein glycans with modulation of reactivity of Gal-1 toward differentiated T_H1- and T_H17- T cells compared with T_H2 cells (*9*). However, Gal-1 can also bind functionally to cell surface glycolipids when suitably presented, as we demonstrated by comparison of splenic T cells from wild-type mice with those from genetically engineered (KO) animals with disrupted GalNAcT gene (GM2/GD2 synthase, *B4galnt1*$^{-/-}$) which lack ganglio-series gangliosides [for details on ganglioside metabolism and nomenclature, see refs. (*22*, *23*)]. Mixed-culture experiments revealed impaired inhibition if the tested Teffs came from KO mice as opposed to wild-type (WT) mice (Figure 1A, right side). Fittingly, binding of labeled Gal-1 to spleen Teffs was markedly weaker when KO mice were the cell source (Figure 1B), analogous to earlier observations with human neuroblastoma cells with reduced GM1 presentation due to blocking the activity of cell surface ganglioside sialidase (S'ase) (*24*). Use of anti-Gal-1 antibody in the mixed cultures abrogated Teff cell suppression (Figure 1A, left side), further confirming the regulatory role of this galectin.

The suppression-inducing member of the ganglio-series in the Teff cell membrane proved to be GM1, a gangliotetraose glycosphingolipid with a single sialic acid attached in α2,3-linkage to the internal galactose (Figure 2). GM1 is rather special in being one of the very few sialoglycoconjugates that is resistant to most forms of vertebrate S'ase, thus facilitating its increase through S'ase reaction on oligosialogangliosides (e.g., GD1a – see Figure 2). This is now recognized as one mechanism for increasing GM1 on the cell surface, mediated by cell membrane-situated S'ase as observed in neuroblastoma cells (*24*, *25*) as well as T cells. Focusing on Teffs, (S'ase) is upregulated upon their activation (*26*), a process thought to account at least in part for the remarkable elevation of GM1 on the cell surface during Teff cell activation (*10*, *27*, *28*).

Of interest was the concurrent elevation of GD1a, metabolic precursor of GM1 (via S'ase), upon T cell activation (*10*). These findings and additional evidence (see below) support the hypothesis that Gal-1 from Tregs engages GM1 on Teffs as its primary counter-receptor in Teff cell suppression. Similar GM1/Gal-1 interaction was observed in the growth regulation of human SK-N-MC neuroblastoma cells (*24*, *29*), further illustrating this as a shared mechanism of Teffs and some neural cells; significantly, microdomain integrity was shown to be relevant for the high-affinity binding (*30*).

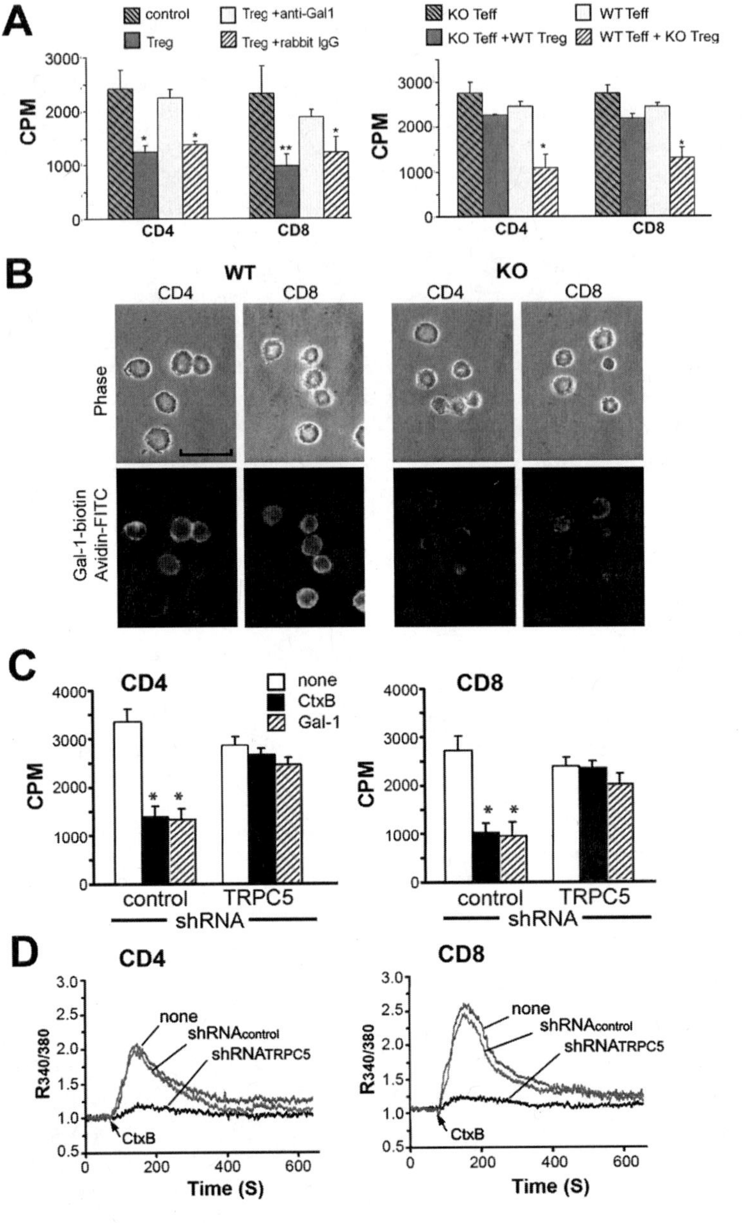

Figure 1. Involvement of ganglio-series gangliosides, galectin-1 (Gal-1) and the TRPC5 Ca^{2+}-channel in effector T cell (Teff) suppression. Reduced effect of regulatory T cells (Treg) on ^{3}H-thymidine incorporation by activated $CD4^{+}/CD8^{+}$ T cells of wild-type mice in the presence of Gal-1-specific antibody (A, left) and by T cells from ganglio-series-deficient (KO) mice (A, right). Different levels of binding of labeled Gal-1 to cells from wild-type (WT) and KO mice revealed the requirement of ganglio-series gangliosides for substantial Gal-1 binding (B).

Knock-down of TRPC5 by short hairpin RNA (shRNA) blocked suppression of activated CD4+ and CD8+ T cells by Gal-1 and CtxB (C). This knock-down effectively precluded Ca^{2+} influx upon CtxB binding to CD4+ and CD8+ T cells, as monitored by fura 2-AM (D). (For further details, please see reference (10)). Abstracted from reference (10) with permission of the Journal of Immunology and the New York Academy of Science (Ledeen et al. 2012. Beyond glycoproteins as galectin counterreceptors: Tumor-effector T cell growth control via ganglioside GM1. Ann NY Acad Sciences 1253:206-221).

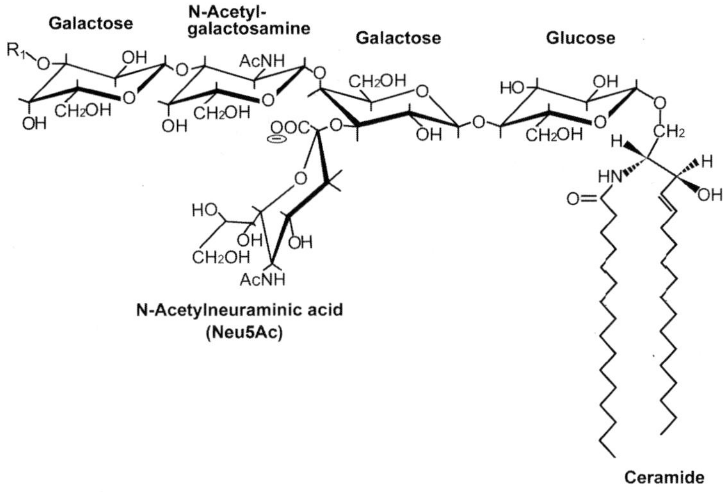

Figure 2. Structure of gangliosides GM1 (R = H) and GD1a (R = Neu5Ac, N-acetylneuraminic acid).

Galectin-1 Interaction with GM1 Promotes Immunosuppression: *In Vivo Evidence*

One line of experimentation has been direct application of the counter-receptors to autoimmune animal models. As outlined above, Gal-1 administration attenuated a number of autoimmune conditions (*9*, *10*, *12–17*). In similar vein, application of GM1, or ganglioside mixtures containing GM1, ameliorated disability in EAE, a widely used model for multiple sclerosis (*31–33*) and experimental autoimmune neuritis, its peripheral nerve counterpart (*34*, *35*). In addition, GM1 reduced the expression of diabetes in the NOD mouse (*36*), a finding that may be correlated with the GM1 deficit that characterizes NOD Teffs (see below). Another general approach has been to observe enhancement of autoimmune pathology in genetically altered mice lacking GM1 or Gal-1. Thus, mice deficient in Gal-1 (*9*), similar to mice lacking GM1 (*10*), showed enhanced EAE disability and neuropathology compared to WT mice.

Parallel Activities of Gal-1 and GM1-Binding Bacterial Toxins

Further insight into the suppression mechanism came in the finding of strikingly parallel activities of Gal-1 and cholera toxin B subunit (CtxB), the latter a protein that binds GM1 with relatively high affinity and specificity (*37*). Detailed structural analysis of binding revealed selection of different conformers of GM1's pentasaccharide by Gal-1 and CtxB, yielding the high-affinity recognition (*38*). The B subunit of *Escherichia coli* heat-labile enterotoxin is structurally and functionally similar to CtxB, and, fittingly, both GM1 cross-linking agents have been shown to effectively suppress a number of autoimmune disorders, in a manner analogous to Gal-1 (*10*, *39–41*).

The mechanistic consequences of GM1 cross-linking were suggested in studies showing that CtxB binding led to Ca^{2+} influx in rat lymphocytes (*42*) and a human leukemic (Jurkat) T cell line (*43*). Equally important, Gal-1 promoted Ca^{2+} influx in a similar manner in Jurkat T cells (*44*). Such influx occurred via a voltage-independent channel (*45*), subsequently shown in a study of NG108-15 neuroblastoma cell differentiation (*46*) to be TRPC5, a member of the canonical subfamily belonging to the transient receptor potential superfamily of signal transduction-gated ion channels (*47*). That this channel is at the heart of the Ca^{2+} influx in T cells in conjunction with T cell suppression was demonstrated by failure of both Teff cell suppression (Figure 1C) and Ca^{2+} influx (Figure 1D) following shRNA knockdown of TRPC5.

Notably, Gal-1 and CtxB showed comparable potency in suppressing proliferation of activated murine Teffs (Figure 1C). The pentavalent nature of CtxB accords with its cross-linking mode of action, an essential feature of its Teff suppression activity. That cross-linking of GM1 rather than mere binding is the *modus operandi* of suppression was indicated in blockage of CtxB- or Gal-1-induced Ca^{2+} influx by non-cross-linking anti-GM1 antibody (*48*); additional evidence came in the observation that IgM but not IgG anti-GM1 antibody induced similar Ca^{2+} influx as CtxB does (*49*).

Signaling Induced by Galectin-1/GM1 Interaction

Further probing into the cross-linking phenomenon revealed a prominent role for a heterodimeric integrin with which GM1 is tightly associated in raft-like microdomains. With Teffs this proved to be β_1 in association with both α_4 and α_5 integrin subunits (*10*), analogous to $\alpha_5\beta_1$ in NG108-15 cells (*46*). Galectin-1 and CtxB thus cross-link GM1 in a manner that results in co-cross-linking of heterodimeric integrin, shown in the latter cells to induce autophosphorylation of associated focal adhesion kinase at Tyr 397 followed by assembly of a signaling complex that includes phospholipase Cγ and phosphoinositide-3 kinase (*46*). The resultant TRPC5 channel activation thus represents Gal-1-induced signaling at a distance, as opposed to direct GM1-TRPC5 association. Although demonstrated more fully in NG108-15 neuroblastoma cells, it appears likely a similar signaling sequence pertains to Teffs in view of the above indicated parallels in neural and immune cell behavior including the similar roles for TRPC5 and heterodimeric integrin.

CD8+ T Cells Show Similar Gal-1/GM1 Interaction

It was of interest that CD8+ T cells (cytotoxic T lymphocytes) showed entirely parallel behavior compared to CD4+ T cells in the above studies. This pertained to activation-induced elevation of GM1, proliferation suppression by Gal-1 and CtxB, GM1 association with $\alpha_4\beta_1$ and $\alpha_5\beta_1$ integrins, and TRPC5-mediated Ca^{2+} influx. This is in line with recognition of CD8+ T cells as major players in autoimmune reactivity (*50–53*). Of particular note, they were shown to express more GM1 than CD4+ T cells (*54*) and experience a higher level of apoptosis with GM1-specific enterotoxin (*54, 55*).

NOD Mouse Pathology and GM1 Deficiency

The hypothesis that Gal-1-induced cross-linking of GM1 mediates autoimmune suppression has found support in a study of the NOD mouse (*48*). This animal is considered a suitable model for the human T1D condition (*56*). It had been previously reported that Teffs from such mice were unresponsive to suppression by Tregs from WT mice (*57*), analogous to Teffs from human T1D patients (*58*), and it thus seemed worth exploring whether this anergy might reflect insufficient GM1 presentation in the Teff cell membrane. This proved to be the case, GM1 presence in NOD CD4+ Teffs being less than half the levels of three other tested strains in both the resting and activated states (Figure 3A); similar deficits were found for GD1a, the above-mentioned metabolic precursor of GM1, and both gangliosides were found reduced to a comparable extent in CD8+ cells as well (*48*).

This was, as noted above, analogous to growth control of the SK-N-MC neuroblastoma cells that was impaired by S'ase inhibition and resulting failure of GM1 elevation (*24, 29*). Mixed-culture experiments substantiated the idea of defective Teffs with insufficient GM1 as the cause of failed suppression (Figure 3B), consistent with the results of GM1 supplementation which significantly restored responsiveness of NOD Teffs to growth inhibition (Figure 3C) and Gal-1-induced Ca^{2+} influx (Figure 3D). GM1 is known to insert spontaneously into the membrane of cultured cells with behavior analogous to that of endogenous GM1 (*59*). Blockade of Gal-1-induced Ca^{2+} influx by non-cross-linking anti-GM1 antibody (Figure 3D) further emphasized the necessity for GM1 cross-linking. TRPC5 channel involvement was supported by the diminished Ca^{2+} influx caused by SK&F96365, a TRP channel inhibitor (*48*).

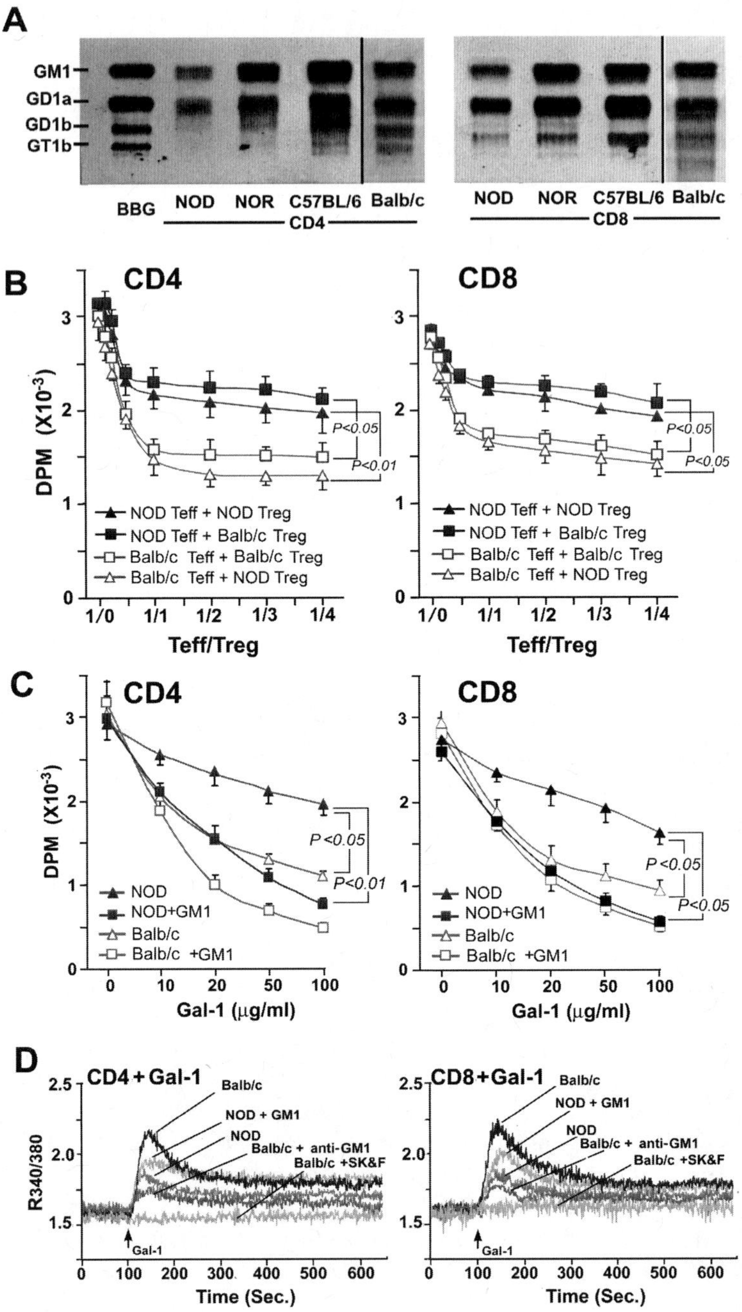

Figure 3. Detection of deficiency in GM1/GD1a in activated effector T cells (Teffs) of NOD mice, its consequence for inter-T cell communication and its amelioration by GM1 replacement in vitro. High-performance thin-layer chromatography using bovine brain ganglioside (BBG) mixture as internal

control revealed a NOD strain-specific defect (A). Experiments with mixed cultures of cells from NOD and BALB/c mice to determine the level of Teff proliferation revealed maintained effectiveness of regulatory T cells (Treg) but impaired responsiveness of Teffs (B). Robust suppression of Balb/c Teffs occurred with galectin-1 (Gal-1) and failed suppression of NOD Teffs was corrected by GM1 pretreatment (C). Involvement of TRPC5 Ca^{2+}-channels (please see also Figure 3D) was evidenced by measuring the Ca^{2+}-influx for these cell populations; TRP channel inhibitor (SK&F) blocked Ca^{2+}-influx, addition of a non-cross-linking anti-GM1 antibody impaired the Gal-1-dependent effect, and pretreatment with GM1 improved the defective signal for activated Teffs from NOD mice (D). (For further details, please see reference (48)). Abstracted from reference (48) with permission from the journal Diabetes; also the New York Academy of Sciences (Ledeen et al. 2012. Beyond glycoproteins as galectin counterreceptors: Tumor-effector T cell growth control via ganglioside GM1. Ann NY Acad Sciences. 1253:206-221).

Conclusions and Future Directions

Galectins are carbohydrate-binding proteins with the defined mission of decoding the biological information encrypted in the "sugar code" [for recent reviews, see refs. (*60*, *61*)]. They are present in virtually all immune cells where they occur either constitutively or through induction. In that sense, they constitute a crucial element in the adaptive immune system that maintains T cell homeostasis and immune tolerance through suppression of autoreactive T cells. Our findings implicate Gal-1 in association with GM1 as key players in that process. A flow scheme summarizing these lines of evidence (Figure 4) indicates Gal-1 cross-linking of GM1, along with GM1-associated integrin(s), as initiating event for signaling in autoimmune suppression. Integrin cross-linking and autophosphorylation builds a signaling complex leading to TRPC5 Ca^{2+} channel activation. Upregulation of S'ase, which converts GD1a to GM1, is one mechanism, along with *de novo* synthesis, that can elevate this Gal-1 counter-receptor on the Teff cell surface. Concurrent activation of Tregs results in upregulation of Gal-1 which finds its GM1 target following release as soluble homodimer and/or as protein presented on the Treg surface. TRPC5 itself is upregulated during Teff activation, thus indicating elevation of all necessary components of this regulatory mechanism (Figure 4).

This would ensure the required amplitude of Ca^{2+} influx for Teff suppression via apoptosis or anergization, failure of which could result from defects of one kind or another in the indicated pathways. As mentioned, insufficient GM1 in the NOD Teff cell membrane resulted in sub-threshold influx of Ca^{2+}, a failure remedied both *in vitro* and *in vivo* by GM1 supplementation. Alternatively, sub-threshold levels of Ca^{2+} influx in that condition could conceivably be remedied with enhanced Gal-1 levels, which may explain the observed suppression of T1D in the NOD mouse by direct application of this galectin (*13*) or by indirect supplementation via Tregs (*2–4*)). Elevation of Gal-1 by these means might compensate for deficient GM1 by more efficient utilization of the GM1 that is present. Although galectins are not considered to have specific protein receptors on the cell surface, in contrast to cytokines or certain hormones, we propose that GM1 does fulfill such a role in lectin-glycan interaction with respect to Teff cell proliferation. Modulation of cell surface glycoconjugate display thus ensures swift regulation *in situ*. These findings suggest the potential advantage in examining other autoimmune conditions for possible points of failure in this proposed mechanism. That in turn could point to potential medical applications based on restoring a threshold level of signaling in patient Teffs to re-establish successful inter-T cell communication.

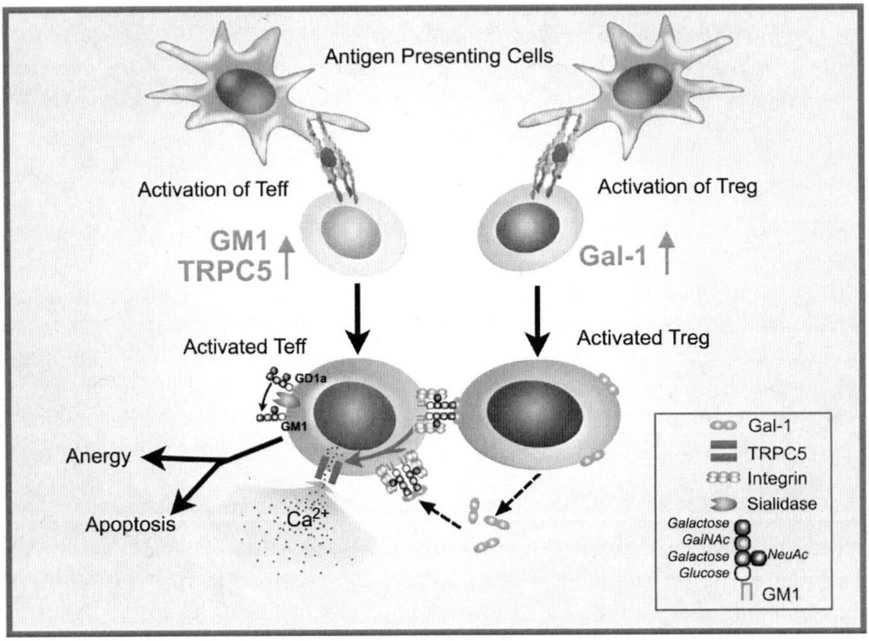

Figure 4. Schematic illustration of inter-T cell communication after activation of effector/regulatory T cells (Teff/Treg) via ganglioside GM1/galectin-1 contact. T cell receptor activation of regulatory T cell (Treg) by antigen presenting cells causes upregulation of galectin-1 (Gal-1) that is expressed on the Treg cell surface and released into the surroundings. As a homodimer it cross-links GM1 which has been elevated through sialidase reaction (and possibly de novo synthesis) in the plasma membrane of Teff following activation of the latter. This induces co-cross-linking of heterodimeric integrin, which is associated with GM1, and this in turn induces a signaling sequence resulting in activation of TRPC5 Ca^{2+} channels. Elevated intracellular Ca^{2+} in Teffs prevents proliferation through anergy and/or apoptosis. Reprinted with permission from the New York Academy of Sciences (Ledeen et al. 2012. Beyond glycoproteins as galectin counterreceptors: Tumor-effector T cell growth control via ganglioside GM1. Ann NY Acad Sciences. 1253:206-221). (see color insert)

Acknowledgments

This study was supported by a grant (RG 3981A) from the National Multiple Sclerosis Society, a grant from the Foundation of Diabetes Research of New Jersey, and funding by the EC (GlycoHIT).

References

1. Sakaguchi, S. $CD4^+$ regulatory T cells for immunologic self-tolerance and negative control of immune responses. *Annu. Rev. Immunol.* **2004**, *22*, 531–562.
2. Tang, Q.; et al. In vitro-expanded antigen-specific regulatory T cells suppress autoimmune diabetes. *J. Exp. Med.* **2004**, *199*, 1455–1465.
3. Staeva-Vieira, T.; Peakman, M.; von Herrath, M Translational mini-review series on type 1 diabetes: Immune-based therapeutic approaches for type 1 diabetes. *Clin. Exp. Immunol.* **2007**, *148*, 17–31.
4. Tarbell, K.V.; et al. Dendritic cell-expanded, islet-specific $CD4^+$ $CD25^+$ $CD62L^+$ regulatory T cells restore normoglycemia in diabetic NOD mice. *J. Exp. Med.* **2007**, *204*, 191–201.
5. Allen, S.E.; et al. Activation-induced FOXP3 in human T effector cells does not suppress proliferation or cytokine production. *Int. Immunol.* **2007**, *19*, 345–354.
6. Tran, D.Q.; Ramsey, H.; Shevach, E.M. Induction of FOXP3 expression in naïve human $CD4^+$FOXP3 T cells by T-cell receptor stimulation is transforming growth factor-beta dependent but does not confer a regulatory phenotype. *Blood* **2007**, *110*, 2983–2990.
7. Kmieciak, M.; et al. Human T cells express CD25 and Foxp3 upon activation and exhibit effector/memory phenotypes without any regulatory/suppressor function. *J. Transl. Med.* **2009**, *7*, 89–95.
8. Garín, M.I.; Chu, C.C.; Golshayan, D.; Cernuda-Morollón, E.; Wait, R.; Lechler, R.I. Galectin-1: A key effector of regulation mediated by CD4+CD25+ T cells. *Blood* **2007**, *109*, 2058–2065.
9. Toscano, M.A.; Bianco, G.A.; Ilarregui, J.M.; et al. Differential glycosylation of T_H1, T_H2 and T_H-17 effector cells selectively regulates susceptibility to cell death. *Nat. Immunol.* **2007**, *8*, 825–834.
10. Wang, J.; Lu, Z.-H.; Gabius, H.-J.; Rohowsky-Kochan, C.; Ledeen, R.W.; Wu, G. Crosslinking of GM1 ganglioside by galectin-1 mediates regulatory T cell activity involving TRPC5 channel activation: possible role in suppressing experimental autoimmune encephalomyelitis. *J. Immunol.* **2009**, *182*, 4036–4045.
11. Kaltner, H.; Gabius, H.-J. A toolbox of lectins for translating the sugar code: the galectin network in phylogenesis and tumors. *Histol. Histopathol.* **2012**, *27*, 397–416.
12. Levi, G.; Tarrab-Hazdai, R.; Teichberg, V.I. Prevention and therapy with electrolectin of experimental autoimmune myasthenia gravis in rabbits. *Eur. J. Immunol.* **1983**, *13*, 500–507.

13. Perone, M.J.; Bertera, S.; Shufesky, W.J.; et al. Suppression of autoimmune diabetes by soluble galectin-1. *J. Immunol.* **2009**, *182*, 2641–2653.
14. Rabinovich, G.A.; Daly, G.; Dreja, H.; et al. Recombinant galectin-1 and its genetic delivery suppress collagen-induced arthritis via T cell apoptosis. *J. Exp. Med.* **1999**, *190*, 385–398.
15. Santucci, L.; Fiorucci, S.; Rubinstein, N.; et al. Galectin-1 suppresses experimental colitis in mice. *Gastroenterology* **2003**, *124*, 1381–1394.
16. Santucci, L.; Fiorucci, S.; Cammilleri, F.; Servillo, G.; Federici, B.; Morelli, A. Galectin-1 exerts immunomodulatory and protective effects on concanavalin A-induced hepatitis in mice. *Hepatology* **2000**, *31*, 399–406.
17. Offner, H.; Celnik, B.; Bringman, T.S.; Casentini-Borocz, D.; Nedwin, G.E.; Vandenbark, A.A. Recombinant human beta-galactoside binding lectin suppresses clinical and histological signs of experimental autoimmune encephalomyelitis. *J. Neuroimmunol.* **1990**, *28*, 177–184.
18. Cooper, D.N.W.; Barondes, S.H. Evidence for export of a muscle lectin from cytosol to extracellular matrix and for a novel secretory mechanism. *J. Cell Biol.* **1990**, *110*, 1681–1691.
19. Gabius, H.-J. Cell surface glycans: The why and how of their functionality as biochemical signals in lectin-mediated information transfer. *Crit. Rev. Immunol.* **2006**, *26*, 43–79.
20. Rappl, G.; Abken, H.; Muche, J.M.; et al. CD4+CD7- leukemic T cells from patients with Sézary syndrome are protected from galectin-1-triggered T cell death. *Leukemia* **2002**, *16*, 840–845.
21. André, S.; Sanchez-Ruderisch, H.; Nakagawa, H; et al. Tumor suppressor $p16^{INK4a}$: Modulator of glycomic profile and galectin-1 expression to increase susceptibility to carbohydrate-dependent induction of anoikis in pancreatic carcinoma cells. *FEBS J.* **2007**, *274*, 3233–3256.
22. Kopitz, J. Glycolipids. In *The Sugar Code: Fundamentals of Glycosciences*; Gabius, H.-J., Ed.; Wiley-VCH: Weinheim, Germany, 2009; pp 177–198.
23. Ledeen, R.W.; Wu, G. Neurobiology Meets Glycosciences. In *The Sugar Code: Fundamentals of Glycosciences*; Gabius, H.-J., Ed.; Wiley-VCH: Weinheim, Germany, 2009; pp 495–516.
24. Kopitz, J.; von Reitzenstein, C.; Burchert, M.; Cantz, M.; Gabius, H.-J. Galectin-1 is a major receptor for ganglioside GM1, a product of the growth-controlling activity of a cell surface ganglioside sialidase, on human neuroblastoma cells in culture. *J. Biol. Chem.* **1998**, *273*, 11205–11211.
25. Schengrund, C.L.; Repman, M.A. Density-dependent changes in gangliosides and sialidase activity of murine neuroblastoma cells. *J. Neurochem.* **1982**, *39*, 940–947.
26. Wang, P.; Zhang, J.; Bian, H.; et al. Induction of lysosomal and plasma membrane-bound sialidases in human T-cells via T-cell receptor. *Biochem. J.* **2004**, *380*, 425–433.
27. Tuosto, L.; Parolini, I.; Schröder, S.; Sargiacomo, M.; Lanzavecchia, A.; Viola, A. Organization of plasma membrane functional rafts upon T cell activation. *Eur. J. Immunol.* **2001**, *31*, 345–349.
28. Brumeanu, T.-D.; Preda-Pais, A.; Stoica, C.; Bona, C.; Casares, S. Differential partitioning and trafficking of GM gangliosides and

cholesterol-rich lipid rafts in thymic and splenic CD4 T cells. *Mol. Immunol.* **2007**, *44*, 530–540.
29. Kopitz, J.; von Reitzenstein, C.; André, S.; Kaltner, H.; Uhl, J.; Ehemann, V.; Cantz, M.; Gabius, H.-J. Negative regulation of neuroblastoma cell growth by carbohydrate-dependent surface binding of galectin-1 and functional divergence from galectin-3. *J. Biol. Chem.* **2001**, *276*, 35917–35923.
30. Kopitz, J.; Bergmann, M.; Gabius, H.-J. How adhesion/growth-regulatory galectins-1 and -3 attain cell specificity: case study defining their target on neuroblastoma cells (SK-N-MC) and marked affinity regulation by affecting microdomain organization of the membrane. *IUBMB Life* **2010**, *62*, 624–628.
31. Shimada, K.; Koh, C.S.; Uemura, K.; Yanagisawa, N. Suppression of experimental allergic encephalomyelitis in Lewis rats by administration of gangliosides. *Cell. Immunol.* **1994**, *154*, 231–239.
32. Sekiguchi, Y.; Ichikawa, M.; Inoue, A.; Itoh, M.; Koh, C.S. Brain-derived gangliosides suppress the chronic relapsing-remitting experimental autoimmune encephalomyelitis in NOD mice induced with myelin oligodendrocyte glycoprotein peptide. *J. Neuroimmunol.* **2001**, *116*, 196–205.
33. Monteiro de Castro, G.; Eduarda, Z.M.; Ventura-Oliveira, D.; Aparecida, V.C.; Ashimine, R.; de Lima Zollner, R. Th1 and Th2 cytokine immunomodulation by gangliosides in experimental autoimmune encephalomyelitis. *Cytokine* **2004**, *26*, 155–163.
34. Ledeen, R.W.; Oderfeld-Nowak, B.; Brosnan, C.F.; Cervone, A. Gangliosides offer partial protection in experimantal allergic neuritis. *Ann. Neurol.* **1990**, *27*, S69–S74.
35. Ponzin, D.; Menegus, A.M.; Kirschner, G.; Nunzi, M.G.; Fiori, M.G.; Raine, C.S. Effects of gangliosides on the expression of autoimmune demyelination in the peripheral nervous system. *Ann. Neurol.* **1991**, *30*, 678–685.
36. Vieira, K.P.; de Almeida e Silva Lima Zollner, A.R.; Malaguti, C.; Vilella, C.A.; de Lima Zollner, R. Ganglioside GM1 effects on the expression of nerve growth factor (NGF), Trk-A receptor, proinflammatory cytokines and on autoimmune diabetes onset in non-obese diabetic (NOD) mice. *Cytokine* **2008**, *42*, 92–104.
37. Fishman, P.H. Role of membrane gangliosides in the binding and action of bacterial toxins. *J. Membr. Biol.* **1982**, *69*, 85–97.
38. Siebert, H.C.; André, S.; Lu, SY; et al. Unique conformer selection of human growth-regulatory lectin galectin-1 for ganglioside GM1 versus bacterial toxins. *Biochemistry* **2003**, *42*, 14762–14773.
39. Williams, N. A.; Stasiuk, L.M.; Nashar, T.O.; Richards, C.M.; Lang, A.K.; Day, M.J.; Hirst, T.R. Prevention of autoimmune disease due to lymphocyte modulation by the B-subunit of *Escherichia coli* heat-labile enterotoxin. *Proc. Natl. Acad. Sci. U.S.A.* **1997**, *94*, 5290–5295.
40. Sobel, D.O.; Yankelevich, B.; Goyal, D.; Nelson, D.; Mazumder, A. The B-subunit of cholera toxin induces immunoregulatory cells and prevents diabetes in the NOD mouse. *Diabetes* **1998**, *47*, 186–191.

41. Salmond, R.J.; Luross, J.A.; Williams, N.A. Immune modulation by the cholera-like enterotoxins. *Expert Rev. Mol. Med.* **2002**, *2002*, 1–16.
42. Dixon, S.J.; Stewart, D.; Grinstein, S.; Spiegel, S. Transmembrane signaling by the B subunit of cholera toxin: increased cytoplasmic free calcium in rat lymphocytes. *J. Cell. Biol.* **1987**, *105*, 1153–1161.
43. Guoy, H.; Detterre, P.; Debre, P.; Bismuth, G. Cell calcium signaling via GM1 cell surface gangliosides in the human Jurkat T cell line. *J. Immunol.* **1994**, *152*, 3271–3281.
44. Walzel, H.; Blach, M.; Hirabayashi, J.; Kasai, K.I.; Brock, J. Involvement of CD2 and CD3 in galectin-1 induced signaling in human Jurkat T cells. *Glycobiology* **2000**, *10*, 131–140.
45. Fang, Y.; Xie, X.; Ledeen, R.W.; Wu, G. Characterization of cholera toxin B subunit-induced Ca^{2+} influx in neuroblastoma cells: evidence for a voltage independent GM1-associated Ca^{2+} channel. *J. Neurosci. Res.* **2002**, *57*, 1–10.
46. Wu, G.; Lu, Z.-H.; Obukhov, A.G.; Nowycky, M.C.; Ledeen, R.W. Induction of calcium influx through TRPC5 channels by cross-linking of GM1 ganglioside associated with α5β1 integrin initiates neurite outgrowth. *J. Neurosci.* **2007**, *27*, 7447–7458.
47. Clapham, D.E.; Runnels, L.W.; Strübing, C. The TRP ion channel family. *Nat. Rev. Neurosci.* **2001**, *2*, 387–396.
48. Wu, G.; Lu, Z.-H.; Gabius, H.-J.; Ledeen, R.W.; Bleich, D. Ganglioside deficiency in effector T cells from NOD mice induces resistance to regulatory T cell suppression. *Diabetes* **2011**, *60*, 2341–2349.
49. Quattrini, A.; Lorenzetti, I.; Sciorati, C.; Corbo, M.; Previtali, S.C.; Feltri, M.L.; Canal, N.; Wrabetz, L.; Nemni, R.; Clementi, E. Human IgM anti-GM1 autoantibodies modulate intracellular calcium homeostasis in neuroblastoma cells. *J. Neuroimmunol.* **2001**, *114*, 213–219.
50. Crawford, M.P.; et al. High prevalence of autoreactive, neuroantigen-specific $CD8^+$ T cells in multiple sclerosis revealed by novel flow cytometric assay. *Blood* **2004**, *103*, 4222–4231.
51. Lassmann, H.; Ransohoff, R.M. The CD4-Th1 model for multiple sclerosis: a critical [correction of crucial] re-appraisal. *Trends Immunol.* **2004**, *25*, 132–137.
52. Walter, U.; Santamaria, P. $CD8^+$ T cells in autoimmunity. *Curr. Opin. Immunol.* **2005**, *17*, 624–631.
53. Coppieters, K.T.; Dotta, F.; Amiran, N.; Campbell, P.D.; Kay, T.W.; Atkinson, M.A.; Roep, B.O.; von Herrath, M.G. Demonstration of islet-autoreactive CD8 T cells in insulitic lesions from recent onset and long-term type 1 diabetes patients. *J. Exp. Med.* **2012**, *209*, 51–60.
54. de Mello Coelho, V.D.; Nguyen, B.; Giri; et al. Quantitative differences in lipid raft components between murine $CD4^+$ and $CD8^+$ T cells. *BMC Immunol.* **2004**, *5*, 2.
55. Nashar, T.O.; Williams, N.A.; Hirst, T.R. Cross-linking of cell surface ganglioside GM1 induces the selective apoptosis of mature $CD8^+$ T lymphocytes. *Int. Immunol.* **1996**, *15*, 731–736.

56. Anderson, M.S.; Bluestone, J.A. The NOD mouse: A model of immune dysregulation. *Annu. Rev. Immunol.* **2005**, *23*, 447–485.
57. D'Alise, A.M.; et al. The defect in T-cell regulation in NOD mice is an effect on the T-cell effectors. *Proc. Natl. Acad. Sci. U.S.A.* **2008**, *105*, 19857–19862.
58. Schneider, A.; Rieck, M.; Sanda, S.; Pihoker, C.; Greenbaum, C.; Buckner, J.H. The effector T cells of diabetic subjects are resistant to regulation via $CD4^+$ $FOXP3^+$ regulatory T cells. *J. Immunol.* **2008**, *181*, 7350–7355.
59. Wu, G.; Ledeen, R.W. Gangliosides as modulators of neuronal calcium. *Prog. Brain Res.* **1994**, *101*, 101–112.
60. Gabius, H.-J., Ed.; *The Sugar Code: Fundamentals of Glycosciences*; Wiley-VCH: Weinheim, Germany, 2009.
61. Gabius, H.-J.; André, S.; Jiménez-Barbero, J.; Romero, A.; Solís, D. From lectin structure to functional glycomics: Principles of the sugar code. *Trends Biochem. Sci.* **2011**, *36*, 298–313.

Chapter 7

How To Build "Lean and Mean" Anti-Tumor T Cells: A Strategic View into the Anti-Carbohydrate Action of Fluorinated Glucosamine Analogs

Charles J. Dimitroff*

Department of Dermatology, Brigham and Women's Hospital, Harvard Medical School, 77 Avenue Louis Pasteur, HIM, Rm. 662, Boston, Massachusetts 02115
***E-mail: cdimitroff@rics.bwh.harvard.edu**

Cell surface N-acetyllactosaminyl glycans have been shown to be key regulators of the vitality and effector function of anti-tumor T cells. When the S-type lectin, galectin-1 (Gal-1), binds N-acetyllactosamines displayed at high levels by distinct membrane glycoproteins on anti-tumor T cells, these cells either undergo apoptosis or adopt an immunoregulatory phenotype. Methods designed to antagonize the expression and function of these galactose – N-acetylglucosamine disaccharides on N- and O-glycans have thus intensified. The hope of such neutralization strategies is to circumvent the consequences of Gal-1-binding and tolerogenic effects to anti-tumor T cells. Because tumors characteristically express an abundance of Gal-1, it has been hypothesized that tumor-derived Gal-1 is a critical determinant in protecting tumor cells from T cell-mediated anti-tumor activity. To date, competitive glycan inhibitors of Gal-1 binding have shown effectiveness towards interfering with Gal-1-mediated effects. Though more recent efforts using fluorinated analogs of glucosamine designed to antagonize the biosynthesis of N-acetyllactosamines in effector/memory T cells have shown great promise for evading Gal-1 control and boosting anti-tumor T cell levels. In this perspective, the history and prospect of fluorinated glucosamine analogs as cancer therapeutics and potential value of eliminating N-acetyllactosamines on anti-tumor T cells to boost anti-tumor immunity is addressed.

Historical View of Fluorinated Glucosamine Analogs in Pharmaceutical Development

Nearly 35-years ago, acetylated and fluorinated derivatives of D-glucosamine were synthesized and evaluated as cytotoxic anti-cancer agents (*1–3*). The intent was to create analogs of natural-occurring hexosamines that could passively enter cancer cells, compete for nucleotide precursors and inhibit ongoing glycoconjugate and RNA/DNA synthesis pathways (*1–3*). This metabolic antagonism could thus potentially alter the expression of cell surface glycoconjugates and/or attenuate cell proliferation. As such, it was proposed that glucosamine analog treatment could change the antigenicity of cancer cell surface and boost immune-mediated mechanisms or simply block cancer growth. Indeed, though evidence suggested that these glucosamine analogs could be metabolized by cancer cells (*1–3*), precisely how they blocked glycan formation or whether nucleotide-sugar analog conjugates were even formed and utilized by glycosyltransferases to incorporate into growing oligosaccharide chains was still unknown.

It was later shown that, at non-growth inhibitory concentrations, the fully acetylated and 4-fluorinated glucosamine analog, 2-acetamido-2,4-dideoxy-1,3,6-tri-O-acetyl-4-fluoro-D-glucopyranose (4-F-GlcNAc), could alter the structure and function of N- and O-glycans on ovarian and colon cancer cell glycoproteins (*2*, *4–8*). These alterations inhibited human ovarian cancer (OCa) and colon cancer (CCa) cell binding to galectin-1 (Gal-1) and endothelial (E)-selectin, respectively (*2*, *4–8*). These results provided hope that modulating N-acetyllactosamine (galactose ß1,4 N-acetylglucosamine) synthesis essential for both Gal-1- and E-selectin-binding activity, could actually interfere with lectin-mediated cell adhesion events critically involved in the metastatic process. In fact, because OCa cell adhesion to the extracellular matrix underlying the peritoneal lining and CCa cell trafficking to liver are, in part, mediated by Gal-1 and E-selectin, respectively, there remains much promise for these sugar analogs to be developed as anti-metastatic therapeutics (*4–18*). Nevertheless, these results offered the experimental rationale for targeting glyco-metabolically active cells distinct from cancer cells, where glycoconjugate processing and function provide key cell behavioral features without posing a significant threat to cell viability.

Subsequent research on fluorinated glucosamine analogs transitioned in intent to altering key glycan-recognition determinants on skin-homing T cells that initiate their entry into skin (*19*). Effector/memory T cells educated to enter dermal tissues require the E-selectin-binding glycan, sialyl Lewis X, for binding E-selectin constitutively expressed on dermal microvessels and for initiating a cascade of adhesive events that facilitates diapedesis. Considering evidence on E-selectin-binding glycan downregulation in 4-F-GlcNAc-treated CCa cells, it was hypothesized that 4-F-GlcNAc treatment could inhibit sialyl Lewis X synthesis on skin-homing T cells and block E-selectin-mediated adhesion to dermal microvessels and recruitment into inflamed skin. Indeed, studies showed that antigen-dependent $CD4^+$ T cell activation in skin-draining lymph nodes triggered sialyl Lewis X biosynthesis that conferred a susceptibility to 4-F-GlcNAc antagonism (*19*, *20*). Treatment with 4-F-GlcNAc reduced the level of sialyl Lewis X and corresponding E-selectin-binding activity, which blunted antigen-dependent T cell-mediated inflammation in the skin (*9–22*). These inhibitory effects were similarly found on human leukemic cells treated with a peracetylated 4-fluorinated N-acetylgalactosamine analog (*23*).

To understand more globally the anti-carbohydrate effects on T cells by fluorinated glucosamine analogs, further evaluations focused on analysis of Gal-1 binding to T cells following 4-F-GlcNAc treatment. Considering Gal-1's key role in binding and inducing apoptosis or immunoregulatory activity in effector $CD4^+$ T cells (*24–30*), understanding the relative difference between inhibition of Gal-1-binding and E-selectin-binding was an important distinction to ascertain. It can be construed that inhibiting the N-acetyllactosamine lattice required for Gal-1-mediated inflammatory silencing of activated/effector T cells may paradoxically offset a deficit in T cell trafficking due to lowering of E-selectin-binding glycans. It was, in fact, demonstrated that the expression of Gal-1-binding glycans on activated $CD4^+$ T cells was more sensitive than E-selectin-binding glycans to 4-F-GlcNAc treatment (*31*). In support of this observation, earlier studies analyzing the specificity of glycoconjugate action showed that 4-F-GlcNAc preferentially limits the synthesis of N-acetyllactosamines in N- and O-glycans on glycoproteins and not on neolactoglycosphingolipids, which can also function as E-selectin-binding glycans (*19–21*, *31–35*).

Collectively, these findings suggested that Gal-1-binding glycans and related triggering of downstream immune tolerogenic pathways may be a more amenable target for 4-F-GlcNAc treatment. This notion posed new questions on how 4-F-GlcNAc can most effectively be used for N-acetyllactosamine antagonism and whether 4-F-GlcNAc should indeed be developed as an anti-inflammatory therapeutic. We have thusly postulated that interfering with the synthesis of Gal-1-binding glycans in effector T cells would be perhaps more applicable in the context of cancer immunotherapy, whereby anti-tumor T cells treated with 4-F-GlcNAc would be resistant to Gal-1-mediated tumor immune evasion (*31*).

Mechanism of Fluorinated Glucosamine Anti-Carbohydrate Action

Early evidence suggested that fully acetylated variants of glucosamine could effectively traverse a cancer cell's plasma membrane and sequester endogenous UTP and CTP pools necessary for steady-state RNA/DNA biosynthesis, which elicited a cytotoxic effect in cancer cells (*2*, *3*). Furthermore, it was found that diversion of endogenous UTP pools by exogenous glucosamine analog treatments could elevate UDP-N-acetylglucosamine levels, thereby lowering native pools of other nucleotide-sugars, such as UDP-galactose and UDP-N-acetylgalactosamine needed for N- and O-glycan extension (*2*, *3*).

Fluorinated glucosamine analogs were synthesized by addition of a fluorine atom, which cannot form a glycosidic bond, at strategic pyranose ring carbons that could antagonize oligosaccharide elongation (*1–3*). As such, by substituting fluorine for a hydroxyl group at the carbon-4 position, it was theorized that, upon entering a cell and incorporation into a growing poly-N-acetyllactosaminyl chain, 4-F-GlcNAc could block glycosidic bonding of a galactose residue at the carbon-4 position. All data on the anti-glycoconjugate effects of 4-F-GlcNAc efficacy subsequently, in fact, indicated that synthesis of (galactose ß1,4 N-acetylglucosamine)$_n$ residues and related sialyl Lewis X moieties were inhibited (*19–22*). More recent structural data provided a more refined assessment in that N-acetyllactosamines and sialyl Lewis X on N-glycans and on core 2 O-glycans were reduced and the content and structural diversity of tri- and tetra-antennary N-glycans and of O-glycans were reduced, while biantennary N-glycans were increased. However, MALDI-TOF mass spectrometry analysis did not reveal any m/z ratios relating to the presence of fluorine atoms in N- and O-glycans released from 4-F-GlcNAc-treated human T cells and leukemic cells, indicating that 4-F-GlcNAc did not in fact incorporate into and truncate glycan chains (*31*). 4-F-GlcNAc treatment also neither affected the expression nor activity of N-acetyllactosamine-synthesizing enzymes or the level of sialyl Lewis X on glycolipids (*31*). As expected though, 4-F-GlcNAc did significantly reduce intracellular levels of UDP-GlcNAc (*31*), which was validated by another group assessing the mechanism of acetylated and fluorinated glucosamine analog action (*36*). What was also noted from this recent work was the first evidence of UDP-4-F-GlcNAc donor sugar in 4-F-GlcNAc-treated cancer cells (*36*).

Cumulatively, data on fluorinated glucosamine analog action and 4-F-GlcNAc anti-carbohydrate efficacy indicate that Gal-1- and E-selectin-binding reductions are not caused by direct 4-F-GlcNAc incorporation into oligosaccharides and consequent chain termination, but rather by shunting endogenous UDP-GlcNAc synthesis towards production of UDP-4-F-GlcNAc (Figure 1).

In that there is no evidence of glycan incorporation of fluorinated analogs, the fluorine residue at the carbon-4 position in UDP-4-F-GlcNAc is likely hindering the ability of N-acetylglucosaminyltransferases to transfer the 4-F-GlcNAc sugar to an oligosaccharide acceptor (*31*, *36*). Alternatively, in addition to titrating out pools of UTP, another potential mode of action is that 4-F-GlcNAc is irreversibly binding and inactivating UDP-acetylglucosamine pyrophosphorylase (UAP) directly. These possibilities need to be investigated further.

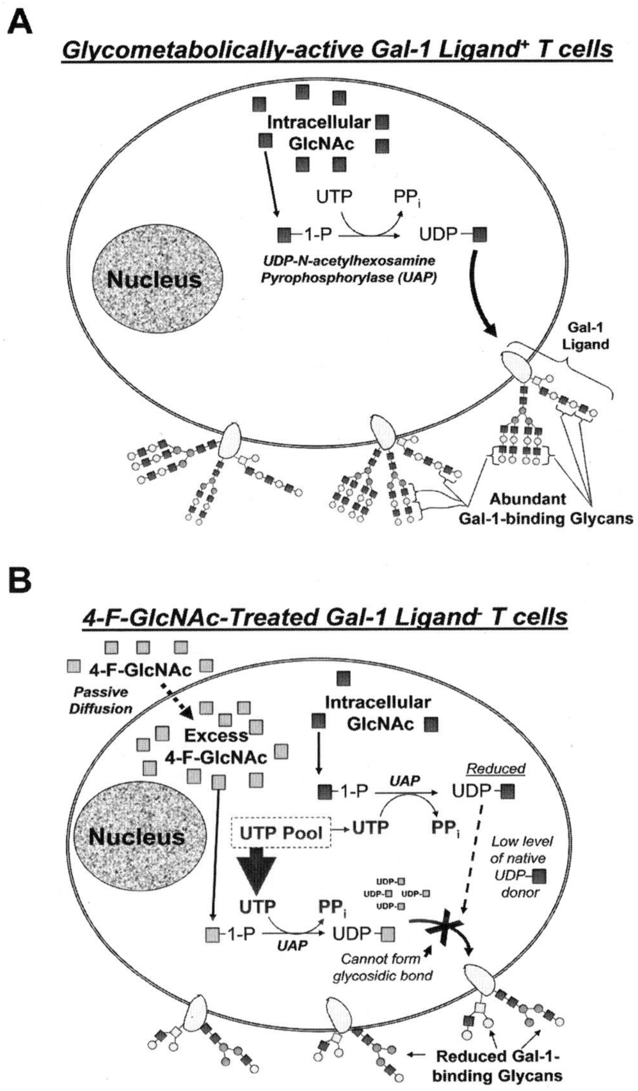

Figure 1. Mechanism of Peracetylated 4-Fluorinated Glucosamine Anti-Carbohydrate Action. (A) T cells actively synthesizing cell surface glycoconjugates are sensitive to glyco-metabolic antagonists, such as fully acetylated 4-F-GlcNAc. (B) Following passive cellular entry and deacetylation of peracetylated 4-fluorinated-glucosamine, 4-F-GlcNAc is phosphorylated and conjugated to UTP by UDP-acetylglucosamine pyrophosphorylase (UAP). Depending on the cytosolic concentration of 4-F-GlcNAc, endogenous UDP-GlcNAc levels are compromised due to sequestration of UTP. This shunting effect causes reductions in N-acetyllactosamines necessary for extending and branching of N- and O-glycan antennae characteristically bound by Gal-1. (see color insert)

Blocking N-acetyllactosamine Synthesis in CD8+ T Cells To Improve Anti-Tumor Immunity

The presence of tumor-infiltrating lymphocytes, in particular, CTLs, and their implication in cancer patient survival and prognosis is not clear (*37–40*). Moreover, adoptive transfer of autologous anti-melanoma CTLs has shown only a modest improvement in patients with advanced disease (*41–43*). These observations suggest that melanomas can innately avert the immune system. Galectins, in particular Gal-1 and Gal-3, have been shown to be produced at high levels by melanoma cells (*44–46*) as well as certain lymphomas, such as Hodgkin's lymphoma (*47–49*) and cutaneous T cell lymphoma (*26*), and found to elicit potent immunosuppressive features (*26*, *48–50*). In fact melanoma-derived Gal-1 has been shown to efficiently subdue the effector function of T helper (Th) 1 and Th17 cell subsets as well as CTLs (*27*, *29*, *50*), all of which express a high level of Gal-1-binding N-acetyllactosamines. Since Gal-1 characteristically binds effector $CD4^+$ T cells with anti-tumor activity and CTLs and causes apoptosis/tolerization, we have hypothesized that reducing Gal-1-binding to N-acetyllactosamines on anti-tumor T cells could significantly elevate anti-tumor T cell immune activity, particularly against tumors that express copious amounts of Gal-1.

Accordingly, most recent efforts in 4-F-GlcNAc development have centered on anti-tumor studies with the intent to lower Gal-1-binding glycans, alleviate Gal-1-dependent immunoregulation boost anti-tumor T cell immunity. Our laboratory has recently accumulated some exciting *in vivo* data on the use of 4-F-GlcNAc to treat melanomas and lymphomas. Melanoma was not only included as a tumor model based on its high Gal-1 expression, but that diminution of E-selectin-binding glycan would be inconsequential. Since microvessels within melanomas do not express E-selectin (*51*), 4-F-GlcNAc-treated T cells could theoretically still infiltrate melanomas while evading Gal-1-dependent control to elicit their effector function. Using non-toxic doses of 4-F-GlcNAc in mice bearing melanoma or lymphoma, we found that tumor growth was grossly attenuated (*52*). These results were, in part, due to 4-F-GlcNAc-dependent sparing of Gal-1-mediated apoptosis of IFN-γ- and IL-17-producing $CD4^+$ T cells and of melanoma specific CTLs by reducing their surface content of Gal-1-binding N-acetyllactosamines. In other words, there was a shift in the effector - regulatory T cell balance towards more Th1 and Th17 cells and more CTLs, and less immune regulating IL-10^+ T cells generated by tumor-derived Gal-1 (*26*, *52*, *53*). These findings reinforced the importance of N-acetyllactosamines in controlling the fate and function of effector $CD4^+$ T cell and CTL subsets and indicated that treating melanomas and lymphomas, which abundantly express Gal-1 and likely other immunosuppressive galectins, with 4-F-GlcNAc could prove to be therapeutically efficacious (*52*). In all, these data highlight the promise of 4-F-GlcNAc to limit tumor growth by boosting T cell-mediated immunity (*53*).

Conclusion and Future Prospects of Fluorinated Glucosamine Analogs

There exists a long standing history on the development of fluorinated glucosamine analogs for the metabolic antagonism of glycoconjugate and DNA/ RNA synthesis. While early studies focused on the merits of cytotoxic-induction in cancer cells by 4-F-GlcNAc, subsequent efforts re-considered these intents and began to evaluate the targeting of glyco-metabolically-active T cells. In this case, the main objective was to selectively target these T cells, which could rapidly uptake glucosamine analogs to antagonize UDP-GlcNAc production and block the synthesis of sialyl Lewis X necessary for E-selectin-mediated trafficking to inflamed skin. During attempts to illuminate the mechanism of 4-F-GlcNAc-glycan alterations and lectin-binding activities, it was appreciated that Gal-1-binding was more efficiently inhibited than E-selectin-binding activity. These results encouraged later efforts to evaluate 4-F-GlcNAc as an inhibitor of Gal-1-binding N-acetyllactosamine synthesis in T cells and blocker of the immunoregulatory control of tumor-derived Gal-1 (Figure 2A).

As such, studies from our laboratory showed that 4-F-GlcNAc elicited potent anti-tumor activity by increasing the quantity of effector T cells and reducing the level of immune regulating IL-10^{+} T cells characteristically generated by tumor-derived Gal-1 (*26*, *52*, *53*) (Figure 2B). However, much skepticism remains as this mode of therapy could theoretically alter glycosylation in other glyco-metabolically-active leukocytes, such as activated antigen-presenting cells and hematopoietic progenitor cells, wherein lectin-binding events are known to affect their immunologic behavior (*54–57*). Future studies are needed to ascertain the relative specificity of anti-glycosylation effects on non-T cells in 4-F-GlcNAc-treated animals.

As a prospective approach, which provides ultimate targeting efficiency, we are beginning efforts to study 4-F-GlcNAc in the setting of adoptive T cell cancer therapy. Adoptive transfer of autologous tumor-specific CTLs as an anti-cancer therapy is a promising, though imperfect, approach to boost anti-tumor immunity (*58–60*). We believe that 4-F-GlcNAc treatment of *in vitro*-expanded tumor Ag-specific CTLs will generate CTLs lacking not only Gal-1-binding N-acetyllactosamines but potentially Gal-9-binding TIM-3 and other immunoregulatory galectin ligands, enhancing their tumoricidal activity due to their insensitivity to galectin(s)-dependent regulation (Figure 2C). Since CTLs express an abundance of N-acetyllactosamines, tailoring 4-F-GlcNAc treatment with this *ex vivo* approach could improve the quantity, longevity and anti-tumor activity of CTLs, particularly against tumors that overexpress Gal-1, Gal-9 and other immunoregulatory galectins. Whereas a neutralizing antibody against a single galectin could help alleviate respective galectin-dependent immunoregulation, 4-F-GlcNAc's ability to potentially inhibit the synthesis of Gal-1, Gal-3 and Gal-9 binding glycans on CTLs could indeed offer a multifaceted strategy, in which multiple galectin regulators are neutralized (*53*). This N-acetyllactosamine reduction strategy could even be advantageous to help boost the potency of cancer vaccines or viral vaccines for other diseases, wherein tumor- and virus-specific CTLs are key regulators of an efficacious immunologic response, though have been shown to be negatively regulated by Gal-9 (*61*, *62*). Moreover, combining 4-F-GlcNAc with a vaccine delivery method, such as skin scarification, can perhaps synergize the efficacy of immunologic response and help maintain protective immunity (*63*, *64*). The mechanism and functional consequences of 4-F-GlcNAc efficacy on CTLs have reinvigorated the prospect of using fluorinated glucosamines as a novel immunotherapeutic adjuvant for treating cancer and for boosting vaccine efficacy against infectious diseases.

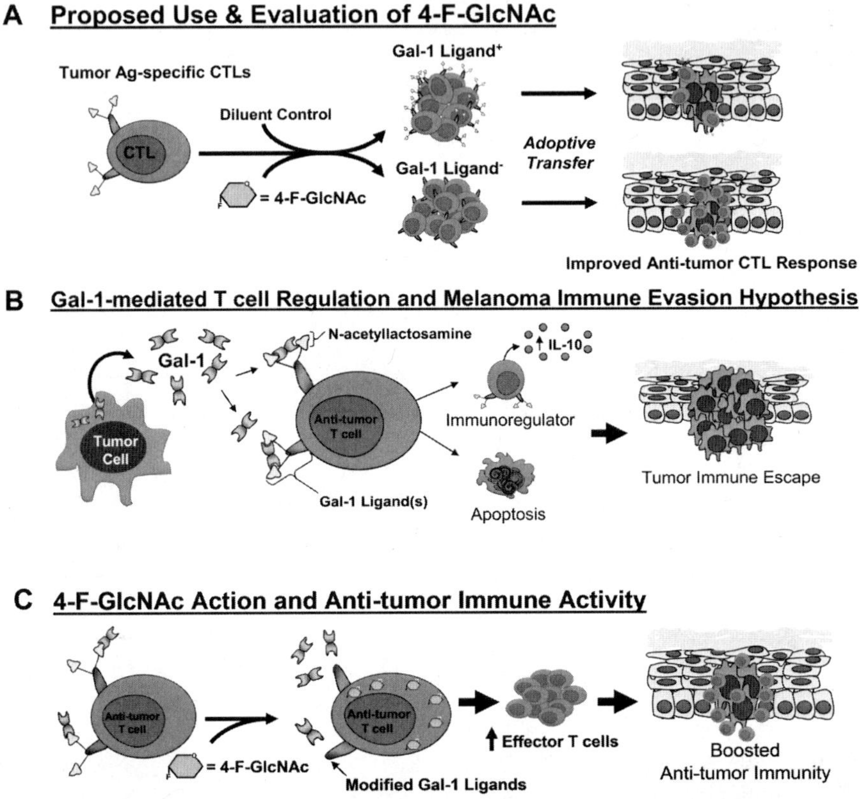

Figure 2. Neutralization of the Gal-1 – Gal-1 ligand axis to Boost Anti-tumor T cell Immunity. (A) A schematic depiction of tumor immune evasion model in which melanoma-derived Gal-1 can antagonize the anti-tumor efficacy of T cells. (B) A cartoon depiction of the metabolic antagonism of Gal-1-binding N-acetyllactosamine synthesis in effector anti-tumor T cells caused by 4-F-GlcNAc and consequent enhancement of anti-tumor immunity. (C) A schematic overview of a novel cancer immunotherapeutic strategy to selectivity target donor CTLs with 4-F-GlcNAc for escaping Gal-1 control and improving the efficacy of adoptive T cell therapy. (see color insert)

Acknowledgments

I thank Drs. Ralph Bernacki, Barbara Woynarowska, Moheswar Sharma, E.V. Chandrasekaran, Khushi Matta and Joseph Lau for their mentorship and early teachings in glycobiology. This work is dedicated to their efforts for opening new research directions in lectin biology and for enhancing our glyco-pathobiological understanding of inflammation and cancer metastasis. Research in the Dimitroff Laboratory is funded by an RO1 AT004628 grant from the National Institutes of Health/National Center for Complementary and Alternative Medicine.

References

1. Bernacki, R.; Porter, C.; et al. Plasma membrane as a site for chemotherapeutic intervention. *Adv. Enzyme Regul.* **1977**, *16*, 217–237.
2. Bernacki, R. J.; Sharma, M.; et al. Biochemical characteristics, metabolism, and antitumor activity of several acetylated hexosamines. *J. Supramol. Struct.* **1977**, *7*, 235–250.
3. Sharma, M.; Bernacki, R. J.; et al. Fluorinated carbohydrates as potential plasma membrane modifiers. Synthesis of 4- and 6-fluoro derivatives of 2-acetamido-2-deoxy-D-hexopyranoses. *Carbohydr. Res.* **1990**, *198*, 205–221.
4. Dimitroff, C. J.; Pera, P.; et al. Cell surface n-acetylneuraminic acid alpha2,3-galactoside-dependent intercellular adhesion of human colon cancer cells. *Biochem. Biophys. Res. Commun.* **1999**, *256*, 631–636.
5. Dimitroff, C. J.; Sharma, A.; et al. Cancer metastasis: A search for therapeutic inhibition. *Cancer Invest.* **1998**, *16*, 279–290.
6. Skrincosky, D. M.; Allen, H. J.; et al. Galaptin-mediated adhesion of human ovarian carcinoma A121 cells and detection of cellular galaptin-binding glycoproteins. *Cancer Res.* **1993**, *53*, 2667–2675.
7. Woynarowska, B.; Dimitroff, C. J.; et al. Inhibition of human HT-29 colon carcinoma cell adhesion by a 4-fluoro-glucosamine analogue. *Glycoconjugate J.* **1996**, *13*, 663–674.
8. Woynarowska, B.; Skrincosky, D. M.; et al. Inhibition of lectin-mediated ovarian tumor cell adhesion by sugar analogs. *J. Biol. Chem.* **1994**, *269*, 22797–22803.
9. Bresalier, R. S.; Byrd, J. C.; et al. Liver metastasis and adhesion to the sinusoidal endothelium by human colon cancer cells is related to mucin carbohydrate chain length. *Int. J. Cancer* **1998**, *76*, 556–562.
10. Gangopadhyay, A.; Lazure, D. A.; et al. Adhesion of colorectal carcinoma cells to the endothelium is mediated by cytokines from CEA stimulated Kupffer cells. *Clin. Exp. Metastasis* **1998**, *16*, 703–712.
11. Gout, S.; Tremblay, P. L.; et al. Selectins and selectin ligands in extravasation of cancer cells and organ selectivity of metastasis. *Clin. Exp. Metastasis* **2008**, *25*, 335–344.
12. Irimura, T.; Ota, M.; et al. Carbohydrate-mediated adhesion of human colon carcinoma cells to human liver sections. *Adv. Exp. Med. Biol.* **2001**, *491*, 403–412.

13. Kitakata, H.; Nemoto-Sasaki, Y.; et al. Essential roles of tumor necrosis factor receptor p55 in liver metastasis of intrasplenic administration of colon 26 cells. *Cancer Res.* **2002**, *62*, 6682–6687.
14. Kruskal, J. B.; Azouz, A.; et al. Hepatic colorectal cancer metastases: Imaging initial steps of formation in mice. *Radiology* **2007**, *243*, 703–711.
15. Opolski, A.; Laskowska, A.; et al. Metastatic potential of human CX-1 colon adenocarcinoma cells is dependent on the expression of sialosyl Le(a) antigen. *Clin. Exp. Metastasis* **1998**, *16*, 673–681.
16. St Hill, C. A.; Farooqui, M.; et al. The high affinity selectin glycan ligand C2-O-sLex and mRNA transcripts of the core 2 beta-1,6-N-acetylglucosaminyltransferase (C2GnT1) gene are highly expressed in human colorectal adenocarcinomas. *BMC Cancer* **2009**, *9*, 79.
17. Tsuiji, H.; Nakatsugawa, S.; et al. Malignant and other properties of human colon carcinoma cells after suppression of sulfomucin production in vitro. *Clin. Exp. Metastasis* **1999**, *17*, 97–104.
18. Weston, B. W.; Hiller, K. M.; et al. Expression of human alpha(1,3)fucosyltransferase antisense sequences inhibits selectin-mediated adhesion and liver metastasis of colon carcinoma cells. *Cancer Res.* **1999**, *59*, 2127–2135.
19. Dimitroff, C. J.; Bernacki, R. J.; et al. Glycosylation-dependent inhibition of cutaneous lymphocyte-associated antigen expression: Implications in modulating lymphocyte migration to skin. *Blood* **2003**, *101*, 602–610.
20. Dimitroff, C. J.; Kupper, T. S.; et al. Prevention of leukocyte migration to inflamed skin with a novel fluorosugar modifier of cutaneous lymphocyte-associated antigen. *J. Clin. Invest.* **2003**, *112*, 1008–1018.
21. Descheny, L.; Gainers, M. E.; et al. Ameliorating skin-homing receptors on malignant T cells with a fluorosugar analog of N-acetylglucosamine: P-selectin ligand is a more sensitive target than E-selectin ligand. *J. Invest. Dermatol.* **2006**, *126*, 2065–2073.
22. Gainers, M. E.; Descheny, L.; et al. Skin-homing receptors on effector leukocytes are differentially sensitive to glyco-metabolic antagonism in allergic contact dermatitis. *J. Immunol.* **2007**, *179*, 8509–8518.
23. Marathe, D. D.; Buffone, A., Jr.; et al. Fluorinated per-acetylated GalNAc metabolically alters glycan structures on leukocyte PSGL-1 and reduces cell binding to selectins. *Blood* **2010**, *115*, 1303–1312.
24. Cedeno-Laurent, F.; Barthel, S. R.; et al. Development of a nascent galectin-1 chimeric molecule for studying the role of leukocyte galectin-1 ligands and immune disease modulation. *J. Immunol.* **2010**, *185*, 4659–4672.
25. Cedeno-Laurent, F.; Opperman, M.; et al. Galectin-1 triggers an immunoregulatory signature in th cells functionally defined by IL-10 expression. *J. Immunol.* **2012**, *188*, 3127–3137.
26. Cedeno-Laurent, F.; Watanabe, R.; et al. Galectin-1 inhibits the viability, proliferation, and Th1 cytokine production of nonmalignant T cells in patients with leukemic cutaneous T-cell lymphoma. *Blood* **2012**, *119*, 3534–3538.
27. Ilarregui, J. M.; Croci, D. O.; et al. Tolerogenic signals delivered by dendritic cells to T cells through a galectin-1-driven immunoregulatory

circuit involving interleukin 27 and interleukin 10. *Nat. Immunol.* **2009**, *10*, 981–991.

28. Perillo, N. L.; Pace, K. E.; et al. Apoptosis of T cells mediated by galectin-1. *Nature* **1995**, *378*, 736–739.
29. Toscano, M. A.; Bianco, G. A.; et al. Differential glycosylation of TH1, TH2 and TH-17 effector cells selectively regulates susceptibility to cell death. *Nat. Immunol.* **2007**, *8*, 825–834.
30. van der Leij, J.; van den Berg, A.; et al. Dimeric galectin-1 induces IL-10 production in T-lymphocytes: An important tool in the regulation of the immune response. *J. Pathol.* **2004**, *204*, 511–518.
31. Barthel, S. R.; et al. Peracetylated 4-fluoro-glucosamine reduces the content and repertoire of N- and O-glycans without direct incorporation. *J. Biol. Chem.* **2011**, *286*, 21717–21731.
32. Barthel, S. R.; et al. Analysis of glycosyltransferase expression in metastatic prostate cancer cells capable of rolling activity on microvascular endothelial (E)-selectin. *Glycobiology* **2008**, *18*, 806–817.
33. Barthel, S. R.; et al. Alpha1,3 fucosyltransferases are master regulators of prostate cancer cell trafficking. *Proc. Natl. Acad. Sci. U.S.A.* **2009**, *106*, 19491–19496.
34. Dimitroff, C. J.; et al. Identification of leukocyte E-selectin ligands, P-selectin glycoprotein ligand-1 and E-selectin ligand-1, on human metastatic prostate tumor cells. *Cancer Res.* **2005**, *65*, 5750–5760.
35. Dimitroff, C. J.; et al. Rolling of human bone-metastatic prostate tumor cells on human bone marrow endothelium under shear flow is mediated by E-selectin. *Cancer Res.* **2004**, *64*, 5261–5269.
36. Nishimura, S. I.; et al. Glycomics for drug discovery: Metabolic perturbation in androgen-independent prostate cancer cells induced by unnatural hexosamine mimics. *Angew. Chem., Int. Ed. Engl.* **2012**, *124*, 1–6.
37. Clemente, C. G.; et al. Prognostic value of tumor infiltrating lymphocytes in the vertical growth phase of primary cutaneous melanoma. *Cancer* **1996**, *77*, 1303–1310.
38. Mihm, M. C., Jr.; et al. Tumor infiltrating lymphocytes in lymph node melanoma metastases: A histopathologic prognostic indicator and an expression of local immune response. *Lab. Invest.* **1996**, *74*, 43–47.
39. Oble, D. A.; et al. Focus on TILs: Prognostic significance of tumor infiltrating lymphocytes in human melanoma. *Cancer Immun.* **2009**, *9*, 3.
40. Liakou, C. I.; et al. Focus on TILs: Prognostic significance of tumor infiltrating lymphocytes in human bladder cancer. *Cancer Immun.* **2007**, *7*, 10.
41. Besser, M. J.; et al. Clinical responses in a phase II study using adoptive transfer of short-term cultured tumor infiltration lymphocytes in metastatic melanoma patients. *Clin. Cancer Res.* **2010**, *16*, 2646–2655.
42. Dudley, M. E.; et al. CD8+ enriched "young" tumor infiltrating lymphocytes can mediate regression of metastatic melanoma. *Clin. Cancer Res.*, *16*, 6122–6131.

43. Dudley, M. E.; et al. Adoptive cell therapy for patients with metastatic melanoma: Evaluation of intensive myeloablative chemoradiation preparative regimens. *J. Clin. Oncol.* **2008**, *26*, 5233–5239.
44. Vereecken, P.; et al. Evaluation of the prognostic significance of serum galectin-3 in American Joint Committee on Cancer stage III and stage IV melanoma patients. *Melanoma Res.* **2009**, *19*, 316–320.
45. Radosavljevic, G.; et al. Deletion of galectin-3 in the host attenuates metastasis of murine melanoma by modulating tumor adhesion and NK cell activity. *Clin. Exp. Metastasis* **2011**, *28*, 451–462.
46. Mourad-Zeidan, A. A.; et al. Expression profiling of Galectin-3-depleted melanoma cells reveals its major role in melanoma cell plasticity and vasculogenic mimicry. *Am. J. Pathol.* **2008**, *173*, 1839–1852.
47. Rodig, S. J.; et al. AP1-dependent galectin-1 expression delineates classical hodgkin and anaplastic large cell lymphomas from other lymphoid malignancies with shared molecular features. *Clin. Cancer Res.* **2008**, *14*, 3338–3344.
48. Juszczynski, P.; et al. The AP1-dependent secretion of galectin-1 by Reed Sternberg cells fosters immune privilege in classical Hodgkin lymphoma. *Proc. Natl. Acad. Sci. U.S.A.* **2007**, *104*, 13134–13139.
49. Gandhi, M. K.; et al. Galectin-1 mediated suppression of Epstein-Barr virus specific T-cell immunity in classic Hodgkin lymphoma. *Blood* **2007**, *110*, 1326–1329.
50. Rubinstein, N.; et al. Targeted inhibition of galectin-1 gene expression in tumor cells results in heightened T cell-mediated rejection: A potential mechanism of tumor-immune privilege. *Cancer Cell* **2004**, *5*, 241–251.
51. Weishaupt, C.; et al. T-cell distribution and adhesion receptor expression in metastatic melanoma. *Clin. Cancer Res.* **2007**, *13*, 2549–2556.
52. Cedeno-Laurent, F.; et al. Metabolic inhibition of galectin-1-binding carbohydrates accentuates anti-tumor immunity. *J. Invest. Dermatol.* **2012**, *132*, 410–420.
53. Cedeno-Laurent, F.; Dimitroff, C. J. Galectins and their ligands: Negative regulators of anti-tumor immunity. *Glycoconjugate J.* **2012**, *29*, 619–625.
54. Rabinovich, G. A.; Croci, D. O. Regulatory circuits mediated by lectin-glycan interactions in autoimmunity and cancer. *Immunity* **2012**, *36*, 322–335.
55. Rabinovich, G. A.; Vidal, M. Galectins and microenvironmental niches during hematopoiesis. *Curr. Opin. Hematol.* **2012**, *18*, 443–451.
56. Sackstein, R. The biology of CD44 and HCELL in hematopoiesis: The 'step 2-bypass pathway' and other emerging perspectives. *Curr. Opin. Hematol.* **2011**, *18*, 239–248.
57. Winkler, I. G. Adhesion to E-selectin promotes growth inhibition and apoptosis of human and murine hematopoietic progenitor cells independent of PSGL-1. *Blood* **2004**, *103*, 1685–1692.
58. Butler, M. O.; et al. A panel of human cell-based artificial APC enables the expansion of long-lived antigen-specific CD4+ T cells restricted by prevalent HLA-DR alleles. *Int. Immunol.* **2010**, *22*, 863–873.

59. Butler, M. O.; et al. Establishment of antitumor memory in humans using in vitro-educated CD8+ T cells. *Sci. Transl. Med.* **2011**, *3*, 80ra34.
60. Butler, M. O.; et al. Long-lived antitumor CD8+ lymphocytes for adoptive therapy generated using an artificial antigen-presenting cell. *Clin. Cancer Res.* **2007**, *13*, 1857–1867.
61. Jin, H. T.; et al. Cooperation of Tim-3 and PD-1 in CD8 T-cell exhaustion during chronic viral infection. *Proc. Natl. Acad. Sci. U.S.A.* **2010**, *107*, 14733–14738.
62. Sharma, S.; et al. T cell immunoglobulin and mucin protein-3 (Tim-3)/ Galectin-9 interaction regulates influenza A virus-specific humoral and CD8 T-cell responses. *Proc. Natl. Acad. Sci. U.S.A.* **2011**, *108*, 19001–19006.
63. Jiang, X.; et al. Skin infection generates non-migratory memory CD8+ T(RM) cells providing global skin immunity. *Nature* **2012**, *483*, 227–231.
64. Kupper, T. S. Old and new: Recent innovations in vaccine biology and skin T cells. *J. Invest. Dermatol.* **2012**, *132*, 829–834.

Chapter 8

Post-Translational Modification of Galectin-3 and Its Role in Biological Function

James C. Byrd, Nachman Mazurek, and Robert S. Bresalier*

Department of Gastrointestinal Medicine and Nutrition,
The University of Texas MD Anderson Cancer Center,
1515 Holcombe Blvd., Houston, Texas 77030
***E-mail: rbresali@mdanderson.org**

The chimeric lectin galectin-3 is subject to structural modifications, primarily in its non-lectin domains, by phosphorylation and proteolysis. These modifications in galectin-3 structure have the potential to alter important biologic functions of intracellular and extracellular galectin-3. We have studied the effect of galectin-3 on the susceptibility of breast and colon cancer cells to death receptor-mediated apoptosis induced by TRAIL. Phosphorylation of intracellular galectin-3 can shift ligand binding from a lectin-carbohydrate to a protein-protein mode, with diverse cellular effects. Phospho-galectin-3 leads to TRAIL sensitivity by human breast cancer cells through induction of PTEN expression. In contrast, extracellular galectin-3 can lead TRAIL resistance in colon cancer cells by inhibiting the TRAIL-dependent clustering and endocytosis of death receptors. The gene for galectin-3, LGALS3 is polymorphic in human populations, and a P64H mutation has been linked to cancer incidence, TRAIL sensitivity, and the susceptibility of the galectin-3 protein to proteolytic cleavage. It is postulated that the truncated protein, which lacks the ability to dimerize, could compete with extracellular full-length galectin-3 act as a dominant-negative inhibitor.

Structure of Galectin-3

Galectins are carbohydrate binding proteins characterized by their affinity for beta-galactosides and by conserved sequences in the carbohydrate-binding site (*1*, *2*). Galectin-3, with a monomer subunit of about 30 kDa, is the only chimeric galectin in mammals. It consists of three structural domains, an N-terminal domain essential for homodimerization, which can be phosphorylated at Ser6, a C-terminal domain containing a single carbohydrate-recognition domain (CRD), and a collagen-like sequence (residues 29-113) linking the N-terminal domain to the CRD (Figure 1).

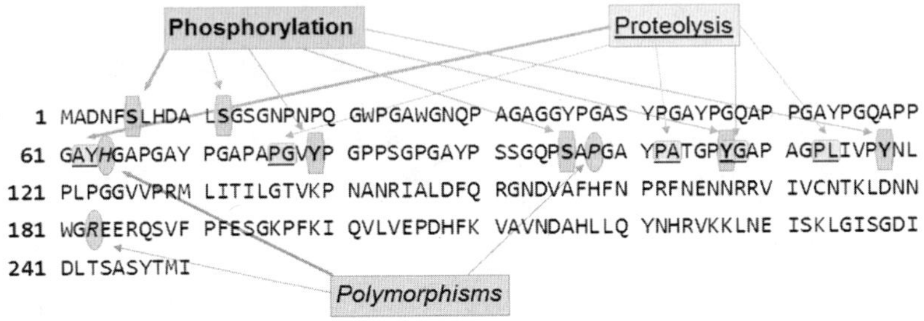

Figure 1. Structure of galectin-3. (see color insert)

Galectin-3 is subject to post-translational processing, primarily in the non-lectin domains. Phosphorylation (*3–11*) and proteolysis (*12–21*) of galectin-3 have been studied with the aim of understanding how these structural modifications affect the biological functions of galectin-3. One important function of galectin-3, particularly in breast and colon cancer, is its role in apoptosis (*8*, *10*, *11*, *22–31*). Phosphorylation of galectin-3 occurs at both serine and tyrosine residues and can have diverse functional effects. The Ser6 phosphorylation of galectin-3 of galectin-3 has been most extensively studied. Proteolysis of full-length galectin-3 can occur at several sites in the collagen-like linker domain. This removal of the N-terminal domain from galectin-3 prevents homodimerization that is necessary for multivalent ligand binding, and the resulting truncated C-terminal galectin-3 can act as an antagonist of full-length galectin-3. Polymorphism of the gene for galectin-3 (LGALS3) results in the expression of galectin-3 with His64 instead of Pro64 and Pro98 instead of Thr98 in a relatively large number of individuals (*24*, *27*, *28*, *32–35*). The relationship of these sequence changes to the phosphorylation and proteolysis of galectin-3 are incompletely understood.

Extracellular and Intracellular Functions of Galectin-3

Galectin-3 has pleiotropic biological functions and has been implicated in cell growth, differentiation, adhesion, RNA processing and malignant transformation. For example, several studies have found a positive relationship between total galectin-3 levels and colon cancer progression (*36–39*). Galectin-3 concentrations are increased in sera from colorectal cancer patients and are higher in those with metastatic disease than in patients with localized tumors (*40*, *41*). Galectin-3 is distributed in the cytoplasm and nucleus, and is present at the cell surface (*2*, *42*), but its specific role in each compartment remains to be determined.

Intracellular (Non-Lectin) Functions of Galectin-3

It is a paradox that the defining characteristic of galectins, carbohydrate binding, is not the basis for some of the most important intracellular functions of galectin-3. Rather, protein-protein interactions are important for many of its intracellular functions. Intracellular ligands for galectin-3 include Bcl-2, synexin, beta-catenin, Sufu , K-Ras, Gemin4, and the transcription factors TTF-1 and TFII-I (*42*). Nuclear galectin-3 participates in mRNA splicing and in regulation of gene transcription. A number of studies have shown that galectin-3 influences gene expression, though few have shown direct interaction on transcription factors (*22*, *43*). Studies from our lab have shown that galectin-3 modulates MUC2 mucin expression in human colon cancer cells at the level of transcription via AP-1 activation (*44*). Galectin-3 transactivates AP-1 by direct interaction with c-Jun and Fra-1, forming a complex at the AP-1 site on the MUC2 promoter. It is not known how the intracellular, non-lectin, functions of galectin-3 are affected by the post-translational processing of galectin-3, but the N-terminal of galectin-3 is essential for some of its protein-protein interactions, such as binding to Bcl-2 and synexin to regulate intrinsic apoptosis (*14*).

Extracellular Functions of Galectin-3

The best-characterized function of secreted galectin-3 is binding to extracellular glycoproteins. Studies from this laboratory have shown that galectin-3 binds to colon cancer mucin (*7*, *45*). Galectin-3 has also been shown to bind LAMP-1 and -2, CEA, Mac-2 binding protein, and laminin (*2*). Other biologically relevant ligands for galectin-3 include DMBT1, IgE, high-affinity IgE receptor, CD32, and cubulin (*2*), and a 40 kDa circulating protein that is an aberrantly glycosylated form of haptoglobin produced by colon cancer cells (*41*).

Extracellular galectin-3 also influences cell/cell and cell/substratum adhesion, invasion and angiogenesis. Galectin-glycan lattices may control the dialog between tumor and tumor-associated stromal and immune cells (*46*). Circulating multimeric soluble galectin-3 induces homotypic aggregation, immune evasion, and enhanced survival, and also promotes homing of blood-borne cells to secondary sites (*47*). Secreted galectin-3 from tumor stromal cells and/or cancer-initiating cells also exhibits immunosuppressive properties and modulates cytokine release (*48*, *49*).

Galectin-3 has been shown to interact with several cell surface glycoprotein receptors. Among these are the binding to beta-integrins (*31*, *50*) and the binding to EGFR/MUC1 complexes (*51*). It has been proposed that multivalent galectin-3 acts as a scaffolding molecule by simultaneously binding glycan ligands on multiple glycoproteins on the cell surface such as growth factor receptors and ECM proteins (*52–55*). Alternatively, it can bind and segregate the same receptors into different membrane domains (*12*).

Phosphorylation of Galectin-3

Early studies of galectin-3 in a variety of cancers focused on it binding to carbohydrates containing the N-acetyl-lactosamine moiety. However, intracellular galectin-3 is subject to phosphorylation, which can modulate its non-lectin functions (Figure 2).

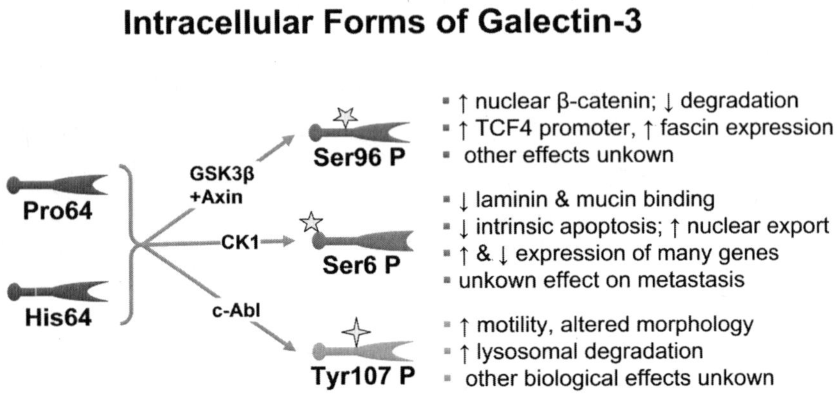

Figure 2. Phosphorlylation of intracellular galectin-3. Note that it is not known whether the P64H or the T98P mutations affect phosphorylation. (see color insert)

Ser6 Phosphorylation of Galectin-3

The casein kinase 1-dependent phosphorylation of serine 6 in the amino-terminal domain of galectin-3 blocks binding of carbohydrates by the C-terminal carbohydrate recognition domain (*7*), while phosphorylation of galectin-3 is necessary for several non-carbohydrate-dependent functions, including its anti-apoptotic activity, its export from the nucleus, and the up-regulation of several genes. This suggests that phosphorylation serves as a switch-board that shifts galectin-3 ligand binding from a lectin-carbohydrate to a protein-protein mode.

Ser96 Phosphorylation

Galectin-3 has been shown to participate in the Wnt signaling pathway by increasing the levels of nuclear beta-catenin and decreasing beta-catenin degradation (*56*). This requires interaction with GSK3beta, and may involve phosphorylation of galectin-3 at residue Ser96 (*57*). In gastric cancer cells, Ser96 phosphorylation of galectin-3 increases TCF4 promoter activity and leads to increased expression of genes, including cyclin D1 and fascin (*22*, *43*).

Tyrosine Phosphorylation

In addition to serine phosphorylation, tyrosine phosphorylation at residue Y107 , Y79 or Y118 has been shown to occur in breast cancer cells, mediated by c-Abl kinase (*3*, *6*). Interference with Y107 phosphorylation alters cell morphology and decreases cell motility (*3*). Also, tyrosine phosphorylation by c-Abl is involved in the lysosomal degradation of galectin-3 (*6*).

Anti-Apoptotic and Pro-Apoptotic Activities of Intracellular Phospho-Galectin-3

Galectins play a significant role in apoptosis and other cellular processes. In particular, galectin-3 may exert anti- or pro-apoptotic activity depending on the cell type and the nature of the stimulus. Cytoplasmic galectin-3 generally functions to decrease intrinsic (mitochondria independent) apoptosis. For example, overexpression of galectin-3 in breast carcinoma renders them resistant to chemotherapeutic drugs (*58*, *59*). The mechanisms by which galectin-3 regulates intrinsic apoptosis are not fully understood. A portion of its anti-apoptotic activity may be attributed to the anti-death motif that is conserved in the Bcl-2 family (*59*). Like Bcl-2, phosphorylation controls the anti-apoptotic function of galectin-3 (*11*). Galectin-3 undergoes phosphorylation at Ser-6 by casein kinase1 (*5*, *7*) and in response to an apoptotic insult phospho-galectin-3 is exported from the nucleus to the cytoplasm, where it maintains mitochondrial homeostasis and blocks cytochrome c release (*10*).

In different cell types, galectin-3 can either increase or decrease extrinsic apoptosis mediated by death receptors. TRAIL, a member of the tumor necrosis factor family, transmits death signals through death domain-containing receptors (*8*). Because TRAIL selectively induces apoptosis in a variety of transformed cells, but not in most normal cells, this pathway is being investigated as a target for therapies, including phase 1 clinical trials of recombinant soluble TRAIL, anti-DR4 antibody, anti-DR5 antibody (*60*). In addition to its direct apoptosis-inducing effect, TRAIL also plays an important role in immune surveillance against tumor initiation, development, and metastasis, suggesting a potential application to cancer therapy (*61–64*). Resistance to TRAIL mediated apoptosis in cancer cells may, however, limit the successes of TRAIL therapy.

We recently found that phospho-galectin-3 plays a pivotal role in the acquisition of TRAIL sensitivity by human breast carcinoma cells (*8*). We identified a TRAIL-induced nonclassical caspase activation cascade mediated by P-Gal3 through induction of PTEN expression and inactivation of the PI3K/Akt survival pathway. The persistent cell death observed in BT549 transfectants expressing P-Gal3 independently of the mitochondria suggests the existence of alternative apoptotic pathways that can bypass the apoptosome and induce apoptotic death. Our results suggest that P-Gal3 regulates PTEN expression at the post-transcriptional level; a finding further supported by the demonstration of coordinate expression of Gal3 and PTEN in both breast cancer cell lines and in a subset of human breast cancer specimens. These findings (*8*) could provide a basis for innovative targeted therapeutic strategies for the activation of PTEN in breast cancer and afford insight into the cellular mechanisms of sensitivity and resistance to apoptosis in cancer cells.

Anti-Apoptotic Activity of Extracellular Galectin-3

Recent results from this lab (*26*) have shown that extracellular galectin-3 can hinder the TRAIL-dependent clustering and endocytosis of DR4 and DR5 death receptors, leading to TRAIL resistance in colon cancer cells (Figure 3). Exposure of LS-LiM6 colon cancer cells to TRAIL results in apoptosis which plateaus at 65% cell death. Residual cells were propagated to yield a TRAIL-resistant cell line, LiM6-TR. Components of apoptotic pathways downstream of caspase-8 activation were similar in LiM6 and LiM6-TR, but TRAIL failed to activate caspase-8 in LiM6-TR, suggesting that DISC formation is deficient. Total protein levels of constituents of the DISC, including DR4, DR5, FADD, FLICE and caspase-8, were not different in LiM6-TR compared to LiM6. However, levels of cell-surface galectin-3 were much higher in LiM6-TR than in LiM6. Internalization of death receptor in LS-LiM6 was blocked in LiM6-TR, but restored by knockdown of galectin-3. Inhibitors of glycosylation sensitized LiM6-TR to TRAIL-dependent apoptosis. These results indicate that galectin-3 binds to the oligosaccharides of DR4 and/or DR5, thus inhibiting the trafficking of death receptors and activation of caspase-8. These results are in contrast to the pro-apoptotic activity of intracellular phospho-galectin-3 leading to TRAIL sensitivity in breast cancer cells, but it is not established to what extent these two results reflect cell type differences or opposing effects of cell-surface vs. intracellular galectin-3.

This anti-apoptotic activity of extracellular galectin-3 represents a novel TRAIL-resistance mechanism in which full-length galectin-3 but not truncated galectin-3 impedes trafficking of death receptors by anchoring them in glycan nanoclusters, blocking the execution of the apoptosis signal. Elevated levels of cell-surface galectin-3 may predict unfavorable outcome to TRAIL-based therapy of colon cancer patients, and small molecule inhibitors of galectin-3 binding could overcome TRAIL resistance. This mechanism affords the prospect of restoration of TRAIL sensitivity, by: (i) decreasing the levels of cell surface galectin-3, (ii) decreasing the extent of glycosylation of death receptors, (iii) removal of the N-terminal domain of galectin-3, or (iv) inhibition of galectin-3/death receptor binding by secreted glycoproteins, oligosaccharides, or small molecule glycomimetics.

Polymorphism of Galectin-3

The gene for galectin-3, LGALS3 is polymorphic in human populations. Three common single nucleotide polymorphisms (snp's) have been identified in the coding region of the galectin-3 gene (Table 1): rs4644 (substituting Cytidine 342 with Adenosine, which changes Proline 64 to Histidine); rs4652 (substituting Adenosine 443 with Cytidine, which changes Threonine 98 to Proline); and rs10148371 (substituting Guanosine 699 with Adenosine, which changes Arginine 183 to Lysine) (*34*, *35*). Of these three snp's, only rs4644 is reported to have functional significance (*27*, *32*).

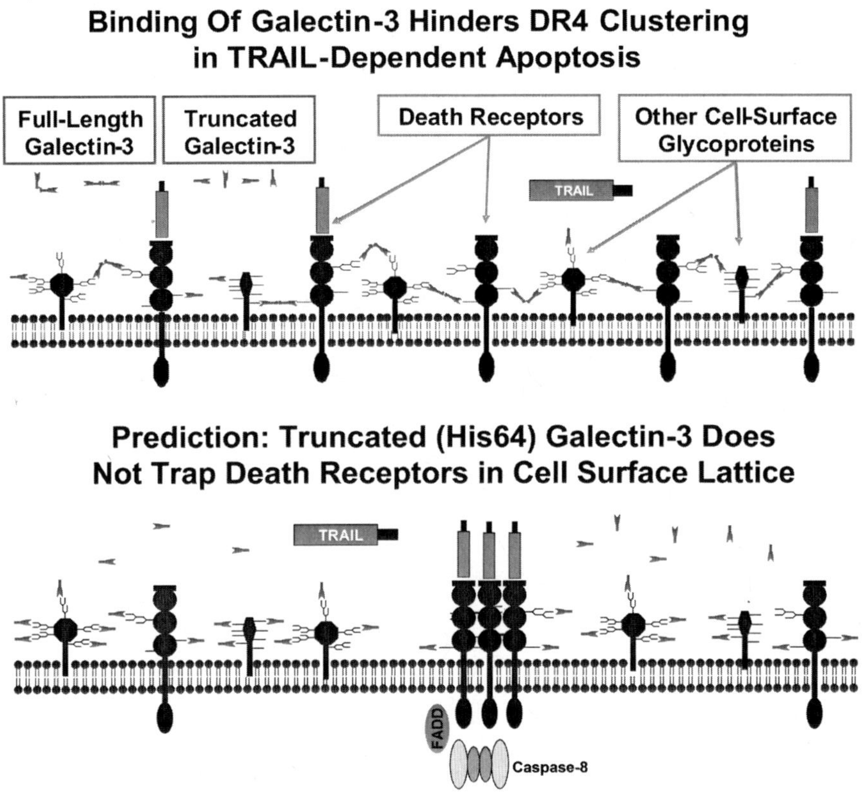

Figure 3. Cell surface galectin-3 confers resistance to TRAIL by impeding trafficking of DR4 death receptors. This model predicts that monovalent truncated galectin-3, resulting from MMP cleavage of His64 galectin-3, would allow TRAIL sensitivity. (see color insert)

Table 1. Coding single nucleotide polymorphisms in LGALS3. (source: dbSNP)

snp ID	*nt change*	*AA change*	*Heterozygosity*	*European*	*Asian*	*African*
rs4644	c.342C>A	P64H	0.414	51% A	18% A	27% A
rs4652	c.443A>C	T98P	0.483	48% C	42% C	82% C
rs10148371	c.699G>A	R183K	0.089	0% A	0% A	12% A

The allele frequency of this polymorphism shows considerable racial variation, with Pro64 galectin-3 much more prevalent in African and Asian populations than in European populations (49% P64, 51% H64). This is intriguing, since African-Americans have higher colon cancer incidence and mortality rates than non-Hispanic whites (*65*). It is not yet known whether expression of His64 galectin-3 is related to colon cancer incidence and progression. In a pilot study (*24*), we examined LGALS3 genotype in eight available cells lines. The preliminary analyses of the genotypes of eight available established colon cancer cell lines revealed a disproportionately high prevalence of homozygotic Pro64 (Caco-2, HCT116, RKO, SW480, LM12, and HT29 cells), and a paucity of cell lines heterozygotic (RSB-1) or homozygotic (KM12) for His64 galectin-3. This suggestive finding (*24*) supports the notion that the P64H mutation could be related to colorectal cancer incidence.

Genotype distribution of rs4644 in Caucasian and Asian populations showed an occurrence of the His64/His64 genotype was significantly higher in breast cancer patients than in controls, indicating that the presence of His64 galectin-3, which is MMP-2/-9 cleavable, could be related to an increased breast cancer incidence and progression (*32*). The His64 galectin-3 has also been reported to be related prostate cancer incidence (*28*), and to predisposition toward rheumatoid arthritis (*33*).

In a recent study, we found that the His64 confers TRAIL sensitivity to breast cancer cells (*27*). When a collection of 9 breast cancer cell lines that express galectin-3 was examined for LGALS3 genotype and sensitivity to TRAIL, 0/5 cell lines that were homozygous for Pro64 galectin-3 were TRAIL sensitive, but 2/2 homozygous His64 cell lines and 1/2 heterozygous cell lines were sensitive to TRAIL. Forced expression of His64 galectin-3 rendered BT549 cells sensitive to TRAIL, but cells expressing Pro64 galectin-3 remained TRAIL-resistant. These results indicate that the naturally occurring P64H mutation in galectin-3 increases sensitivity to death receptor-mediated apoptosis. The conclusion could be relevant to disparities in breast cancer outcomes across population groups, and could guide design of future clinical trials of TRAIL-based therapies.

Proteolysis of Galectin-3

The association of His64 galectin-3 with disease incidence and TRAIL sensitivity may be related to sequence-dependent proteolytic cleavage. The gene product of the functional germline mutation (rs4644) substituting proline with histidine (H64 allele) is susceptible to matrix metalloprotease cleavage which may produce a truncated protein (21 kDa, Gal3C), lacking the ability to homodimerize and thus the potential to act as a cross-linker. Indeed, it was reported that purified recombinant galectin-3 bearing the H64 but not the P64 is cleaved by purified MMP-2 or -9 to produce a 21 kDa truncated protein (*18*). Furthermore, the 21 kDa truncated protein could be detected in both total lysates and conditioned media of the galectin-3-null human breast carcinoma cells (Bt-549) expressing the H64 protein but not the P64 variant (*32*).

Truncation of Galectin-3 by Proteolysis

Extracellular galectin-3 is subject to cleavage by matrix metalloproteinases (MMPs) to produce a truncated protein that retains carbohydrate-binding activity, but loses the ability to oligomerize. Specific sites of proteolysis that have been identified (Figure 1) include Ala62-Tyr63 (MMP2, MMP7, MMP9, MMP13, and MT1-MMP), with additional minor sites of cleavage at Gly32-Ala33 (MMP2), at Pro92-Ser93 and Pro102-Ala103 (MMP13), and at Pro76-Gly77 and Pro113-Leu114 (MMP7) (*20*). Prostate specific antigen (*21*) cleaves galectin-3 at a unique site, Tyr107-Gly108. Phosphorylation of Tyr107 inhibits this cleavage (*4*). Susceptibility of galectin-3 to enzymatic cleavage at Ala62-Tyr63 depends on substituting amino acid Pro64 with His64 (*13*, *18*). The resulting 21 kDa truncated protein can be detected in lysates and media of BT549 human breast cancer cells expressing the H64 protein but not the P64 form (*16*, *32*). Collagenase cleavage of galectin-3 at Pro113-Leu114 provides a readily available, albeit non-physiological, truncated galectin-3, Gal-3C (*19*).

Biological Consequences of Proteolytic Cleavage

Oligomeric galectin-3 modulates functions critical to the development and maintenance of the tumor phenotype, including cell adhesion, migration, invasion, angiogenesis, immune function, and apoptosis (*19*, *66–68*). It is postulated that the truncated protein, which lacks the ability to dimerize, competes with extracellular full-length galectin-3 and inhibits crosslinking, acting as a dominant-negative inhibitor (Figure 3). Gal-3C has been shown to inhibit tumor growth, angiogenesis, and metastasis, and has the potential to modulate immunoadjuvant therapy that targets EGFR, VEGF, or death receptors (*15*, *17*, *23*). While carbohydrate-specific galectin-3 inhibitors are being tested in clinical trials as potential cancer therapies, truncated galectin-3 also has therapeutic potential.

Significance of the Post-Translational Modification of Galectin-3 in Its Biological Function

The modifications in galectin-3 structure resulting from phosphorylation, proteolysis and polymorphism have the potential to alter important biologic functions of galectin-3, including modulation of the susceptibility of breast and colon cancer cells to death receptor-mediated apoptosis. Understanding these modifications could help to develop new diagnostic, prognostic, and therapeutic approaches to a number of diseases. For example, immunohistochemical detection for phospho-galectin-3 might be more cancer-specific than staining for total galectin-3. Similarly, proteolytically truncated galectin-3, besides being a competitive inhibitor, might also serving a diagnostic marker, since its production requires expression of full-length galectin-3 and matrix metalloproteases, both of which are cancer-associated.

References

1. Cooper, D. N. W. Galectinomics: Finding themes in complexity. *Biochim. Biophys. Acta* **2002**, *1572*, 209–231.
2. Byrd, J. C.; Bresalier, R. S. Galectin-3 in the Progression and Metastasis of Colorectal Neoplasia. In *Galectins*; Klyosov, A. A., Witzak, Z. J., Platt, D., Eds.; John Wiley and Sons: Newark, NJ, 2009; pp 221–232.
3. Balan, V.; Nangia-Makker, P.; Jung, Y. S.; Wang, Y.; Raz, A. Galectin-3: A novel substrate for c-Abl kinase. *Biochim. Biophys. Acta* **2010**, *1803*, 1198–1205.
4. Balan, V.; Nangia-Makker, P.; Kho, D. H.; Wang, Y.; Raz, A. Tyrosine-phosphorylated galectin-3 protein is resistant to prostate-specific antigen (PSA) cleavage. *J. Biol. Chem.* **2012**, *287*, 5192–5198.
5. Huflejt, M. E.; Turck, C. W.; Lindstedt, R.; Barondes, S. H.; Leffler, H. L-29, a soluble lactose-binding lectin, is phosphorylated on serine 6 and serine 12 in vivo and by casein kinase I. *J. Biol. Chem.* **1993**, *268*, 26712–26718.
6. Li, X.; Ma, Q.; Wang, J.; Liu, X.; Yang, Y.; Zhao, H.; Wang, Y.; Jin, Y.; Zeng, J.; Li, J.; Song, L.; Li, X.; Li, P.; Qian, X.; Cao, C. c-Abl and Arg tyrosine kinases regulate lysosomal degradation of the oncoprotein galectin-3. *Cell Death Differ.* **2010**, *17*, 1277–1287.
7. Mazurek, N.; Conklin, J; Byrd, J. C.; Raz, A.; Bresalier, R. S. Phosphorylation of the beta-galactoside-binding protein galectin-3 modulates binding to its ligands. *J. Biol. Chem.* **2000**, *275*, 36311–36315.
8. Mazurek, N.; Sun, Y. J.; Liu, K. F.; Gilcrease, M. Z.; Schober, W.; Nangia-Makker, P.; Raz, A.; Bresalier, R. S. Phosphorylated galectin-3 mediates tumor necrosis factor-related apoptosis-inducing ligand signaling by regulating phosphatase and tensin homologue deleted on chromosome 10 in human breast carcinoma cells. *J. Biol. Chem.* **2007**, *282*, 21337–21348.
9. Mazurek, N.; Sun, Y. J.; Price, J.; Ramdas, L.; Schoher, W.; Nangia-Makker, P.; Raz, A.; Bresalier, R. S. Phosphorylation of galectin-3 contributes to malignant transformation of human epithelial cells via modulation of unique sets of genes. *Cancer Res.* **2005**, *65*, 10767–10775.
10. Takenaka, Y.; Fukumori, T.; Yoshii, T.; Oka, N.; Hidenori, I.; Kim, H.-R.; Bresalier, R. S.; Raz, A. Phosphorylation of the N-terminal domain of galectin-3 regulates its cellular localization and anti-apoptotic function in response to chemotherapeutic drugs. *Mol. Cell. Biol.* **2004**, *24*, 4395–4406.
11. Yoshi, T.; Fukumori, T.; Honjo, Y.; Inohara, H.; Kim, H. R. C.; Raz, A Galectin-3 phosphorylation is required for its anti-apoptotic function and cell cycle arrest. *J. Biol. Chem.* **2002**, *277*, 6852–6857.
12. Earl, L. A.; Bi, S.; Baum, L. G. Galectin multimerization and lattice formation is regulated by linker region structure. *Glycobiology* **2011**, *21*, 6–12.
13. Fry, S. A.; Van den Steen, P. E.; Royle, L.; Wormald, M. R.; Leathem, A. J.; Opdenakker, G.; McDonnell, J. M.; Dwek, R. A.; Rudd, P. M. Cancer-associated glycoforms of gelatinase B exhibit a decreased level of binding to galectin-3. *Biochemistry* **2006**, *45*, 15249–15258.

14. Gong, H. C.; Honjo, Y.; Nangia-Makker, P.; Hogan, V.; Mazurek, N.; Bresalier, R. S.; Raz, A. The NH2 terminus of galectin-3 governs cellular compartmentalization and functions in cancer cells. *Cancer Res.* **1999**, *59*, 6239–6245.
15. John, C. M.; Leffler, H.; Kahl-Knuttsson, B.; Svensson, I.; Jarvis, G. A. Truncated galectin-3 inhibits tumor growth and metastasis in orthotopic nude mouse model of human breast cancer. *Clin. Cancer Res.* **2003**, *9*, 2374–2383.
16. Nangia-Makker, P.; Raz, T.; Tait, L.; Hogan, V.; Fridman, R.; Raz, A. Galectin-3 cleavage: A novel surrogate marker for matrix metalloproteinase activity in growing breast cancers. *Cancer Res.* **2007**, *67*, 11760–11768.
17. Nangia-Makker, P.; Wang, Y.; Raz, T.; Tait, L.; Balan, V.; Hogan, V.; Raz, A. Cleavage of galectin-3 by matrix metalloproteases induces angiogenesis in breast cancer. *Int. J. Cancer* **2010**, *127*, 2530–2541.
18. Ochieng, J.; Fridman, R.; Nangia-Makker, P.; Kleiner, D. E.; Liotta, L. A.; Stetler-Stevenson, W. G.; Raz, A. Galectin-3 is a novel substrate for human matrix metalloproteinases-2 and -9. *Biochemistry* **1994**, *33*, 14109–14114.
19. Ochieng, J.; Green, B.; Evans, S.; James, O.; Warfield, P. Modulation of the biological functions of galectin-3 by matrix metalloproteinases. *Biochim. Biophys. Acta* **1998**, *1379*, 97–106.
20. Puthenedam, M.; Wu, F.; Shetye, A.; Michaels, A.; Rhee, K. J.; Kwon, J. H. Matrilysin-1 (MMP7) cleaves galectin-3 and inhibits wound healing in intestinal epithelial cells. *Inflammatory Bowel Dis.* **2011**, *17*, 260–267.
21. Saraswati, S.; Block, A. S.; Davidson, M. K.; Rank, R. G.; Mahadevan, M.; Diekman, A. B. Galectin-3 is a substrate for prostate specific antigen (PSA) in human seminal plasma. *Prostate* **2011**, *71*, 197–208.
22. Cheong, T. C.; Shin, J. Y.; Chun, K. H. Silencing of galectin-3 changes the gene expression and augments the sensitivity of gastric cancer cells to chemotherapeutic agents. *Cancer Sci.* **2010**, *101*, 94–102.
23. Hoyer, K. K.; Pang, M.; Gui, D.; Shintaku, I. P.; Kuwabara, I.; Liu, F. T.; Said, J. W.; Baum, L. G.; Teitell, M. A. An anti-apoptotic role for galectin-3 in diffuse large B-cell lymphomas. *Am. J. Pathol.* **2004**, *164*, 893–902.
24. Mazurek, N.; Byrd, J. C.; Sun, Y. J.; Bresalier, R. S. Galectin-3 sequence polymorphisms dictate TRAIL sensativity or resistance of human breast and colon cancer cells. *Proc. Am. Assoc. Cancer Res.* **2009**, *50*, 27.
25. Mazurek, N.; Byrd, J. C.; Sun, Y. J.; Bresalier, R. S. Nuclear galectin-3 confers tumor necrosis factor-related apoptosis-inducing ligand (TRAIL) resistance to colon cancer cells by inhibiting caspase-8 activation. *Gastroenterology* **2009**, *136* (Suppl 1), A756.
26. Mazurek, N.; Byrd, J. C.; Sun, Y.; Hafley, M.; Ramirez, K.; Burks, J.; Bresalier, R. S. Cell-surface galectin-3 confers resistance to TRAIL by impeding trafficking of death receptors in metastatic colon adenocarcinoma cells. *Cell Death Differ.* **2012**, *19*, 523–533.
27. Mazurek, N.; Byrd, J. C.; Sun, Y.; Ueno, S.; Bresalier, R. S. A galectin-3 sequence polymorphism confers TRAIL sensitivity to human breast cancer cells. *Cancer* **2011**, *117*, 4375–4380.

28. Meyer, A.; Coinac, I.; Bogdanova, N.; Dubrowinskaja, N.; Turmanov, N.; Haubold, S.; Schürmann, P.; Imkamp, F.; von Klot, C.; Merseburger, A. S.; Machtens, S.; Bremer, M.; Hillemanns, P.; Kuczyk, M. A.; Karstens, J. H.; Serth, J.; Dörk, T. Apoptosis gene polymorphisms and risk of prostate cancer: A hospital-based study of German patients treated with brachytherapy. *Urol Oncol* **2011**, [Epub ahead of print] PMID:21396839.
29. Oka, N.; Nakahara, S.; Takenaka, Y.; Fukumori, T.; Hogan, V.; Kanayama, H. O.; Yanagawa, T.; Raz, A. Galectin-3 inhibits tumor necrosis factor-related apoptosis-inducing ligand-induced apoptosis by activating Akt in human bladder carcinoma cells. *Cancer Res.* **2005**, *65*, 7546–7553.
30. Yu, F.; Finley, R. L., Jr; Raz, A.; Kim, H. R. Galectin-3 translocates to the perinuclear membranes and inhibits cytochrome c release from the mitochondria. A role for synexin in galectin-3 translocation. *J. Biol. Chem.* **2002**, *277*, 15819–15827.
31. Zhuo, Y.; Chammas, R.; Bellis, S. L. Sialylation of beta1 integrins blocks cell adhesion to galectin-3 and protects cells against galectin-3-induced apoptosis. *J. Biol. Chem.* **2008**, *283*, 22177–22185.
32. Balan, V.; Nangia-Makker, P.; Schwartz, A. G.; Jung, Y. S.; Tait, L.; Hogan, V.; Raz, T.; Wang, Y.; Yang, Z. Q.; Wu, G. S.; Guo, Y.; Li, H.; Abrams, J.; Couch, F. J.; Lingle, W. L.; Lloyd, R. V.; Ethier, S. P.; Tainsky, M. A.; Raz, A. Racial disparity in breast cancer and functional germ line mutation in galectin-3 (rs4644): A pilot study. *Cancer Res.* **2008**, *68*, 10045–10050.
33. Hu, C. Y.; Chang, S. K.; Wu, C. S.; Tsai, W. I.; Hsu, P. N. Galectin-3 gene (LGALS3) +292C allele is a genetic predisposition factor for rheumatoid arthritis in Taiwan. *Clin. Rheumatol.* **2011**, *30*, 1227–1233.
34. Martins, L.; Leoni, S.; Friguglietti, C.; Ward, L.; Kulcsar, M.; Kimura, E. Polymorphism on codon 98 of the galectin-3 gene are not associated to benign and malignant thyroid tumors. *Arq. Bras. Endocrinol. Metab.* **2006**, *50*, 1075–1081.
35. Poirier, O.; Nicaud, V.; Vionnet, N.; Raoux, S.; Tarnow, L.; Vlassara, H.; Parving, H.; Cambien, F. Polymorphism screening of four genes encoding advanced glycation end-product putative receptors association study with nephropathy in type 1 diabetic patients. *Diabetes* **2001**, *50*, 1214–1218.
36. Schoeppner, H. L.; Raz, A.; Ho, S. B.; Bresalier, R. S. Expression of an endogenous galactose-binding lectin correlates with neoplastic progression in the colon. *Cancer* **1995**, *75*, 2818–2826.
37. Irimura, T.; Matsushita, Y.; Sutton, R. C.; Carralero, D.; Ohannesian, D. W.; Cleary, K. R.; Ota, D. M.; Nicolson, G. L.; Lotan, R. Increased content of an endogenous lactose-binding lectin in human colorectal carcinoma progressed to metastatic stages. *Cancer Res.* **1991**, *51*, 387–393.
38. Hittelet, A.; Legendre, H.; Nagy, N.; Bronckart, Y.; Pector, J. C.; Salmon, I.; Yeaton, P.; Gabius, H. J.; Kiss, R.; Camby, I. Upregulation of galectins-1 and -3 in human colon cancer and their role in regulating cell migration. *Int. J. Cancer* **2003**, *103*, 370–379.
39. Inufusa, H.; Nakamura, M.; Adachi, T.; Aga, M.; Kurimoto, M.; Nakatani, Y.; Wakano, T.; Miyake, M.; Okuno, K.; Shiozaki, H.; Yasutomi, M. Role of

galectin-3 in adenocarcinoma liver metastasis. *Int. J. Oncol.* **2001**, *19*, 913–919.

40. Iurisci, I.; Tinari, N.; Natoli, C.; Angelucci, D.; Cianchetti, E.; Iacobelli, S. Concentration of galectin-3 in the sera of normal controls and cancer patients. *Clin. Cancer Res.* **2000**, *6*, 1389–1393.
41. Bresalier, R. S.; Byrd, J. C.; Tessler, D.; Lebel, J.; Koomen, J.; Hawke, D.; Half, E.; Liu, K. F.; Mazurek, N.; Mazurek, N. A circulating ligand for galectin-3 is a haptoglobin-related glycoprotein elevated in individuals with colon cancer. *Gastroenterology* **2004**, *127*, 741–748.
42. Hausdek, K. C.; Spronnk, K. J.; Voss, P. G.; Patterson, R. J.; Wang, J. L.; Arnoys, E. J. Dynamics ofgalectin-3 in the nucleus and cytoplasm. *Biochim. Biophys. Acta* **2010**, *1800*, 181–189.
43. Kim, S. J.; Choi, I. J.; Cheong, T. C.; Lee, S. J.; Lotan, R.; Park, S. H.; Chun, K. H. Galectin-3 increases gastric cancer cell motility by up-regulating fascin-1 expression. *Gastroenterology* **2010**, *138*, 1035–1045.
44. Song, S.; Byrd, J. C.; Mazurek, N.; Liu, K.; Koo, J. S.; Bresalier, R. S. Galectin-3 modulates MUC2 mucin expression in human colon cancer cells at the level of transcription via AP-1 activation. *Gastroenterology* **2005**, *129*, 1581–1591.
45. Bresalier, R. S.; Byrd, J. C.; Wang, L.; Raz, A. Colon cancer mucin: A new ligand for the beta-galactoside binding protein galectin-3. *Cancer Res.* **1996**, *56*, 4354–4357.
46. Thiemann, S.; Baum, L. G. The road less traveled: Regulation of leukocyte migration across vascular and lymphatic endothelium by galectins. *J. Clin. Immunol.* **2011**, *3*, 2–9.
47. Nangia-Makker, P.; Balan, V.; Raz, A Regulation of tumor progression by extracellular galectin-3. *Cancer Microenviron.* **2008**, *1*, 43–51.
48. Wei, J.; Barr, J.; Kong, L. Y.; Wang, Y.; Wu, A.; Sharma, A. K.; Gumin, J.; Henry, V.; Colman, H.; Sawaya, R.; Lang, F. F.; Heimberger, A. B. Glioma-associated cancer-initiating cells induce immunosuppression. *Clin. Cancer Res.* **2010**, *16*, 461–473.
49. Filer, A.; Bik, M.; Parsonage, G. N.; Fitton, J.; Trebilcock, E.; Howlett, K.; Cook, M.; Raza, K.; Simmons, D. L.; Thomas, A. M.; Salmon, M.; Scheel-Toellner, D.; Lord, J. M.; Rabinovich, G. A.; Buckley, C. D. Galectin 3 induces a distinctive pattern of cytokine and chemokine production in rheumatoid synovial fibroblasts via selective signaling pathways. *Arthritis Rheum.* **2009**, *60*, 1604–1614.
50. Al-Awqati, Q Terminal differentiation in epithelia: The role of integrins in hensin polymerization. *Annu. Rev. Physiol.* **2011**, *73*, 401–412.
51. Merlin, J.; Stechly, L.; de Beaucé, S.; Monté, D.; Leteurtre, E.; van Seuningen, I.; Huet, G.; Pigny, P. Galectin-3 regulates MUC1 and EGFR cellular distribution and EGFR downstream pathways in pancreatic cancer cells. *Oncogene* **2011**, *30*, 2514–2525.
52. Markowska, A. I.; Liu, F. T.; Panjwani, N. Galectin-3 is an important mediator of VEGF- and bFGF-mediated angiogenic response. *J. Exp. Med.* **2010**, *207*, 1981–1993.

53. Guo, H. B.; Johnson, H.; Randolph, M.; Lee, I.; Pierce, M. Knockdown of GnT-Va expression inhibits ligand-induced downregulation of the epidermal growth factor receptor and intracellular signaling by inhibiting receptor endocytosis. *Glycobiology* **2009**, *19*, 547–559.
54. Shalom-Feuerstein, R.; Plowman, S. J.; Rotblat, B.; Ariotti, N.; Tian, T.; Hancock, J. F.; Kloog, Y. K-ras nanoclustering is subverted by overexpression of the scaffold protein galectin-3. *Cancer Res.* **2008**, *68*, 6608–6616.
55. Dermotte, N.; Wieers, G.; Van Der Smissen, P.; Moser, M.; Schmidt, C.; Thielemans, K.; Squifflet, J. L.; Weynand, B.; Carrasco, J.; Lurquin, C.; Courtoy, P. J.; van der Bruggen, P. A galectin-3 ligand corrects the impaired function of human CD4 and CD8 tumor-infiltrating lymphocytes and favors tumor rejection in mice. *Cancer Res.* **2010**, *70*, 7476–7488.
56. Song, S.; Mazurek, N.; Liu, C.; Sun, Y.; Ding, Q. Q.; Liu, K.; Hung, M. C.; Bresalier, R. S. Galectin-3 mediates nuclear beta-catenin accumulation and Wnt signaling in human colon cancer cells by regulation of glycogen synthase kinase-3beta activity. *Cancer Res.* **2009**, *69*, 1343–1349.
57. Shimura, T; Takenaka, Y.; Fukumori, T.; Tsutsumi, S.; Okada, K.; Hogan, V.; Kikuchi, A.; Kuwano, H.; Raz, A. Implication of galectin-3 in Wnt signaling. *Cancer Res.* **2005**, *65*, 3535–3537.
58. Choi, J. H.; Chun, K. H.; Raz, A.; Lotan, R. Inhibition of N-(4-hydroxyphenyl)retinamide-induced apoptosis in breast cancer cells by galectin-3. *Cancer Biol. Ther.* **2004**, *3*, 447–452.
59. Akahani, S.; Nangia-Makker, P.; Inohara, H.; Kim, H. R.; Raz, A. Galectin-3: A novel antiapoptotic molecule with a functional BH1 (NWGR) domain of Bcl-2 family. *Cancer Res.* **1997**, *57*, 5272–5276.
60. Cretney, E.; Takeda, K.; Smytha, M. J. Cancer: Novel therapeutic strategies that exploit the TNF-related apoptosis-inducing ligand (TRAIL)/TRAIL receptor pathway. *Int. J. Biochem. Cell Biol.* **2007**, *39*, 280–286.
61. Cretney, E.; Takeda, K.; Yagita, H.; Glaccum, M.; Peschon, J. J.; Smyth, M. J. Increased susceptibility to tumor initiation and metastasis in TNF-related apoptosis-inducing ligand-deficient mice. *J. Immunol.* **2002**, *168*, 1356–1361.
62. Takeda, K.; Hayakawa, Y.; Smyth, M. J.; Kayagaki, N.; Yamaguchi, N.; Kakuta, S.; Iwakura, Y.; Yagita, H.; Okumura, K. Involvement of tumor necrosis factor-related apoptosis-inducing ligand in surveillance of tumor metastasis by liver natural killer cells. *Nat. Med.* **2001**, *7*, 94–100.
63. Aza-Blanc, P.; Cooper, C. L.; Wagner, K.; Batalov, S.; Deveraux, Q. L.; Cooke, M. P. Identification of modulators of TRAIL-induced apoptosis via RNAi-based phenotypic screening. *Mol. Cell.* **2003**, *12*, 627–637.
64. Kendrick, J. E.; Estes, J. M.; Straughn, J. M.; Alvarez, R. D.; Buchsbaum, D. J. Tumor necrosis factor-related apoptosis-inducing ligand (TRAIL) and its therapeutic potential in breast and gynecologic cancers. *Gynecol. Oncol.* **2007**, *106*, 614–621.
65. Laiyemo, A. O.; Doubeni, C.; Pinsky, P. F.; Doria-Rose, V. P.; Bresalier, R.; Lamerato, L. E.; Crawford, E. D.; Kvale, P.; Fouad, M.; Hickey, T.; Riley, T.; Weissfeld, J.; Schoen, R. E.; Marcus, P. M.; Prorok, P. C.; Berg, C. D. Race

and colorectal cancer disparities: Health-care utilization vs different cancer susceptibilities. *J. Natl. Cancer Inst.* **2010**, *102*, 538–546.
66. Dhirapong, A.; Lleo, A.; Leung, P.; Gershwin, M. E.; Liu, F. T. The immunological potential of galectin-1 and -3. *Autoimmun. Rev.* **2009**, *8*, 360–363.
67. Dumic, J.; Dabelic, S.; Flögel, M. Galectin-3: An open-ended story. *Biochim. Biophys. Acta* **2006**, *1760*, 616–635.
68. Fukumori, T.; Kanayama, H. O.; Raz, A. The role of galectin-3 in cancer drug resistance. *Drug Resist. Updates* **2007**, *10*, 101–108.

Galectin Mechanisms and Therapeutic Approaches in Cancer

Chapter 9

The Role of Galectin-3 in Malignant Melanoma

Gordana Radosavljevic,[1] Ivan Jovanovic,[1] Jelena Pantic,[1] Nada Pejnovic,[1] Nebojsa Arsenijevic,[1] Daniel K. Hsu,[2] and Miodrag L. Lukic*,[1]

[1]Center for Molecular Medicine and Stem Cell Research, Faculty of Medicine Science, University of Kragujevac, Svetozara Markovica 69, 34000 Kragujevac, Serbia
[2]Department of Dermatology, School of Medicine, University of California Davis, Sacramento, California 95816, United States
***E-mail: miodrag.lukic@medf.kg.ac.rs**

Mechanisms by which Galectin-3 participate in regulation of innate and acquired immune responses include adhesion of neutrophils, chemoattraction of monocytes/macrophages and activation of mast cells and T-cell survival. We have demonstrated proinflammatory effects of Galectin-3 in several experimental models of T-cell-mediated inflammatory and autoimmune diseases. Galectin-3 is also expressed in malignant cells and is involved in tumor development and progression as well as tumor immune escape. Using Galectin-3-deficient mice and malignant melanoma model we recently showed that the expression of Galectin-3 in the host cells facilitate establishment of metastasis in the lung. Mechanisms contributing to resistance to melanoma in Galectin-3-deficient mice appear to be the lower tumor cell adhesion and modulation of immune responses. Galectin-3-deficient mice had higher serum levels of IFN-gamma and IL-17 and a decrease in the percentage and total number of regulatory $CD4^{+}Foxp3^{+}$T cells compared to wild-type mice. Protective effects of Galectin-3 deficiency on metastatic melanoma spread was dependent on NK cells and associated with an enhanced cytotoxic activity of splenic NK cells *in vitro* and increased frequency of effective cytotoxic CD27^{high}CD11b^{high} NK cells as well as immature CD27^{high}CD11b^{low}NK cells *in vivo*. Thus, target inhibition of Galectin-3 expression can prevent melanoma metastasis by decreasing tumor cell adhesion and by enhancing NK cell-mediated anti-tumor immune response.

Introduction

Galectins, a family of evolutionarily conserved carbohydrate-binding proteins, are defined by homologous carbohydrate recognition domains (CRDs) and affinity for β-galactosides (*1*, *2*). Presently, 15 mammalian galectins have been identified and classified into three distinct groups based on their structures and number of CRDs they include: proto-type, chimera type and tandem repeat type galectins (*2–4*). There are no specific receptors for individual galectins, but they bind to a set of cell surface or extracellular matrix glycoproteins that contain suitable oligosaccharides (*4*). As different members of galectin family have specific distribution, expression patterns and binding ability, they exert different modulatory functions in various physiological and pathological processes (*5*).

Galectin-3 is a unique chimera-type member of galectin family which contains three structural domains: (i.) an NH2-terminal domain with a serine phosphorylation site that participate in regulation of intracellular signaling; (ii.) collagen-like sequence, sensitive to matrix metalloproteinase MMP-2 and MMP-9-induced proteolysis; and (iii.) a COOH-terminal domain containing a single CRD with Asp-Trp-Gly-Arg amino acid sequence (NWGR) responsible for the anti-apoptotic action of Galectin-3 (*6–10*). Similarly to other galectins, Galectin-3 is present both inside and outside cells (*11–13*) and interacts with numerous intracellular and extracellular ligands. Galectin-3 upon binding to multivalent carbohydrates can form pentamers that modulate intracellular signaling cascade (*14*). In general, extracellular Galectin-3 acts as an adhesion molecule by cross-linking adjacent cells or cells and extracellular matrix components (*15*) and has chemokine-like functions in recruitment of macrophages and neutrophils (*16*). Intracellular Galectin-3 has been shown to exert diverse cellular functions including pre-mRNA splicing (*17*), regulation of cell growth and cell cycle progression and apoptosis (*18*). In addition, cytoplasmic Galectin-3 is anti-apoptotic, whereas nuclear and extracellular Galectin-3 is pro-apoptotic molecule (*10*, *19*, *20*). The ability of Galectin-3 to function as a potent modulator of immune responses has attracted much attention.

The Role of Galectin-3 in Immunoregulation

Galectin-3 is expressed in many immunocompetent and inflammatory cells, either constitutively or in an inducible fashion, suggesting its pleiotropic functions in regulating innate and acquired immune response (*21*). Galectin-3 may regulate immune response through its ability to modulate immune cell activation, differentiation, migration and apoptosis [reviewed in (*21–23*)].

Mechanisms by which Galectin-3 may participate in regulation of innate immune response are activation and adhesion of neutrophils (*24*), chemoattraction of monocytes/macrophages (*16*), opsonization of apoptotic neutrophils (*25*) and activation of mast cells (*26*). Further, Galectin-3 can stimulate important pathways involved in the innate immune response including oxidative burst in neutrophils (*27*) and mast cell degranulation (*26*).

T cells play a central role in the acquired immune response. An important role for Galectin-3 in regulation of T-cell receptor signaling was studied by Demetriou and colleagues (*28*) who suggested that Galectin-3 might play an inhibitory role in T-cell activation by forming complexes with TCR glycans, therefore limiting TCR clustering necessary for initiation of TCR-mediated signaling. Several studies have demonstrated that Galectin-3 is also involved in T-cell apoptosis. For example, intracellular Galectin-3 inhibits (*10*), whereas extracellular Galectin-3 induces T-cell apoptosis (*29*).

It has been suggested that although lack of Galectin-3 does not affect differentiation and maturation of dendritic cells (DCs), it greatly influences the magnitude, but not the nature of the acquired immune response (*30*). This view has been challenged by our data of dendritic cell phenotypes during induction of experimental autoimmune encephalomyelitis (EAE) in Gal-3 deficient mice (*31*). Breuilh et al. (*30*) showed that Galectin-3 modulates immune response during helminthic infection and that its expression in dendritic cells controls the magnitude of T-cell priming. We have shown important associations of Galectin-3 with various pathological conditions using several experimental models of T-cell-mediated inflammatory and autoimmune diseases. Our recent study in Galectin-3-deficient mice strongly indicates that Galectin-3 plays an important pro-inflammatory role in Con-A-induced hepatitis by promoting the activation of T lymphocytes, NKT cells and DCs, secretion of pro-inflammatory cytokines and prevention of M2 macrophage polarization and mononuclear cell apoptosis which result in severe liver injury (*32*).

Galectin-3 is also involved in immune-mediated pancreatic β-cell damage and is required for MLD-STZ induced diabetes by promoting the expression of pro-inflammatory IFN-gamma, TNF-alpha and IL-17 as well as iNOS in immune and accessory effector cells (*33*). Interestingly, Galectin-3 may exert protective effect in obesity induced type 2 diabetes (unpublished data). Namely, we found increased body weight, amount of visceral adipose tissue and fasting blood glucose levels in Gal-3$^{-/-}$ mice fed high-fat diet which was accompanied with adipose tissue inflammation as reflected by increased proportion of Type 1 T and NKT lymphocytes and pro-inflammatory macrophages, and reduced percentages of CD4$^+$CD25$^+$FoxP3$^+$ regulatory T cells. Also pancreatic islet inflammation with marked infiltration of mononuclear cells, higher NLRP3 inflammasome and IL-1ß expression and increased accumulation of advanced glycation endproducts (AGE) and upregulation of receptor for AGE (RAGE) was found in obese Gal-3$^{-/-}$ mice.

These data suggest important immunoregulatory and protective roles for Gal-3 in metabolic disorders including type 2 diabetes, which could be of therapeutic importance. We showed that Galectin-3 promotes Th1- and Th17-type cytokine response in a model of autoimmune neuroinflammation (*31*). Recent findings also demonstrate that Galectin-3 is able to activate immune and inflammatory signaling events through phosphorylation of various transcriptional factors, suggesting that Galectin-3 exerts cytokine-like regulatory actions, amplifying the inflammatory cascade in the brain (*34*).

In addition to immunoregulatory roles in various inflammatory and autoimmune diseases, Galectin-3 is also expressed in malignant cells and is involved in tumor development and progression as well as tumor immune escape. In the current review, we focus on the role of Galectin-3 in tumor biology, as evaluated in malignant melanoma.

The Role of Galectin-3 in Tumors

Tumor-associated Galectin-3 may play a significant role in different processes important for tumorigenesis and tumor progression through its involvement in regulation of cell proliferation, apoptosis, cell adhesion, invasion, angiogenesis and metastasis (*4*, *18*).

Presence of Galectin-3 inside cells promotes malignant cell transformation by stimulating cell growth and inhibiting apoptosis (*18*). Some studies suggest that increased expression of this lectin may be necessary for malignant transformation of at least some cell types, since inhibition of Galectin-3 expression in cells of human MDA-MB-435 breast cancer cells and thyroid papillary carcinoma, resulted in the loss of the malignant cell phenotype and slower tumor growth (*35*, *36*). These findings were confirmed in experiments in which transfection of normal thyroid follicular cells by Galectin-3 cDNA induced their malignant cell transformation (*37*).

Galectin-3 can trigger malignant cell transformation by interacting with essential components of signalling pathways such as oncogenic Ras proteins (*38*) since it preferentially binds to K-Ras and causes activation of phosphatidylinositol 3-kinase (PI3K) and Raf1 thus modulating gene expression at the transcriptional level (*38*, *39*). Additional mechanism by which Galectin-3 may participate in tumorigenesis is its action on regulators of cell cycle (*18*, *40*). It has been reported that Galectin-3 downregulates expression of cyclin E and cyclin A and upregulates expression of cell cycle inhibitors p21 (WAF1) and p27 (KIP1) (*41*). Other studies have shown that Galectin-3 by interacting with β-catenin enhances the expressions of cyclin D and c-myc and promotes cell cycle progression (*40*, *42*). Human MDA-MB-435 breast cancer cells transfected with antisense Galectin-3 cDNA have reduced proliferative capacity, indicating the important role for Galectin-3 in the proliferation of malignant cells (*43*).

Galectin-3 has a role in tumor progression by regulating apoptosis. Overexpression of intracellular Galectin-3 in aggressive form of B cell lymphomas protected these cells from apoptosis (*44*). Matarrese et al. (*45*) demonstrated that intracellular Galectin-3 maintains mitochondrial integrity and block release of pro-apoptotic factors, thereby preventing apoptotic cell death. Another mechanism by which Galectin-3 might exert anti-apoptotic action is its interaction with Bcl-2 [reviewed in (*18*)]. Several studies have indicated that overexpression of Galectin-3 protects malignant cells from apoptosis after the loss of cell anchorage (anoikis) (*41*, *46*) that also underlies anticancer drug resistance (*45*, *47*), which is considered to be a hallmark of metastatic phenotype (*48*, *49*).

Outside the cell, galectin-3 plays a pivotal role in different steps of tumor progression and metastasis such as cell adhesion, promotion of survival of anchorage dependent cells, invasiveness and migration of metastatic cells (*46*, *50–52*). Cell surface-associated Galectin-3 expressed on tumor cells stimulates homotypic cell-cell adhesion resulting in the formation of tumor emboli allowing survival of malignant cells during hematogeneous dissemination (*18*, *53*, *54*). This lectin also stimulates the binding of tumor cells to different components of extracellular matrix (heterotypic interaction), and thus accelerates tumor invasion and metastasis (*18*, *52*). In addition, high levels of circulating Galectin-3 in cancer patients are associated with higher incidence of metastasis in distant organs (*55*). There are evidence that Galectin-3 may bind to a number of substrates such as Thomsen-Fridenreich antigen and transmembrane mucin protein MUC1 (*56*, *57*).

Galectin-3 has been shown to promote motility and invasiveness of malignant cells, and also to affect metastases by exerting its effect on tumor angiogenesis (*18*). Accumulation of Galectin-3 in lung cancer cells is associated with enhanced cell motility and invasiveness *in vitro* (*58*). In addition, Galectin-3 has a role in controlling tumor cell migration and therefore tumor cell invasion by modulating activation or expression of integrins (*18*, *46*). Galectin-3 also participates in angiogenesis by stimulating the migration of endothelial cells *in vitro* (*59*). Beside this, it has been reported that Galectin-3 stimulates angiogenesis in vivo that resulted in breast cancer growth in nude mice. It seems that through interaction with αvβ3 integrin, this lectin mediates vascular endothelial growth factor (VEGF) and basic fibroblast growth factor (bFGF) - mediated angiogenesis (*60*).

Finally, clinical evidence has shown that expression of Galectin-3 is altered in malignant cells (*61*). Overexpression of Galectin-3 in human tumors generally correlates with tumor progression and metastasis (*61*). However, the expression of Galectin-3 has been shown to increase (*62*) or decrease (*63*) with progression of colorectal carcinoma. Also, decreased expression of this molecule in tumor tissue has been associated with higher metastatic capacity of breast carcinoma cells (*64*). It seems that Galectin-3 expression is dependent on the organ or tissue, and may be modulated by tumor- or tissue specific factors (*61*). Additionally, Galectin-3 can modulate the effects of matrix metalloproteinases, so that activity of this lectin in various processes of tumor progression is under control of the enzymes present in the tumor microenvironment (*65*).

The Role of Galectin-3 in Human Melanoma

Human melanoma is the most aggressive form of skin cancer that originates in malignant melanocytes. Malignant transformation of melanocytes is multistep process that involves activation of multiple oncogenes (e.g. N-Ras and BRAF) and the inactivation of tumor suppressor genes (e.g. PTEN and $p16^{IKN4A}$), resulting in "unplanned" proliferation of melanoma cells which also become immortal and able to invade and metastasize to other tissues (*66–68*).

Although the data from studies describing the role of Galectin-3 in the pathogenesis of malignant melanoma are conflicting, the general conclusion is that Galectin-3 could modulate melanoma progression and metastasis. It was demonstrated that expression of Galectin-3 is upregulated in primary and metastatic melanoma lesions compared with benign nevi, suggesting that its overexpression correlates with metastatic progression of human melanoma and poor clinical outcome (*69*). Further, melanocytes accumulation of Galectin-3, particularly in the nucleus, is associated with melanoma progression. It seems that this translocation of Galectin-3 to nucleus of malignant melanocytes results in a more aggressive tumor behavior, as it acts as a survival factor and renders melanocytes resistant to apoptosis induced by anoikis and chemotherapeutic agents (*69*).

Similarly, Galectin-3 expression was shown to be higher in malignant compared to benign tumor lesions (*70*). The nuclecytoplasmic pattern of Galectin-3 expression is associated with probability of malignant phenotype and poor prognostic impact on patient's outcome (*70*). There are data that expression of Galectin-3 also correlates with lymphatic invasion and distant metastasis, suggesting its pivotal role in lymphogenous metastasis (*71*). Furthermore, some studies have reported that serum level of Galectin-3 is higher in patients with advanced melanoma (*55*, *72*).

Studies using xenograft melanoma model in nude mice with human melanoma cell lines have shown that Galectin-3 expression was lower in metastatic melanoma lesions than in thin primary lesions which was inversely correlated with tumor aggressiveness (*73*). Given the role of Galectin-3 in adhesion interactions, it seems that the progressive decrease of Galectin-3 levels may act as a trigger for metastatic dissemination of melanocytes (*73*). The results from clinical study demonstrated higher Galectin-3 expression in thin primary melanomas compared to benign nevi, and a progressive fall in Galectin-3 expression between thin primary melanomas, thicker melanomas and metastatic lesions, suggesting that Galectin-3 might be a marker for melanoma progression (*74*).

Metastatic phenotype of melanoma is associated with high invasive potential, ability of melanocytes to survive and to colonize distant organs, effective tumor angiogenesis and high plasticity of melanocytes (*68*, *75*). For example, highly aggressive melanocytes have the capacity to produce "vasculogenic mimicry" (vasculogenic channels lined by melanoma cells) by expressing endothelium- and epithelium-associated markers, and to form a vasculogenic-like network *in vitro* (*76*). The study using human melanoma cell lines has demonstrated that Galectin-3 exerts pro-tumorigenic and pro-metastatic properties by promoting tumor angiogenesis and melanoma cell "vasculogenic mimicry" (*77*).

Galectin-3 might play an important role in tumor immunity by regulating the survival of immune cells in tumor microenvironment. It has been demonstrated that expression of Galectin-3 in human melanoma biopsies correlated with apoptosis of tumor-associated lymphocytes (*78*), therefore contributing to tumor immune escape.

The existing information suggests that Galectin-3 might be a potential therapeutic target in treatment of malignant tumors.

The Role of Galectin-3 in Murine B16-F1 Melanoma Metastasis

A series of experimental and clinical evidence indicate that Galectin-3 on the surface of tumor cells as well as circulating Galectin-3 have regulatory roles in tumor progression and metastasis, but the role of Galectin-3 in regulating anti-tumor immunity and metastatic process *in vivo* still remains a puzzle. Using Galectin-3-deficient mice we recently provided evidence that expression of Galectin-3 in the host also facilitate establishment of metastasis in B16-F1 malignant melanoma model (*79*). In fact, Galectin-3 deficient mice were significantly protected against the development of metastatic melanoma reflected by decreased number and size of melanoma colonies in the lung.

Based on these findings, we suggest that expression of Galectin-3 on the host cells could be critical for promoting lung tumorigenesis as well as metastasis. Similar conclusion has been drown from the study of NNK-induced lung tumorogenesis in Galectin-3 deficient mice (*80*). Additionally, we demonstrated that one of the mechanisms contributing to resistance of Galectin-3-deficient mice is lower tumor cell adhesion. In this context, our results from *in vitro* assays showed that deletion of Galectin-3 decreased number of attached malignant cells in lung tissue sections (*79*). We assume that endothelial Galectin-3 may be pivotal for the adhesion of tumor cells through its interaction with numerous carbohydrate ligands expressed on tumor cells (*54*, *81*, *82*), thus participating in the formation of metastatic foci in target tissue (*83*).

Recent study demonstrated that Galectin-3 by segregation of CD8 from TCR molecule (*84*) caused anergy of tumor-specific cytotoxic T lymphocytes (CTLs), suggesting that Galectin-3 in tumor microenvironment could impair T-cell mediated anti-tumor immunity *in vivo* (*85*). Our study showed that deletion of Galectin-3 in the C57BL/6 mice inhibited formation of metastasis by modifying anti-melanoma immune response (*79*). We found that Galectin-3-deficient mice had higher serum levels of IFN-gamma and IL-17 compared to wild-type C57BL/6 (WT) mice. Further, injection of melanoma cells resulted in a significant increase in the percentage and total number of regulatory $CD4^{+}Foxp3^{+}$T cells in WT mice, but not in Galectin-3-deficient mice.

Most importantly, we noticed that protective effects of Galectin-3 deficiency on metastatic melanoma spread was dependent on NK cells and associated with an enhanced cytotoxic activity of splenic NK cells *in vitro* and increased frequency of effective cytotoxic $CD27^{high}CD11b^{high}$NK cells as well as immature $CD27^{high}CD11b^{low}$NK cells in the spleen. On the other side, we showed that WT mice had increased percentage of $CD27^{low}CD11b^{high}$ less functionally exhausted NK cells as well as NK cells bearing inhibitory KLRG1 receptor (*79*). We postulated that metastatic melanoma spread in WT mice was mainly associated with decreased cytotoxic capacity of NK cells most probably due to increased expansion of suppressive $CD4^{+}Foxp3^{+}$ T regulatory cells in spleens. Also, an inverse correlation between NK cell activity and expansion of regulatory T cells has been demonstrated in cancer patients (*86*), indicating that regulatory T cells might hamper NK cell function (*87*, *88*).

Our findings indicate that expression of Galectin-3 on the host cells may facilitate melanoma metastasis by affecting tumor cell adhesion and by modulating mainly innate anti-tumor immune response (*79*). Thus, target inhibition of Galectin-3 expression can prevent melanoma metastasis by decreasing tumor cell adhesion and by enhancing NK cell-mediated anti-tumor immune response.

Effects of Galectin-3 Inhibition *in Vitro*

Given the important roles for Galectin-3 in modulating numerous processes relevant for tumorogenesis and tumor progression, this lectin could be considered as one of molecular targets in the therapy of malignant diseases.

Inhibitory effects by certain Galectin-3 inhibitors on growth and metastasis in cancer cell lines have been demonstrated. Thus, treatment of B16-F1 and UV-237 with a monoclonal antibody against tumor cell surface lectins before their intravenous injection strongly inhibits experimental lung metastasis of melanoma and fibrosarcoma cells (*89*). The Galectin-3C is a soluble recombinant galectin that binds carbohydrates and competes with endogenous Galectin-3 for carbohydrate binding sites. It has been shown that Galectin-3C significantly decreased the tumor growth and metastasis of breast MDA-MB-535 carcinoma in a mouse orthotopic model (*90*). The pH-modified citrus pectin (MCP), a competitive inhibitor for natural ligands of Galectin-3, has been shown to affect homotypic aggregation of B16-F1 melanoma cells (*91*, *92*), angiogenesis and tumor cells adhesion to endothelial cells *in vitro* (*93*). In addition, injection of B16-F1 melanoma cells with MCP resulted in a marked decrease of experimental metastasis in the lung tissue (*92*).

Recently, Galectin-3 has sparked interest for developing synthetic selective inhibitors. Thus, thiodigalactoside diester Td131_1 preferentially binds and inhibits Galectin-3, because it has a high affinity and specificity for this lectin due to the specific interactions of its two ester moieties with Arg^{144} and Arg^{186} of Galectin-3 (*94*). Data from Lin et al (*95*) demonstrated that treatment of papillary thyroid cancer cell lines and human ex vivo papillary thyroid cancer with Td131_1 results in their enhanced sensitivity to chemotherapeutic drug such as doxorubicin. It seems that Td131_1 activates apoptosis and improves the sensitivity of papillary thyroid cancer cells to radiotherapy and to chemotherapy in a synergistic fashion, suggesting that Galectin-3 inhibitor is a promising agent for advanced tumors that are refractory to conventional therapies. Interestingly, pre-treatment of C57BL/6 mice with selective inhibitor of Galectin-3 (TD139) led to attenuation of liver injury in Concanavalin A-induced hepatitis model *in vivo* (*32*).

These observations clearly indicate that blockade of Galectin-3 might result in therapeutic benefits in cancer metastasis as well as in autoimmune and inflammatory diseases.

Acknowledgments

This study is supported by grants: ON175069, ON175071 and ON175103 from Ministry of Education and Science, and from the Faculty of Medical Science, University of Kragujevac (project JP 01/10), Serbia.

References

1. Cooper, D. N. Galectinomics: Finding themes in complexity. *Biochim. Biophys. Acta* **2002**, *1572*, 209–231.
2. Leffler, H.; Carlsson, S.; Hedlund, M.; Qian, Y.; Poirier, F. Introduction to galectins. *Glycoconjugate J.* **2004**, *19*, 433–440.
3. Cooper, D. N.; Barondes, S. H. God must love galectins; he made so many of them. *Glycobiology* **1999**, *9*, 979–984.
4. Yang, R. Y.; Rabinovich, G. A.; Liu, F. T. Galectins: Structure, function and therapeutic potential. *Expert Rev. Mol. Med.* **2008**, *544* (10), e17.
5. Liu, F. T.; Yang, R. Y.; Hsu, D. K. Galectins in acute and chronic inflammation. *Ann. N.Y. Acad. Sci.* **2012**, DOI: 10.1111/j.1749-6632.2011.06386.x.
6. Herrmann, J.; Turck, C. W.; Atchison, R. E.; Huflejt, M. E.; Poulter, L.; Gitt, M. A.; Burlingame, AL; Barondes, S. H.; Leffler, H. Primary structure of the soluble lactose binding lectin L-29 from rat and dog and interaction of its non-collagenous proline-, glycine-, tyrosine-rich sequence with bacteria and tissue collagenase. *J. Biol. Chem.* **1993**, *268*, 26704–26711.
7. Barondes, S. H.; Cooper, D. N.; Gitt, M. A.; Leffler, H. Galectins: Structure and function of a large family of animal lectins. *J. Biol. Chem.* **1994**, *269*, 20807–20810.
8. Gong, H. C.; Honjo, Y.; Nangia-Makker, P.; Hogan, V.; Mazurak, N.; Bresalier, R. S.; Raz, A. The NH2 terminus of galectin-3 governs cellular compartmentalization and functions in cancer cells. *Cancer Res.* **1999**, *59*, 6239–6245.
9. Ochieng, J.; Green, B.; Evans, S.; James, O.; Warfield, P. Modulation of the biological functions of galectin-3 by matrix metalloproteinases. *Biochim. Biophys. Acta* **1998**, *1379*, 97–106.
10. Yang, R. Y.; Hsu, D. K.; Liu, F. T. Expression of galectin-3 modulates T-cell growth and apoptosis. *Proc. Natl. Acad. Sci. U.S.A.* **1996**, *93*, 6737–6742.
11. Sato, S.; Hughes, R. C. J. Regulation of secretion and surface expression of Mac-2, a galactoside-binding protein of macrophages. *J. Biol. Chem.* **1994**, *269*, 4424–4430.
12. Moutsatsos, I. K.; Wade, M.; Schindler, M.; Wang, J. L. Endogenous lectins from cultured cells: Nuclear localization of carbohydrate-binding protein 35 in proliferating 3T3 fibroblasts. *Proc. Natl. Acad. Sci. U.S.A.* **1987**, *84*, 6452–6456.
13. Perillo, N. L.; Marcus, M. E.; Baum, L. G. Galectins: Versatile modulators of cell adhesion, cell proliferation, and cell death. *J. Mol. Med.* **1998**, *76*, 402–412.
14. Ahmad, N.; Gabius, H. J.; André, S.; Kaltner, H.; Sabesan, S.; Roy, R; Liu, B.; Macaluso, F.; Brewer, C. F. Galectin-3 precipitates as a pentamer with synthetic multivalent carbohydrates and forms heterogeneous cross-linked complexes. *J. Biol. Chem.* **2004**, *279*, 10841–10847.
15. Dumic, J.; Dabelic, S.; Flögel, M. Galectin-3: An open-ended story. *Biochim. Biophys. Acta* **2006**, *1760*, 616–635.

16. Sano, H.; Hsu, D. K.; Yu, L.; Apgar, J. R.; Kuwabara, I.; Yamanaka, T.; Hirashima, M.; Liu, F. T. Human galectin-3 is a novel chemoattractant for monocytes and macrophages. *J. Immunol.* **2000**, *165*, 2156–2164.
17. Dagher, S. F.; Wang, J. L.; Patterson, R. J. Identification of galectin-3 as a factor in pre-mRNA splicing. *Proc. Natl. Acad. Sci. U.S.A.* **1995**, *92*, 1213–1217.
18. Liu, F. T.; Rabinovich, G. A. Galectins as modulators of tumour progression. *Nat. Rev. Cancer* **2005**, *5*, 29–41.
19. Califice, S.; Castronovo, V.; Bracke, M.; van den Brûle, F. Dual activities of galectin-3 in human prostate cancer: Tumor suppression of nuclear galectin-3 vs tumor promotion of cytoplasmic galectin-3. *Oncogene* **2004**, *23*, 7527–7536.
20. Nakahara, S.; Oka, N.; Raz, A. On the role of galectin-3 in cancer apoptosis. *Apoptosis* **2005**, *10*, 267–275.
21. Chen, H. Y.; Liu, F. T.; Yang, R. Y. Roles of galectin-3 in immune responses. *Arch. Immunol. Ther. Exp.* **2005**, *53* (6), 497–504.
22. Henderson, N. C.; Sethi, T. The regulation of inflammation by galectin-3. *Immunol.Rev.* **2009**, *230*, 160–171.
23. Hsu, D. K.; Chen, H. Y.; Liu, F. T. Galectin-3 regulates T-cell functions. *Immunol. Rev.* **2009**, *230*, 114–127.
24. Kuwabara, I.; Liu, F. T. Galectin-3 promotes adhesion of human neutrophils to laminin. *J. Immunol.* **1996**, *156*, 3939–3944.
25. Karlsson, A.; Christenson, K.; Matlak, M.; Björstad, Å.; Brown, K. L.; Telemo, E.; Salomonsson, E.; Leffler, H.; Bylund, J. Galectin-3 functions as an opsonin and enhances the macrophage clearance of apoptotic neutrophils. *Glycobiology* **2009**, *19*, 16–20.
26. Frigeri, L. G.; Zuberi, R. I.; Liu, F. T. Epsilon BP, a beta-galactoside-binding animal lectin, recognizes IgE receptor (Fc epsilon RI) and activates mast cells. *Biochemistry* **1993**, *32*, 7644–7649.
27. Yamaoka, A.; Kuwabara, I.; Frigeri, L. G.; Liu, F. T. A human lectin, galectin-3 (epsilon bp/Mac-2), stimulates superoxide production by neutrophils. *J. Immunol.* **1995**, *154*, 3479–3487.
28. Demetriou, M.; Granovsky, M.; Quaggin, S.; Dennis, J. W. Negative regulation of T-cell activation and autoimmunity by Mgat5 N-glycosylation. *Nature* **2001**, *409*, 733–739.
29. Fukumori, T.; Takenaka, Y.; Yoshii, T.; Kim, H. R. C.; Hogan, V.; Inohara, H.; Kagawa, S.; Raz, A. CD29 and CD7 mediate galectin-3- induced type II T-cell apoptosis. *Cancer Res.* **2003**, *63*, 8302–8311.
30. Breuilh, L.; Vanhoutte, F.; Fontaine, J.; van Stijn, C. M.; Tillie-Leblond, I.; Capron, M.; Faveeuw, C.; Jouault, T.; van Die, I.; Gosset, P.; Trottein, F. Galectin-3 modulates immune and inflammatory responses during helminthic infection: Impact of galectin-3 deficiency on the functions of dendritic cells. *Infect. Immun.* **2007**, *75*, 5148–5157.
31. Jiang, H. R.; Al Rasebi, Z.; Mensah-Brown, E.; Shahin, A.; Xu, D.; Goodyear, C. S.; Fukada, S. Y.; Liu, F. T.; Liew, F. Y.; Lukic, M. L. Galectin- 3 deficiency reduces the severity of experimental autoimmune encephalomyelitis. *J. Immunol.* **2009**, *182*, 1167–1173.

32. Volarevic, V.; Milovanovic, M.; Ljujic, B.; Pejnovic, N.; Arsenijevic, N.; Nilsson, U.; Leffler, H.; Lukic, M. L. Galectin-3 deficiency prevents concanavalin A- induced hepatitis in mice. *Hepatology* **2011**, DOI: 10.1002/hep.25542.
33. Mensah-Brown, E. P.; Al Rabesi, Z.; Shahin, A.; Al Shamsi, M.; Arsenijevic, N.; Hsu, D. K.; Liu, F. T.; Lukic, M. L. Targeted disruption of the galectin-3 gene results in decreased susceptibility to multiple low dose streptozotocin-induced diabetes in mice. *Clin. Immunol.* **2009**, *130*, 83–88.
34. Jeon, S. B.; Yoon, H. J.; Chang, C. Y.; Koh, H. S.; Jeon, S. H.; Park, E. J. Galectin-3 exerts cytokine-like regulatory actions through the JAK-STAT pathway. *J. Immunol.* **2010**, *185*, 7037–7046.
35. Honjo, Y.; Nangia-Makker, P.; Inohara, H.; Raz, A. Downregulation of galectin-3 suppresses tumorigenicity of human breast carcinoma cells. *Clin. Cancer Res.* **2001**, *7*, 661–668.
36. Yoshii, T.; Inohara, H.; Takenaka, Y.; Honjo, Y.; Akahani, S.; Nomura, T.; Raz, A.; Kubo, T. Galectin-3 maintains the transformed phenotype of thyroid papillary carcinoma cells. *Int. J. Oncol.* **2001**, *18*, 787–792.
37. Takenaka, Y.; Inohara, H.; Yoshii, T.; Oshima, K.; Nakahara, S.; Akahani, S.; Honjo, Y.; Yamamoto, Y.; Raz, A.; Kubo, T. Malignant transformation of thyroid follicular cells by galectin-3. *Cancer Lett.* **2003**, *195*, 111–119.
38. Elad-Sfadia, G.; Haklai, R.; Balan, E.; Kloog, Y. Galectin-3 augments K-Ras activation and triggers a Ras signal that attenuates ERK but not phosphoinositide 3-kinase activity. *J. Biol. Chem.* **2004**, *279*, 34922–34930.
39. Ashery, U.; Yizhar, O.; Rotblat, B.; Elad-Sfadia, G.; Barkan, B.; Haklai, R.; Kloog, Y. Spatiotemporal organization of Ras signaling: Rasosomes and the galectin switch. *Cell. Mol. Neurobiol.* **2006**, *26*, 471–495.
40. Shimura, T.; Takenaka, Y.; Fukumori, T.; Tsutsumi, S.; Okada, K.; Hogan, V.; Kikuchi, A.; Kuwano, H.; Raz, A. Implication of galectin-3 in Wnt signaling. *Cancer Res.* **2005**, *65*, 3535–3537.
41. Kim, H. R.; Lin, H. M.; Biliran, H.; Raz, A. Cell cycle arrest and inhibition of anoikis by galectin-3 in human breast epithelial cells. *Cancer Res.* **1999**, *59*, 4148–4154.
42. Shimura, T.; Takenaka, Y.; Tsutsumi, S.; Hogan, V.; Kikuchi, A.; Raz, A Galectin-3, a novel binding partner of beta-catenin. *Cancer Res.* **2004**, *64*, 6363–6367.
43. Vandenbrule, F.; Bellahcene, A.; Jackers, P; Liu, F.; Sobel, M.; Castronovo, V. Antisense galectin-3 alters thymidine incorporation in human MDA-MB435 breast cancer cells. *Int. J. Oncol.* **1997**, *11*, 261–264.
44. Hoyer, K. K.; Pang, M.; Gui, D.; Shintaku, I. P.; Kuwabara, I.; Liu, F. T.; Said, J. W.; Baum, L. G.; Teitell, M. A. An anti-apoptotic role for galectin-3 in diffuse large B-cell lymphomas. *Am. J. Pathol.* **2004**, *164*, 893–902.
45. Matarrese, P.; Tinari, N.; Semeraro, M. L.; Natoli, C.; Iacobelli, S.; Malorni, W. Galectin-3 overexpression protects from cell damage and death by influencing mitochondrial homeostasis. *FEBS Lett.* **2000a**, *473*, 311–315.
46. Matarrese, P.; Fusco, O.; Tinari, N.; Natoli, C.; Liu, F. T.; Semeraro, ML; Malorni, W.; Iacobelli, S. Galectin-3 overexpression protects from apoptosis by improving cell adhesion properties. *Int. J. Cancer* **2000b**, *85*, 545–554.

47. Fukumori, T.; Kanayama, H. O.; Raz, A. The role of galectin-3 in cancer drug resistance. *Drug Resist. Updates* **2007**, *10*, 101–108.
48. Méhes, G.; Witt, A.; Kubista, E.; Ambros, P. F. Circulating breast cancer cells are frequently apoptotic. *Am. J. Pathol.* **2001**, *159*, 17–20.
49. Kerbel, R. S.; Kobayashi, H.; Graham, C. H. Intrinsic or acquired drug resistance and metastasis: Are they linked phenotypes? *J. Cell. Biochem.* **1994**, *56*, 37–47.
50. Le Marer, N.; Hughes, R. C. Effects of the carbohydrate-binding protein galectin-3 on the invasiveness of human breast carcinoma cells. *J. Cell. Physiol.* **1996**, *168*, 51–58.
51. van Den Brûle, F. A.; Buicu, C.; Sobel, M. E.; Liu, F. T.; Castronovo, V. Galectin-3, a laminin-binding protein fails to modulate adhesion of human melanoma cells to laminin. *Neoplasma* **1995**, *42*, 215–219.
52. Inohara, H.; Raz, A. Functional evidence that cell surface galectin-3 mediates homotypic cell adhesion. *Cancer Res.* **1995**, *55*, 3267–3271.
53. Rabinovich, G. A.; Cumashi, A.; Bianco, G. A.; Ciavardelli, D.; Iurisci, I; D'Egidio, M.; Piccolo, E.; Tinari, N.; Nifantiev, N. E.; Iacobelli, S. Synthetic lactulose amines: Novel class of anticancer agents that induce tumor-cell apoptosis and inhibit galectin-mediated homotypic cell aggregation and endothelial cell morphogenesis. *Glycobiology* **2006**, *16*, 210–220.
54. Khaldoyanidi, S. K.; Glinsky, V. V.; Sikora, L.; Glinskii, A. B.; Mossine, V. V.; Quinn, T. P.; Glinsky, G. V.; Sriramarao, P. MDA-MB-435 human breast carcinoma cell homo- and heterotypic adhesion under flow conditions is mediated in part by Thomsen-Friedenreich antigen-galectin-3 interactions. *J. Biol. Chem.* **2003**, *278*, 4127–4134.
55. Iurisci, I.; Tinari, N.; Natoli, C.; Angelucci, D.; Cianchetti, E.; Iacobelli, S. Concentrations of galectin-3 in the sera of normal controls and cancer patients. *Clin. Cancer Res.* **2000**, *6*, 1389–1393.
56. Glinsky, V. V.; Huflejt, M. E.; Glinsky, G. V.; Deutscher, S. L.; Quinn, T. P. Effects of Thomsen-Friedenreich antigen-specific peptide P-30 on beta-galactoside-mediated homotypic aggregation and adhesion to the endothelium of MDA-MB-435 human breast carcinoma cells. *Cancer Res.* **2000**, *60*, 2584–2588.
57. Zhao, Q.; Barclay, M.; Hilkens, J.; Guo, X.; Barrow, H.; Rhodes, J. M.; Yu, L. G. Interaction between circulating galectin-3 and cancer associated MUC1 enhances tumour cell homotypic aggregation and prevents anoikis. *Mol. Cancer* **2010**, *9*, 154.
58. O'Driscoll, L.; Linehan, R.; Liang, Y. H.; Joyce, H.; Oglesby, I.; Clynes, M. Galectin-3 expression alters adhesion, motility and invasion in a lung cell line (DLKP), in vitro. *Anticancer Res.* **2002**, *22*, 3117–3125.
59. Nangia-Makker, P.; Honjo, Y.; Sarvis, R.; Akahani, S.; Hogan, V.; Pienta, K. J.; Raz, A. Galectin-3 induces endothelial cell morphogenesis and angiogenesis. *Am. J. Pathol.* **2000**, *156*, 899–909.
60. Markowska, A. I.; Liu, F.-T.; Panjwani, N. Galectin-3 is an important mediator of VEGF- and bFGF-mediated angiogenic response. *J. Exp. Med.* **2010**, *207*, 1981–1993.

61. Danguy, A.; Camby, I.; Kiss, R. Galectins and cancer. *Biochim. Biophys. Acta* **2002**, *1572*, 285–293.
62. Schoeppner, H. L.; Raz, A.; Ho, S. B.; Bresalier, R. S. Expression of an endogenous galactose-binding lectin correlates with neoplastic progression in the colon. *Cancer* **1995**, *75*, 2818–2826.
63. Lotz, M. M.; Andrews, C. W.; Korzelius, C. A., Jr; Lee, E. C.; Steele, G. D.; Clarke, A., Jr; Mercurio, A. M. Decreased expression of Mac-2 (carbohydrate binding protein 35) and loss of its nuclear localization are associated with the neoplastic progression of colon carcinoma. *Proc. Natl. Acad. Sci. U.S.A.* **1993**, *90*, 3466–3470.
64. Castronovo, V.; Van Den Brûle, F. A.; Jackers, P.; Clausse, N.; Liu, F. T.; Gillet, C.; Sobel, M. E. Decreased expression of galectin-3 is associated with progression of human breast cancer. *J. Pathol.* **1996**, *179*, 43–48.
65. Nangia-Makker, P.; Balan, V.; Raz, A. Regulation of tumor progression by extracellular galectin-3. *Cancer Microenviron.* **2008**, *1*, 43–51.
66. Fisher, D. E.; Kwong, L. N.; Chin, L Melanoma. In *DeVita, Hellman, and Rosenberg's Cancer Principles & Practice of Oncology*, 8th ed.; Lippincott Williams & Wilkins: New York, 2008; Chapter 48, pp 1889−1965.
67. Hsu, M. Y.; Meier, F.; Herlyn, M. Melanoma development and progression: A conspiracy between tumor and host. *Differentiation* **2002**, *70*, 522–536.
68. Villanueva, J.; Herlyn, M. Melanoma and tumor microenvironment. *Curr. Oncol. Rep.* **2008**, *10*, 439–446.
69. Prieto, V. G.; Mourad-Zeidan, A. A.; Melnikova, V.; Johnson, M. M.; Lopez, A.; Diwan, A. H.; Lazar, A. J.; Shen, S. S.; Zhang, P. S.; Reed, J. A.; Gershenwald, J. E.; Raz, A.; Bar-Eli, M. Galectin-3 expression is associated with tumor progression and pattern of sun exposure in melanoma. *Clin. Cancer Res.* **2006**, *12*, 6709–6715.
70. Abdou, A. G.; Hammam, M. A.; Farargy, S. E.; Farag, A. G.; El Shafey, E. N.; Farouk, S.; Elnaidany, N. F. Diagnostic and prognostic role of galectin 3 expression in cutaneous melanoma. *Am. J. Dermatopathol.* **2010**, *32*, 809–814.
71. Buljan, M.; Šitum, M.; Tomas, D.; Milošević, M.; Krušlin, B. Prognostic value of galectin-3 in primary cutaneous melanoma. *J. Eur. Acad. Dermatol. Venereol.* **2011**, *25*, 1174–1181.
72. Vereecken, P.; Zouaoui Boudjeltia, K.; Debray, C.; Awada, A.; Legssyer, I.; Sales, F.; Petein, M.; Vanhaeverbeek, M.; Ghanem, G.; Heenen, M. High serum galectin-3 in advanced melanoma: Preliminary results. *Clin. Exp. Dermatol.* **2006**, *31*, 105–109.
73. Vereecken, P.; Debray, C.; Petein, M.; Awada, A.; Lalmand, M. C.; Laporte, M.; Van Den Heule, B; Verhest, A.; Pochet, R.; Heenen, M. Expression of galectin-3 in primary and metastatic melanoma: Immunohistochemical studies on human lesions and nude mice xenograft tumors. *Arch. Dermatol. Res.* **2005**, *296*, 353–358.
74. Brown, E. R.; Doig, T.; Anderson, N.; Brenn, T.; Doherty, V.; Xu, Y.; Bartlett, J. M.; Smyth, J. F.; Melton, D. W. Association of galectin-3 expression with melanoma progression and prognosis. *Eur. J. Cancer* **2011**DOI: 10.1016./j.ejca.2011.09.003.

75. Hendrix, M. J.; Seftor, E. A.; Hess, A. R.; Seftor, R. E. Vasculogenic mimicry and tumour-cell plasticity: Lessons from melanoma. *Nat. Rev. Cancer* **2003**, *3*, 4114–4121.
76. Maniotis, A. J.; Folberg, R.; Hess, A.; Seftor, E. A.; Gardner, L. M.; Pe'er, J.; Trent, J. M.; Meltzer, P. S.; Hendrix, M. J. Vascular channel formation by human melanoma cells in vivo and in vitro: Vasculogenic mimicry. *Am. J. Pathol.* **1999**, *155*, 739–752.
77. Mourad-Zeidan, A. A.; Melnikova, V. O.; Wang, H.; Raz, A.; Bar-Eli, M. Expression profiling of Galectin-3-depleted melanoma cells reveals its major role in melanoma cell plasticity and vasculogenic mimicry. *Am. J. Pathol.* **2008**, *173*, 1839–1852.
78. Zubieta, M. R.; Furman, D.; Barrio, M.; Bravo, A. I.; Domenichini, E.; Mordoh, J. Galectin-3 expression correlates with apoptosis of tumor-associated lymphocytes in human melanoma biopsies. *Am. J. Pathol.* **2006**, *168*, 1666–1675.
79. Radosavljevic, G.; Jovanovic, I.; Majstorovic, I.; Mitrovic, M.; Lisnic, V. J.; Arsenijevic, N.; Jonjic, S.; Lukic, M. L. Deletion of galectin-3 in the host attenuates metastasis of murine melanoma by modulating tumor adhesion and NK cell activity. *Clin. Exp. Metastasis* **2011**, *28*, 451–462.
80. Abdel-Aziz, H. O.; Murai, Y.; Takasaki, I.; Tabuchi, Y.; Zheng, H. C.; Nomoto, K.; Takahashi, H.; Tsuneyama, K.; Kato, I; Hsu, D. K.; Liu, F. T.; Hiraga, K.; Takano, Y. Targeted disruption of the galectin-3 gene results in decreased susceptibility to NNK-induced lung tumorigenesis: An oligonucleotide microarray study. *J. Cancer Res. Clin. Oncol.* **2008**, *134*, 777–788.
81. Glinsky, V. V.; Glinsky, G. V.; Rittenhouse-Olson, K.; Huflejt, M. E.; Glinskii, O. V.; Deutscher, S. L.; Quinn, T. P. The role of Thomsen-Friedenreich antigen in adhesion of human breast and prostate cancer cells to the endothelium. *Cancer Res.* **2001**, *61*, 4851–4857.
82. Krishnan, V.; Bane, S. M.; Kawle, P. D.; Naresh, K. N.; Kalraiya, R. D. Altered melanoma cell surface glycosylation mediates organ specific adhesion and metastasis via lectin receptors on the lung vascular endothelium. *Clin. Exp. Metastasis* **2005**, *22*, 11–24.
83. Dittmar, T.; Heyder, C.; Gloria-Maercker, E.; Hatzmann, W.; Zänker, K. S. Adhesion molecules and chemokines: The navigation system for circulating tumor (stem) cells to metastasize in an organ specific manner. *Clin. Exp. Metastasis* **2008**, *25*, 11–32.
84. Demotte, N.; Stroobant, V.; Courtoy, P. J.; Van Der Smissen, P.; Colau, D.; Luescher, I. F.; Hivroz, C.; Nicaise, J.; Squifflet, J. L.; Mourad, M.; Godelaine, D.; Boon, T.; van der Bruggen, P. Restoring the association of the T cell receptor with CD8 reverses anergy in human tumor-infiltrating lymphocytes. *Immunity* **2008**, *28*, 414–424.
85. Demotte, N.; Wieërs, G.; Van Der Smissen, P.; Moser, M.; Schmidt, C.; Thielemans, K.; Squifflet, J. L.; Weynand, B.; Carrasco, J.; Lurquin, C.; Courtoy, P. J.; van der Bruggen, P. A galectin-3 ligand corrects the impaired function of human CD4 and CD8 tumor-infiltrating lymphocytes and favors tumor rejection in mice. *Cancer Res.* **2010**, *70*, 7476–7488.

86. Ghiringhelli, F.; Ménard, C.; Terme, M.; Flament, C.; Taieb, J.; Chaput, N.; Puig, P. E.; Novault, S.; Escudier, B.; Vivier, E.; Lecesne, A.; Robert, C.; Blay, J. Y.; Bernard, J.; Caillat-Zucman, S.; Freitas, A.; Tursz, T.; Wagner-Ballon, O.; Capron, C.; Vainchencker, W.; Martin, F.; Zitvogel, L. CD4+CD25+ regulatory T cells inhibit natural killer cell functions in a transforming growth factor-beta-dependent manner. *J. Exp. Med.* **2005**, *202*, 1075–1085.
87. Ralainirina, N.; Poli, A.; Michel, T.; Poos, L.; Andrès, E.; Hentges, F.; Zimmer, J. Control of NK cell functions by CD4+CD25+ regulatory T cells. *J. Leukoc. Biol.* **2007**, *81*, 144–153.
88. Smyth, M. J.; Teng, M. W.; Swann, J.; Kyparissoudis, K.; Godfrey, D. I.; Hayakawa, Y. CD4+CD25+ regulatory T cells suppress NK cell-mediated immunotherapy of cancer. *J. Immunol.* **2006**, *176*, 1582–1587.
89. Meromsky, L.; Lotan, R.; Raz, A. Implications of endogenous tumor cell surface lectins as mediators of cellular interactions and lung colonization. *Cancer Res.* **1986**, *46*, 5270–5275.
90. John, C. M.; Leffler, H.; Kahl-Knutsson, B.; Svensson, I.; Jarvis, G. A. Truncated galectin-3 inhibits tumor growth and metastasis in orthotopic nude mouse model of human breast cancer. *Clin. Cancer Res.* **2003**, *9*, 2374–2383.
91. Inohara, H.; Raz, A. Effects of natural complex carbohydrate (citrus pectin) on murine melanoma cell properties related to galectin-3 functions. *Glycoconjugate J.* **1994**, *11*, 527–532.
92. Platt, D.; Raz, A. Modulation of the lung colonization of B16-F1 melanoma cells by citrus pectin. *J. Natl. Cancer Inst.* **1992**, *84*, 438–442.
93. Nangia-Makker, P.; Hogan, V.; Honjo, Y.; Baccarini, S.; Tait, L.; Bresalier, R.; Raz, A. Inhibition of human cancer cell growth and metastasis in nude mice by oral intake of modified citrus pectin. *J. Natl. Cancer Inst.* **2002**, *94*, 1854–1862.
94. Delaine, T.; Cumpstey, I.; Ingrassia, L.; Le Mercier, M.; Okechukwu, P.; Leffler, H.; Kiss, R.; Nilsson, U. J. Galectin-inhibitory thiodigalactoside ester derivatives have antimigratory effects in cultured lung and prostate cancer cells. *J. Med. Chem.* **2008**, *51*, 8109–8114.
95. Lin, C. I.; Whang, E. E.; Donner, D. B.; Jiang, X.; Price, B. D.; Carothers, A. M.; Delaine, T.; Leffler, H.; Nilsson, U. J.; Nose, V.; Moore, F. D., Jr.; Ruan, D. T. Galectin-3 targeted therapy with a small molecule inhibitor activates apoptosis and enhances both chemosensitivity and radiosensitivity in papillary thyroid cancer. *Mol. Cancer Res.* **2009**, *7*, 1655–1662.

Chapter 10

Galectins as Novel Targets for the Treatment of Malignant Gliomas

Herwig M. Strik*,[1] and Matthias Ocker[2]

[1]Department of Neurology and Medical School, University of Marburg, Baldingerstrasse, D-35043 Marburg, Germany
[2]Institute for Surgical Research, Medical School, University of Marburg, Baldingerstrasse, D-35043 Marburg, Germany
***E-mail: strik@med.uni-marburg.de**

The treatment of brain tumors is associated with important limitations, not only because complete surgical resection is impossible, but also because blood-brain barrier protects the brain from external substances and is permeable only for small-molecular, lipophilic substances. The most common malignant brain tumors, glioblastomas, are associated with a grim prognosis of approximately 12 months in unselected series. In addition to special aspects associated with their intracranial localization, gliomas have a marked resistance against antiapoptotic stimuli. A high migratory potential, intense neoangiogenesis and a strong immunosuppressive environment also contribute to the usually rapid proliferation in spite of all therapeutic efforts. An ideal anti-glioma compound should be orally available, small-molecular and lipophilic and modulate several or all of the known factors proliferation, apoptosis resistance, angiogenesis and immune escape. Among other molecular factors, carbohydrate-binding galectins -1, -3, -4 and -8 – are known to be expressed in malignant gliomas. Galectin -1 and -3 have been shown to be associated with proliferation, apoptosis-resistance and migration. Effects on angiogenesis and immune escape may also exist. Intra- or extracellular modulation of galectin functions therefore appears to be a promising strategy for the treatment of malignant gliomas.

Introduction

The most common malignant brain tumor, glioblastoma multiforme, is also the most aggressively growing, classified as grade IV by WHO. The median survival in unselected series still does not exceed approx. 12 months (*1*) and 14-17 months in large chemotherapy trials (*2*, *3*). Neither operation nor ionizing irradiation or systemic antineoplastic treatment are able to cure patients suffering from this disease.

Several biological features are known to contribute to the poor response to antineoplastic treatment and aggressive growth of these tumors. One prominent characteristic of gliomas is a marked resistance against apoptosis-inducing stimuli (*4*). Mutations of p53, for example, are found in numerous glioblastomas and cause a deficiency in cell death (*5*). The balance between pro- and antiapoptotic factors, called the apoptotic rheostat, is shifted towards antiapoptotic functions such as upregulation of anti-apoptotic and downregulation of pro-apoptotic members of the B-cell lymphoma 2 (BCL-2) protein family (*6*). A comparison of individual tumors even showed an additional anti-apoptotic shift during the development from primary to recurrent disease. Such mechanisms may contribute to the resistance against radiotherapy or chemotherapy and lead to even increased protection during the course of the disease. Conventional tumor therapy like chemotherapy or ionizing irradiation aims at inducing apoptosis. Therefore, suppression of antiapoptotic stimuli may enhance the effect of such treatments (*7*).

Alkylating agents are most often applied to treat malignant gliomas. ACNU (nimustine), BCNU (carmustine) or CCNU (lomustine) efficiently pass through the blood-brain barrier and have been effective in numerous studies. The combination of ACNU with cytarabinoside (Ara-C) or etoposide (VM26) achieved a median overall survival of approx. 17 months, which is still among the best results in large multicenter trials (*2*). The hematotoxicity observed with these combinations, however, was considerable.

Another alkylating agent, temozolomide, is an orally available imidazotetrazine derivative with good penetration through the blood-brain barrier and favorable toxicity profile. In a large multicenter trial, addition of temozolomide was significantly more effective than radiotherapy alone (*3*).

Ever since this study was published, efforts have been made to further enhance the effect of this chemotherapeutic agent. Dose-dense application of temozolomide aims at depleting MGMT, an important anti-alkylating molecule that is able to revert the effect of temozolomide (*8*). The effect of this strategy, however, is limited and more efficient inhibition of apoptosis-resistance desired.

Another important feature of malignant gliomas is a marked potential for migration and invasion (*9*). Since glioma cells can migrate up to several centimeters from the main tumor localization (*10*), local treatment strategies like surgery or radiotherapy are not able to cure patients. Systemic chemotherapy will probably be less effective in the infiltration zone surrounding the tumor because the blood-brain barrier is intact in this region, as opposed to the main tumor bulk, and migrating cell have a reduced proliferation rate, so a reduced response to radiation and chemotherapy has to be expected (*11*). Inhibition of migration and invasion of glioma cells might therefore enhance the effect of local tumor treatment. For example, matrix metalloproteinases like MMP-2 and -9 and integrins like $\alpha_V\beta_3$ have been shown to markedly influence glioma cell migration (*12*) and might therefore be suitable targets for future therapeutic intervention.

One crucial feature of cells to form a well-functioning tumor tissue is to gain sufficient blood supply. An important role for glioma angiogenesis has been proven for hypoxia-inducible factor-1α (HIF-1α), transforming growth factor beta (TGF-β), basic fibroblast growth factor (bFGF) and – most importantly – vascular endothelial growth factor (VEGF) (*13*). Conversely, anti-angiogenic endostatin is downregulated during the malignant transformation of human gliomas (*14*). After first discouraging results, numerous studies have shown promising results with the anti-VEGF antibody bevacizumab (*15*), proving the importance of this strategy.

A further prominent feature of malignant gliomas is the abundant infiltration with up to 30% of monocytes/microglial cells (*16*) without apparent tumor cell phagocytosis. These monocytic cells may probably be modulated towards chronic inflammatory M2 macrophages. These could promote tumor growth through the production of specific cytokines. Mainly immunosuppressive growth factors like interleukin (IL)-4, IL13 and IL10 have been found in human gliomas, while proinflammatory cytokines like IL12, tumor necrosis factor α (TNFα) or interferon γ (IFN-γ) were absent (*17*). Moreover, other immunosuppressive factors like CD70, HLA-G or HLA-E (*18*, *19*) – and possibly also other, yet unknown factors - contribute to the immune escape of malignant gliomas (*18*, *20*). On the other hand, immune cells are capable of destroying glioma cells after activation *in vitro,* indicating that immune therapies might be effective but seem to be inhibited by the immunosuppressive milieu of gliomas (*21*, *22*).

Biology of Galectins

Galectins are members of the lectin family of proteins with a high affinity to β-galactosides (*23*, *24*). Today, 15 galectin members have been identified that contain highly conserved carbohydrate-recognition domains (CRD) of about 130 amino acids and are divided into three groups based on the structure of the CRD (*25*, *26*). Like other lectins, galectins are commonly expressed in various tissues and exert a variety of biological functions dependent on their ability to bind intracellular and extracellular glycoconjugates, including extracellular matrix components like laminin or fibronectin (*27*).

Physiologically, galectins are expressed in lymphatic (lymph nodes, thymus, spleen) and epithelial tissues (liver, lung, breast) but also on endothelial cells, brain and inflammatory cells like macrophages (*24*). As galectins can be localized in the nucleus and/or the cytoplasm (*28*) as well as on the extracellular cell surface, the biologic effects are heterogeneous, too, ranging from effects on RNA splicing to cell adhesion and survival signaling (*27*, *29–33*). These effects are commonly also linked to oncogenic properties of cells, i.e. enhanced cell proliferation, migration, immune evasion and resistance to apoptotic stimuli (*34*,

35). Consequently, enhanced expression of e.g. galectin-1 and galectin-3 has been observed during cancer development and metastasis (*36*).

During malignant progression, a shift in localization from nucleus to cytoplasm has been described for these galectins, too (*37*). The exact mechanisms, how galectins contribute to malignant transformation and progression are not completely understood but several lines of evidence suggest that galectins can modulate and activate growth-factor related signaling via activation of the Ras-Raf-MAPK and PI3K pathways and regulation of downstream target gene transcription (*38*, *39*). This activation of the survival pathway via MAPK by galectin-3 has also been linked to its anti-apoptotic properties (*40*). Galectin-3 also has homology to the potent anti-apoptotic molecule bcl-2 and is able to block changes in mitochondrial membrane potential, thus preventing cytochrome c release and intrinsic apoptosis induction (*41*, *42*). Interestingly, galectin-3 does also have pro-apoptotic properties indicating a strong context-dependency of this molecule in cancer cells (*43*).

Angiogenesis is considered a hallmark of tumor growth and prerequisite for metastasis. Galectin-3 has been demonstrated to increase motility of endothelial cells and to promote capillary growth by interaction of galectin-3 with integrins and other cell surface molecules (*44–46*). This mechanism is also related to the known functions of esp. galectin-3 during cell adhesion and metastasis formation. Here, overexpression of galectin-3 facilitates adhesion to extracellular matrix components (e.g. fibronectin or laminin) or integrins (*34*, *41*, *47*). In line with this model, high levels of galectin-3 have been detected in patients with metastatic diseases compared to healthy controls (*48*). This leads to enhanced adhesion of cancer cells to endothelial cells, supports the aggregation of tumor cells and prevents anoikis during metastatic spread (*49*, *50*).

Galectins expressed at the cell surface have been attributed immunosuppressive properties by inducing apoptosis in monocytes and T cells (*51*) or suppressing production of IL5 (*52*) and inhibiting differentiation of B cells (*34*, *53–55*). These mechanisms thus contribute to the putative evasion of tumor cells of the immune response. Overall galectins are thus able to promote tumor growth on various levels, i.e. intracellular signaling, extracellular adhesion and matrix interaction and immune surveillance.

Galectins in Malignant Gliomas

Several studies demonstrated an overexpression of galectin-1 and galectin-3 in various malignant glioma cell lines (*56*, *57*) and in specimens from human tumor samples (*58*). Galectin levels correlated significantly with angiogenesis, malignant potential and overall survival of glioma patients (*59–64*). Interestingly, the expression of galectin-1 and galectin-3 is also associated with WHO grading and increases with progression (*65*, *66*).

In experimental settings, inhibition of galectins by siRNA lead to decreased proliferation, invasion and angiogenesis (*67*, *68*). Additionally, knockdown of galectin-1 increased the immune rejection of glioma xenografts and also impaired the endoplasmic reticulum stress response, leading to enhanced sensitivity towards chemotherapy using temozolomide (*69–71*).

Overall, the biological functions related to galectins as well as the currently available experimental and clinical data give a clear rationale for further development of galectin-inhibiting therapy approaches. The distinct roles of galectins on tumor cells, endothelial cells, extracellular stroma components and immune cells gives the opportunity to target and influence several hallmarks of cancer development and progression simultaneously to achieve improved treatment responses and prolonged overall survival for patients with malignant glioma. An ideal compound to modulate galectins in malignant gliomas would be small-molecular and lipophilic in order to pass the blood-brain barrier and orally available to allow for continuous application and combination with other treatment strategies like conventional chemotherapy.

References

1. DeAngelis, L. M.; Burger, P. C.; Green, S. B.; Cairncross, J. G. Malignant glioma: Who benefits from adjuvant chemotherapy? *Ann. Neurol.* **1998**, *44*, 691–695.
2. Weller, M.; Muller, B.; Koch, R.; Bamberg, M.; Krauseneck, P. Neuro-Oncology Working Group 01 trial of nimustine plus teniposide versus nimustine plus cytarabine chemotherapy in addition to involved-field radiotherapy in the first-line treatment of malignant glioma. *J. Clin. Oncol.* **2003**, *21*, 3276–3284.
3. Stupp, R.; Mason, W. P.; van den Bent, M. J.; Weller, M.; Fisher, B.; Taphoorn, M. J.; Belanger, K.; Brandes, A. A.; Marosi, C; Bogdahn, U.; et al. Radiotherapy plus concomitant and adjuvant temozolomide for glioblastoma. *N. Engl. J. Med.* **2005**, *352*, 987–996.
4. Bogler, O.; Weller, M. Apoptosis in gliomas, and its role in their current and future treatment. *Front. Biosci.* **2002**, *7*, e339–353.
5. Ohgaki, H.; Dessen, P.; Jourde, B.; Horstmann, S.; Nishikawa, T.; Di Patre, P. L.; Burkhard, C.; Schuler, D.; Probst-Hensch, N. M.; Maiorka, P. C.; et al. Genetic pathways to glioblastoma: A population-based study. *Cancer Res.* **2004**, *64*, 6892–6899.
6. Strik, H.; Deininger, M.; Streffer, J.; Grote, E.; Wickboldt, J.; Dichgans, J.; Weller, M.; Meyermann, R. BCL-2 family protein expression in initial and recurrent glioblastomas: Modulation by radiochemotherapy. *J. Neurol., Neurosurg. Psychiatry* **1999**, *67*, 763–768.
7. Ocker, M.; Höpfner, M. Apoptosis-Modulating Drugs for Improved Cancer Therapy. *Eur. Surg. Res.* **2012**, *48*, 111–120.
8. Hegi, M. E.; Diserens, A. C.; Gorlia, T.; Hamou, M. F.; de Tribolet, N.; Weller, M.; Kros, J. M.; Hainfellner, J. A.; Mason, W.; Mariani, L.; et al. MGMT gene silencing and benefit from temozolomide in glioblastoma. *N. Engl. J. Med.* **2005**, *352*, 997–1003.
9. Bolteus, A. J.; Berens, M. E.; Pilkington, G. J. Migration and invasion in brain neoplasms. *Curr. Neurol. Neurosci. Rep.* **2001**, *1*, 225–232.

10. Kelly, P. J.; Daumas-Duport, C.; Kispert, D. B.; Kall, B. A.; Scheithauer, B. W.; Illig, J. J. Imaging-based stereotaxic serial biopsies in untreated intracranial glial neoplasms. *J. Neurosurg.* **1987**, *66*, 865–874.
11. Evan, G.; Littlewood, T. A matter of life and cell death. *Science* **1998**, *281*, 1317–1322.
12. Wild-Bode, C.; Weller, M.; Wick, W. Molecular determinants of glioma cell migration and invasion. *J. Neurosurg.* **2001**, *94*, 978–984.
13. Fischer, I.; Gagner, J. P.; Law, M.; Newcomb, E. W.; Zagzag, D. Angiogenesis in gliomas: Biology and molecular pathophysiology. *Brain Pathol.* **2005**, *15*, 297–310.
14. Strik, H. M.; Schluesener, H. J.; Seid, K.; Meyermann, R.; Deininger, M. H. Localization of endostatin in rat and human gliomas. *Cancer* **2001**, *91*, 1013–1019.
15. Kunnakkat, S.; Narayana, A. Bevacizumab in the treatment of high-grade gliomas: An overview. *Angiogenesis* **2011**, *14*, 423–430.
16. Graeber, M. B.; Scheithauer, B. W.; Kreutzberg, G. W. Microglia in brain tumors. *Glia* **2002**, *40*, 252–259.
17. Parney, I. F.; Farr-Jones, M. A.; Chang, L. J.; Petruk, K. C. Human glioma immunobiology in vitro: Implications for immunogene therapy. *Neurosurgery* **2000**, *46*, 1169–1177discussion 1177-1168.
18. Wischhusen, J.; Jung, G.; Radovanovic, I.; Beier, C.; Steinbach, J. P.; Rimner, A.; Huang, H.; Schulz, J. B.; Ohgaki, H.; Aguzzi, A.; et al. Identification of CD70-mediated apoptosis of immune effector cells as a novel immune escape pathway of human glioblastoma. *Cancer Res.* **2002**, *62*, 2592–2599.
19. Wischhusen, J.; Schneider, D.; Mittelbronn, M.; Meyermann, R.; Engelmann, H.; Jung, G.; Wiendl, H.; Weller, M. Death receptor-mediated apoptosis in human malignant glioma cells: Modulation by the CD40/CD40L system. *J. Neuroimmunol.* **2005**, *162*, 28–42.
20. Wiendl, H.; Mitsdoerffer, M.; Hofmeister, V.; Wischhusen, J.; Bornemann, A.; Meyermann, R.; Weiss, E. H.; Melms, A.; Weller, M. A functional role of HLA-G expression in human gliomas: An alternative strategy of immune escape. *J. Immunol.* **2002**, *168*, 4772–4780.
21. Steiner, H. H.; Bonsanto, M. M.; Beckhove, P.; Brysch, M.; Geletneky, K.; Ahmadi, R.; Schuele-Freyer, R.; Kremer, P.; Ranaie, G.; Matejic, D.; et al. Antitumor vaccination of patients with glioblastoma multiforme: A pilot study to assess feasibility, safety, and clinical benefit. *J. Clin. Oncol.* **2004**, *22*, 4272–4281.
22. De Vleeschouwer, S.; Fieuws, S.; Rutkowski, S.; Van Calenbergh, F.; Van Loon, J.; Goffin, J.; Sciot, R.; Wilms, G.; Demaerel, P.; Warmuth-Metz, M.; et al. Postoperative adjuvant dendritic cell-based immunotherapy in patients with relapsed glioblastoma multiforme. *Clin. Cancer Res.* **2008**, *14*, 3098–3104.
23. Leffler, H.; Carlsson, S.; Hedlund, M.; Qian, Y.; Poirier, F. Introduction to galectins. *Glycoconjugate J.* **2004**, *19*, 433–440.
24. Yang, R. Y.; Rabinovich, G. A.; Liu, F. T. Galectins: Structure, function and therapeutic potential. *Expert Rev. Mol. Med.* **2008**, *10*, e17.

25. Barondes, S. H.; Castronovo, V.; Cooper, D. N.; Cummings, R. D.; Drickamer, K.; Feizi, T.; Gitt, M. A.; Hirabayashi, J.; Hughes, C.; Kasai, K.; et al. Galectins: A family of animal beta-galactoside-binding lectins. *Cell* **1994**, *76*, 597–598.
26. Barondes, S. H.; Cooper, D. N.; Gitt, M. A.; Leffler, H. Galectins. Structure and function of a large family of animal lectins. *J. Biol. Chem.* **1994**, *269*, 20807–20810.
27. Liu, F. T.; Patterson, R. J.; Wang, J. L. Intracellular functions of galectins. *Biochim. Biophys. Acta* **2002**, *1572*, 263–273.
28. Davidson, P. J.; Davis, M. J.; Patterson, R. J.; Ripoche, M. A.; Poirier, F.; Wang, J. L. Shuttling of galectin-3 between the nucleus and cytoplasm. *Glycobiology* **2002**, *12*, 329–337.
29. Dagher, S. F.; Wang, J. L.; Patterson, R. J. Identification of galectin-3 as a factor in pre-mRNA splicing. *Proc. Natl. Acad. Sci. U.S.A.* **1995**, *92*, 1213–1217.
30. Hsu, DK; Liu, FT Regulation of cellular homeostasis by galectins. *Glycoconj J* **2004**, *19*, 507–515.
31. Ochieng, J.; Furtak, V.; Lukyanov, P. Extracellular functions of galectin-3. *Glycoconjugate J.* **2004**, *19*, 527–535.
32. Patterson, R. J.; Wang, W.; Wang, J. L. Understanding the biochemical activities of galectin-1 and galectin-3 in the nucleus. *Glycoconjugate J.* **2004**, *19*, 499–506.
33. Wang, J. L.; Gray, R. M.; Haudek, K. C.; Patterson, R. J. Nucleocytoplasmic lectins. *Biochim. Biophys. Acta* **2004**, *1673*, 75–93.
34. Liu, F. T.; Rabinovich, G. A. Galectins as modulators of tumour progression. *Nat. Rev. Cancer* **2005**, *5*, 29–41.
35. Newlaczyl, A. U.; Yu, L. G. Galectin-3: A jack-of-all-trades in cancer. *Cancer Lett.* **2011**, *313*, 123–128.
36. Danguy, A.; Camby, I.; Kiss, R. Galectins and cancer. *Biochim. Biophys. Acta* **2002**, *1572*, 285–293.
37. Sanjuan, X.; Fernandez, P. L.; Castells, A.; Castronovo, V.; van den Brule, F.; Liu, F. T.; Cardesa, A.; Campo, E. Differential expression of galectin 3 and galectin 1 in colorectal cancer progression. *Gastroenterology* **1997**, *113*, 1906–1915.
38. Paz, A.; Haklai, R.; Elad-Sfadia, G.; Ballan, E.; Kloog, Y. Galectin-1 binds oncogenic H-Ras to mediate Ras membrane anchorage and cell transformation. *Oncogene* **2001**, *20*, 7486–7493.
39. Elad-Sfadia, G.; Haklai, R.; Balan, E.; Kloog, Y. Galectin-3 augments K-Ras activation and triggers a Ras signal that attenuates ERK but not phosphoinositide 3-kinase activity. *J. Biol. Chem.* **2004**, *279*, 34922–34930.
40. Takenaka, Y.; Fukumori, T.; Yoshii, T.; Oka, N.; Inohara, H.; Kim, H. R.; Bresalier, R. S.; Raz, A. Nuclear export of phosphorylated galectin-3 regulates its antiapoptotic activity in response to chemotherapeutic drugs. *Mol. Cell Biol.* **2004**, *24*, 4395–4406.
41. Matarrese, P.; Tinari, N.; Semeraro, M. L.; Natoli, C.; Iacobelli, S.; Malorni, W. Galectin-3 overexpression protects from cell damage and death by influencing mitochondrial homeostasis. *FEBS Lett.* **2000**, *473*, 311–315.

42. Yu, F.; Finley, R. L., Jr.; Raz, A.; Kim, H. R. Galectin-3 translocates to the perinuclear membranes and inhibits cytochrome c release from the mitochondria. A role for synexin in galectin-3 translocation. *J. Biol. Chem.* **2002**, *277*, 15819–15827.
43. Califice, S.; Castronovo, V.; Bracke, M.; van den Brule, F. Dual activities of galectin-3 in human prostate cancer: Tumor suppression of nuclear galectin-3 vs tumor promotion of cytoplasmic galectin-3. *Oncogene* **2004**, *23*, 7527–7536.
44. Nangia-Makker, P.; Honjo, Y.; Sarvis, R.; Akahani, S.; Hogan, V.; Pienta, K. J.; Raz, A. Galectin-3 induces endothelial cell morphogenesis and angiogenesis. *Am. J. Pathol.* **2000**, *156*, 899–909.
45. Fukushi, J.; Makagiansar, I. T.; Stallcup, W. B. NG2 proteoglycan promotes endothelial cell motility and angiogenesis via engagement of galectin-3 and alpha3beta1 integrin. *Mol. Biol. Cell* **2004**, *15*, 3580–3590.
46. Markowska, A. I.; Liu, F. T.; Panjwani, N. Galectin-3 is an important mediator of VEGF- and bFGF-mediated angiogenic response. *J. Exp. Med.* **2010**, *207*, 1981–1993.
47. Ochieng, J.; Leite-Browning, M. L.; Warfield, P. Regulation of cellular adhesion to extracellular matrix proteins by galectin-3. *Biochem. Biophys. Res. Commun.* **1998**, *246*, 788–791.
48. Iurisci, I.; Tinari, N.; Natoli, C.; Angelucci, D.; Cianchetti, E.; Iacobelli, S. Concentrations of galectin-3 in the sera of normal controls and cancer patients. *Clin. Cancer Res.* **2000**, *6*, 1389–1393.
49. Khaldoyanidi, S. K.; Glinsky, V. V.; Sikora, L.; Glinskii, A. B.; Mossine, V. V.; Quinn, T. P.; Glinsky, G. V.; Sriramarao, P. MDA-MB-435 human breast carcinoma cell homo- and heterotypic adhesion under flow conditions is mediated in part by Thomsen-Friedenreich antigen-galectin-3 interactions. *J Biol Chem* **2003**, *278*, 4127–4134.
50. Zhao, Q.; Barclay, M.; Hilkens, J.; Guo, X.; Barrow, H.; Rhodes, J. M.; Yu, L. G. Interaction between circulating galectin-3 and cancer-associated MUC1 enhances tumour cell homotypic aggregation and prevents anoikis. *Mol. Cancer* **2010**, *9*, 154.
51. Perillo, N. L.; Pace, K. E.; Seilhamer, J. J.; Baum, L. G. Apoptosis of T cells mediated by galectin-1. *Nature* **1995**, *378*, 736–739.
52. Cortegano, I.; del Pozo, V.; Cardaba, B.; de Andres, B.; Gallardo, S.; del Amo, A.; Arrieta, I.; Jurado, A.; Palomino, P.; Liu, F. T.; et al. Galectin-3 down-regulates IL-5 gene expression on different cell types. *J. Immunol.* **1998**, *161*, 385–389.
53. Liu, F. T. Galectins: A new family of regulators of inflammation. *Clin. Immunol.* **2000**, *97*, 79–88.
54. Acosta-Rodriguez, E. V.; Montes, C. L.; Motran, C. C.; Zuniga, E. I.; Liu, F. T.; Rabinovich, G. A.; Gruppi, A. Galectin-3 mediates IL-4-induced survival and differentiation of B cells: Functional cross-talk and implications during *Trypanosoma cruzi* infection. *J. Immunol.* **2004**, *172*, 493–502.
55. Rabinovich, G. A.; Toscano, M. A.; Ilarregui, J. M.; Rubinstein, N. Shedding light on the immunomodulatory properties of galectins: Novel regulators

of innate and adaptive immune responses. *Glycoconjugate J.* **2004**, *19*, 565–573.

56. Kuklinski, S.; Pesheva, P.; Heimann, C.; Urschel, S.; Gloor, S.; Graeber, S.; Herzog, V.; Pietsch, T.; Wiestler, O. D.; Probstmeier, R. Expression pattern of galectin-3 in neural tumor cell lines. *J. Neurosci. Res.* **2000**, *60*, 45–57.
57. Jung, T. Y.; Jung, S.; Ryu, H. H.; Jeong, Y. I.; Jin, Y. H.; Jin, S. G.; Kim, I. Y.; Kang, S. S.; Kim, H. S. Role of galectin-1 in migration and invasion of human glioblastoma multiforme cell lines. *J. Neurosurg.* **2008**, *109*, 273–284.
58. Strik, H. M.; Kolodziej, M.; Oertel, W.; Basecke, J. Glycobiology in malignant gliomas: Expression and functions of galectins and possible therapeutic options. *Curr. Pharm. Biotechnol.* **2011**.
59. Bresalier, R. S.; Yan, P. S.; Byrd, J. C.; Lotan, R.; Raz, A. Expression of the endogenous galactose-binding protein galectin-3 correlates with the malignant potential of tumors in the central nervous system. *Cancer* **1997**, *80*, 776–787.
60. Yamaoka, K.; Mishima, K.; Nagashima, Y.; Asai, A.; Sanai, Y.; Kirino, T. Expression of galectin-1 mRNA correlates with the malignant potential of human gliomas and expression of antisense galectin-1 inhibits the growth of 9 glioma cells. *J. Neurosci. Res.* **2000**, *59*, 722–730.
61. Strik, H. M.; Deininger, M. H.; Frank, B.; Schluesener, H. J.; Meyermann, R. Galectin-3: Cellular distribution and correlation with WHO-grade in human gliomas. *J. Neurooncol.* **2001**, *53*, 13–20.
62. Camby, I.; Belot, N.; Lefranc, F.; Sadeghi, N.; de Launoit, Y.; Kaltner, H.; Musette, S.; Darro, F.; Danguy, A.; Salmon, I.; et al. Galectin-1 modulates human glioblastoma cell migration into the brain through modifications to the actin cytoskeleton and levels of expression of small GTPases. *J. Neuropathol. Exp. Neurol.* **2002**, *61*, 585–596.
63. Deininger, M. H.; Trautmann, K.; Meyermann, R.; Schluesener, H. J. Galectin-3 labeling correlates positively in tumor cells and negatively in endothelial cells with malignancy and poor prognosis in oligodendroglioma patients. *Anticancer Res.* **2002**, *22*, 1585–1592.
64. Le Mercier, M.; Fortin, S.; Mathieu, V.; Kiss, R.; Lefranc, F. Galectins and gliomas. *Brain Pathol.* **2010**, *20*, 17–27.
65. Camby, I.; Belot, N.; Rorive, S.; Lefranc, F.; Maurage, C. A.; Lahm, H.; Kaltner, H.; Hadari, Y.; Ruchoux, M. M.; Brotchi, J.; et al. Galectins are differentially expressed in supratentorial pilocytic astrocytomas, astrocytomas, anaplastic astrocytomas and glioblastomas, and significantly modulate tumor astrocyte migration. *Brain Pathol.* **2001**, *11*, 12–26.
66. Rorive, S.; Belot, N.; Decaestecker, C.; Lefranc, F.; Gordower, L.; Micik, S.; Maurage, C. A.; Kaltner, H.; Ruchoux, M. M.; Danguy, A.; et al. Galectin-1 is highly expressed in human gliomas with relevance for modulation of invasion of tumor astrocytes into the brain parenchyma. *Glia* **2001**, *33*, 241–255.
67. Strik, H. M.; Schmidt, K.; Lingor, P.; Tonges, L.; Kugler, W.; Nitsche, M.; Rabinovich, G. A.; Bahr, M. Galectin-1 expression in human glioma cells: Modulation by ionizing radiation and effects on tumor cell proliferation and migration. *Oncol. Rep.* **2007**, *18*, 483–488.

68. Fortin, S.; Le Mercier, M.; Camby, I.; Spiegl-Kreinecker, S.; Berger, W.; Lefranc, F.; Kiss, R. Galectin-1 is implicated in the protein kinase C epsilon/vimentin-controlled trafficking of integrin-beta1 in glioblastoma cells. *Brain Pathol.* **2010**, *20*, 39–49.
69. Rubinstein, N.; Alvarez, M.; Zwirner, N. W.; Toscano, M. A.; Ilarregui, J. M.; Bravo, A.; Mordoh, J.; Fainboim, L.; Podhajcer, O. L.; Rabinovich, G. A. Targeted inhibition of galectin-1 gene expression in tumor cells results in heightened T cell-mediated rejection; A potential mechanism of tumor-immune privilege. *Cancer Cell* **2004**, *5*, 241–251.
70. Le Mercier, M.; Mathieu, V.; Haibe-Kains, B.; Bontempi, G.; Mijatovic, T.; Decaestecker, C.; Kiss, R.; Lefranc, F. Knocking down galectin 1 in human hs683 glioblastoma cells impairs both angiogenesis and endoplasmic reticulum stress responses. *J. Neuropathol. Exp. Neurol.* **2008**, *67*, 456–469.
71. Le Mercier, M.; Fortin, S.; Mathieu, V.; Roland, I.; Spiegl-Kreinecker, S.; Haibe-Kains, B.; Bontempi, G.; Decaestecker, C.; Berger, W.; Lefranc, F.; et al. Galectin 1 proangiogenic and promigratory effects in the Hs683 oligodendroglioma model are partly mediated through the control of BEX2 expression. *Neoplasia* **2009**, *11*, 485–496.

Chapter 11

Dynamic Tuning of Galectins and Their Binding Sites During Mammary Tumor Progression and Metastasis

Joana T. de Oliveira and Fátima Gärtner*

Institute of Molecular Pathology and Immunology (IPATIMUP), and Instituto de Ciências Biomédicas de Abel Salazar (ICBAS), University of Porto, Porto, Portugal
***E-mail: fgartner@ipatimup.pt**

Galectins are essentially bridging molecules and as such their biological effect will be dependent on their levels of expression, binding sites availability on their ligands, presence of other competitive galectins or even members of other families of endogenous lectins. Classically, glycosylation patterns were believed to be fairly constant in cells of the same tissue origin and the process was not thought to be a quickly modulated one able to transduce external signals. Nevertheless, a growing amount of data now suggests glycosylation to be a much more dynamic microenvironment-related mechanism. The consequent formation of different glycans alters the array of lectins which are able to recognize them. Therefore, rather discrete and transient changes in interacting glycans, glycan carriers and glycan receptors may profoundly influence the fate of an invasive tumor cell and ultimately its ability to metastasize to distant sites. This mini-review will focus on the dynamic interplay between galectins and their binding sites in a spontaneous model of mammary tumor progression and invasion, canine mammary tumors (CMT).

Introduction

Integrins (*1*), cadherins (*2–7*), caveolins (*8*), metalloproteinases (*9*), hormone receptors (*10*), growth factors (*11*), growth factor receptors (*12*) and mucins (*13*, *14*) putatively modulate the interactions between mammary tumour cells and their surrounding microenvironment, at least in part, by their well-known interplay with galectin-3 *via* its carbohydrate recognition domain [reviewed in (*15*)]. However, the interplay between these ligands and galectin-3 has been shown to be modulated not only by the levels of expression of the lectin but also by differential glycosylation of the ligands in several settings (*16–20*).

Galectins' Levels of Expression: Adapting to Presenting Microenvironments in CMT Progression

Galectin-3 is down-regulated during the process of malignant transformation of canine mammary glands. Its expression being significantly decreased in malignant when compared with benign canine mammary tumors (CMT) (*21*). Galectin-3 is a marker of progression in other types of tumors presenting increased expression in non-aggressive tumors and being reduced in aggressive ones, the opposite having also been observed (*22–25*). Galectin-1 is on the other hand overexpressed in malignant CMT, and found in the nucleus and cytoplasm of tumor cells (*21*). Several examples of dynamic and differential expression of galectins-1 and -3 in physiological and pathological contexts suggesting they play opposing roles can be found in the literature (*26–28*). Among other examples, in lymphoma cells, galectin-1 induces apoptosis while galectin-3 induces cell-cell aggregation (*29*) and blocks the execution of the cell surface apoptotic signal (*30*).

In accordance to its pro-adhesive effects, it comes as no surprise that galectin-3 is highly expressed by vessel-invading tumor cell subpopulations in both primary and metastatic CMT while in well-established metastatic lesions, there is galectin-3 staining almost only in tumor cells surrounding necrotic areas, a pattern resembling that observed in the primary malignant CMT (*21*). On the opposite galectin-1 is down-regulated in tumour emboli and up-regulated in well-established primary and metastatic lesions (unpublished results by the authors of this paper). Accordingly, galectin-1 serum levels are not elevated in cancer patients (*31*) while those of galectin-3 have been found to be increased (*32*).

Cytoplasmic staining of galectin-3 is associated with increased aggressiveness in CMT whereas significant down-regulation of nuclear galectin-3 expression is observed in malignant when compared with benign tumors (*21*). The cytoplasmic subcellular distribution of galectin-3 is an important feature related to malignancy and is suggested to be responsible for increasing apoptosis resistance of tumor cells that migrate and/or are shed into the circulation (*33–35*). Indeed, xenografts from a CMT cell line with an *in vitro* homogeneous cytoplasmic-only expression of galectin-3, quickly metastasize. However, a heterogeneous pattern with specific galectin-3 positive areas is observed in well-established xenografts suggesting a role for microenvironment in the regulation of galectin-3 expression. In primary tumor xenografts, cells staining for galectin-3 were specifically located in necrosis-surrounding regions and tumor emboli, as observed in spontaneously occurring malignant CMT. Likewise, metastatic lesions displayed low galectin-3 expression which was mainly present in necrosis-surrounding areas and inside tumor vessels (*21*).

The reasons why intravascular tumor cells consistently overexpress galectin-3 when compared to sedentary tumor cells still need clarification. However a few hypothesis are to be considered. Galectin-3 is a hypoxia regulated protein (*36*). Hypoxia also leads to activation of epidermal growth factor receptor (EGFR) kinase function and hence may enhance tumor cell migration (*37*, *38*). Interestingly, EGFR expression is up-regulated in CMT intravascular tumor cells and viable cells adjacent to necrotic areas paralleling that of galectin-3. This indicates a possible joint role of EGFR and galectin-3 in the survival and invasion process of tumor cells under stress conditions in malignant CMT (*39*). Adding to that, high level of activity in necrotic areas was found when analyzing EGFR by autoradiography (Berns and Rutteman, unpublished data, Department of Clinical Sciences of Companion Animals, Faculty of Veterinary Medicine, Utrecht University, the Netherlands) and its levels were significantly associated to the presence of necrosis in CMT (*39*).

Since vessel-invading tumor cells express both galectin-3 and EGFR, the hypothesis that tumor cells which intravasate, are mainly those exposed to stress conditions seems very plausible. Furthermore, as galectin-3, EGFR has also been associated to angiogenesis which could in addition aid in providing an escape pathway for these stress-exposed cells (*15*, *40*).

Another line of thinking arises from the fact that galectin-3 expression has been associated to cell differentiation in several contexts (*41*). Epithelial to mesenchymal transition (EMT) has been suggested to be crucial for cells to acquire invasive characteristics, migrate throughout the ECM and ultimately intravasate (*42*, *43*). In the absence of galectin-3 there is decreased TGFβ-induced EMT, myofibroblast activation and collagen production with reduced β-catenin phosphorylation and translocation to the nucleus (*44*). Accordingly, in low galectin-3-expressing malignant CMT, there is little nuclear expression of β-catenin (*45*, *46*). This further points to galectin-3 re-expression being implicated in acquisition of aggressive characteristics in stress-exposed cells, such as those under hypoxic conditions.

Mixed type malignant CMT (carcinosarcomas) present a common histogenesis between epithelial and mesenchymal cells (*47*). These mixed malignant mammary tumours are considered a naturally occurring model of EMT [reviewed in (*48*)]. Galectin-1 was consistently co-expressed with mesenchymal while galectin-3, when present, was co-expressed with epithelial markers in this natural model of EMT (unpublished data). However, the differentiation status of galectin-3-positive intravascular tumor cells could not always be associated with loss or gain of membrane expression of E-cadherin since both E-cadherin-negative and E-cadherin-positive tumor emboli were found in malignant CMT.

Interestingly however, β-catenin expression was often found at the cell membrane, in contact sites between some intravascular tumor cells indicating a correct assembly of the adherens junctions complex at these sites (*21*). Since the hallmark of EMT is loss of E-cadherin expression (*49*), current findings do not support the assumption that all intravascular tumor cells found in CMT have undergone complete EMT and/or the inverse process mesenchymal to epithelial transition (MET) but rather point to the presence of several cells in hybrid states inside vessels (*21*). The isolated expression either of anti-adhesion, lymph node metastasis-associated, glycan Sialyl Lewis X (*50*) or the adherens junction E-cadherin at the cell surface of CMT emboli cells, seems to corroborate this assumption (*51*). Despite this it is the authors' opinion that MET is crucial for cell-cell aggregation inside vessels insuring anoikis survival for the 2% of the circulating tumor cells that in fact successfully arrive at distant sites and metastasize (*52*). Thus overexpression of galectin-3 seems to be a characteristic of potentially metastatic tumor cells in malignant CMT but does not appear to be exclusively associated to a differentiation status.

Glycosylation of Galectin-Ligands: Modulating Galectin-Mediated CMT Cell-Cell Adhesion

Mucins have been associated to malignancy (*13*, *14*, *53*) and are important carriers of tumour-associated glycan antigens (*54*, *55*). Variable glycoforms of MUC1 have been found to be involved in carcinogenesis (*56*, *57*). MUC1 is involved in cell-cell aggregation, (its sialylation being particularly important for the mucin's anti-aggregation effect) (*58*, *59*); and cell-ECM adhesion (*58*, *60*, *61*) in which MUC1 specific O-glycosylation plays a relevant role (*62*). MUC1 is overexpressed and significantly associated to vascular invasion and distant metastases in malignant CMT (*21*, *39*).

In primary tumour cells, the mucin is present in a cytoplasmic vesicular pattern and all around the cell membrane. This high level of MUC1 expression is significantly associated with the above mentioned galectin-3 generalized down-regulation. Furthermore, the two molecules are not co-expressed in primary tumor sedentary cells (*39*). Despite the described overexpression of its well-known ligand, galectin-3-binding sites are expressed at the tumor cell surface only in moderately differentiated tumor areas, their expression being low in the majority of sedentary primary tumor cells. However, in malignant CMT, intravascular tumor cells and tumor vasculature strongly express galectin-3-binding sites pointing to the existence of galectin-3-mediated cell–cell interactions, which could thus facilitate anoikis survival and metastatic spread (*21*, *63*). Interestingly, in these vessel-invading cell tumor subpopulations MUC1 expression is focally localized at the cell membrane where it co-expresses with galectin-3 (*39*).

Different glycosylation patterns of MUC1 mucin in normal mucosa and colon cancer tissues correlate well with galectin-3-binding sites expression (*64*). Sialylation thus acts as an important on/off switch mechanism modifying galectin-3 binding to its ligands during tumor progression in malignant CMT. The differential presence of α2, 6- linked sialic acid in sedentary tumor cells and certain tumor subpopulations, such as invasive fronts, may account for differences observed in galectin-3-binding site expression and modulate galectin-3-mediated adhesion between tumor cells at these locations (*39*). Up- or down-regulating of sialyltransferases is a well-known mechanism of motility tuning, turning galectin-3-binding positive cells into negative ones and *vice-versa*, allowing cells to migrate in a physiological context. Indeed there is an increase of both galectin-1 and -3 binding following alpha 2,6 neuraminidase treatment of glycans at the cell surface *in vitro* (*65*).

The Thomsen-Friedenreich antigen (T antigen) is one of the most common glycoforms of MUC1 found in breast cancer patients. MUC1 interaction with galectin-3 *in vitro* via T antigen, causes clustering of the mucin at the cell surface with consequent exposure of smaller adhesion molecules. This has been proven to increase E-cadherin mediated cell-cell adhesion and ICAM-1 mediated cell-endothelial adhesion (*17*, *66*). A similar effect has been observed for galectins-2, 4 and -8 by interaction with MUC1 *via* T antigen (*31*). Most cells of primary malignant CMT show high levels of sialylated T antigen when compared to the un-substituted form of the antigen which is expressed in low levels and is often negative. However, surprisingly, intravascular tumor cells express mainly the unsubstituted form of the T antigen. This allows a proven physical interaction *in vivo* between galectin-3 and MUC1-carried T antigen, therefore supporting an important role in metastasis (*39*). Alterations in the glycosylation patterns of its ligands, namely increased disialylated core 1 O-glycan structures, have been implied to alter galectin-3 affinity at the cell surface with consequent differences in cell biological behaviour (*67*).

Core 1 biosynthesis is dependent on the activity of core 1 beta1,3 Gal-transferase (*68*) which has been found to be impaired by mutations in the molecular chaperone Cosmc leading to increased expression of Tn and sialyl Tn antigens (*69*). In order to have the unsubstituted core 1 (T antigen), there must not be action of ST6GalNacI and II (*70*). The action of these enzymes leads to the biosynthesis of Sialyl Tn and/or Sialyl-6T antigen. ST6GalNAc-I is the key-enzyme leading to sialyl-Tn biosynthesis in MUC1-Tn glycoform (*71*) while ST6GalNAc-II sialylates better the T antigen (*70*). MUC1 is also a natural carrier of Sialyl Tn (*72*). It is of note that ST6GalNacI and II enzymes perform very fast (*70*). Their subcellular localization has been suggested to influence their activity in breast cancer cells (*73*) as has the tumour microenvironment which was found to importantly modulate Sialyl-Tn expression (*74*).

Galectin-3 has been implicated in the apical sorting of several proteins (*75*) but in the absence of galectin-3 there is still apical targeting of MUC1. However, this can be blocked by overexpression of an alpha 2,6 sialyltransferase (*76*) further corroborating the importance of sialylation in the interplay between MUC1 and the galectins family. In a normal context MUC1 is localized at the apical cell membrane while EGFR is localized basolaterally. MUC1-EGFR interaction in a non-tumour context is a sign of temporary polarization disruption and mediates cell survival programs. These are thought to be persistently present in several types of carcinoma where there is loss of polarization with permanent interaction of transmembrane mucins and growth factor receptors (*77*). In breast cancer cells this interaction is at least in part mediated by galectin-3. *In vitro* and *in vivo* results show the lectin's co-expression with both of its ligands in intravascular tumour cells, further supporting its importance for cell survival in this context (*39*, *78*).

Microenvironment seems therefore to play a vital role in the availability of ligands for galectin-3-binding in CMT. This is corroborated in the CMT metastatic cell line which shows a homogeneous expression of galectin-3-binding sites *in vitro* (*21*) which turns to a heterogeneous one in tumor xenografts (*39*). Also, galectin-3-binding site expression is low in the vast majority of sedentary primary tumor cells to the opposite of invasive fronts where it is high akin to spontaneously occurring CMT. In addition, binding of galectin-3 is again increased, following neuraminidase treatment in galectin-3-binding sites negative areas, resembling the observations in the spontaneous model (*39*). Other than downregulation of sialyltransferases which can at least in part mask galectin-3-ligands in these cells, there may be higher activity in invading tumor cells of specific glycosyltranferases (*79*) some of which responsible for assembling ligands for galectin-3, such as the metastasis-related GnTV and concomitant lower activity of competitive GnTIII, which leads to the production of N-glycans not recognized by the lectin (*80*, *81*) Indeed, recently GnT-III-mediated glycosylation, was found to be altered upon EMT/MET-inducing microenvironment changes (*82*).

Glycosylation of Galectin-Ligands: Modulating Galectin-Mediated CMT Cell-ECM Adhesion

Downregulation of galectin-3-binding sites in the ECM parallels the malignant transformation of canine mammary glands. In fact, galectin-3-binding sites are significantly decreased in the ECM of malignant tissue when compared with that of normal-adjacent glands. In most benign lesions the ECM also presents strong expression of galectin-3-binding sites. A coordinated decrease of galectin-3-binding sites in the ECM may further account for the loss of galectin-3-mediated cell–ECM adhesion in the tumor microenvironment (*21*). The decreased galectin-3 binding to the ECM is attributable, at least in part, to binding sites occupancy by other galectins and altered stromal glycosylation. Although there are substantial differences in the type of glycans recognized by galectins-1 and 3 they often compete for the same ligands (*83*). Galectin-3 affinity for the T antigen, for instance, is two times higher than that of galectin-1 (*84*). These differences might account at least in part for their divergent biological functions.

Galectin-1 is scattered throughout the tumor stroma and could thus be leading to galectin-3-binding site occupancy (*21*). The decrease in galectin-3-binding sites is also most likely due to differential ECM glycosylation in malignant CMT. Sialylation is a prevalent type of glycosylation in tumour cells but not in the ECM of malignant CMT (*85*). However, in normal adjacent mammary tissue, both ECA and PNA bind to matrix glycoproteins in tissue stroma and gland mucus secretion in addition to the apical border of luminal cells while in the ECM of malignant CMT, there is a striking decrease in ECA- and PNA-binding sites pointing to an overall decrease in galactosylation (*21*).

Collagen glycosylation is known to affect tumor cell adhesion to and spreading on collagen IV (*86*). In normal mammary glands, the collagen-galactosylating enzyme, GLT25D1 (*87*), is expressed with slightly higher levels than in benign CMT. However, the enzyme expression levels decrease considerably in malignant CMT (*21*). Galectin-3 knockdown causes a decrease in GLT25D1 mRNA levels *in vitro*. This suggests that downregulation of galectin- 3 may be at least partially responsible for the decreased GLT25D1 mRNA expression levels found in spontaneously occurring malignant CMT (*21*).

Concluding Remarks

Circulating tumour cells (*88*), micrometastases (*89*) and well-established metastases (*90*) may coexist in the patient. In these, changes in the expression of galectins, glycans and the glycoproteins which carry them are at least in part microenvironment related. Galectin-3 has been shown to play a crucial role in cancer drug resistance [reviewed in (*91*)]. Inhibition of galectin-3/T antigen interaction was shown to reduce experimental metastatic disease (*92*). However, other galectins seem to be able to step up and perform its functions. Novel potential specific galectin inhibitors and galectin-targeted therapy are increasingly being studied (*93–95*) but there is an increasing need to broaden their galectin-specter of action and take into account the relevance of the glycosylation status of their ligands in other to achieve therapeutic efficacy.

References

1. Restucci, B.; De Vico, G.; Maiolino, P. Expression of beta 1 integrin in normal, dysplastic and neoplastic canine mammary gland. *J. Comp .Pathol.* **1995**, *113* (2), 165–173.
2. Gama, A.; Paredes, J.; Milanezi, M. F.; Reis-Filho, J. S.; Gärtner, F.; Schmitt, F. C. P-cadherin expression in canine lactating mammary gland. *J. Cell, Biochem.* **2002**, *86* (3), 420–421.
3. Reis, A. L.; Carvalheira, J.; Schmitt, F. C.; Gärtner, F. Immunohistochemical study of the expression of E-cadherin in canine mammary tumours. *Vet. Rec.* **2003**, *152* (20), 621–624.
4. Gama, A.; Paredes, J.; Albergaria, A.; Gärtner, F.; Schmitt, F. P-cadherin expression in canine mammary tissues. *J. Comp. Pathol.* **2004**, *130* (1), 13–20.
5. Sarli, G.; Preziosi, R.; De Tolla, L.; Brunetti, B.; Benazzi, C. E-cadherin immunoreactivity in canine mammary tumors. *J. Vet. Diagnostic Invest.* **2004**, *16*, 542–547.
6. Matos, A. J.; Lopes, C.; Carvalheira, J.; Santos, M.; Rutteman, G. R.; Gärtner, F. E-cadherin expression in canine malignant mammary tumours: Relationship to other clinico-pathological variables. *J. Comp. Pathol.* **2006**, *134* (2–3), 182–189.
7. Nowak, M.; Madej, J. A.; Podhorska-Okolow, M.; Dziegiel, P. Expression of extracellular matrix metalloproteinase (MMP-9), E-cadherin and proliferation-associated antigen Ki-67 and their reciprocal correlation in canine mammary adenocarcinomas. *In vivo* **2008**, *22*, 463–470.

8. Pereira, P. D.; Lopes, C. C.; Matos, A. J.; Cortez, P. P.; Gärtner, F.; Medeiros, R.; Lopes, C. Caveolin-1 in diagnosis and prognosis of canine mammary tumours: Comparison of evaluation systems. *J. Comp. Pathol.* **2010**, *143* (2–3), 87–93.
9. Santos, A.; Lopes, C.; Frias, C.; Amorim, I.; Vicente, C.; Gärtner, F.; Matos, A. Immunohistochemical evaluation of MMP-2 and TIMP-2 in canine mammary tumours: A survival study. *Vet. J.* **2011**, *190* (3), 396–402.
10. Geraldes, M.; Gärtner, F.; Schmitt, F. Immunohistochemical study of hormonal receptors and cell proliferation in normal canine mammary glands and spontaneous mammary tumours. *Vet. Rec.* **2000**, *146* (14), 403–406.
11. Santos, A. A.; Oliveira, J. T.; Lopes, C. C.; Amorim, I. F.; Vicente, C. M.; Gärtner, F. R.; Matos, A. J. Immunohistochemical expression of vascular endothelial growth factor in canine mammary tumours. *J. Comp. Pathol.* **2010**, *143* (4), 268–275.
12. Gama, A.; Gärtner, F.; Alves, A.; Schmitt, F. Immunohistochemical expression of Epidermal Growth Factor Receptor (EGFR) in canine mammary tissues. *Res. Vet. Sci.* **2009**, *87* (3), 432–437.
13. de Oliveira, J. T.; Pinho, S. S.; de Matos, A. J.; Hespanhol, V.; Reis, C. A.; Gärtner, F. MUC1 expression in canine malignant mammary tumours and relationship to clinicopathological features. *Vet. J.* **2009**, *182* (3), 491–493.
14. Tavares, C.; de Oliveira, J. T.; Lopes, C.; Carvalheira, J.; de Matos, A. J.; Rutteman, G. R.; Reis, CA; Gärtner, F. Mucin 6 and Tn antigen expression in canine mammary tumours: Correlation with pathological features. *J. Comp. Pathol.* **2012**, Epub ahead of print; DOI: 10.1016/j.jcpa.2012.03.007.
15. Nangia-Makker, P.; Balan, V.; Raz, A. Regulation of tumor progression by extracellular galectin-3. *Cancer Microenviron.* **2008**, *1*, 43–51.
16. Fry, S. A.; Van den Steen, P. E.; Royle, L.; Wormald, M. R.; Leathem, A. J.; Opdenakker, G.; McDonnell, J. M.; Dwek, R. A.; Rudd, P. M. Cancer-associated glycoforms of gelatinase B exhibit a decreased level of binding to galectin-3. *Biochemistry* **2006**, *45* (51), 15249–15258.
17. Yu, L. G.; Andrews, N.; Zhao, Q.; McKean, D.; Williams, J. F.; Connor, L. J.; Gerasimenko, O. V.; Hilkens, J.; Hirabayashi, J.; Kasai, K.; Rhodes, J. M. Galectin-3 interaction with Thomsen-Friedenreich disaccharide on cancer-associated MUC1 causes increased cancer cell endothelial adhesion. *J. Biol. Chem.* **2007**, *282* (1), 773–781.
18. Goetz, J. G.; Joshi, B.; Lajoie, P.; Strugnell, S. S.; Scudamore, T.; Kojic, L. D.; Nabi, I. R. Concerted regulation of focal adhesion dynamics by galectin-3 and tyrosine-phosphorylated caveolin-1. *J. Cell Biol.* **2008**, *180* (6), 1261–1275.
19. Zhuo, Y.; Chammas, R.; Bellis, S. L. Sialylation of beta1 integrins blocks cell adhesion to galectin-3 and protects cells against galectin-3-induced apoptosis. *J. Biol. Chem.* **2008**, *283*, 22177–22185.
20. Markowska, A. I.; Jefferies, K. C.; Panjwani, N. Galectin-3 protein modulates cell surface expression and activation of vascular endothelial growth factor receptor 2 in human endothelial cells. *J. Biol. Chem.* **2011**, *286* (34), 29913–29921.

21. de Oliveira, J. T.; de Matos, A. J.; Gomes, J.; Vilanova, M.; Hespanhol, V.; Manninen, A.; Rutteman, G.; Chammas, R.; Gärtner, F.; Bernardes, E. S. Coordinated expression of galectin-3 and galectin-3-binding sites in malignant mammary tumors: Implications for tumor metastasis. *Glycobiology* **2010**, *20* (11), 1341–1352.
22. Brown, E. R.; Doig, T.; Anderson, N.; Brenn, T.; Doherty, V.; Xu, Y.; Bartlett, J. M.; Smyth, J. F.; Melton, D. W. Association of galectin-3 expression with melanoma progression and prognosis. *Eur. J. Cancer* **2011**, *48* (6), 865–874.
23. Buljan, M.; Šitum, M.; Tomas, D.; Milošević, M.; Krušlin, B. Prognostic value of galectin-3 in primary cutaneous melanoma. *J. Eur. Acad. Dermatol. Venereol.* **2010**, *25* (10), 1174–1181.
24. Canesin, G.; Gonzalez-Peramato, P.; Palou, J.; Urrutia, M.; Cordón-Cardo, C.; Sánchez-Carbayo, M. Galectin-3 expression is associated with bladder cancer progression and clinical outcome. *Tumour Biol.* **2010**, *31* (4), 277–285.
25. Ege, C. B.; Akbulut, M.; Zekioğlu, O.; Ozdemir, N. Investigation of galectin-3 and heparanase in endometrioid and serous carcinomas of the endometrium and correlation with known predictors of survival. *Arch. Gynecol. Obstet.* **2011**, *284* (5), 1231–1239.
26. Froehlich, R.; Hambruch, N.; Haeger, J. D.; Dilly, M.; Kaltner, H.; Gabius, H. J.; Pfarrer, C. Galectin fingerprinting detects differences in expression profiles between bovine endometrium and placentomes as well as early and late gestational stages. *Placenta* **2012**, *33* (3), 195–201.
27. Gál, P.; Vasilenko, T.; Kostelníková, M.; Jakubco, J.; Kovác, I.; Sabol, F.; André, S.; Kaltner, H.; Gabius, H. J.; Smetana, K., Jr Open wound healing in vivo: Monitoring binding and presence of adhesion/growth-regulatory galectins in rat skin during the course of complete re-epithelialization. *Acta Histochem. Cytochem.* **2011**, *44* (5), 191–199.
28. Kopitz, J.; Ballikaya, S.; André, S.; Gabius, H. J. Ganglioside GM1/galectin-dependent growth regulation in human neuroblastoma cells: Special properties of bivalent galectin-4 and significance of linker length for ligand selection. *Neurochem. Res.* **2012**, *37* (6), 1267–1276.
29. Suzuki, O.; Hirsch, B.; Abe, M.; Dürkop, H.; Stein, H. Galectin-1-mediated cell death is increased by CD30-induced signaling in anaplastic large cell lymphoma cells but not in Hodgkin lymphoma cells. *Lab Invest.* **2012**, *92* (2), 191–199, DOI:10.1038/labinvest.2011.151.
30. Mazurek, N.; Byrd, J. C.; Sun, Y.; Hafley, M.; Ramirez, K.; Burks, J.; Bresalier, R. S. Cell-surface galectin-3 confers resistance to TRAIL by impeding trafficking of death receptors in metastatic colon adenocarcinoma cells. *Cell Death Differ.* **2012**, *19* (3), 523–33, DOI:10.1038/cdd.2011.123.
31. Barrow, H.; Guo, X.; Wandall, H. H.; Pedersen, J. W.; Fu, B.; Zhao, Q.; Chen, C.; Rhodes, J. M.; Yu, L. G. Serum galectin-2, -4, and -8 are greatly increased in colon and breast cancer patients and promote cancer cell adhesion to blood vascular endothelium. *Clin. Cancer Res.* **2011**, *17* (22), 7035–7046.

32. Iurisci, I.; Tinari, N.; Natoli, C.; Angelucci, D.; Cianchetti, E.; Iacobelli, S. Concentrations of galectin-3 in the sera of normal controls and cancer patients. *Clin. Cancer Res.* **2000**, *6* (4), 1389–1393.
33. Califice, S.; Castronovo, V.; Bracke, M.; van den Brûle, F. Dual activities of galectin-3 in human prostate cancer: Tumor suppression of nuclear galectin-3 vs tumor promotion of cytoplasmic galectin-3. *Oncogene* **2004**, *23*, 7527–7536.
34. Glinsky, V. V.; Raz, A. Modified citrus pectin anti-metastatic properties: One bullet, multiple targets. *Carbohydr. Res.* **2009**, *344* (14), 1788–1791.
35. Cheong, T. C.; Shin, J. Y.; Chun, K. H. Silencing of galectin-3 changes the gene expression and augments the sensitivity of gastric cancer cells to chemotherapeutic agents. *Cancer Sci.* **2010**, *101* (1), 94–102.
36. Greijer, A. E.; van der Groep, P.; Kemming, D.; Shvarts, A.; Semenza, G. L.; Meijer, G. A.; van de Wiel, MA; Belien, J. A.; van Diest, P. J.; van der Wall, E. Up-regulation of gene expression by hypoxia is mediated predominantly by hypoxia-inducible factor 1 (HIF-1). *J. Pathol.* **2005**, *206* (3), 291–304.
37. Bockhorn, M.; Jain, R. K.; Munn, L. L. Active versus passive mechanisms in metastasis: Do cancer cells crawl into vessels, or are they pushed? *Lancet Oncol.* **2007**, *8*, 444–448.
38. Wang, X.; Schneider, A. HIF-2alpha-mediated activation of the epidermal growth factor receptor potentiates head and neck cancer cell migration in response to hypoxia. *Carcinogenesis* **2010**, *31*, 1202–1210.
39. de Oliveira, J. T.; de Matos, A. J.; Santos, A. L.; Pinto, R.; Gomes, J.; Hespanhol, V.; Chammas, R.; Manninen, A.; Bernardes, E. S.; Albuquerque Reis, C.; Rutteman, G.; Gärtner, F. Sialylation regulates galectin-3/ligand interplay during mammary tumour progression: A case of targeted uncloaking. *Int. J. Dev. Biol.* **2011**, *55* (7–9), 823–834.
40. Soares, R.; Guo, S.; Gärtner, F.; Schmitt, F. C.; Russo, J. 17 beta-estradiol-mediated vessel assembly and stabilization in tumor angiogenesis requires TGF beta and EGFR crosstalk. *Angiogenesis* **2003**, *6* (4), 271–281.
41. Betka, J.; Plzák, J.; Smetana, K., Jr; Gabius, H. J. Galectin-3, an endogenous lectin, as a tool for monitoring cell differentiation in head and neck carcinomas with implications for lectin-glycan functionality. *Acta Otolaryngol.* **2003**, *123* (2), 261–263.
42. Sethi, S.; Macoska, J.; Chen, W.; Sarkar, F. H. Molecular signature of epithelial-mesenchymal transition (EMT) in human prostate cancer bone metastasis. *Am. J. Transl. Res.* **2010**, *3* (1), 90–99.
43. Ding, W.; You, H.; Dang, H.; LeBlanc, F.; Galicia, V.; Lu, S. C.; Stiles, B.; Rountree, C. B. Epithelial-to-mesenchymal transition of murine liver tumor cells promotes invasion. *Hepatology* **2010**, *52* (3), 945–953.
44. Mackinnon, A. C.; Gibbons, M. A.; Farnworth, S. L.; Leffler, H.; Nilsson, U. J.; Delaine, T.; Simpson, A. J.; Forbes, S. J.; Hirani, N.; Gauldie, J; Sethi, T. Regulation of transforming growth factor-β1-driven lung fibrosis by galectin-3. *Am. J. Respir. Crit. Care Med.* **2012**, *185* (5), 537–546.
45. de Matos, A. J.; Lopes, C. C.; Faustino, A. M.; Carvalheira, J. G.; Rutteman, G. R.; Gärtner, F. E-cadherin, beta-catenin, invasion and lymph

node metastases in canine malignant mammary tumours. *APMIS* **2007**, *115* (4), 327–334.

46. Gama, A.; Paredes, J.; Gärtner, F.; Alves, A.; Schmitt, F. Expression of E-cadherin, P-cadherin and beta-catenin in canine malignant mammary tumours in relation to clinicopathological parameters, proliferation and survival. *Vet. J.* **2008**, *177* (1), 45–53.
47. Gärtner, F.; Geraldes, M.; Cassali, G.; Rema, A.; Schmitt, F. DNA measurement and immunohistochemical characterization of epithelial and mesenchymal cells in canine mixed mammary tumours: Putative evidence for a common histogenesis. *Vet. J.* **1999**, *158* (1), 39–47.
48. Cardiff, R. D. The pathology of EMT in mouse mammary tumorigenesis. *J. Mammary Gland Biol. Neoplasia* **2010**, *15* (2), 225–233.
49. Perl, A. K.; Wilgenbus, P.; Dahl, U.; Semb, H.; Christofori, G. A causal role for E-cadherin in the transition from adenoma to carcinoma. *Nature* **1998**, *392*, 190–193.
50. Pinho, S. S.; Matos, A. J.; Lopes, C.; Marcos, N. T.; Carvalheira, J.; Reis, C. A.; Gärtner, F. Sialyl Lewis x expression in canine malignant mammary tumours: Correlation with clinicopathological features and E-cadherin expression. *BMC Cancer* **2007**, *7*, 124.
51. Pinho, S. S.; Reis, C. A.; Gärtner, F.; Alpaugh, M. L. Molecular plasticity of E-cadherin and sialyl lewis x expression, in two comparative models of mammary tumorigenesis. *PLoS One* **2009**, *4* (8), e6636.
52. Chambers, A. F.; Groom, A. C.; MacDonald, I. C. Dissemination and growth of cancer cells in metastatic sites. *Nat. Rev .Cancer* **2002**, *2*, 563–572.
53. Reis, C. A.; David, L.; Carvalho, F.; Mandel, U.; de Bolós, C.; Mirgorodskaya, E.; Clausen, H.; Sobrinho-Simões, M. Immunohistochemical study of the expression of MUC6 mucin and co-expression of other secreted mucins (MUC5AC and MUC2) in human gastric carcinomas. *J. Histochem. Cytochem.* **2000**, *48* (3), 377–388.
54. Carvalho, F.; David, L.; Aubert, J. P.; López-Ferrer, A.; De Bolós, C.; Reis, C. A.; Gärtner, F.; Peixoto, A.; Alves, P.; Sobrinho-Simões, M. Mucins and mucin-associated carbohydrate antigens expression in gastric carcinoma cell lines. *Virchows Arch.* **1999**, *435* (5), 479–485.
55. Pinto, R.; Carvalho, A. S.; Conze, T.; Magalhães, A.; Picco, G.; Burchell, J. M.; Taylor-Papadimitriou, J.; Reis, C. A.; Almeida, R.; Mandel, U.; Clausen, H.; Söderberg, O.; David, L. Identification of new cancer biomarkers based on aberrant mucin glycoforms by in situ proximity ligation. *J. Cell. Mol. Med.* **2011**, DOI:10.1111/j.1582-4934.2011.01436.x.
56. Reis, C. A.; David, L.; Seixas, M.; Burchell, J.; Sobrinho-Simões, M. Expression of fully and under-glycosylated forms of MUC1 mucin in gastric carcinoma. *Int. J. Cancer* **1998**, *79* (4), 402–410.
57. Santos-Silva, F.; Fonseca, A.; Caffrey, T.; Carvalho, F.; Mesquita, P.; Reis, C.; Almeida, R.; David, L.; Hollingsworth, M. A. Thomsen-Friedenreich antigen expression in gastric carcinomas is associated with MUC1 mucin VNTR polymorphism. *Glycobiology* **2005**, *15* (5), 511–517.
58. Ligtenberg, M. J.; Buijs, F.; Vos, H. L.; Hilkens, J. Suppression of cellular aggregation by high levels of episialin. *Cancer Res* **1992**, *52* (8), 2318–2324.

59. Wesseling, J.; van der Valk, S. W.; Hilkens, J A mechanism for inhibition of E-cadherin-mediated cell-cell adhesion by the membrane-associated mucin episialin/MUC1. *Mol. Biol. Cell* **1996**, *7* (4), 565–577.
60. Wesseling, J.; van der Valk, S. W.; Vos, H. L.; Sonnenberg, A.; Hilkens, J. Episialin (MUC1) overexpression inhibits integrin-mediated cell adhesion to extracellular matrix components. *J .Cell. Biol.* **1995**, *129* (1), 255–265.
61. Kondo, K.; Kohno, N.; Yokoyama, A.; Hiwada, K. Decreased MUC1 expression induces E-cadherin-mediated cell adhesion of breast cancer cell lines. *Cancer Res.* **1998**, *58* (9), 2014–2019.
62. Satoh, S.; Hinoda, Y.; Hayashi, T.; Burdick, M. D.; Imai, K.; Hollingsworth, M. A. Enhancement of metastatic properties of pancreatic cancer cells by MUC1 gene encoding an anti-adhesion molecule. *Int. J. Cancer* **2000**, *88* (4), 507–518.
63. Inohara, H.; Raz, A. Functional evidence that cell surface galectin-3 mediates homotypic cell adhesion. *Cancer Res.* **1995**, *55* (15), 3267–3271.
64. Saeland, E.; Belo, A. I.; Mongera, S.; van Die, I.; Meijer, G. A.; van Kooyk, Y. Differential glycosylation of MUC1 and CEACAM5 between normal mucosa and tumour tissue of colon cancer patients. *Int. J .Cancer* **2011**, *131* (1), 117–128, DOI:10.1002/ijc.26354.
65. Stowell, S. R.; Arthur, C. M.; Mehta, P.; Slanina, K. A.; Blixt, O.; Leffler, H.; Smith, D. F.; Cummings, R. D. Galectin-1, -2, and -3 exhibit differential recognition of sialylated glycans and blood group antigens. *J. Biol. Chem.* **2008**, *283* (15), 10109–10123.
66. Zhao, Q.; Guo, X.; Nash, G. B.; Stone, P. C.; Hilkens, J.; Rhodes, J. M.; Yu, L. G. Circulating galectin-3 promotes metastasis by modifying MUC1 localization on cancer cell surface. *Cancer Res.* **2009**, *69*, 6799–6806.
67. Antonopoulos, A.; Demotte, N.; Stroobant, V.; Haslam, S. M.; van der Bruggen, P.; Dell, A. Loss of effector function of human cytolytic T lymphocytes is accompanied by major alterations in N- and O-glycosylation. *J. Biol. Chem.* **2012**, *287* (14), 11240–11251.
68. Brockhausen, I.; Yang, J.; Dickinson, N.; Ogata, S.; Itzkowitz, S. H. Enzymatic basis for sialyl-Tn expression in human colon cancer cells. *Glycoconjugate J.* **1998**, *15* (6), 595–603.
69. Ju, T.; Lanneau, G. S.; Gautam, T.; Wang, Y.; Xia, B.; Stowell, S. R.; Willard, M. T.; Wang, W.; Xia, J. Y.; Zuna, R. E.; Laszik, Z.; Benbrook, D. M.; Hanigan, M. H.; Cummings, R. D. Human tumor antigens Tn and sialyl Tn arise from mutations in Cosmc. *Cancer Res.* **2008**, *68* (6), 1636–1646.
70. Marcos, N. T.; Pinho, S.; Grandela, C.; Cruz, A.; Samyn-Petit, B.; Harduin-Lepers, A.; Almeida, R.; Silva, F.; Morais, V.; Costa, J; Kihlberg, J.; Clausen, H.; Reis, C. A. Role of the human ST6GalNAc-I and ST6GalNAc-II in the synthesis of the cancer-associated sialyl-Tn antigen. *Cancer Res.* **2004**, *64* (19), 7050–7057.
71. Marcos, N. T.; Bennett, E. P.; Gomes, J.; Magalhaes, A.; Gomes, C.; David, L.; Dar, I.; Jeanneau, C.; DeFrees, S.; Krustrup, D.; Vogel, L. K.; Kure, E. H.; Burchell, J.; Taylor-Papadimitriou, J.; Clausen, H.; Mandel, U.; Reis, C. A. ST6GalNAc-I controls expression of sialyl-Tn antigen in gastrointestinal tissues. *Front. Biosci. (Elite Ed)* **2011**, *3*, 1443–1455.

72. Burdick, M. D.; Harris, A.; Reid, C. J.; Iwamura, T.; Hollingsworth, M. A. Oligosaccharides expressed on MUC1 produced by pancreatic and colon tumor cell lines. *J. Biol. Chem.* **1997**, *272* (39), 24198–24202.
73. Sewell, R.; Bäckström, M.; Dalziel, M.; Gschmeissner, S.; Karlsson, H.; Noll, T.; Gätgens, J.; Clausen, H.; Hansson, G. C.; Burchell, J.; Taylor-Papadimitriou, J. The ST6GalNAc-I sialyltransferase localizes throughout the Golgi and is responsible for the synthesis of the tumor-associated sialyl-Tn O-glycan in human breast cancer. *J. Biol. Chem.* **2006**, *281* (6), 3586–3594.
74. Brockhausen, I.; Yang, J.; Lehotay, M.; Ogata, S.; Itzkowitz, S. Pathways of mucin O-glycosylation in normal and malignant rat colonic epithelial cells reveal a mechanism for cancer-associated Sialyl-Tn antigen expression. *Biol. Chem.* **2001**, *382* (2), 219–232.
75. Mattila, P. E.; Youker, R. T.; Mo, D.; Bruns, J. R.; Cresawn, K. O.; Hughey, R. P.; Ihrke, G.; Weisz, O. A. Multiple biosynthetic trafficking routes for apically secreted proteins in MDCK cells. *Traffic* **2012**, *13* (3), 433–442, DOI:10.1111/j.1600-0854.2011.01315.x.
76. Kinlough, C. L.; Poland, P. A.; Gendler, S. J.; Mattila, P. E.; Mo, D.; Weisz, O. A.; Hughey, R. P. Core-glycosylated mucin-like repeats from MUC1 are an apical targeting signal. *J. Biol. Chem.* **2011**, *286* (45), 39072–39081.
77. Kufe, D. W. Mucins in cancer: Function, prognosis and therapy. *Nat. Rev. Cancer* **2009**, *9*, 874–885.
78. Ramasamy, S.; Duraisamy, S.; Barbashov, S.; Kawano, T.; Kharbanda, S.; Kufe, D. The MUC1 and galectin-3 oncoproteins function in a microRNA-dependent regulatory loop. *Mol. Cell.* **2007**, *27*, 992–1004.
79. Gomes, J.; Marcos, N. T.; Berois, N.; Osinaga, E.; Magalhães, A.; Pinto-de-Sousa, J.; Almeida, R.; Gärtner, F.; Reis, C. A. Expression of UDP-N-acetyl-D-galactosamine: Polypeptide N-acetylgalactosaminyltransferase-6 in gastric mucosa, intestinal metaplasia, and gastric carcinoma. *J. Histochem. Cytochem.* **2009**, *57* (1), 79–86.
80. Nangia-Makker, P.; Honjo, Y.; Sarvis, R.; Akahani, S.; Hogan, V.; Pienta, K. J.; Raz, A. Galectin-3 induces endothelial cell morphogenesis and angiogenesis. *Am. J. Pathol.* **2000**, *156* (3), 899–909.
81. Pinho, S. S.; Reis, C. A.; Paredes, J.; Magalhães, A. M.; Ferreira, A. C.; Figueiredo, J.; Xiaogang, W.; Carneiro, F.; Gärtner, F.; Seruca, R. The role of N-acetylglucosaminyltransferase III and V in the post-transcriptional modifications of E-cadherin. *Hum. Mol. Genet.* **2009**, *18* (14), 2599–2608.
82. Pinho, S. S.; Oliveira, P.; Cabral, J.; Carvalho, S.; Huntsman, D.; Gärtner, F.; Seruca, R.; Reis, C. A.; Oliveira, C. Loss and recovery of Mgat3 and GnT-III mediated E-cadherin N-glycosylation is a mechanism involved in epithelial-mesenchymal-epithelial transitions. *PLoS One* **2012**, *7* (3), e33191.
83. Song, X.; Xia, B.; Stowell, S. R.; Lasanajak, Y.; Smith, D. F.; Cummings, R. D. Novel fluorescent glycan microarray strategy reveals ligands for galectins. *Chem. Biol.* **2009**, *16* (1), 36–47.
84. Bian, C. F.; Zhang, Y.; Sun, H.; Li, D. F.; Wang, D. C. Structural basis for distinct binding properties of the human galectins to Thomsen-Friedenreich antigen. *PLoS One* **2011**, *6* (9), e25007.

85. Pinho, S. S.; Osório, H.; Nita-Lazar, M.; Gomes, J.; Lopes, C.; Gärtner, F.; Reis, C. A. Role of E-cadherin N-glycosylation profile in a mammary tumour model. *Biochem. Biophys. Res. Commun.* **2009**, *379*, 1091–1096.
86. Lauer-Fields, J. L.; Malkar, N. B.; Richet, G.; Drauz, K.; Fields, G. B. Melanoma cell CD44 interaction with the alpha 1(IV)1263-1277 region from basement membrane collagen is modulated by ligand glycosylation. *J. Biol. Chem.* **2003**, *278* (16), 14321–14330.
87. Schegg, B.; Hülsmeier, A. J.; Rutschmann, C.; Maag, C.; Hennet, T. Core glycosylation of collagen is initiated by two beta (1-O) galactosyltransferases. *Mol. Cell. Biol.* **2009**, *29*, 943–952.
88. da Costa, A.; Oliveira, J. T.; Gärtner, F.; Kohn, B.; Gruber, A. D.; Klopfleisch, R. Potential markers for detection of circulating canine mammary tumor cells in the peripheral blood. *Vet. J.* **2011**, *190* (1), 165–168.
89. Matos, A. J.; Faustino, A. M.; Lopes, C.; Rutteman, G. R.; Gärtner, F. Detection of lymph node micrometastases in malignant mammary tumours in dogs by cytokeratin immunostaining. *Vet. Rec.* **2006**, *158* (18), 626–30.
90. Misdorp, W. Tumours of the Mammary Gland. In *Tumours in Domestic Animals*, 4th ed.; Meuten, D. J., Ed.; Iowa State Press: Ames, IA, 2002; pp 575–606.
91. Turner, J. G.; Dawson, J; Sullivan, D. M. Nuclear export of proteins and drug resistance in cancer. *Biochem. Pharmacol.* **2012**, *83* (8), 1021–1032.
92. Glinskii, O. V.; Sud, S.; Mossine, V. V.; Mawhinney, T. P.; Anthony, D. C.; Glinsky, G. V.; Pienta, K. J.; Glinsky, V. V. Inhibition of Prostate cancer bone metastasis by synthetic TF antigen mimic/galectin-3 inhibitor lactulose-l-leucine. *Neoplasia* **2012**, *14* (1), 65–73.
93. Collins, P. M.; Oberg, C. T.; Leffler, H.; Nilsson, U. J.; Blanchard, H. Taloside inhibitors of galectin-1 and galectin-3. *Chem. Biol. Drug Des.* **2012**,, *79* (3), 339–346, DOI:10.1111/j.1747-0285.2011.01283.x.
94. Yang, Y.; Zhou, Z.; He, S.; Fan, T.; Jin, Y.; Zhu, X.; Chen, C.; Zhang, Z. R.; Huang, Y. Treatment of prostate carcinoma with (galectin-3)-targeted HPMA copolymer-(G3-C12)-5-Fluorouracil conjugates. *Biomaterials* **2012**, *33* (7), 2260–2271.
95. Kopansky, E.; Shamay, Y.; David, A. Peptide-directed HPMA copolymer-doxorubicin conjugates as targeted therapeutics for colorectal cancer. *J. Drug Target* **2011**, *19* (10), 933–943.

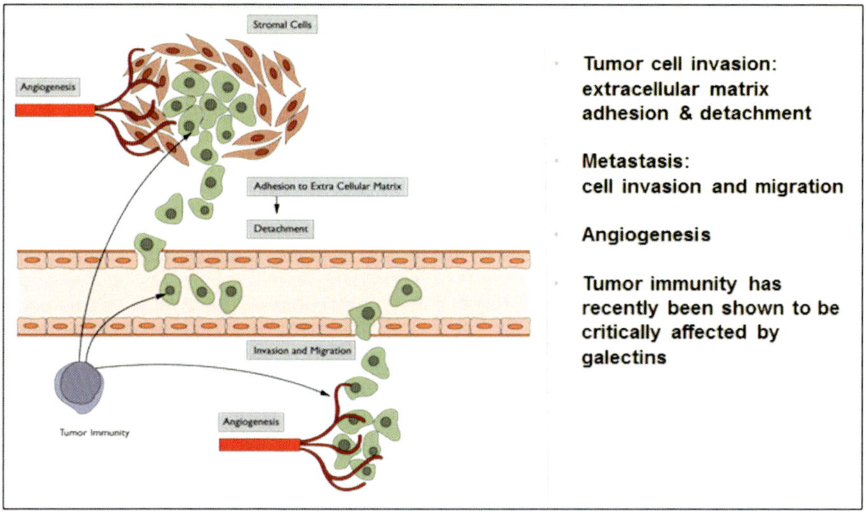

Figure 2. The major areas in cancer biology where galectins may function in the extracellular environment. (Chapter 1)

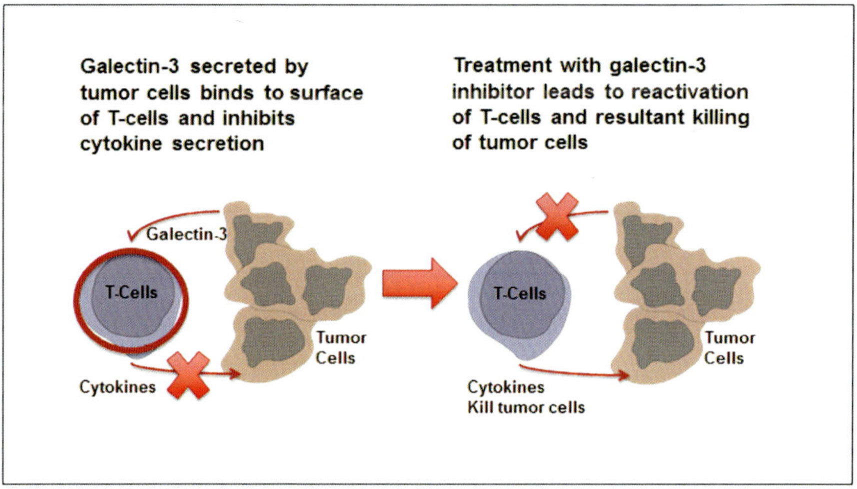

Figure 3. The "galectin effect", illustrating the hypothesis that tumor-secreted galectin-3 binds to cytotoxic T cells and renders them anergic, unable to kill tumor cells. (Chapter 1)

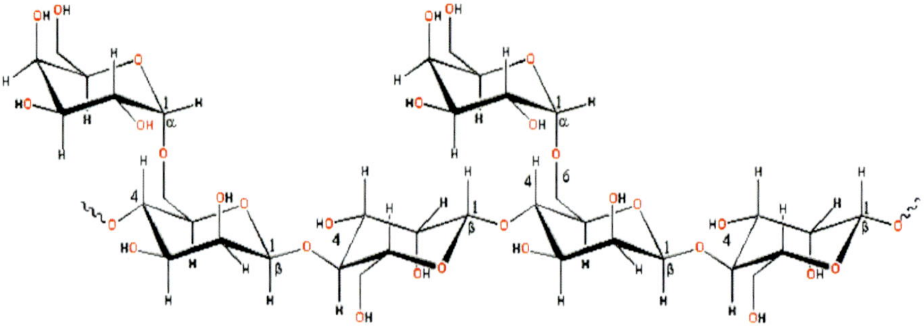

Figure 4. Structure of the basic repeating building block of DAVANAT. Each DAVANAT® molecule consists of 54 such units (ref 119). (Chapter 1)

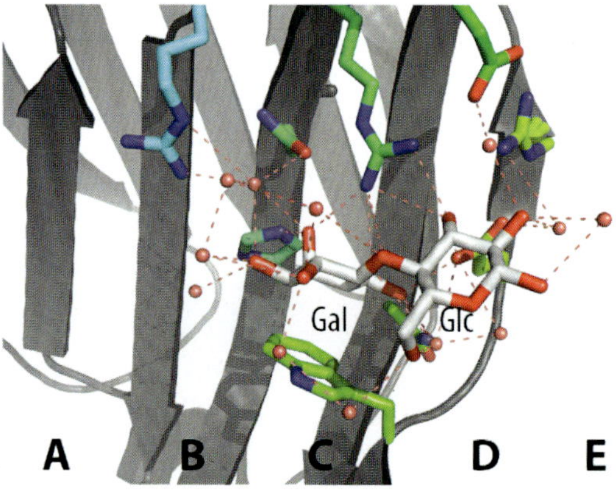

Figure 1. An ultra-high resolution (0.86Å) X-ray structure of galectin-3 in complex with lactose (ref 10) showing the core β-D-galactoside situated in sub-site C and the D-glucose in sub-site D. Sub-sites A-B and E protrudes beyond gal-HO3 and glc-HO1, respectively, and are unoccupied. (Chapter 2)

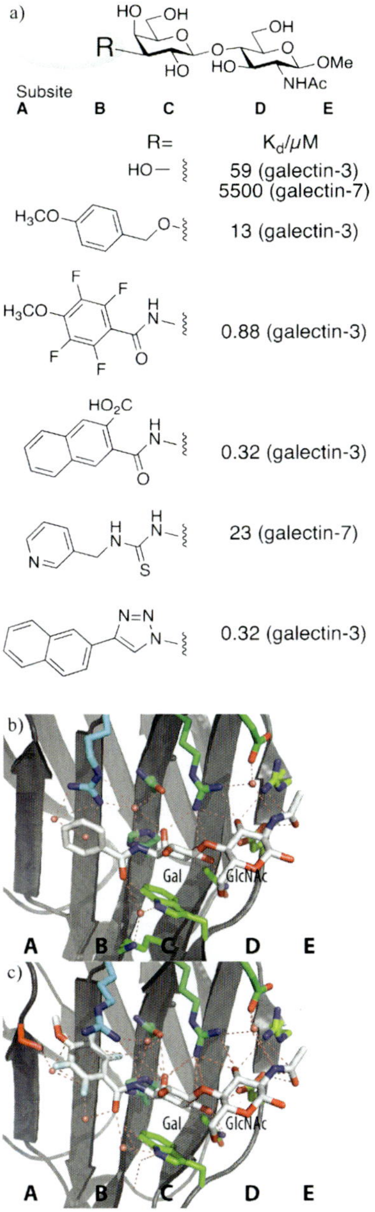

Figure 2. a) Derivatives of N-acetyllactosamine carrying aromatic moieties at O3′ or C3′ interacting favorably in galectin sub-sites A-B. K_d values are determined by a competitive fluorescence polarization assay (refs 11, 12). X-ray structure of galectin-3 co-crystallized with a b) 3′-benzamido-LacNAc derivative (ref 10) and a c) 3′-(2,3,5,6-tetrafluoro-4-methoxy)-benzamido-LacNAc derivative (ref 13) (Chapter 2).

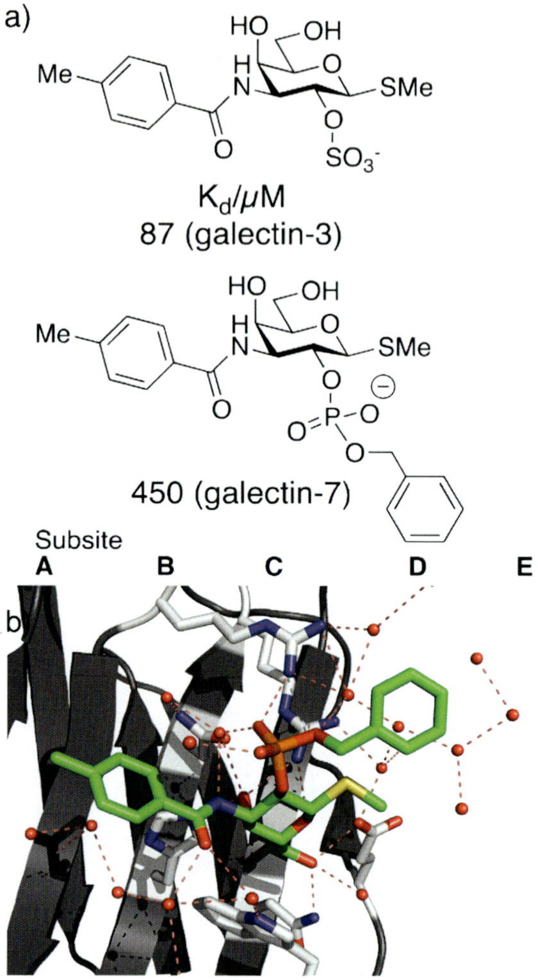

Figure 7. a) 2,3-Disubstituted galactosides interacting with sub-sites perpendicular to the A-E sub-sites. b) A 2-O-benzylphosphate in complex with galectin-7. (Chapter 2)

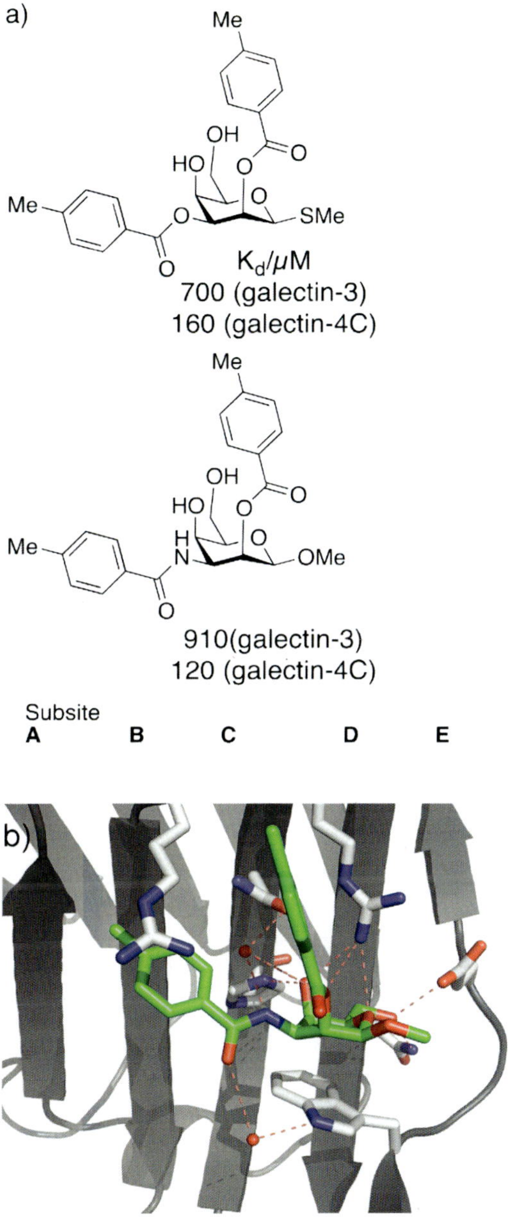

Figure 8. a) 2,3-Disubstituted talosides interacting with sub-sites perpendicular to the A-E sub-sites. b) A 2,3-disubstituted taloside in complex with galectin-3. (Chapter 2)

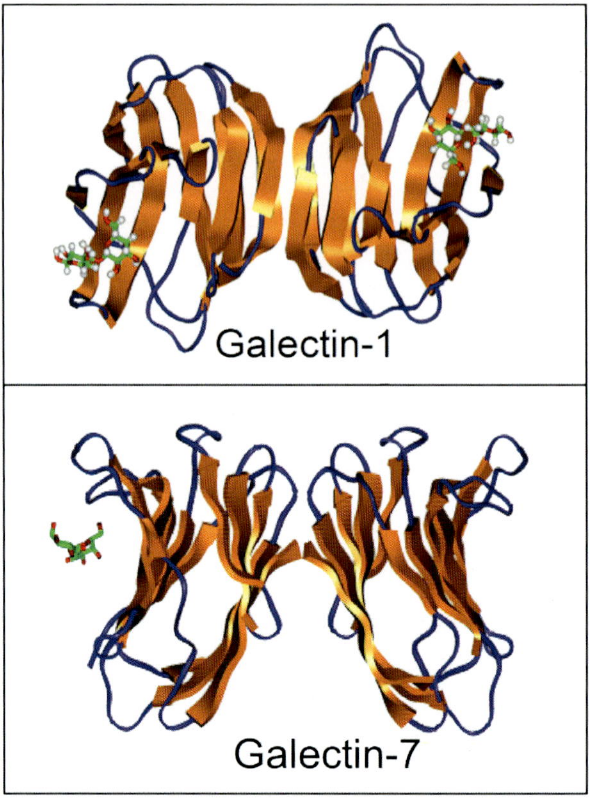

Figure 1. The structure of prototype galectin-1 dimer (PDB access code 1gzw) (upper panel) and prototype galectin-7 dimer (PDB access code 1bkz) (lower panel). The carbohydrate binding site in each monomer subunit (upper panel) or in one of the monomer subunits in the dimer (lower panel) is indicated by a lactose molecule shown as a ball-and-stick structure in green. (Chapter 3)

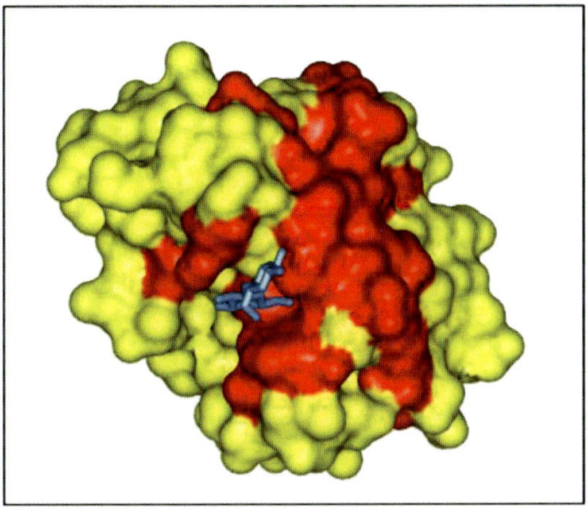

Figure 2. A space filling model of the surface of galectin-1 (PDB access code 1gzw) is shown in yellow, with the anginex interaction site in red, and a molecule of lactose at its binding site in blue (Nesmelova et al, unpublished results). (Chapter 3)

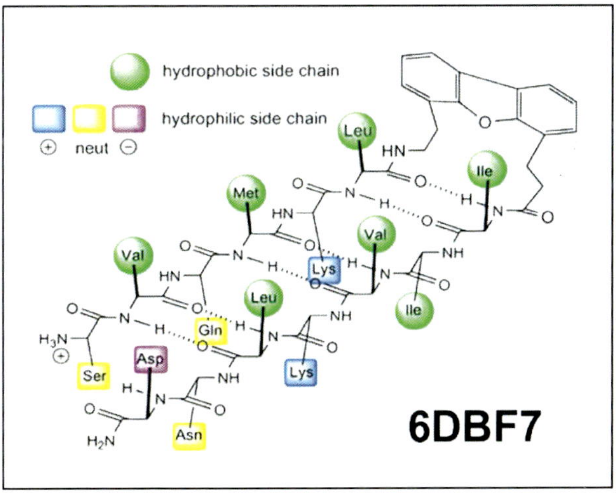

Figure 3. A cartoon structure of 6DBF7. The dibenzofuran moiety is shown head-on at the top right, and polar residues on the hydrophilic side of the amphipathic β-sheet are highlighted with squares and non-polar residues on the hydrophobic side of the amphipathic β-sheet are highlighted with circles. (Chapter 3)

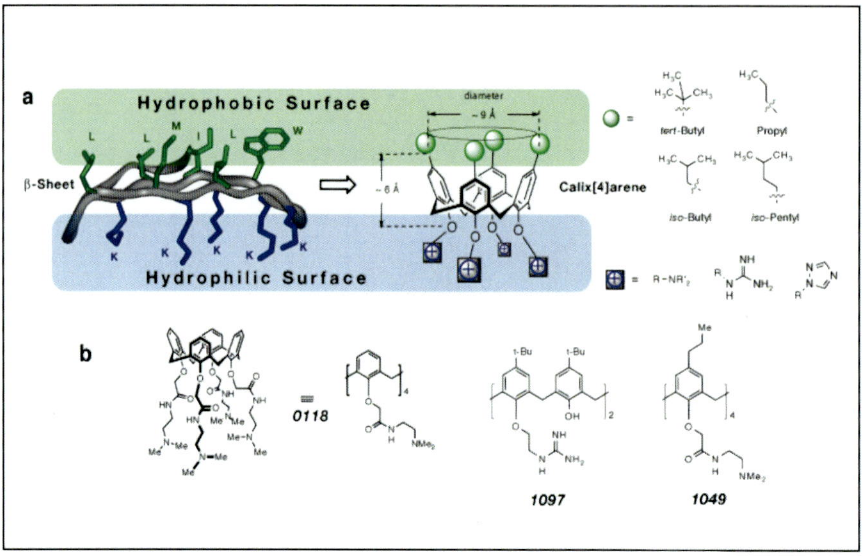

Figure 4. (A) The design concept for β-sheet topomimetics of anginex is shown, with topological features influencing the choice of the calix[4]arene scaffold for arraying hydrophobic and hydrophilic substituents to mimic the structural and compositional characteristics of anginex. In the folded structure of anginex, hydrophobic and hydrophilic surfaces, as well as specific amino acid residues in one letter code, are indicated. The calix[4]arene scaffold is shown to scale, and hydrophobic (t-Bu = tert-butyl; Me = methyl) and basic group chemical substituents that were used on the two faces of the calix[4]arene scaffold are indicated. (B) Two structural representations of the tetra-amine compound 0118 and two related analogs, diguanidine 1097 and inactive tetraamine 1049 are shown. (Chapter 3)

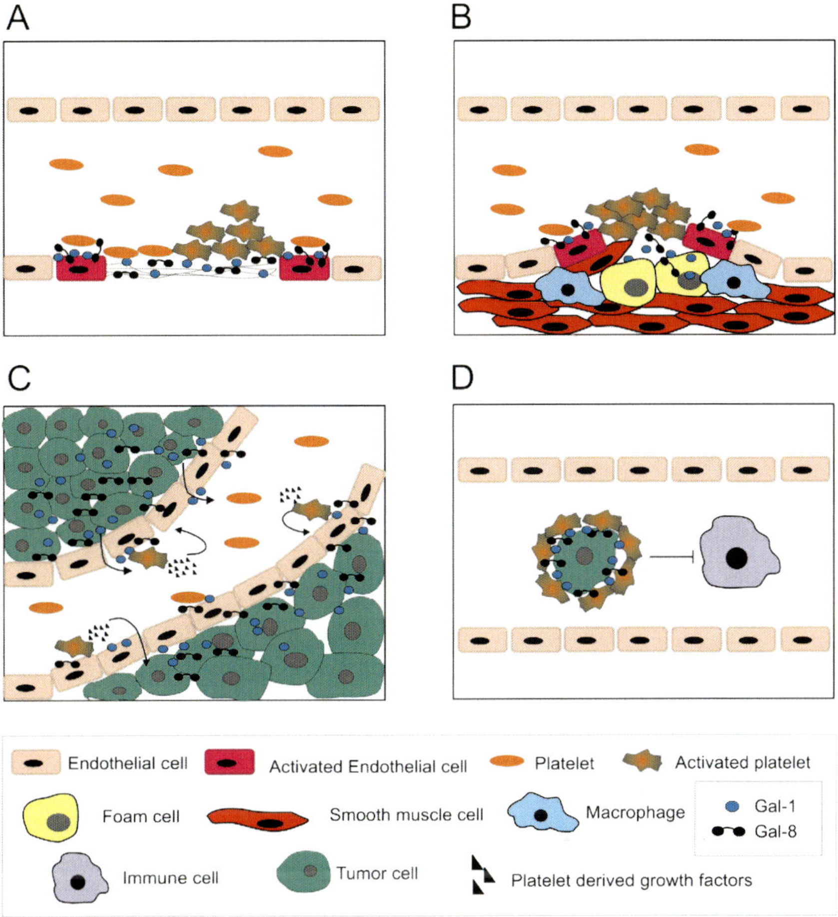

Figure 1. Potential Galectins roles in physiopathological platelet responses. A- When endothelial injury occurs, platelets could recognize Gal-1 and Gal-8 present in the surface of activated endothelial cells and in the exposed subendothelial extracellular matrix. Galectins would be able to trigger platelet adhesion, spreading and thrombus formation. B- Galectins might be involved in atheroma plaque formation and progression. When plaque rupture occurs platelets may bind to galectins present in the plaque and in the activated endothelium thus enhancing thrombus formation. C- Tumor cells overexpress Gal-1 and Gal-8. The lectins are released or exposed in the tumor cell surface and this might activate platelets which release the content of their granules that is rich in growth factors that can promote tumor development and angiogenesis. D- A circulating tumor cell that express Gal-1 and Gal-8 on its surface can bind platelets, thus forming heterotypic aggregates which may possibly protect tumor cells against immune attack, favouring metastasis. (Chapter 5)

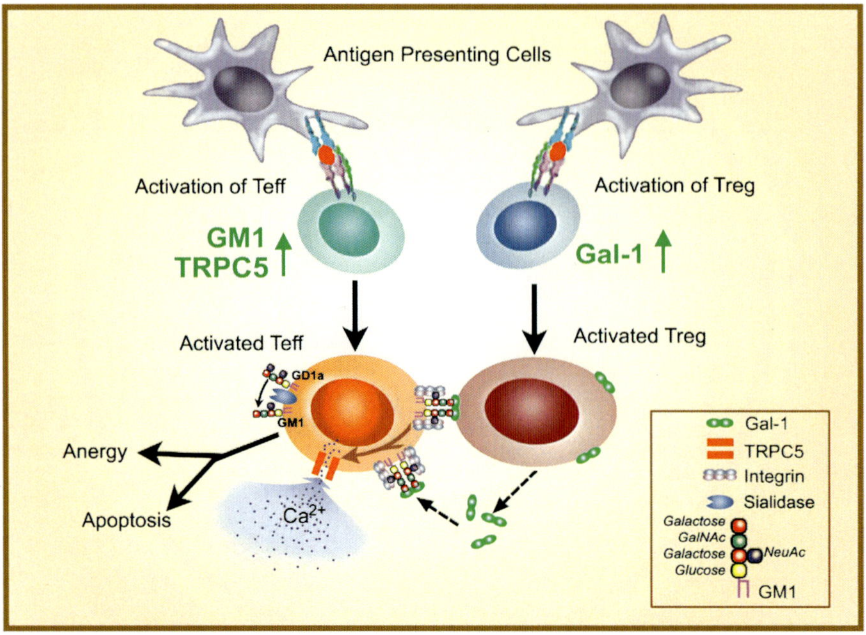

Figure 4. Schematic illustration of inter-T cell communication after activation of effector/regulatory T cells (Teff/Treg) via ganglioside GM1/galectin-1 contact. T cell receptor activation of regulatory T cell (Treg) by antigen presenting cells causes upregulation of galectin-1 (Gal-1) that is expressed on the Treg cell surface and released into the surroundings. As a homodimer it cross-links GM1 which has been elevated through sialidase reaction (and possibly de novo synthesis) in the plasma membrane of Teff following activation of the latter. This induces co-cross-linking of heterodimeric integrin, which is associated with GM1, and this in turn induces a signaling sequence resulting in activation of TRPC5 Ca^{2+} channels. Elevated intracellular Ca^{2+} in Teffs prevents proliferation through anergy and/or apoptosis. Reprinted with permission from the New York Academy of Sciences (Ledeen et al. 2012. Beyond glycoproteins as galectin counterreceptors: Tumor-effector T cell growth control via ganglioside GM1. Ann NY Acad Sciences. 1253:206-221). (Chapter 6)

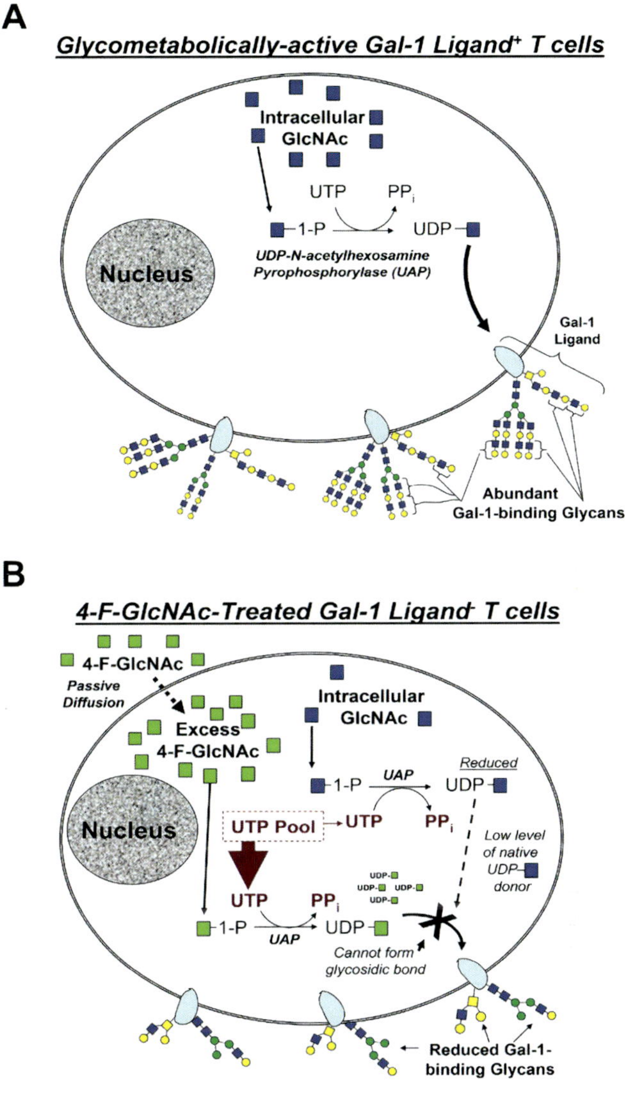

Figure 1. Mechanism of Peracetylated 4-Fluorinated Glucosamine Anti-Carbohydrate Action. (A) T cells actively synthesizing cell surface glycoconjugates are sensitive to glyco-metabolic antagonists, such as fully acetylated 4-F-GlcNAc. (B) Following passive cellular entry and deacetylation of peracetylated 4-fluorinated-glucosamine, 4-F-GlcNAc is phosphorylated and conjugated to UTP by UDP-acetylglucosamine pyrophosphorylase (UAP). Depending on the cytosolic concentration of 4-F-GlcNAc, endogenous UDP-GlcNAc levels are compromised due to sequestration of UTP. This shunting effect causes reductions in N-acetyllactosamines necessary for extending and branching of N- and O-glycan antennae characteristically bound by Gal-1. (Chapter 7)

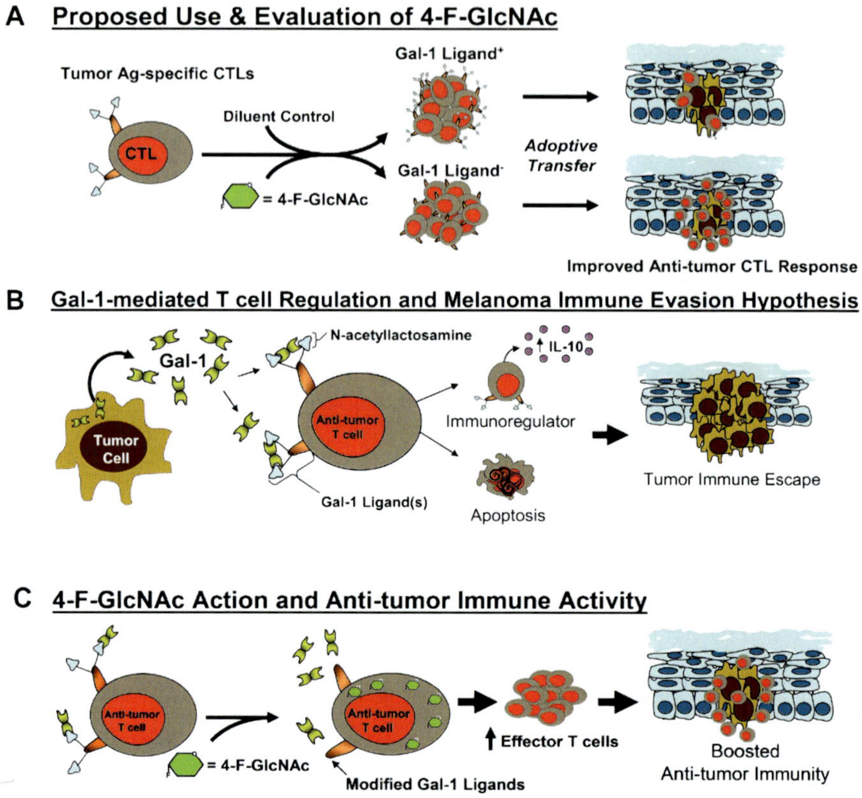

Figure 2. Neutralization of the Gal-1 – Gal-1 ligand axis to Boost Anti-tumor T cell Immunity. (A) A schematic depiction of tumor immune evasion model in which melanoma-derived Gal-1 can antagonize the anti-tumor efficacy of T cells. (B) A cartoon depiction of the metabolic antagonism of Gal-1-binding N-acetyllactosamine synthesis in effector anti-tumor T cells caused by 4-F-GlcNAc and consequent enhancement of anti-tumor immunity. (C) A schematic overview of a novel cancer immunotherapeutic strategy to selectivity target donor CTLs with 4-F-GlcNAc for escaping Gal-1 control and improving the efficacy of adoptive T cell therapy. (Chapter 7)

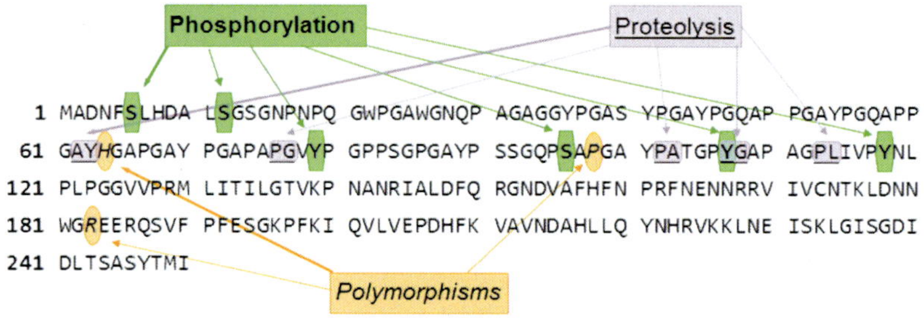

Figure 1. Structure of galectin-3. (Chapter 8)

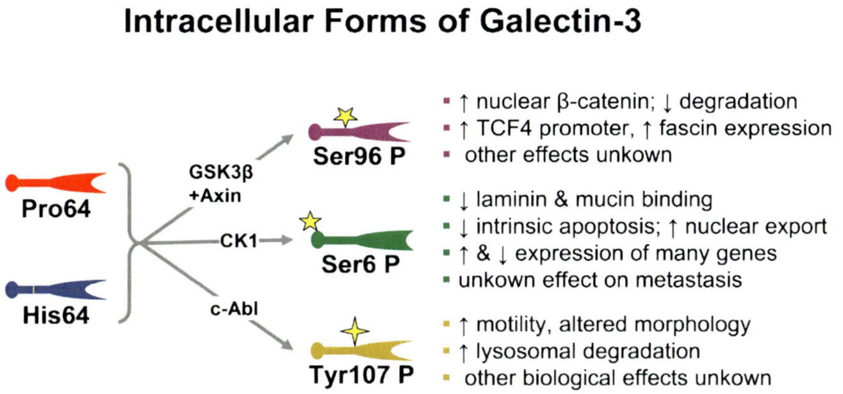

Figure 2. Phosphorlylation of intracellular galectin-3. Note that it is not known whether the P64H or the T98P mutations affect phosphorylation. (Chapter 8)

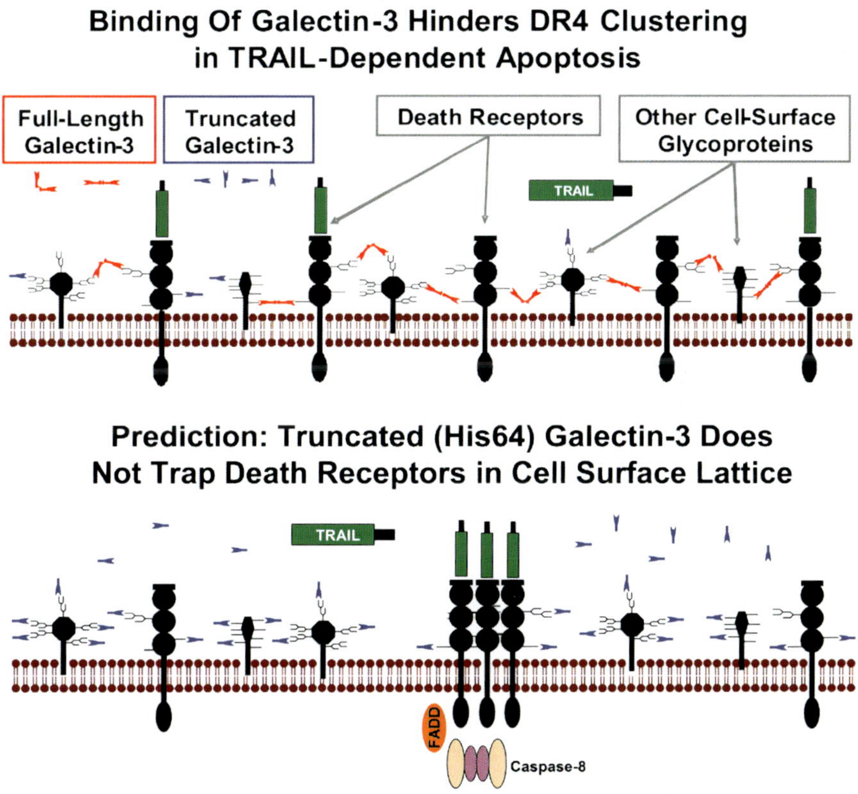

Figure 3. Cell surface galectin-3 confers resistance to TRAIL by impeding trafficking of DR4 death receptors. This model predicts that monovalent truncated galectin-3, resulting from MMP cleavage of His64 galectin-3, would allow TRAIL sensitivity. (Chapter 8)

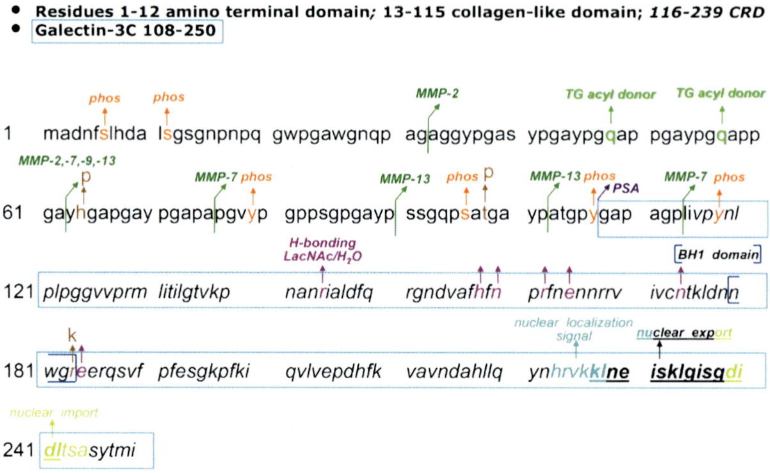

Figure 1. The primary amino acid sequence of recombinant human galectin-3 (Gal-3) notated using various colors or styles of font as to sites of phosphorylation, proteolytic digestion, transglutamination, genetic polymorphism, hydrogen bonds to lactose or N-acetyllactosamine ligands, and nuclear localization. (Chapter 12)

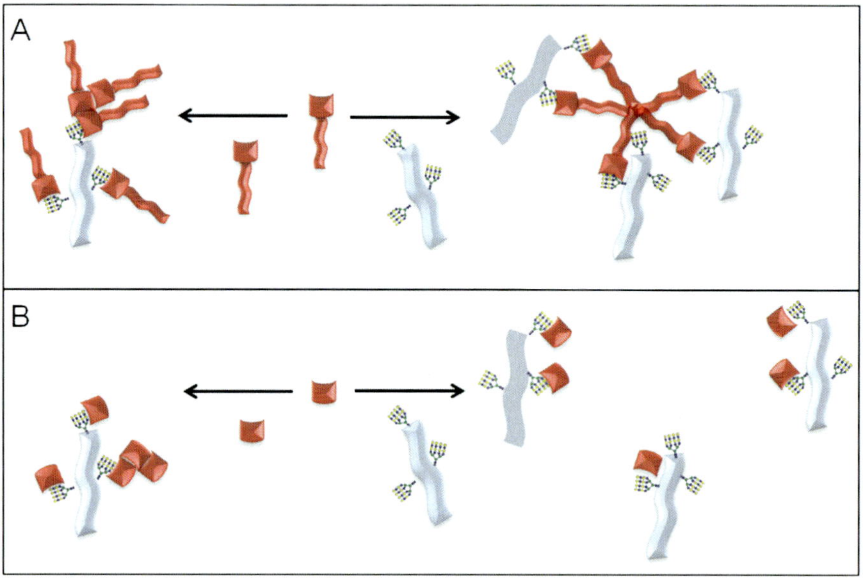

Figure 2. Schematic (A) showing the Gal-3 (red) multimeric binding (right) to the N-glycans (galactose, yellow circle; N-acetylhexosamine, blue square; mannose, green circle; colors/symbols according to the Nomenclature Committee Consortium for Functional Glycomics) of glycoproteins resulting in receptor clustering. C-terminal multimerization (left) is thought to occur when there is high concentration of Gal-3 relative to its carbohydrate ligands. Schematic (B) illustrating the binding of Gal-3C (red) to the N-glycans of glycoproteins

(right side) does not result in receptor clustering. C-terminal multimerization (left) similar to that which has been postulated to occur with Gal-3 also is likely to occur with Gal-3C. (Chapter 12)

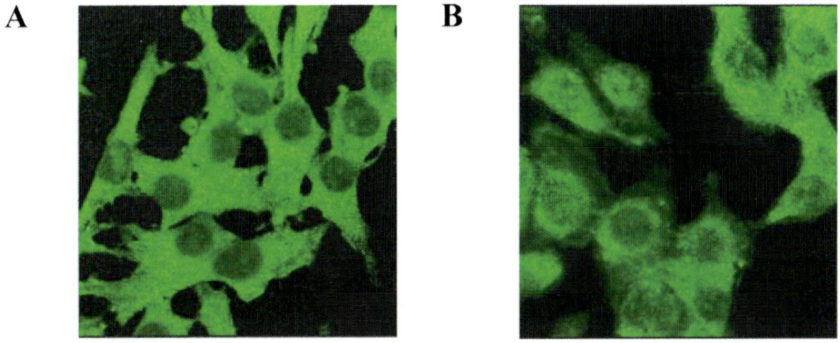

Figure 3. Images from confocal microscopy of MDA-MB-435 cells after incubation with Gal-3-FITC (A) and Gal-3C-FITC (B). More intense fluorescence is associated with the cytoplasm than the nucleus in cells treated with either Gal-3- or Gal-3C-FITC, although the difference in intensity between the two cellular locations is somewhat more dramatic with Gal-3-FITC. In addition, the cells incubated with Gal-3C-FITC have a more rounded shape and fewer cellular processes are apparent compared to the cells incubated with Gal-3-FITC. (Chapter 12)

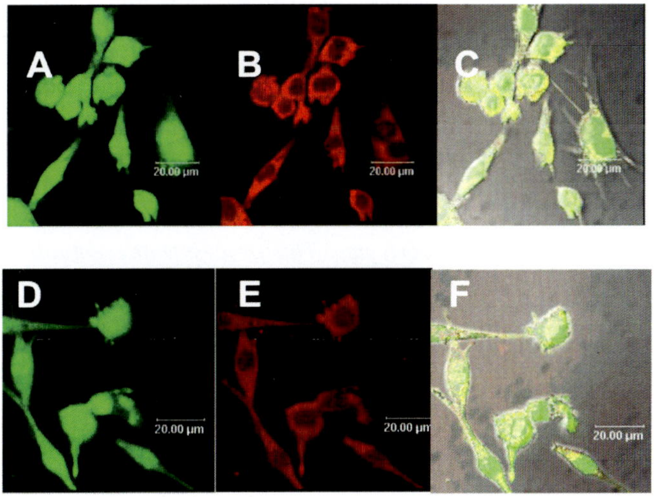

Figure 5. Confocal photomicrographs of MDA-MB-435 cells growing on microscope slides and incubated with Gal-3 (A-C) or -3C (D-F) labeled with FITC (green) or stained with antibody to caveolin-1 (red). Yellow/green overlays of the FITC and caveolin-1 images (C, F) are also shown. The FITC-labeled Gal-3 and -3C are clearly observed in cell nuclei and cytoplasm. Caveolin-1 is localized in the cytoplasm. (Chapter 12)

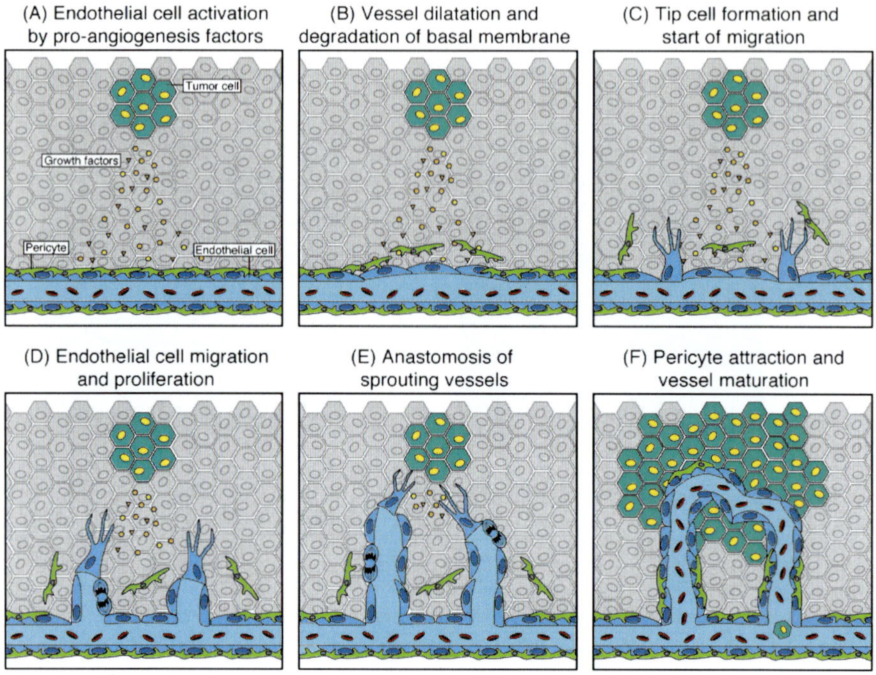

Figure 1. Tumor angiogenesis Schematic representation of the different steps of the angiogenesis cascade. First, tumor cells under metabolic stress, e.g. hypoxia, secrete growth factors that activate endothelial cells in nearby capillaries (A). The activated endothelial cells produce proteases which degrade the basal membrane, accompanied by vessel dilatation and pericyte detachment (B). Next, endothelial tip cells start to move in the direction of the growth factor gradient (C). The continuous proliferating and migrating endothelial cells form tube-like structures (D) which grow towards the tumor cells (E). Eventually the growing sprouts anastomose and a functional vessel is formed by depositing a new basal membrane and attraction of pericytes. This process will eventually allow the tumor to grow and also will facilitate tumor metastasis (F). (Chapter 13)

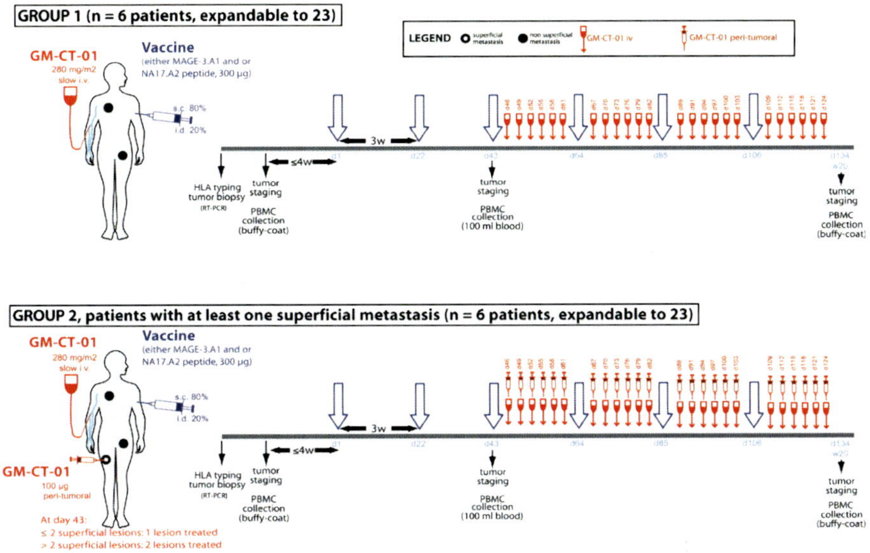

Figure 1. Treatment plan of the clinical trial involving GM-CT-01. Treatment allocation: Patients will be divided in two treatment arms. Both will run in parallel. Patients with at least one measurable lesion will be assigned to ***group 1*** *and will receive the following treatment: peptide vaccinations and systemic GM-CT-01 injections. Patients with at least one measurable and at least one superficial metastasis will be assigned in priority to* ***group 2*** *and will receive the following treatment: peptide vaccinations, systemic GM-CT-01 administrations and peri-tumoral administration of GM-CT-01 in one or two superficial metastases. (Chapter 16)*

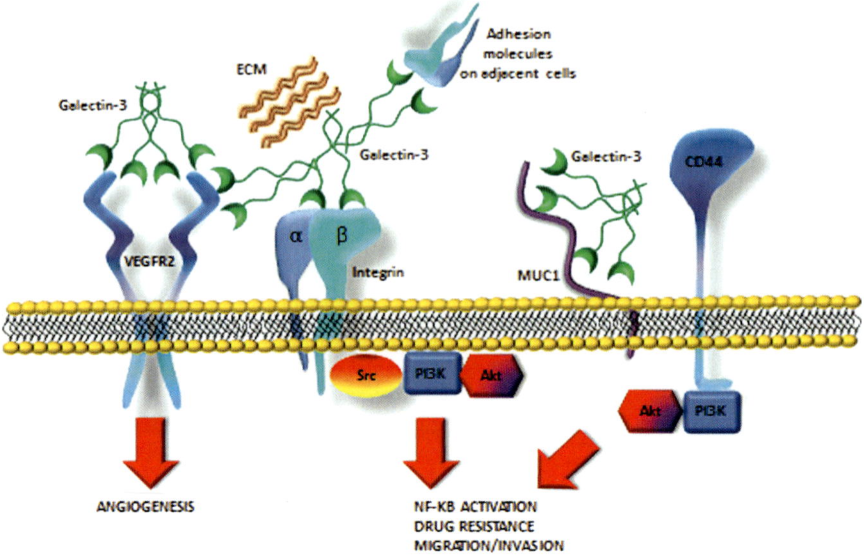

Figure 1. Main interactions between Gal-3 and molecules relevant in MM pathobiology. (Chapter 17)

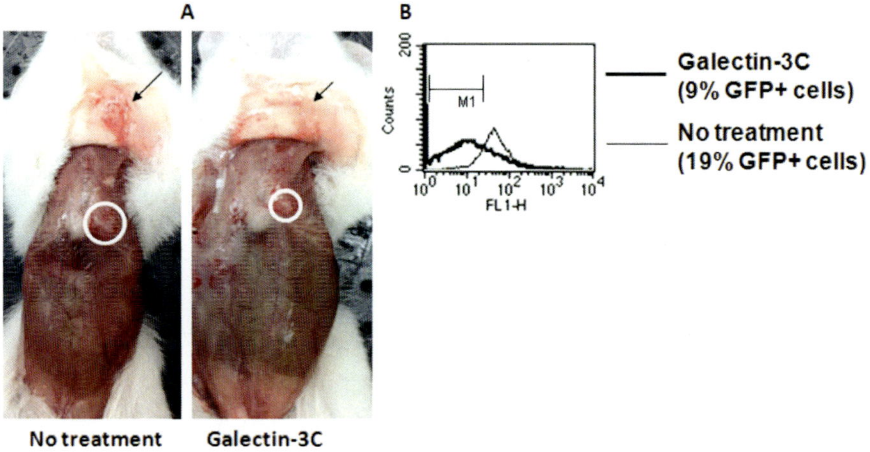

Figure 2. Representative results of Gal-3C treatment outcome on in vivo MM-induced angiogenesis. A) White circles mark the subcutaneous tumors. The arrows show the macroscopic evidence of sub-cutaneous capillaries. B) Flow-cytometry assessment of GFP-expressing HUVEC cells in tumor masses. The frequency of positive cells is shown. (Chapter 17)

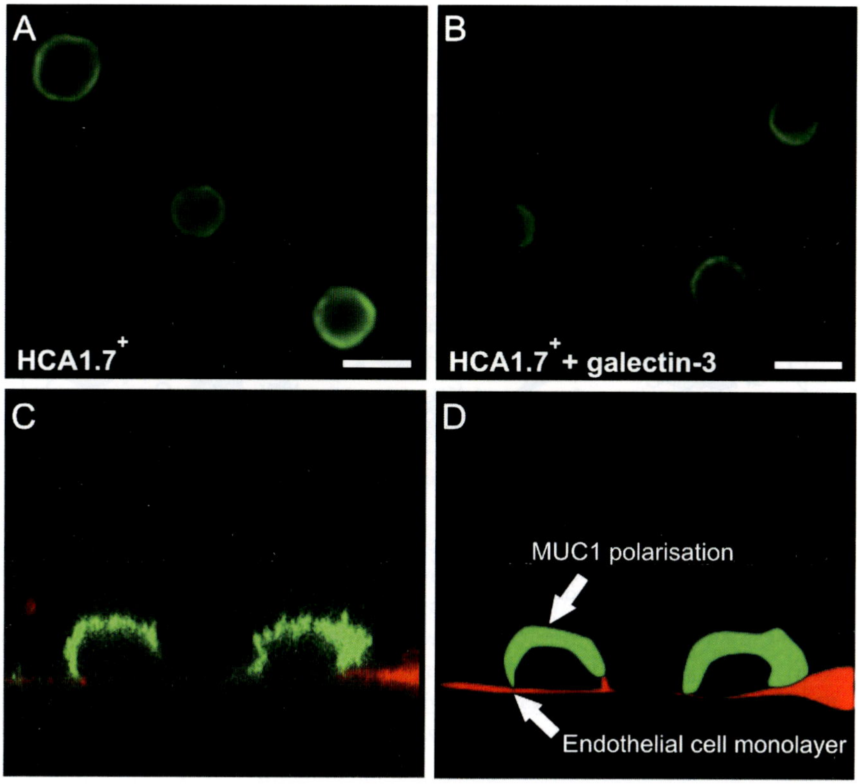

Figure 1. Galectin-3-MUC1 interaction induces MUC1 cell surface localisation. MUC1 immunohistochemistry shows homogenous MUC1 cell surface localization (A) but polarization (B) in response to galectin-3 binding (B) in the MUC1 positively-transfected HCA1.7$^+$, a derivative of human breast epithelial HBL-100 cells. Confocal images (C) of galectin-3-treated HCA1.7$^+$ cells in the xz plane showing absence of MUC1 (green) at the HCA1.7+ and HUVEC (red) contact points. A schematic representation of this heterotypic epithelial-endothelial adhesion illustrates the absence of MUC1 at the cell-cell junction (D). (Chapter 18)

Chapter 12

Galectin-3C: Human Lectin for Treatment of Cancer

Gary A. Jarvis,[1,2] Leonardo Mirandola,[3] Yu Yuefei,[3] Everardo Cobos,[3,4] Maurizio Chiriva-Internati,[3,4] and Constance M. John*,[1,5]

[1]Center for Immunochemistry, Veterans Affairs Medical Center, 4150 Clement Street, San Francisco, California 94121
[2]Department of Laboratory Medicine, University of California, San Francisco, California 94143
[3]Department of Internal Medicine at the Division of Hematology & Oncology, Texas Tech University Health Sciences Center and Southwest Cancer Treatment and Research Center, Lubbock, Texas 79415
[4]Laura W. Bush Institute for Women's Health and Center for Women's Health and Gender-Based Medicine, Amarillo, Texas 79106
[5]MandalMed, 665 3rd Street, Suite 250, San Francisco, California 94107
***E-mail: connie@mandalmed.com**

A summary is provided of the compelling data supporting galectin-3, as a target for cancer therapy, and for the clinical development of a truncated form of human galectin-3, termed galectin-3C, for cancer. Lacking the N-terminal domain of galectin-3 that facilitates its multimerization when bound to carbohydrate ligands, galectin-3C functions as an inhibitor of the galectin-3 crosslinking mediated by the N-terminal domain that can be induced by multivalent oligosaccharides and glycoconjugates intra- or extracellularly, on cell surfaces, or in extracellular matrices. Numerous studies show that galectin-3 plays a key role in tumorigenicity and metastasis and is a novel target for the development of cancer therapeutics. Data presented indicate that galectin-3C can be localized in a carbohydrate-dependent manner similar to most information reported regarding galectin-3. Exogenous galectin-3C facilitated anoikis in human breast cells, illustrating an effect it is expected to produce in vivo by reducing cell-cell or cell-ECM adhesion of metastatic cells. Based on the activity of galectin-3, we postulate that galectin-3C also inhibits the metastatic process by preventing integrin activation and focal adhesion turnover. The data described provide evidence of the important functions of galectin-3 in the processes of metastasis and tumorigenicity, and the potential therapeutic effect of inhibiting the activity of galectin-3 with galectin-3C. Galectin-3 has a complex, multi-faceted role that is critical in the relationship between the cells of various types of malignancies and the microenvironment, and further development of galectin-3C as a clinical candidate for cancer treatment is warranted.

Introduction

The goal of this review is to provide an overview of the rationale for and the data supporting the human lectin, galectin (Gal)-3, as a target for cancer therapy, and for the clinical development of a proprietary N-terminally truncated form of human Gal-3 as a therapeutic agent for cancer. In addition, we aim to point out the salient features, potential advantages,and challenges in terms of understanding the mechanism of action of Gal-3 or Gal-3C, and the development of the latter as a novel therapeutic agent for cancer.

We have shown that Gal-3C has promising anticancer activity. Twice a day intramuscular (i.m.) injection of Gal-3C reduced the growth of tumors and metastasis in an orthotopic xenograft mouse model of breast cancer (*1*). Recently, we reported that continuous administration of Gal-3C using an osmotic pump reduced tumor growth in an non-obese diabetic severe combined immunodeficiency (NOD-SCID) mouse model of multiple myeloma and facilitated the anticancer activity of bortezomib (Velcade™) (*2*). The average tumor volume of bortezomib-treated animals was 19.6% and of Gal-3C treated animals was 13.5% of the average volume of the untreated controls at day 35. The combination of Gal-3C with bortezomib produced the greatest effect, reducing the mean tumor volume in treated animals by 94% compared to the untreated controls at day 35 (*2*). Our in vitro data showed that Gal-3C inhibited chemotaxis and invasion of U266 MM cells induced by stromal cell-derived factor (SDF)-1α, and that combined treatment by Gal-3C with bortezomib resulted in a synergistically reduced human umbilical cord vascular endothelial cell migration by approximately 70%. Recent reports from other laboratories on the significant anti-angiogenic activity of Gal-3C (*3*, *4*) support our results. We aim to test Gal-3C in clinical trials for treatment of multiple myeloma that has a median survival rate of only 5 years and is considered incurable.

One of the challenges in the development of Gal-3C for treatment of cancer has been the identification of its major molecular mechanism or mechanisms of anti-cancer activity some of which remain incompletely understood. Some functions of Gal-3 have been elucidated only recently. In addition, however, a relatively wide range of activities have been attributed to Gal-3 that, in some instances, has produced the opposite effect in different cell types or under different conditions. For example, Gal-3 has been shown to stimulate cell migration (*2*, *5–7*) or cellular adhesion (*8–10*), and to have anti-apoptotic (*9*, *11–16*) or pro-apoptotic (*17*, *18*) activity depending on factors such as cell type, subcellular localization, and post-translational modifications.

The affinity of lectins for their carbohydrate ligands is often less than that of receptors with ligands that are other proteins or small molecules. In addition, for the galectins avidity is important due to the multimeric binding to ligands. Thus, concentration dependent effects may be an important determinant. However there is little known about the regulation of the localization of the galectins in general and of Gal-3 specifically (*19*). The potential biological importance of galectin concentration is highlighted by the prognostic significance of the serum levels of Gal-3 for risk of death from cardiac failure (*20*, *21*).

What is the relationship between the structure and function of galectin-3 and galectin-3C?

Gal-3 is a member of a family of mammalian carbohydrate-binding proteins (lectins) that are defined by affinity for β-galactosides and structural similarity. All galectins bind lactose and *N*-acetyllactosamine, but vary in their affinity and specificity for β-galactoside-expressing glycoconjugates (*22*, *23*). Gal-3 is composed of three distinct structural motifs: a short amino terminal region, a sequence rich in G-X-Y tandem repeats characteristic of the collagen supergene family, and a carboxyl-terminus of about 135 amino acids containing the globular carbohydrate recognition domain (CRD). There is close homology between Gal-3 proteins of different species, but the number of *N*-terminal tandem repeats and, hence, the sizes of the proteins vary (*24*). Recombinant human Gal-3 (Figure 1) has 250 amino acid residues (*25*).

The X-ray crystal structure of Gal-3C, in complex with lactose and *N*-acetyllactosamine, was reported previously and showed that the CRD was composed of five- and six-stranded β-sheets arranged in a β-sandwich. The binding site for the disaccharide ligand (lactose or *N*-acetyllactosamine) was in a shallow pocket over β-strands S4−S6. The β-galactose moiety was the most tightly bound and interacted via hydrogen bonds with amino acids in strands S4−S5 (His-158, Asn-160, Arg-162, Asn-174, and Glu-184) (*26*). Recently the high- to ultra-high resolution crystal structures of Gal-3C in the ligand-free state and in complex with lactose or glycerol was solved, and revealed that the positions of water and carbohydrate oxygen atoms were similar in all three states, (*27*).

The affinity of Gal-3 and Gal-3C and other galectins for various oligosaccharides was compared using frontal affinity chromatography that revealed greater affinity for branched or repeated unit ligands (*28*). In addition, the thermodynamic properties of human Gal-3 (*29*), and murine Gal-3 and the murine CRD have been investigated (*30*). The binding properties of the CRD domain of galectin-3 were shown to be similar to those of the intact molecule.

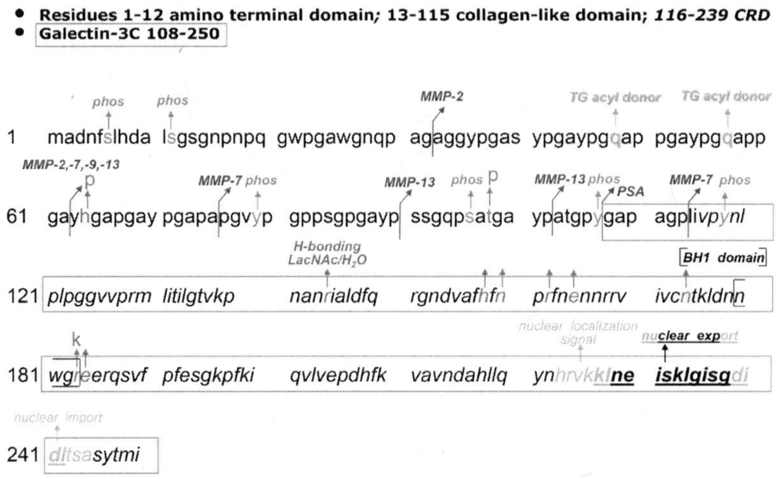

Figure 1. The primary amino acid sequence of recombinant human galectin-3 (Gal-3) notated using various colors or styles of font as to sites of phosphorylation, proteolytic digestion, transglutamination, genetic polymorphism, hydrogen bonds to lactose or N-acetyllactosamine ligands, and nuclear localization. (see color insert)

Intact Gal-3 is isolated as a monomer but can undergo multimerization that potentiates its binding through the *C*-terminal carbohydrate recognition domain (CRD) to multivalent carbohydrates or glycoconjugates inducing glycoprotein precipitation and cell agglutination, and the *N*-terminal domain of the protein is required for this multimerization (*31–35*). Data from precipitation studies indicate that Gal-3 can form pentamers when binding to multivalent carbohydrate ligands (*36*). The multimerization of Gal-3 mediated by the *N*-terminal domain is thought to be important in numerous biological activities that play a role in cancer including effects on cell adhesion and migration (*9*, *37–40*), angiogenesis (*3*, *41*, *42*), growth factor signaling (*43*, *44*), and intracellular protein trafficking in epithelial cells (*45*, *46*).

The galectins including Gal-3 are thought to play a role in innate immune functions in infections particularly parasitic ones and allergies (*47–52*) which helps to explain the disparate activities of Gal-3 in mediating Th-2 adaptive immunity, promoting rapid repair mechanisms by stimulating the migration of monocytes and macrophages, wound-healing and fibrosis responses, and inducing angiogenesis (*6*, *41*, *53–56*). It has been proposed that the pattern recognition of mammalian lectins such as Gal-3 in innate immunity can be generally classified as density-dependent glycan recognition because since both the glycans and the lectins are multivalent, concentration and avidity may be more significant than the affinity for a specific binding site (*35*).

Extracellular Gal-3 is a substrate for enzymatic digestion by several members of the family of matrix metalloproteinases (MMPs) that affects its functionality. MT1-MMP, MMP-2, -9 and -13 cleave the A^{62}-Y^{63} bond which abrogates hemagglutination and multimerization of Gal-3 while increasing the potential for carbohydrate binding (*57–60*). Recently, it has been shown that MMP-7 (matrilysin-1) cleaves Gal-3 at 3 sites including A^{62}-Y^{63}, and also P^{76}-G^{77}, and P^{113}-L^{114}, and that MMP-7 cleavage inhibited Gal-3-mediated wound healing in a scratch assay with T84 intestinal epithelial cells (*61*). MMP-13 proteolytic cleavage sites in gal-3 have been identified as including P^{90}-S^{91}, and P^{102}-A^{103}, in addition to A^{62}-Y^{63} (*59*). An alternative site that is apparently susceptible to MMP-2 cleavage, G^{32}-A^{33}, also has been reported (*62*). It has been proposed that cleavage of extracellular Gal-3 by MMPs may play a critical role in tumorigenicity (*63*).

Gal-3 can be phosphorylated on S^6 by casein kinase 1 (CK1), a modification that has been reported to reduce the affinity of Gal-3 for its carbohydrate ligands, colon cancer mucin and laminin, and to be required for the tumorigenicity of Gal-3, to promote its transport from the nucleus into the cytoplasm, inhibition of anoikis, and inhibition of drug-induced cell death (*14*, *64–67*). In addition, Y^{79}, T^{107}, and Y^{108} can be phosphorylated by c-Abl (*16*). In mouse fibroblasts, tyrosine phosphorylation and secretion of Gal-3 were dependent on expression of calpain 4, the common small regulatory subunit of the calpain system that affects cell adhesion and migration (*68*). Data show that glycogen synthase kinase-3 (GSK-3ß) can phosphorylate Gal-3 that contains the GBK-3ß binding motif, SGQPS, at amino acid residues 92-96 containing the kinase substrate motif, S^{96} (*69*, *70*). Gal-3 also can be multimerized by transglutaminase that catalyzes cross-linking between glutamine and other amino acid residues (*71*, *72*).

Variants at three single nucleotide polymorphism (SNP) sites of the human Gal-3 gene *LGALS3* have been identified and found to have significance in cancer (*73–76*). One polymorphism rs4644, LGALS3 +191 A>C, changes residue 64 from histidine to proline (Gal-3 64 H to P). The homozygous allele for H^{64} is correlated with disparity in risk of breast cancer among Caucasian compared to Asian women, being expressed by 12% and 5% of Caucasian and Asian women, and 37% and 82% of breast cancer patients, respectively. Interestingly, expression of H^{64} Gal-3 in BT-549 human breast carcinoma cells significantly increased their tumorigenicity and angiogenic potential when injected in nude mice compared to P^{64} Gal-3-expressing cells. H^{64} Gal-3 expression in the BT-549 cells increased resistance to induction of apoptosis by cisplatin. The H64 lectin is cleaved at the A^{62}-T^{63} bond by MMPs. In contrast, the P^{64} lectin was not susceptible to MMP cleavage at the A^{62}-T^{63} bond, but was cleaved at G^{32}-A^{33} (*73*, *74*). Gal-3 H^{64} recently was shown to enhance nuclear accumulation of β-catenin in gastric cancer cells (*77*).

Another SNP, rs4652, LGALS3 +292 A>C, alters residue 98 such that in place of threonine, a proline is expressed (Gal-3 98 T to P). Expression of the CC genotype of Gal-3 +292 for P^{98} was correlated with non-responsiveness to platinum-based chemotherapy, and significantly reduced survival among 320 Stage III or IV non-small cell lung cancer patients (*76*).

A third SNP, rs10148371, causes the substitution of R^{183} in the NWGR anti-apoptotic domain with K (*78*). Stable expression of the mutant protein in colon carcinoma cells increased the sensitivity to drug-induced apoptosis, and a small increase in expression of the lysine-encoding genotype in males with colorectal cancer was detected (*78*).

The LGALS3 gene has been mapped to human chromosome 14 at region 14q21-22 (*79*), and the promoter region has been characterized (*80*). The promoter activity of the second intron of LGALS3 was found to be down-regulated by wild-type but not a mutated form of p53 (*81*). Analysis of the methylation of the Gal-3 promoter in prostate adenocarcinoma revealed that it was nearly unmethylated in normal and benign hyperplasia tissues, variously methylated in stage I, heavily methylated in stage II, and lightly methylated in stages III and IV, and suggested that a LGALS3 gene methylation-specific PCR assay could be diagnostic for the stage of prostate carcinoma (*82*).

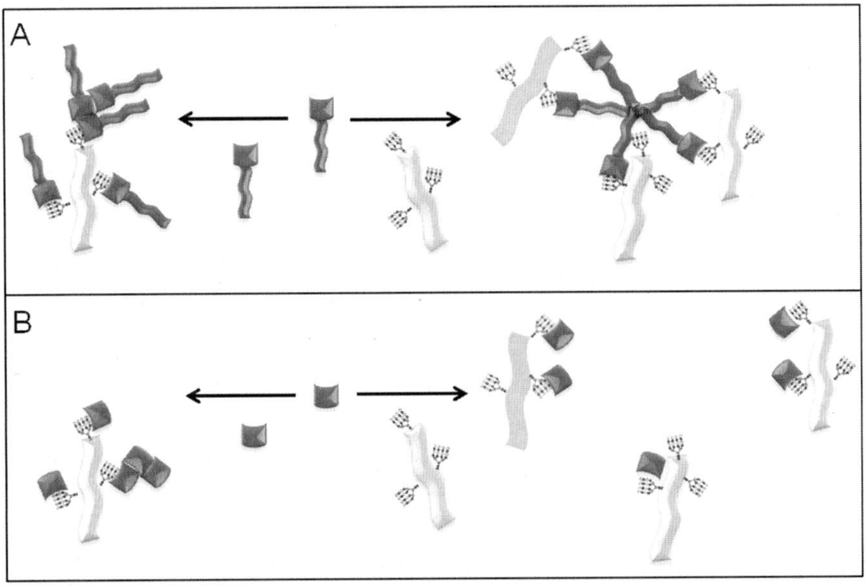

Figure 2. Schematic (A) showing the Gal-3 (red) multimeric binding (right) to the N-glycans (galactose, yellow circle; N-acetylhexosamine, blue square; mannose, green circle; colors/symbols according to the Nomenclature Committee Consortium for Functional Glycomics) of glycoproteins resulting in receptor clustering. C-terminal multimerization (left) is thought to occur when there is high concentration of Gal-3 relative to its carbohydrate ligands. Schematic (B) illustrating the binding of Gal-3C (red) to the N-glycans of glycoproteins (right side) does not result in receptor clustering. C-terminal multimerization (left) similar to that which has been postulated to occur with Gal-3 also is likely to occur with Gal-3C. (see color insert)

Human galectin-3C (Gal-3C) is composed of the *C*-terminal 143 amino acids of human Gal-3 (Figure 2). Gal-3C can be produced by exhaustive collagenase digestion of Gal-3 (*1*, *32*), and has been found to be produced *in vivo* by the chymotrypsin-like serine protease, prostate specific antigen (*4*, *83*). Lacking the *N*-terminal domain that facilitates the multimerization of Gal-3 when bound to carbohydrate ligands, Gal-3C (Figure 2B) functions as an inhibitor of the Gal-3-mediated crosslinking that can be induced by multivalent oligosaccharides and glycoconjugates intra- or extracellularly, on cell surfaces, or in extracellular matrices. However, there are data indicating that the interactions of the *C*-terminal domain of Gal-3 can induce its multimerization (*24*, *84*, *85*). Recently using a fluorescence anisotropy assay it was confirmed that the *C*-terminal hemophilic binding can induce oligomerization (*84*), and based on the data a new model was proposed wherein carbohydrate binding nucleates CRD-mediated oligomerization of Gal-3 (*86*) as similarly depicted in the schematic shown in the left hand side of Figure 2.

Where are galectin-3 and galectin-3C localized and distributed?

Gal-3 is widely expressed in epithelial cells, and some immune cells, macrophages, neutrophils, mast cells, sensory neurons, and in many malignant tumors. Depending on the cell type, after its cytoplasmic synthesis galectin-3 can be localized in the cytoplasm and/or nucleus, and can be both absorbed and secreted by cells (*19*, *87–92*). Lacking an *N*-terminal signaling sequence, Gal-3 can be secreted by non-classical mechanisms and is absorbed by cells in a carbohydrate-dependent or -independent manner (*87*, *93–97*). The *N*-terminus has been implicated in secretion of human Gal-3 as it was abrogated by deletion the of the *N*-terminal 11 amino acids (*93*). Gal-3 can shuttle between the nucleus and the cytoplasm; it can be exported from the nucleus of one cell, be transported through the cytoplasm, and be imported into the nucleus of another cell (*92*).

Localization of Gal-3 in both the nucleus and cytoplasm must represent some balance between nuclear import and export mechanisms, and the factors that determine its retention in either compartment (*19*). There are data regarding amino acid residues of Gal-3 critical for the nuclear localization but some aspects of this process are not clear (*19*). Findings indicate that when Gal-3 is phosphorylated at S^6, the major site of phosphorylation in vivo, the protein can be exported from the nucleus to the cytoplasm where it can protect cells from drug-induced apoptosis in response to apoptotic insults (*66*). Accordingly, it has been reported that expression of a mutant Gal-3 lacking the first 11-amino acids from the *N*-terminus in human breast carcinoma BT-549 cells led to abolishment of the secretion of the *N*-terminally truncated Gal-3, loss of nuclear localization, and reduced carbohydrate-mediated functions compared with the wild-type protein (*66*). However, in a subsequent study it was found that nuclear import of murine Gal-3 in mouse 3T3 fibroblasts was unaffected by deleting the amino half of the protein (*98*). Accumulation of Gal-3 in the nucleus of cells treated with leptomycin B suggested that nuclear export may be mediated by interactions with exportin-1 (CRM1) (*98*).

Studies of mutant proteins lacking the *C*-terminal 10 amino acids or with site-directed mutations in the IXLT nuclear localization domain (residues 240-243 of the human protein), first found in the *Drosophila* protein Dsh (dishevelled), suggest that IXLT sequence is critical for nuclear import (*98*). A leucine-rich nuclear export signal in Gal-3 (residues 227-242 of the human protein) that overlaps with the IXLT sequence has been reported to be important for nuclear export (*99*). Another overlapping domain important for Gal-3 nuclear location was identified at residues 223-228, and is similar to nuclear localization signal domains of proteins such as p-53 and c-myc (*100*). Mutant Gal-3 (R224A) had impaired nuclear translocation that was dependent on expression of importin-β and accelerated degradation (*100*).

In human breast cancer cells, rapid secretion of Gal-3 could be induced by incubation with fetuin or by loss of cell anchorage suggesting that secretion was regulated by adhesive processes (*101*, *102*). Gal-3 facilitated its own uptake in the macrophage-type cells by mechanisms not entirely clear but dependent on the *N*-terminal domain (*97*). One possibility proposed is that endocytosis of Gal-3 results from its clustering and activation of cell- surface integrins that induces their translocation (*40*, *95*).

Interactions of Gal-3 in the nucleus and cytoplasm have been recently reviewed (*19*). In the nucleus Gal-3, acts as a pre-mRNA splicing factor and is associated with ribonucleoprotein complexes (*103–106*). Nuclear Gal-3 interacts with Gemin4 (*107*, *108*). Sufu (Suppressor of fused) that is a negative regulator of the Hedgehog pathway apparently can bind to Gal-3 in both the nucleus and cytoplasm, and can act to prevent its nuclear localization (*109*). In the cytoplasm Gal-3 can inhibit apoptosis (*14*, *15*, *110*, *111*), induce AKT phosphorylation leading to the inactivation of GSK-3β and increased nuclear levels of β-catenin degradation and induction of Wnt signaling (*69*, *112–115*), and can interact with activated GTP-bound K-Ras (*116*, *117*).

Cytoplasmic Gal-3 also functions in the carbohydrate-dependent apical sorting of proteins. A prototypical characteristic of epithelial cells is polarization of the plasma membrane into apical and basolateral surfaces. Apical sorting of proteins can occur through utilization of sphingolipid/cholesterol-enriched membrane microdomains (lipid rafts) or through non-raft mechanisms, and the carbohydrate-dependent apical sorting of non-raft dependent proteins by Gal-3 has been demonstrated (*45*, *46*, *96*). Both Gal-3 and apical glycoproteins were identified in high molecular weight clusters that formed minutes after exit of the trans-Golgi network in polarized epithelial cells suggesting that multimerization of the glycoproteins was mediated by the *N*-terminal domain of Gal-3 (*45*).

To investigate cellular uptake and subcellular localization, we labeled Gal-3 and Gal-3C with fluorescein isothiocyanate (FITC) and analyzed the intracellular localization of Gal-3C-FITC and Gal-3-FITC in MDA-MB-435 cancer cells using confocal microscopy. The MDA-MB-435 cells were incubated with Gal-3C-FITC and Gal-3-FITC for 2 hours, washed with 50 mM lactose, and then imaged. As shown in Figure 3 below, localization of both proteins was seen primarily in the cytoplasm with lesser intensity fluorescence observed associated with the nuclei.

A 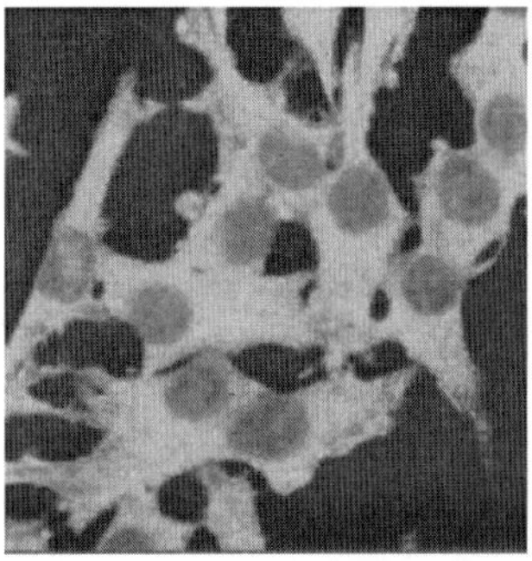 B 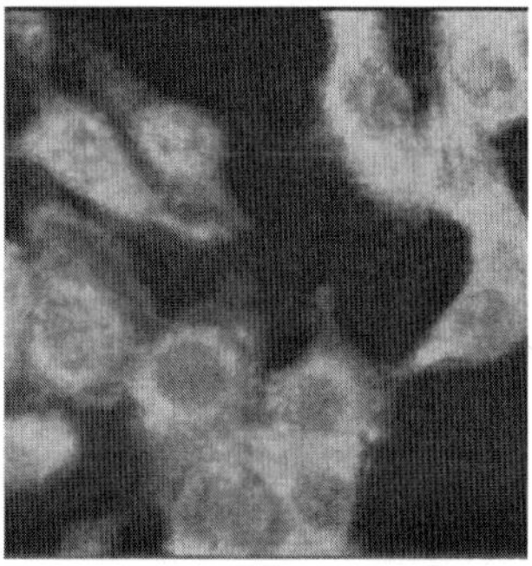

Figure 3. Images from confocal microscopy of MDA-MB-435 cells after incubation with Gal-3-FITC (A) and Gal-3C-FITC (B). More intense fluorescence is associated with the cytoplasm than the nucleus in cells treated with either Gal-3- or Gal-3C-FITC, although the difference in intensity between the two cellular locations is somewhat more dramatic with Gal-3-FITC. In addition, the cells incubated with Gal-3C-FITC have a more rounded shape and fewer cellular processes are apparent compared to the cells incubated with Gal-3-FITC. (see color insert)

Interestingly, the cells incubated with Gal-3C-FITC were more rounded in shape and had fewer cellular processes compared to the cells incubated with Gal-3-FITC. This is consistent with the role of Gal-3 in promoting cellular adhesion by increasing binding to ECM molecules, expression of integrins, and remodeling of the actin cytoskeleton (*9*, *118–121*).

To determine if Gal-3C was endocytosed by the MDA-MB-435 cells, flow cytometry was performed before and after washing the cells with PBS containing 50 mM lactose to remove cell surface lectin, treating with trypsin, and washing twice again with 50 mM lactose. The results showed that Gal-3C was internalized by the cells (Figure 4A), and that the endocytosis of Gal-3C-FITC could be inhibited by the presence of 50 mM lactose demonstrating the carbohydrate dependence of uptake (Figure 4B).

To ascertain whether Gal-3C-FITC could be secreted after being endocytosed, the MDA-MB-435 cells were incubated with Gal-3C-FITC for 2 h, washed, and then fixed or not, followed by a second 2-h incubation period. The results (Figure 4C) demonstrated that without fixation, the levels of Gal-3C-FITC were significantly reduced in this time frame suggesting that the internalized FITC-labeled Gal-3C was secreted by the cells. Some of the decrease in Gal-3C-FITC could be due to intracellular degradation. However, this is likely to be a slow process as a previous study examining both the cell-associated and protein secreted by Madin-Darby canine kidney cells showed using ^{35}S labeled-Gal-3 that only about 15% of the protein was degraded intracellularly in 24 h (*93*).

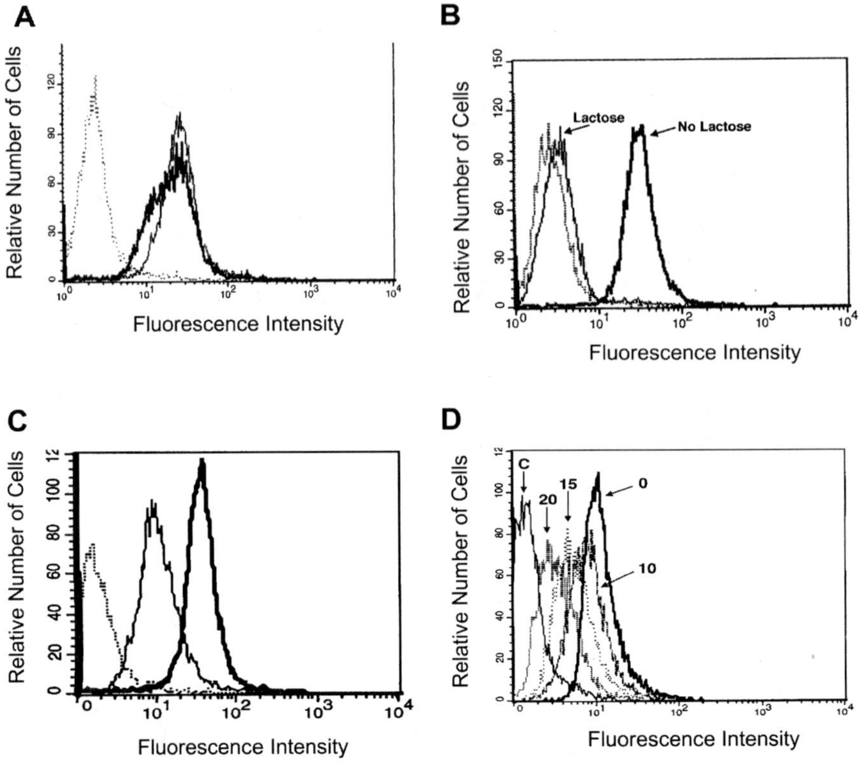

Figure 4. Uptake of Gal-3C-FITC by MDA-MB-435 cells. (A) Cells were incubated with Gal-3C FITC for 2 hours after which they were analyzed by flow cytometry. The two histograms on the right are cells washed with or without 50 mM lactose following the incubation with Gal-3C-FITC. Control cells are represented by the histogram on the left. (B) Lactose inhibits uptake of Gal-3C-FITC. The histogram on the right is MDA-MB-435 cells after incubation with Gal-3C-FITC or Gal-3C-FITC containing 50 mM lactose for 2 h. The lactose inhibited the uptake of Gal-3C-FITC. The farthest left histogram represents the control cells. (C) Endocytosed Gal-3C FITC is secreted. The histogram on the far right is for cells incubated with Gal-3C-FITC for 2 h, followed by two washes with PBS, then fixation. The middle histogram represents cells treated in the same manner, followed by room temperature incubation for 2 h, two washes, and then analysis without fixation. The histogram on the far left represents control cells. Endocytosis of Gal-3C-FITC is inhibitable by filipin (D) Gal-3C-FITC uptake by MDA-MB-435 cells in the presence or absence of filipin at 10, 15, or 20 μg/ml after incubation for 2 h.

We next investigated whether uptake of Gal-3C-FITC might occur via caveolae. One pathway for endocytosis is through caveolae that are membrane invaginations, and there are data suggesting that uptake of Gal-3 occurs through these invaginations (*95*). We tested whether treatment with filipin, an inhibitor of caveolae (*122*, *123*), could block the uptake of Gal-3C-FITC. As filipin exhibited some degree of toxicity at higher concentrations, only viable cells were analyzed based on co-staining with propidium iodide. As shown in Figure 4D, our results indicate that filipin, an inhibitor of caveolae, reduced uptake of Gal-3C-FITC in a dose-dependent manner, and suggest that in MDA-MB-435 cells the major pathway for this uptake is through a caveolae-dependent mechanism. This result is consistent with the filipin-mediated inhibition of Gal-3 endocytosis that was previously observed in breast cancer cells (*95*).

A recent detailed analysis of uptake of Gal-3 and the Gal-3 CRD (amino acids 114–250) clearly revealed that more than one type of cellular uptake of Gal-3 can occur. Study of human THP-1 monocytic cells differentiated into naïve (M0), classical (M1) or alternatively activated (M2) macrophage-like cells revealed that in M1 cells Gal-3 uptake was carbohydrate independent and inhibited only by chlorpromazine which uncouples clathrin-dependent uptake, or by interference with the *N*-terminal domain of Gal-3, while in M2 cells uptake was carbohydrate-dependent but also involved the *N*-terminal domain (*97*).

The data we have presented suggest that cellular localization, and carbohydrate-dependent secretion, and endocytosis of Gal-3C are quite similar to some reports on Gal-3 (*92*, *93*, *95*, *102*) but differ from a finding that the N-terminal domain is critical (*124*). However, nuclear localization of an *N*-terminally truncated form of human Gal-3 was previously reported (*95*).

Our data (Figure 4C) demonstrating uptake of Gal-3C FITC followed by its apparent rapid secretion by MDA-MB-435 cells are similar to results in the study of macrophages showing galectin-3 is rapidly endocytosed and is not degraded but rather enters a pool of intracellular recycling Gal-3 (*97*). In previous work, we found the elimination half-life of ^{35}S-labeled Gal-3C in the serum and cellular fraction of the blood to be 3 and 4.3 h, respectively (*1*). However, some results show that Gal-3C may be longer-lived in some intracellular compartments (*86*),

Caveolins are membrane scaffold proteins of caveolae that play a role in signal transduction. We performed confocal microscopy on MDA-MB-435 cells that had been incubated with Gal-3-FITC and Gal-3C-FITC and immunostained for caveolin-1 (Figure 5). The results show that Gal-3- and Gal-3C-FITC can be detected in both the cytoplasm and the nucleus of the cells (Figure 5A), whereas caveolin-1 was much more highly-associated with the cytoplasm (Figure 5B), such that the cytoplasm is yellow-colored in the merged image and the nuclear localization of Gal-3C-FITC is revealed by the green-tint of the nucleus (Figure 5C).

Abundant expression of caveolin-1 in the cytoplasm of the MDA-MB-435 cells concurrent with the presence of exogenous Gal-3-FITC and Gal-3C-FITC (Figure 5) is in accord with the previously reported functional interaction of caveolin-1 with Gal-3 to stabilize focal adhesion (FA) kinase within FAs promoting their disassembly and turnover in MDA-MB-435 cells (*120*). In differentiated thyroid cancer where Gal-3 is recognized as the single most accurate marker, Gal-3 and caveolin-1 were found function synergistically to promote FA signaling and cell migration (*125*).

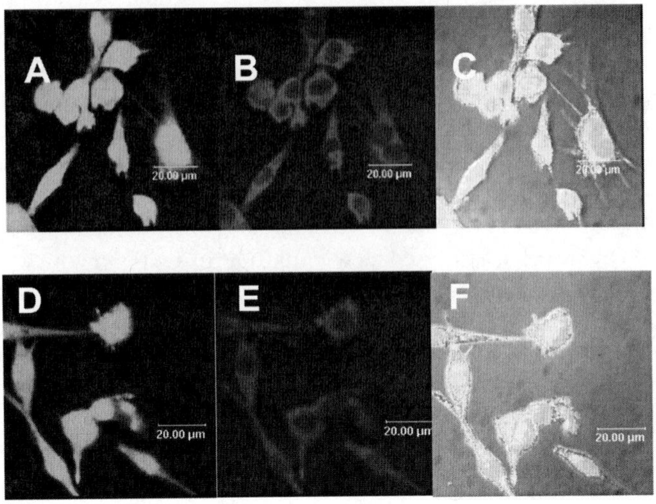

Figure 5. Confocal photomicrographs of MDA-MB-435 cells growing on microscope slides and incubated with Gal-3 (A-C) or -3C (D-F) labeled with FITC (green) or stained with antibody to caveolin-1 (red). Yellow/green overlays of the FITC and caveolin-1 images (C, F) are also shown. The FITC-labeled Gal-3 and -3C are clearly observed in cell nuclei and cytoplasm. Caveolin-1 is localized in the cytoplasm. (see color insert)

In terms of biodistribution of exogenous Gal-3C, our previous data showed that in mice there is greater localization in the liver, kidneys, and spleen compared to the heart or lungs (*1*). Recently, it has been shown that Gal-3 is present in human seminal plasma and that prostate specific antigen (PSA) which is a Zn^{2+}-sensitive chymotrypsin-like serine protease secreted by prostatic epithelium that normally functions in liquefaction of semen after ejaculation, cleaves Gal-3 between T^{107} and G^{108} yielding Gal-3C (*83*). Furthermore, T^{107} previously was shown to be phosphorylated by c-Abl and dephosphoryated by PTEN, and phosphorylated T^{107} was found to be resistant to PSA cleavage (*4*, *16*). Interestingly, both the 1-107 and the 108-250 (Gal-3C) amino acid fragments, unlike full-length Gal-3, inhibited chemotaxis of cultured prostate cancer cells and capillary tube formation of HUVEC cells (*4*). The data imply that in addition to the levels of PSA that are used as a prognostic indicator in prostate cancer, the ratio of phosphorylated to dephosphorylated Gal-3 might be used as a complementary value to that of PSA for prognosis of prostate cancer. The fact that Gal-3C is produced in vivo in some human prostate cancer patients indicates that the protein is unlikely to be highly immunogenic which is relevant to its therapeutic utilization.

Does the expression of galectin-3 in cancer support development of galectin-3C as an anticancer agent?

Gal-3 has been found to be overexpressed in many types of cancer including thyroid, melanoma, colon, gastric, renal, and non-small cell lung cancer. Analyses of Gal-3 expression revealed significantly higher levels in serum (*126*, *127*) and urine (*128*) of patients with various types of cancer including bladder, lung, breast, gastrointestinal, ovarian, cervical, bladder, melanoma, and Hodgkin's lymphoma.

Correlations of Gal-3 expression with stage and/or metastatic potential of several types of cancer have been reported. There is good evidence that cytoplasmic Gal-3 expression is anti-apoptotic and that its cytoplasmic expression in some types of cancer increases drug resistance (*129*, *130*). In addition, there are data suggesting that at least in some types of cancer, such as prostate, tongue, and melanoma, nuclear Gal-3 inhibits tumor promotion which is increased upon its translocation to the cytoplasm (*14*, *131*, *132*).

Lung cancer which is the second leading cause of cancer among men and women in the USA, is categorized into small cell (SCLC) and non-small cell lung cancer (NSCLC). SCLC often is already metastatic when diagnosed and although responsive to initial chemotherapy, resistance often develops upon relapse. Although NSCLC is less likely to have metastasized before presentation, it is also less sensitive to chemotherapy. Immunostaining revealed the expression of Gal-3 to be markedly different in SCLC and NSCLC carcinomas, with only minimal or absent expression in SCLC specimens suggesting that Gal-3 may be important in the response of lung tumors to chemotherapy (*133*). Examining Gal-3 immunoexpression in 94 NSCLC cases revealed that survival was significantly increased among patients whose tumors did not express Gal-3 (*134*). Also, a recent study in 320 NSCLC patients found that those with the A or AA genotype at a single nucleotide polymorphism (SNP) site in Gal-3, rs4652 (Gal-3 +292 A>C), that changes the threonine at residue 98 to a proline (98 Thr to 98 Pro) had significantly longer survival than those with the CC genotype (*76*).

Gal-3 binds to colon cancer mucin in a manner that can be significantly inhibited by desialylation (*135*). Immunohistochemical staining for Gal-3 in 117 primary lesions and 16 liver metastases of colorectal cancer revealed greater expression than in normal mucosa. Increased levels of Gal-3 expression in the primary lesions were correlated with progression of clinical stage, liver and lymph node metastasis, and venous invasion (*136*). Groups with strongly positive galectin-3 expression have a significantly poorer prognosis in terms of disease-free survival invasion (*136*, *137*).

The use of Gal-3 expression as a marker of malignancy is gaining credibility in thyroid cancers (*138*, *139*). More than 30 recent studies have shown that Gal-3 is highly expressed in papillary thyroid cancer compared to relative to normal thymocytes (*140*). Gal-3 is more highly expressed in early stages of papillary carcinoma, and its expression intensity decreases during tumor progression (*141*). Cytoplasmic galectin-3 expression was observed in papillary thyroid (82%), follicular (33%), medullary (9%) carcinomas but not in anaplastic carcinomas. Galectin-3 nuclear expression was observed in papillary thyroid (62%) and follicular carcinomas (33%) but not in medullary, anaplastic carcinomas (*115*).

Primary lesions of papillary carcinoma with metastasis expressed higher levels of Gal than those without metastases, but the expression of Gal-3 was significantly decreased in metastatic lesions in the lymph nodes compared with primary lesions (*142*).

Immunohistochemical analysis of 98 human breast lesions showed the expression of Gal-3 was significantly down-regulated in ductal carcinoma in situ and in invasive ductal carcinoma, particularly when infiltrating axillary lymph nodes (*143*). Examination of Gal-3 mRNA expression in breast tumors and xenografts revealed elevated levels and protein in the luminal epithelial cells of normal and benign ducts, decreased expression in low grade ductal carcinoma in situ, and re-expression in peripheral tumor cells in invasive carcinoma (*144*). Comprehensive expression profiles using breast tumor tissue microarrays found that the nuclear expression of Gal-3 in luminal epithelial cells correlated with a shorter overall survival in a subset of patients (*145*).

Median levels in the urine of ovarian cancer patients were ~2-fold ($P = 0.003$) and 10-fold ($P = 0.008$) higher than in urine of the healthy controls (*128*). A recent ovarian study that analyzed the expression of Gal-3 by immunohistochemistry in 71 patients (54 serous, 13 endometrioid,and 4 mucinous ovarian carcinomas) found that there was shorter progression free survival of patients with high levels compared to those with low levels (*146*).

Hoyer et al. found overexpression of Gal-3 in specific B-cell neoplasms, diffuse large B-cell lymphoma (DLBCL), primary effusion lymphoma (PEL), and multiple myeloma (MM) (*13*). Overexpression of Gal-3 in Burkitt lymphoma cells increased resistance to Fas-mediated apoptosis, and Gal-3-positive PEL cells that were genetically modified to express an *N*-terminally truncated Gal-3 similar to Gal-3C were more sensitive to induction of Fas-dependent apoptosis (*13*).

The bone marrow microenvironment provides a sanctuary for multiple myeloma cells and chronic myelogenous leukemia (CML) cells. Gal-3 was upregulated by co-culture of CML cells with HS-5 bone marrow stromal cells, and Gal-3 overexpression promoted the long-term lodgement of CML cells in the bone marrow (*147*).

The location-dependent functionality of Gal-3 adds to the challenge in correlating its expression with tumorigenicity and metastasis. However, the levels of extracellular Gal-3 are the subject of studies of its serum levels. Serum levels of Gal-3 are significantly higher in melanoma patients compared to healthy volunteers (*148*), and melanocytes accumulate galectin-3 with tumor progression (*149*). Serum levels in patients with thyroid tumors (*150*), pancreatic carcinomas (*150*), head and neck squamous cell carcinomas (*151*), breast and colorectal cancers (*152*) were elevated compared to healthy controls. Patients with hepatocellular carcinoma (HCC) had higher serum levels of Gal-3 compared to those with chronic liver disease, and a higher expression of nuclear Gal-3 in the tumors was correlated with markedly worse prognosis (*153*).

In summary, the complexity of the localization and distribution of Gal-3 increases the difficulty of correlating its expression with the occurrence and progression of cancer. Nonetheless, there are compelling data showing that the expression of Gal-3 in the cytoplasm and extracellularly increases in many types of cancer, and that the regulated localization of Gal-3 plays an important role in tumorigenicity and metastasis which supports Gal-3 as a target for cancer therapy. Our data regarding Gal-3C indicate that it can be localized in a carbohydrate-dependent manner similar to some of the localization of Gal-3, including apparent transport into the nucleus. Further study is required to elucidate the relationship between the subcellular localization of Gal-3C and efficacy in cancer.

What is the role of galectin-3 in metastasis? Will galectin-3C be therapeutic for cancer as an anti-metastatic agent?

An early observation in the galectin field was that many tumor cells express galectins on their surface that could be cross-linked by exogenous glycoproteins and then aggregate tumor cells and lead to tumor metastasis (*154*). The finding that hematogenous cancer metastases originate from intravascular growth of endothelium-attached rather than extravasated cancer cells highlights the key role of tumor-endothelial cell interactions in cancer metastases (*155*). The report that this critical interaction is mediated by Gal-3 provides one rationale for targeting it in inhibition of metastasis (*156*). Altered glycosylation of glycoproteins and glycolipids is one of the molecular changes that accompany malignant transformation (*157*). Tumor growth and metastasis was suppressed in mice deficient inbeta-1,6-*N*-acetylglcosaminyltrasferase V (Mgat5), an enzyme that catalyzes the addition of 1,6GlcNAc to form tri- and tetra antenna-like oligosaccharides that are often modified further to form polylactosamines that are high affinity ligands of Gal-3 (*158–160*).

Gal-3 binds to a number of glycosylated molecules that are strongly implicated in carcinogenesis, tumorigenicity, angiogenesis and/or metastasis such as laminin (*161*, *162*), carcinoembryonic antigen (CEA) (*163*), Thomsen-Friedenreich (TF) antigen (*156*, *164*), Mac-2-binding protein (*8*, *37*, *165*), lyosome-associated membrane proteins (LAMPS) (*166*), and integrins including $\alpha1\beta1$ (*38*), $\alpha5\beta1$ (*40*, *43*), and $\alpha5\beta3$ (*3*), $\alpha3\beta1$ (*121*, *167*, *168*). Gal-3 can promote $\alpha5\beta1$ integrin remodeling in FA (*43*), and has been found to modulate the expression of integrins (*118*). We showed that Gal-3C can inhibit $\alpha v\beta3$ integrin clustering on human umbilical cord vascular endothelial cells (HUVEC) (*2*).

Mucins (MUC) are large membrane-bound or secreted *O*-linked glycoproteins that protect and lubricate the luminal surfaces of ducts (*169*). MUC1, MUC4, and MUC16 (formerly CA-125) have been shown to be aberrantly overexpressed in various malignancies including cystic fibrosis and cancer. MUC1 binds to Gal-3 (*170*, *171*), and this interaction facilitates enhanced homotypic aggregation of cancer cells and increases their survival in anchorage-independent conditions (*172*). Gal-1 (*173*) and Gal-3 (*174*) have been reported to bind MUC16 that is a prognostic indicator in ovarian cancer (*175*, *176*) and is important in adhesion of ovarian cancer cells (*177*).

The interaction of surface Gal-3 with serum glycoproteins appears to promote aggregation of tumor cells in circulation (*178*). Blocking the adhesive interactions of cancer cells facilitates a type of apoptosis induced by loss of cell anchorage that is termed anoikis. By inducing homotypic aggregation and, thereby, protecting circulating cells from anoikis, Gal-3 plays a role in the survival of tumor cells until arrival and establishment at distant metastatic sites (*8*).

We tested the ability of Gal-3C to facilitate anoikis that was induced in two cancer cell lines by culturing them on polyHEMA-coated tissue culture dishes to prevent cell adhesion. To prepare the dishes, PolyHEMA (Sigma Aldrich, St. Louis, MO) was solubilized in methanol (50 mg/ml), and then diluted in ethanol to 10 mg/ml, and 4-ml of the solution was used to coat 100-mm petri dishes followed by drying in a biosafety cabinet with two repetitions. The cells (1.5×10^6) were cultured for 3 days on the polyHEMA-coated dishes with media containing Gal-3 or Gal-3C. The data (Figure 6) demonstrated that Gal-3C increased and Gal-3 reduced anoikis in both cell types. These results illustrate in vitro one type of effect that Gal-3C is expected to produce in vivo by increasing the anoikis of metastatic cancer cells by reducing either cell-cell or cell-ECM adhesion.

There is evidence that other galectins, such as Gal-1 (*179*) are tumorigenic. Being composed of the Gal-3 carbohydrate recognition domain, Gal-3C could be viewed as a "pan galectin inhibitor" because it has more affinity for some cancer-associated carbohydrates than most galectins. For example, Gal-3C has reportedly more affinity for $LacNAc_2$, (K_D = 4.8 μM), $LacNAc_3$, (0.87 μM) and $LacNAc_5$, (0.43 μM) than Gal-1 (K_D = 50, 45, and 39 μM, respectively) and has similar or more affinity than Gal-8 (K_D = 3.5, 9.6 and 1.6 μM, respectively) (*28*). The TF antigen (Galβ1-3GalNAcα1-O-Ser/Thr) is the main glycan on O-linked mucins that are common in tumor-associated glycosylation – occurring in over 90% of cancers. The affinity of Gal-3 for the TF antigen was recently shown to be more than 2 orders of magnitude higher than that of Gal-1 (*180*).

Expression of recombinant Gal-3 in weakly metastatic fibrosarcoma cells resulted in an increased incidence of experimental lung metastases in syngeneic and nude mice (*181*). Increased expression of Gal-3 from antisense DNA in human colon cancer cells also increased metastases, and a reduction in Gal-3 expression was associated with decreased liver colonization and spontaneous metastasis in athymic nude mice (*182*).

Modified citrus pectin (MCP) is a high molecular weight naturally-occurring complex carbohydrate that is thought to bind to and thereby inhibit galectins and especially Gal-3 (*183*). MCP blocked vascular endothelial growth factor (VEGF)-induced migration of multiple myeloma cells, and inhibited metastasis in several mouse models of cancer (*183–186*). Inclusion of inhibitors of Gal-3 such as MCP or antibody to TF-antigen or Gal-3, in solution with DU-145 human prostate and MDA-MB-435 cancer cells blocked more than 90% of their deposition 3 h after injection in the tail vein of mice (*164*) Upregulation of MMP-1 by Gal-3 apparently facilitates cell motility (*187*, *188*).

In a recent in vitro analysis, we found that 2.0 μg/ml Gal-3C inhibited more than 60% of the chemotaxis of U266 multiple myeloma cells stimulated by the chemokine, stem cell-derived factor(SDF)-1α in vitro (*2*). Our previous in vivo studies with Gal-3C revealed promising anti-metastatic activity in a xenograft MDA-MB-435 model of human breast cancer (*1*). Nude mice were treated with Gal-3C after MDA-MB-435 mammary fat pad tumors were palpable (>100 mm^3). Gal-3C was administered twice a day by i.m. injection of a dose of 5 mg/kg for 90 days and controls (n = 20) received vehicle only. Tumor volume ($W^2 \times L/2$, where W is the smallest dimension) was assessed weekly with calipers. Metastases were analyzed microscopically at autopsy by fluorescence imaging and by (H and E) analysis of paraffin-embedded tissues. Eleven out of twenty control mice compared to only four of the twenty mice in the Gal-3C group developed axillary lymph node metastasis ($p = 0.022$).

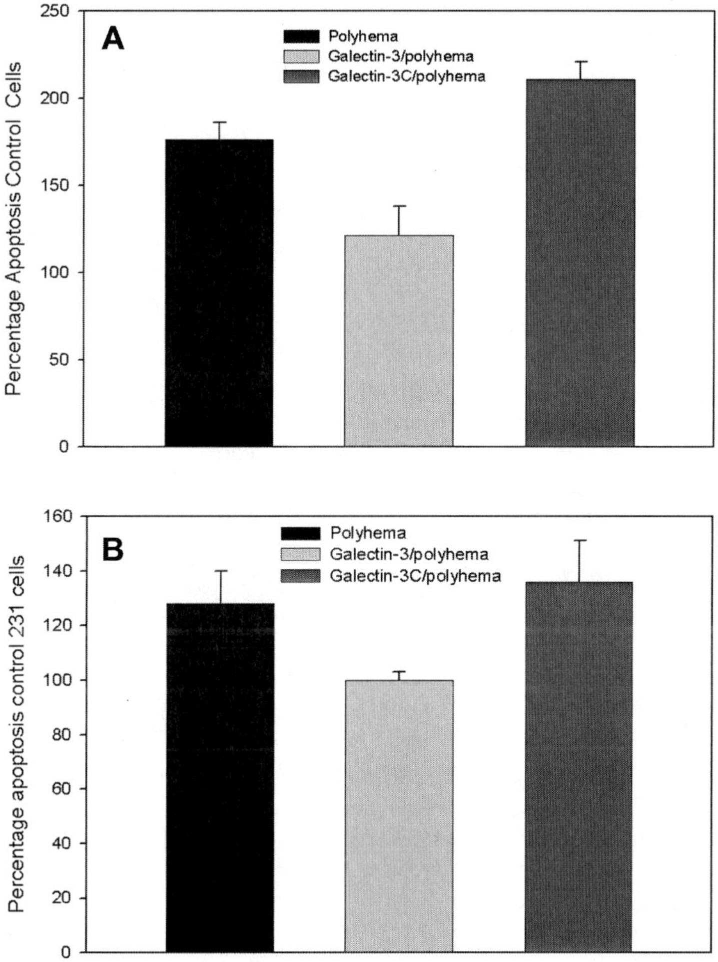

Figure 6. Anoikis (apoptosis induced by loss of cell anchorage) in MDA-MB-435 (A) and MDA-MB-231 (B) cells cultured on plates coated with polyHEMA. Polyhema-induced anoikis was inhibited by galectin-3 (1 µg/ml) and increased by galectin-3C (1 µg/ml). Apoptosis was detected as fluorescence of a substrate of caspase 3/7 using a kit available from Promega. Graphs represent duplicate wells with SD. Similar results were obtained in separate experiments and other cell lines.

We postulate that another mechanism whereby Gal-3C can inhibit chemotaxis of cancer cells and metastasis is by inhibiting the activation of integrins and turnover of FAs. A wide array of dynamic morphogenetic processes including cell adhesion and migration are regulated by integrin signaling. Galectins bind the *N*-glycans of some integrins and have been described as regulating integrin-mediated adhesion to the ECM (*38*, *121*). FAs are bidirectional sensors that are thought to enable cells to integrate intracellular and extracellular cues to respond appropriately to their environment. Recent data show that the galectin lattice alone can induce turnover of FAs. Gal-3 and tyrosine phosphorylated caveolin-1, which is expressed by plasma cells (*189*), can interdependently promote tumor cell migration (*120*, *190*). Gal-3, the MGAT5/Gal-3 lattice, and tyrosine phosphorylated caveolin-1 act together via integrin aggregation to regulate FAs and induce cell migration (*3*, *120*, *121*, *167*, *190*).

FAs mediate the interaction between ECM and cytoskeletal proteins leading to actomyosin contraction and actin polymerization that are required for cell migration and that play important roles in metastasis. Integrin clustering induces autophosphorylation of FA kinase, which forms a high affinity binding site for SH2-contining protein such as the Src family kinases, PI3K, Grb7, and phospholipase Cγ. Activation of FAK and PI3K leads to F-actin instability and the translocation of integrins to fibrillar adhesions (*40*). Recent data show that the promigratory activity of Gal-3 is dependent on activation of PI3K (*191*).

Investigation of the relationship between the adhesive and migratory potential of human ovarian cancer cells on laminin fibers in vitro showed that the extent of directed migration was dependent on cell polarity and FA expression, and that weakly adherent cells were more metastatic (*192*). These data highlight the potential significance of Gal-3 in regulating metastasis since it is thought to play an important role in cell adhesion, cell polarity, and the turnover of FAs (*43*, *96*, *102*, *120*, *130*, *172*, *191*, *193*, *194*).

Silencing expression of Gal-3 in animal models of cancers such as in prostate (*195*) and breast (*196*) reduced tumor growth and metastasis. However, results apparently contradictory to postulated roles for Gal-3 in cancer were obtained when galectin-3$^{(-/-)}$ mutant mice were crossed with genetic mouse models of intestinal cancer, *Apc^{Min}* and *Apc^{1638N}*, and a mouse mammary gland model, *PyMT*. Gal-3 was not a rate-limiting factor in tumorigenicity in these mice (*197*). This very likely was due to activity of other members of the galectin family, and the more than 1.3 fold up- or down-regulation of the expression of 22 glycosyltransferases (*55*). Gal-3 expression was significant in a study of the susceptibility to lung cancer induced by a powerful carcinogen, 4-(methylnitrosamino)-1-(3-pyridyle)-1-butanone (NNK) which revealed a decrease (28.6 vs 52.1%, $P < 0.05$) in tumors in Gal-3$^{-/-}$ deficient compared to wild-type (Gal-3$^{+/+}$) mice at 32 weeks (*198*). In addition, a recent study in a B16F1 model of melanoma revealed that lung metastases were 5-fold lower ($P<0.05$), and the average metastatic colony size was less ($P<0.05$) in Gal-3$^{(-/-)}$ mutant mice compared to WT mice (*199*).

The data described above provide striking evidence of the important role of Gal-3 in the process of metastasis, and the potential therapeutic effect of inhibiting metastasis with Gal-3C. However, despite its centrality in the lethality of most cancers there is no precedent for the development of a therapeutic agent that specifically acts by inhibition of the metastatic process. Nonetheless, given its importance in malignancy the potential to develop an inhibitor of metastasis must not be casually ignored. In any case, due to its novelty the development of an anti-cancer agent that is purported to act primarily as an inhibitor of metastasis could present unique challenges in clinical development.

How does galectin-3 affect the development of tumors and does galectin-3C have potential for inhibition of solid tumor?

Gal-3 has been shown to be important in a number of signal transduction pathways that are critical in cancer and tumorigenicity as has been described in a number of recent reviews (*129*, *200–202*). There is direct evidence that Gal-3 is required for expression of the transformed phenotype of tumors. Inhibition of Gal-3 expression caused breast carcinoma and thyroid papillary carcinoma cells to lose the transformed phenotypes in cell culture (*196*, *203*). Transfection of Gal-3 cDNA into a normal thyroid follicular cell line induced a transformed phenotype (*204*).

Gal-3 is thought to inhibit apoptosis at multiple sites (*11*, *205*, *206*) and has been reported to affect the extrinsic mitochondria-independent pathway of apoptosis induced by extracellular ligand binding and activation of caspase-8 (*13*, *207*), and the intrinsic intracellular pathway mediated by the release of cytochrome c (*111*, *208*, *209*). Even though Gal-3 is not a member of the Bcl-2 family, it contains the NWGR motif at residues 180-183 that is conserved in the BH1 domain of the *bcl-2* family, and it has 48% sequence similarity with Bcl-2 (*205*). Substitution of the G182 residue with A in the NWGR motif abrogates its antiapoptotic activity (*11*, *12*).

A close correlation has been found between the expression of Gal-3, malignancy, tumorigenicity and *K-Ras* that is the most frequently mutated of the Ras (*H, N* and *K*) genes in human cancers. These Ras proteins bind guanine nucleotides and when in the activated GTP-bound state, activate effectors such as Raf and PI3K that regulate cell proliferation, differentiation, and death. Interaction of S^6 phosphorylated Gal-3 in the cytoplasm with K-Ras stabilizes its active GTP-bound form (*67*, *116*, *210*).

Aberrant activation of the wingless-type(Wnt) signal transduction pathway that results in gene transcription by beta-catenin is thought to play a central role in the biology of cancer, and to be affected by Gal-3. Beta-catenin shuttles between the nucleus and the cytosol depending on its phosphorylation state, and the stimulation by beta-catenin of expression of cyclin D1 and c-myc has been shown to be dependent on Gal-3 (*113*). More recent data show that inhibition of Wnt-2 and Gal-3 synergistically induced apoptosis in colorectal cells (*114*), and suggested that Gal-3 mediates Wnt signaling at least partially by preventing the degradation of beta-catenin (*112*).

Both the EGF and the TGF-β1 receptors are crosslinked at the cell surface by Gal-3 binding to Mgat5-modified *N*-glycans on the receptors, and delaying constitutive endocytosis (*160*). VEGF-A and its receptors, particularly the glycoprotein VEGF receptor 2 (VEGF-R2) are critical for induction of angiogenesis.Interaction on the cell membrane between Gal-3 and VEGF-R2 was found to be dependent on the expression of Mgat5, and knockdown of either Gal-3 or Mgat5 increased the level of internalized VEGF-R2 indicating that Gal-3 clustering of the VEGF-R2 facilitates angiogenic signaling also by reducing its constitutive endocytosis (*42*). Gal-3 induces and inhibition of Gal-3 with MCP or Gal-3C blocks capillary tubular formation of human umbilical vascular endothelial cells (HUVEC) in vitro (*2–4*, *183*). β-lactose and Gal-3C reduced VEGF- and bFGF-mediated angiogenesis in vitro and the angiogenic response is reduced in Gal-3 knockdown cells and Gal3(-/-) animals (*3*).

Avastin (bevacizumab), the first anti-angiogenic agent, is a recombinant humanized monoclonal antibody approved for treatment of metastatic colorectal cancer by the FDA in 2004, and later also approved for treatment of NSCLC, metastatic renal cell cancer, and recurrent glioblastoma multiforme. It binds to and neutralizes the activity of VEGF, thus, inhibits the activation of the VEGF receptor. However, there are serious adverse side effects from bevacizumab that include severe or fatal hemorrhage/ bleeding, wound healing complications, gastrointestinal perforation, arterial thromboembolism, and congestive heart failure (*211*). We postulate that Gal-3C may have a lower risk of adverse side effects given its differing mechanism of inhibition of VEGF-mediated signaling, the viability of Gal-3 knockout mice (*212–214*), and our lack of observation of apparent adverse side effects in mice treated with Gal-3C (*1*). In addition, Gal-3C may have advantages in reducing adverse side effects from chemotherapeutic agents when used in combination therapies due to potential beneficial effects on the fibrotic response from damage to internal organs including in the heart (*20*), liver (*215*), lung (*44*), and kidney (*216*).

There have been several studies showing that inhibition of Gal-3 or of its ligands reduced the growth of primary tumors. Treatment of nude mice in an orthotopic xenograft MDA-MB-435 model of human breast cancer with 1% modified citrus pectin in the drinking water from one week prior to until day 35 after injection of MDA-MB-435 cells reduced tumor volume to 30% that of control animals (*183*). Reduction in the expression of Gal-3 in PC-3 prostate cancer cells by small interfering RNA (siRNA) inhibited cell migration and invasion, cell proliferation, anchorage-independent colony formation. The average weight of the PC-3 tumors with Gal-3 knockdown in nude mice was less than 40% that of the controls (*195*). Knockdown of the expression of Gal-3 N-glycan ligands by inhibition of Mgat5 with siRNA in human lung adenocarcinoma cells expressing the CD133 stem cell marker reduced their growth in vitro and in xenografts (*217*).

We found that inhibition of Gal-3 by treatment with Gal-3C significantly reduced average tumor volume in established MDA-MB-435 xenograft human breast tumors in the study described above (*1*). At day 90, the mean tumor volume of the treated mice was 49% that of the control group (P =0.003). In two treated mice the tumor disappeared by the end of the study even though it was about ten times the original size at day 40-60. We found that the elimination half-life of Gal-3C was only 3 h in the mice and, therefore, with sustained delivery of the protein that would maintain therapeutic concentrations of the protein it may be possible to achieve a greater response in terms of effect on tumor volume.

Subsequently using an osmotic pump for continuous delivery of Gal-3C in an NOD-SCID subcutaneous model of MM, we showed that the average tumor volume of the Gal-3C treated animals was only 13.5% that of the untreated controls at day 35 (*2*).

In summary, there are numerous studies indicating that Gal-3 promotes the growth of tumors and that inhibiting Gal-3 with agents such as MCP or Gal-3C could have therapeutic anti-tumor effects (*202*). Most solid tumors are treated by a combination of approaches including surgery, chemotherapy with one or more agents, and/or radiation. There is evidence that Gal-3 increases resistance to chemotherapeutic agents such as cisplatin, doxorubicin, etoposide, and gemcitabine (*129*, *140*, *218*, *219*). GCS-100, a form of modified citrus pectin, overcame bortezomib resistance and enhanced dexamethasone-induced apoptosis in multiple myeloma cells in vitro (*186*). Our data indicate that Gal-3C can facilitate the in vivo anti-tumor effect of bortezomib in multiple myeloma (*2*). Additional in vitro mechanistic and animal studies of combination therapy of anti-Gal-3 agents with chemo- or radiotherapy are warranted and are expected to provide relevant data regarding potential clinical application in treatment of solid tumors.

Conclusion

There have been a number of studies indicating that Gal-3 plays a dynamic role in the processes of tumorigenesis and metastasis, and showing that inhibitors of Gal-3 such as MCP or Gal-3C could have important therapeutic potential in cancer. Although much has been learned in the last decade about the effect of Gal-3 in cancer that is thought to be dependent on its variable localization, phosphorylation, enzymatic digestion, concentration, and the concentration of its ligands, there are aspects of the biology that remain to be more fully elucidated (*16*, *74*, *92*, *220*, *221*). These include how the localization and expression of Gal-3 are regulated, and the relationship between and triggers for the signal transduction cascades that involve Gal-3, which functions of Gal-3 are most significant in vivo, and to what extent inhibitors of Gal-3 will be therapeutic as single agents and in combination therapy in human cancer. There are challenges in designing experiments to elucidate the role of Gal-3 as it affects both extracellular interactions of cancer cells with the microenvironment, as well as intracellular functioning of oncogenes, regulation of cellular polarity and migratory potential, and inflammatory signaling.

Overall, the data show that Gal-3 has a complex, multi-faceted role that is critical in the relationship between cells of various malignancies and their microenvironment. Inhibiting Gal-3 directly such as with Gal-3C is expected to produce differing therapeutic effects compared to inhibitors of a single downstream effector such as PI3K (*222*) that is increasingly recognized as a target for cancer therapy (*223*). Based on endogenous expression in humans, preliminary animal experiments, the body of data regarding Gal-3 knockout mice, it is expected that Gal-3C will have a relatively low profile of adverse side effects. These facts together with the novelty of its mechanism of action as an inhibitor of Gal-3, the similarity to Gal-3 in its biodistribution, its potential to directly inhibit metastasis which plays such a profound role in most cancers, and promising preliminary data in xenograft models of breast cancer and multiple myeloma strongly support further development of Gal-3C as a clinical candidate for cancer treatment.

Acknowledgments

The work was supported by grant awards from the National Institutes of Health (CA135862 to C.M.J. and M.C.-I., CA092801 to C.M.J.) and a United States Department of the Army Breast Cancer Research Program Grant (DAMD17-98-1-8326 to G.A.J.).

References

1. John, C. M.; Leffler, H.; Kahl-Knutsson, B.; Svensson, I.; Jarvis, G. A. Truncated galectin-3 inhibits tumor growth and metastasis in orthotopic nude mouse model of human breast cancer. *Clin. Cancer Res.* **2003**, *9*, 2374–2383.
2. Mirandola, L.; Yu, Y.; Chui, K.; Jenkins, M. R.; Cobos, E.; John, C. M.; Chiriva-Internati, M. Galectin-3C inhibits tumor growth and increases the anticancer activity of bortezomib in a murine model of human multiple myeloma. *PLoS One* **2011**, *6*, e21811.
3. Markowska, A. I.; Liu, F. T.; Panjwani, N. Galectin-3 is an important mediator of VEGF- and bFGF-mediated angiogenic response. *J. Exp. Med.* **2010**, *207*, 1981–1993.
4. Balan, V.; Nangia-Makker, P.; Kho, D. H.; Wang, Y.; Raz, A. Tyrosine-phosphorylated galectin-3 protein is resistant to prostate-specific antigen (PSA) cleavage. *J. Biol. Chem.* **2012**, *287*, 5192–5198.
5. Le Marer, N.; Hughes, R. C. Effects of the carbohydrate-binding protein galectin-3 on the invasiveness of human breast carcinoma cells. *J. Cell. Physiol.* **1996**, *168*, 51–58.
6. Sano, H.; Hsu, D. K.; Yu, L.; Apgar, J. R.; Kuwabara, I.; Yamanaka, T.; Hirashima, M.; Liu, F. T. Human galectin-3 is a novel chemoattractant for monocytes and macrophages. *J. Immunol.* **2000**, *165*, 2156–2164.
7. Kobayashi, T.; Shimura, T.; Yajima, T.; Kubo, N.; Araki, K.; Tsutsumi, S.; Suzuki, H.; Kuwano, H.; Raz, A. Transient gene silencing of galectin-3 suppresses pancreatic cancer cell migration and invasion through degradation of beta-catenin. *Int. J. Cancer* **2011**, *129*, 2775–2786.
8. Inohara, H.; Akahani, S.; Koths, K.; Raz, A. Interactions between galectin-3 and Mac-2-binding protein mediate cell-cell adhesion. *Cancer Res.* **1996**, *56*, 4530–4534.
9. Matarrese, P.; Fusco, O.; Tinari, N.; Natoli, C.; Liu, F. T.; Semeraro, M. L.; Malorni, W.; Iacobelli, S. Galectin-3 overexpression protects from apoptosis by improving cell adhesion properties. *Int. J. Cancer* **2000**, *85*, 545–554.

10. Sato, S.; Ouellet, N.; Pelletier, I.; Simard, M.; Rancourt, A.; Bergeron, M. G. Role of galectin-3 as an adhesion molecule for neutrophil extravasation during streptococcal pneumonia. *J. Immunol.* **2002**, *168*, 1813–1822.
11. Akahani, S.; Nangia-Makker, P.; Inohara, H.; Kim, H. R.; Raz, A. Galectin-3: A novel antiapoptotic molecule with a functional BH1 (NWGR) domain of Bcl-2 family. *Cancer Res.* **1997**, *57*, 5272–5276.
12. Kim, H. R.; Lin, H. M.; Biliran, H.; Raz, A. Cell cycle arrest and inhibition of anoikis by galectin-3 in human breast epithelial cells. *Cancer Res.* **1999**, *59*, 4148–4154.
13. Hoyer, K. K.; Pang, M.; Gui, D.; Shintaku, I. P.; Kuwabara, I.; Liu, F. T.; Said, J. W.; Baum, L. G.; Teitell, M. A. An anti-apoptotic role for galectin-3 in diffuse large B-cell lymphomas. *Am. J. Pathol.* **2004**, *164*, 893–902.
14. Takenaka, Y.; Fukumori, T.; Yoshii, T.; Oka, N.; Inohara, H.; Kim, H. R.; Bresalier, R. S.; Raz, A. Nuclear export of phosphorylated galectin-3 regulates its antiapoptotic activity in response to chemotherapeutic drugs. *Mol. Cell. Biol.* **2004**, *24*, 4395–4406.
15. Oka, N.; Nakahara, S.; Takenaka, Y.; Fukumori, T.; Hogan, V.; Kanayama, H. O.; Yanagawa, T.; Raz, A. Galectin-3 inhibits tumor necrosis factor-related apoptosis-inducing ligand-induced apoptosis by activating Akt in human bladder carcinoma cells. *Cancer Res.* **2005**, *65*, 7546–7553.
16. Balan, V.; Nangia-Makker, P.; Jung, Y. S.; Wang, Y.; Raz, A. Galectin-3: A novel substrate for c-Abl kinase. *Biochim. Biophys. Acta* **2010**, *1803*, 1198–1205.
17. Fukumori, T.; Takenaka, Y.; Yoshii, T.; Kim, H. R.; Hogan, V.; Inohara, H.; Kagawa, S.; Raz, A. CD29 and CD7 mediate galectin-3-induced type II T-cell apoptosis. *Cancer Res.* **2003**, *63*, 8302–8311.
18. Stowell, S. R.; Qian, Y.; Karmakar, S.; Koyama, N. S.; Dias-Baruffi, M.; Leffler, H.; McEver, R. P.; Cummings, R. D. Differential roles of galectin-1 and galectin-3 in regulating leukocyte viability and cytokine secretion. *J. Immunol.* **2008**, *180*, 3091–3102.
19. Haudek, K. C.; Spronk, K. J.; Voss, P. G.; Patterson, R. J.; Wang, J. L.; Arnoys, E. J. Dynamics of galectin-3 in the nucleus and cytoplasm. *Biochim. Biophys. Acta* **2009**, *1800*, 181–189.
20. Lok, D. J.; Van Der Meer, P.; de la Porte, P. W.; Lipsic, E.; Van Wijngaarden, J.; Hillege, H. L.; van Veldhuisen, D. J. Prognostic value of galectin-3, a novel marker of fibrosis, in patients with chronic heart failure: Data from the DEAL-HF study. *Clin. Res. Cardiol.* **2011**, *99*, 323–328.
21. de Boer, R. A.; van Veldhuisen, D. J.; Gansevoort, R. T.; Muller Kobold, A. C.; van Gilst, W. H.; Hillege, H. L.; Bakker, S. J.; van der Harst, P. The fibrosis marker galectin-3 and outcome in the general population. *J. Intern. Med.* **2012**, *272*, 55–64.
22. Barondes, S. H.; Cooper, D. N.; Gitt, M. A.; Leffler, H. Galectins. Structure and function of a large family of animal lectins. *J. Biol. Chem.* **1994**, *269*, 20807–20810.
23. Rabinovich, G. A. Galectins: An evolutionarily conserved family of animal lectins with multifunctional properties; a trip from the gene to clinical therapy. *Cell Death Differ.* **1999**, *6*, 711–721.

24. Barboni, E. A.; Bawumia, S.; Henrick, K.; Hughes, R. C. Molecular modeling and mutagenesis studies of the N-terminal domains of galectin-3: Evidence for participation with the C-terminal carbohydrate recognition domain in oligosaccharide binding. *Glycobiology* **2000**, *10*, 1201–1208.
25. Oda, Y.; Leffler, H.; Sakakura, Y.; Kasai, K.; Barondes, S. H. Human breast carcinoma cDNA encoding a galactoside-binding lectin homologous to mouse Mac-2 antigen. *Gene* **1991**, *99*, 279–283.
26. Seetharaman, J.; Kanigsberg, A.; Slaaby, R.; Leffler, H.; Barondes, S. H.; Rini, J. M. X-ray crystal structure of the human galectin-3 carbohydrate recognition domain at 2.1-A resolution. *J. Biol. Chem.* **1998**, *273*, 13047–13052.
27. Saraboji, K.; Hakansson, M.; Genheden, S.; Diehl, C.; Qvist, J.; Weininger, U.; Nilsson, U. J.; Leffler, H.; Ryde, U.; Akke, M.; Logan, D. T. The carbohydrate-binding site in galectin-3 is preorganized to recognize a sugarlike framework of oxygens: Ultra-high-resolution structures and water dynamics. *Biochemistry* **2012**, *51*, 296–306.
28. Hirabayashi, J.; Hashidate, T.; Arata, Y.; Nishi, N.; Nakamura, T.; Hirashima, M.; Urashima, T.; Oka, T.; Futai, M.; Muller, W.; Yagi, F.; Kasai, K. Oligosaccharide specificity of galectins: A search by frontal affinity chromatography. *Biochim. Biophys. Acta* **2002**, *1572*, 232–254.
29. Bachhawat-Sikder, K.; Thomas, C. J.; Surolia, A. Thermodynamic analysis of the binding of galactose and poly-N-acetyllactosamine derivatives to human galectin-3. *FEBS Lett.* **2001**, *500*, 75–79.
30. Ahmad, N.; Gabius, H. J.; Sabesan, S.; Oscarson, S.; Brewer, C. F. Thermodynamic binding studies of bivalent oligosaccharides to galectin-1, galectin-3, and the carbohydrate recognition domain of galectin-3. *Glycobiology* **2004**, *14*, 817–825.
31. Hsu, D. K.; Zuberi, R. I.; Liu, F. T. Biochemical and biophysical characterization of human recombinant IgE-binding protein, an S-type animal lectin. *J. Biol. Chem.* **1992**, *267*, 14167–14174.
32. Massa, S. M.; Cooper, D. N.; Leffler, H.; Barondes, S. H. L-29, an endogenous lectin, binds to glycoconjugate ligands with positive cooperativity. *Biochemistry* **1993**, *32*, 260–267.
33. Morris, S.; Ahmad, N.; Andre, S.; Kaltner, H.; Gabius, H. J.; Brenowitz, M.; Brewer, F. Quaternary solution structures of galectins-1, -3, and -7. *Glycobiology* **2004**, *14*, 293–300.
34. Boscher, C.; Dennis, J. W.; Nabi, I. R. Glycosylation, galectins and cellular signaling. *Curr. Opin. Cell. Biol.*, *23*, 383–392.
35. Dam, T. K.; Brewer, C. F. Lectins as pattern recognition molecules: The effects of epitope density in innate immunity. *Glycobiology* **2010**, *20*, 270–279.
36. Ahmad, N.; Gabius, H. J.; Andre, S.; Kaltner, H.; Sabesan, S.; Roy, R.; Liu, B.; Macaluso, F.; Brewer, C. F. Galectin-3 precipitates as a pentamer with synthetic multivalent carbohydrates and forms heterogeneous cross-linked complexes. *J. Biol. Chem.* **2004**, *279*, 10841–7.
37. Sasaki, T.; Brakebusch, C.; Engel, J.; Timpl, R. Mac-2 binding protein is a cell-adhesive protein of the extracellular matrix which self-assembles into

ring-like structures and binds beta1 integrins, collagens and fibronectin. *EMBO J.* **1998**, *17*, 1606–1613.
38. Ochieng, J.; Leite-Browning, M. L.; Warfield, P. Regulation of cellular adhesion to extracellular matrix proteins by galectin-3. *Biochem. Biophys. Res. Commun.* **1998**, *246*, 788–791.
39. Hughes, R. C. Galectins as modulators of cell adhesion. *Biochimie* **2001**, *83*, 667–676.
40. Lagana, A.; Goetz, J. G.; Cheung, P.; Raz, A.; Dennis, J. W.; Nabi, I. R. Galectin binding to Mgat5-modified N-glycans regulates fibronectin matrix remodeling in tumor cells. *Mol. Cell. Biol.* **2006**, *26*, 3181–3193.
41. Nangia-Makker, P.; Honjo, Y.; Sarvis, R.; Akahani, S.; Hogan, V.; Pienta, K. J.; Raz, A. Galectin-3 induces endothelial cell morphogenesis and angiogenesis. *Am. J. Pathol.* **2000**, *156*, 899–909.
42. Markowska, A. I.; Jefferies, K. C.; Panjwani, N. Galectin-3 protein modulates cell surface expression and activation of vascular endothelial growth factor receptor 2 in human endothelial cells. *J. Biol. Chem.* **2011**, *286*, 29913–29921.
43. Dennis, J. W.; Lau, K. S.; Demetriou, M.; Nabi, I. R. Adaptive regulation at the cell surface by N-glycosylation. *Traffic* **2009**, *10*, 1569–1578.
44. Mackinnon, A. C.; Gibbons, M. A.; Farnworth, S. L.; Leffler, H.; Nilsson, U. J.; Delaine, T.; Simpson, A. J.; Forbes, S. J.; Hirani, N.; Gauldie, J.; Sethi, T. Regulation of TGF-beta1 driven lung fibrosis by galectin-3. *Am. J. Respir. Crit. Care Med.* **2012**, *185*, 537–546.
45. Delacour, D.; Greb, C.; Koch, A.; Salomonsson, E.; Leffler, H.; Le Bivic, A.; Jacob, R. Apical sorting by galectin-3-dependent glycoprotein clustering. *Traffic* **2007**, *8*, 379–388.
46. Delacour, D.; Cramm-Behrens, C. I.; Drobecq, H.; Le Bivic, A.; Naim, H. Y.; Jacob, R. Requirement for galectin-3 in apical protein sorting. *Curr. Biol.* **2006**, *16*, 408–414.
47. Truong, M. J.; Gruart, V.; Kusnierz, J. P.; Papin, J. P.; Loiseau, S.; Capron, A.; Capron, M. Human neutrophils express immunoglobulin E (IgE)-binding proteins (Mac- 2/epsilon BP) of the S-type lectin family: Role in IgE-dependent activation. *J. Exp. Med.* **1993**, *177*, 243–248.
48. Liu, F. T.; Hsu, D. K.; Zuberi, R. I.; Kuwabara, I.; Chi, E. Y.; Henderson, W. R., Jr. Expression and function of galectin-3, a beta-galactoside-binding lectin, in human monocytes and macrophages. *Am. J. Pathol.* **1995**, *147*, 1016–1028.
49. Capron, M.; Soussi Gounni, A.; Morita, M.; Truong, M. J.; Prin, L.; Kinet, J. P.; Capron, A. Eosinophils: From low- to high-affinity immunoglobulin E receptors. *Allergy* **1995**, *50*, 20–23.
50. Kimata, H. Enhancement of IgE production in B cells by neutrophils via galectin-3 in IgE-associated atopic eczema/dermatitis syndrome. *Int. Arch. Allergy Immunol.* **2002**, *128*, 168–170.
51. Bernardes, E. S.; Silva, N. M.; Ruas, L. P.; Mineo, J. R.; Loyola, A. M.; Hsu, D. K.; Liu, F. T.; Chammas, R.; Roque-Barreira, M. C. *Toxoplasma gondii* infection reveals a novel regulatory role for galectin-3 in the interface of innate and adaptive immunity. *Am. J. Pathol.* **2006**, *168*, 1910–1920.

52. Vasta, G. R. Roles of galectins in infection. *Nat. Rev. Microbiol.* **2009**, *7*, 424–438.
53. MacKinnon, A. C.; Farnworth, S. L.; Hodkinson, P. S.; Henderson, N. C.; Atkinson, K. M.; Leffler, H.; Nilsson, U. J.; Haslett, C.; Forbes, S. J.; Sethi, T. Regulation of alternative macrophage activation by galectin-3. *J. Immunol.* **2008**, *180*, 2650–2658.
54. Henderson, N. C.; Mackinnon, A. C.; Farnworth, S. L.; Poirier, F.; Russo, F. P.; Iredale, J. P.; Haslett, C.; Simpson, K. J.; Sethi, T. Galectin-3 regulates myofibroblast activation and hepatic fibrosis. *Proc. Natl. Acad. Sci. U.S.A* **2006**, *103*, 5060–5065.
55. Saravanan, C.; Cao, Z.; Head, S. R.; Panjwani, N. Detection of differentially expressed wound-healing-related glycogenes in galectin-3-deficient mice. *Invest. Ophthalmol. Vis. Sci.* **2009**, *50*, 5690–5696.
56. Lin, H. M.; Moon, B. K.; Yu, F.; Kim, H. R. Galectin-3 mediates genistein-induced G(2)/M arrest and inhibits apoptosis. *Carcinogenesis* **2000**, *21*, 1941–1945.
57. Ochieng, J.; Fridman, R.; Nangia-Makker, P.; Kleiner, D. E.; Liotta, L. A.; Stetler-Stevenson, W. G.; Raz, A. Galectin-3 is a novel substrate for human matrix metalloproteinases-2 and -9. *Biochemistry* **1994**, *33*, 14109–14114.
58. Ochieng, J.; Green, B.; Evans, S.; James, O.; Warfield, P. Modulation of the biological functions of galectin-3 by matrix metalloproteinases. *Biochim. Biophys. Acta* **1998**, *1379*, 97–106.
59. Guevremont, M.; Martel-Pelletier, J.; Boileau, C.; Liu, F. T.; Richard, M.; Fernandes, J. C.; Pelletier, J. P.; Reboul, P. Galectin-3 surface expression on human adult chondrocytes: A potential substrate for collagenase-3. *Ann. Rheum. Dis.* **2004**, *63*, 636–643.
60. Toth, M.; Osenkowski, P.; Hesek, D.; Brown, S.; Meroueh, S.; Sakr, W.; Mobashery, S.; Fridman, R. Cleavage at the stem region releases an active ectodomain of the membrane type 1 matrix metalloproteinase. *Biochem. J.* **2005**, *387*, 497–506.
61. Puthenedam, M.; Wu, F.; Shetye, A.; Michaels, A.; Rhee, K. J.; Kwon, J. H. Matrilysin-1 (MMP7) cleaves galectin-3 and inhibits wound healing in intestinal epithelial cells. *Inflamm. Bowel Dis.* **2011**, *17*, 260–267.
62. Nangia-Makker, P.; Raz, T.; Tait, L.; Hogan, V.; Fridman, R.; Raz, A. Galectin-3 cleavage: a novel surrogate marker for matrix metalloproteinase activity in growing breast cancers. *Cancer Res.* **2007**, *67*, 11760–11768.
63. Nangia-Makker, P.; Balan, V.; Raz, A. Regulation of tumor progression by extracellular galectin-3. *Cancer Microenviron.* **2008**, *1*, 43–51.
64. Huflejt, M. E.; Turck, C. W.; Lindstedt, R.; Barondes, S. H.; Leffler, H. L-29, a soluble lactose-binding lectin, is phosphorylated on serine 6 and serine 12 in vivo and by casein kinase I. *J. Biol. Chem.* **1993**, *268*, 26712–26718.
65. Mazurek, N.; Conklin, J.; Byrd, J. C.; Raz, A.; Bresalier, R. S. Phosphorylation of the beta-galactoside-binding protein galectin-3 modulates binding to its ligands. *J. Biol. Chem.* **2000**, *275*, 36311–36315.
66. Yoshii, T.; Fukumori, T.; Honjo, Y.; Inohara, H.; Kim, H. R.; Raz, A. Galectin-3 phosphorylation is required for its anti-apoptotic function and cell cycle arrest. *J. Biol. Chem.* **2002**, *277*, 6852–6857.

67. Levy, R.; Biran, A.; Poirier, F.; Raz, A.; Kloog, Y. Galectin-3 mediates cross-talk between K-Ras and Let-7c tumor suppressor microRNA. *PLoS One* **2011**, *6*, e27490.
68. Menon, S.; Kang, C. M.; Beningo, K. A. Galectin-3 secretion and tyrosine phosphorylation is dependent on the calpain small subunit, Calpain 4. *Biochem. Biophys. Res. Commun* **2011**, *410*, 91–96.
69. Shimura, T.; Takenaka, Y.; Fukumori, T.; Tsutsumi, S.; Okada, K.; Hogan, V.; Kikuchi, A.; Kuwano, H.; Raz, A. Implication of galectin-3 in Wnt signaling. *Cancer Res.* **2005**, *6*, 3535–3537.
70. Kim, S. J.; Choi, I. J.; Cheong, T. C.; Lee, S. J.; Lotan, R.; Park, S. H.; Chun, K. H. Galectin-3 increases gastric cancer cell motility by up-regulating fascin-1 expression. *Gastroenterology* **2010**, *138*, 1035–1045, e1–2.
71. van den Brule, F. A.; Liu, F. T.; Castronovo, V. Transglutaminase-mediated oligomerization of galectin-3 modulates human melanoma cell interactions with laminin. *Cell Adhes. Commun.* **1998**, *5*, 425–435.
72. Mehul, B.; Bawumia, S.; Hughes, R. C. Cross-linking of galectin 3, a galactose-binding protein of mammalian cells, by tissue-type transglutaminase. *FEBS Let.t* **1995**, *360*, 160–164.
73. Balan, V.; Nangia-Makker, P.; Schwartz, A. G.; Jung, Y. S.; Tait, L.; Hogan, V.; Raz, T.; Wang, Y.; Yang, Z. Q.; Wu, G. S.; Guo, Y.; Li, H.; Abrams, J.; Couch, F. J.; Lingle, W. L.; Lloyd, R. V.; Ethier, S. P.; Tainsky, M. A.; Raz, A. Racial disparity in breast cancer and functional germ line mutation in galectin-3 (rs4644): A pilot study. *Cancer Res.* **2008**, *68*, 10045–10050.
74. Nangia-Makker, P.; Wang, Y.; Raz, T.; Tait, L.; Balan, V.; Hogan, V.; Raz, A. Cleavage of galectin-3 by matrix metalloproteases induces angiogenesis in breast cancer. *Int. J. Cancer* **2010**, *127*, 2530–2541.
75. Hu, C. Y.; Chang, S. K.; Wu, C. S.; Tsai, W. I.; Hsu, P. N. Galectin-3 gene (LGALS3) +292C allele is a genetic predisposition factor for rheumatoid arthritis in Taiwan. *Clin. Rheumatol.* **2011**, *30*, 1227–1233.
76. Wu, F.; Hu, N.; Li, Y.; Bian, B.; Xu, G.; Zheng, Y. Galectin-3 genetic variants are associated with platinum-based chemotherapy response and prognosis in patients with NSCLC. *Cell. Oncol. (Dordrecht)* **2012**, *35*, 175–180.
77. Kim, S. J.; Shin, J. Y.; Cheong, T. C.; Choi, I. J.; Lee, Y. S.; Park, S. H.; Chun, K. H. Galectin-3 germline variant at position 191 enhances nuclear accumulation and activation of beta-catenin in gastric cancer. *Clin. Exp. Metastasis* **2011**, *28*, 743–750.
78. Nangia-Makker, P.; Kato, I.; Raz, T.; ; Vitaly, B.; Raz, A. Galectin-3 SNP rs10148371 in the Anti-Death Motif NWGR Is Related to the Colon Cancer Incidence in African Americans. ACR 103rd Annual Meeting 2012. *Cancer Res.* Chicago, IL., Abstract 2017.
79. Raimond, J.; Zimonjic, D. B.; Mignon, C.; Mattei, M.; Popescu, N. C.; Monsigny, M.; Legrand, A. Mapping of the galectin-3 gene (LGALS3) to human chromosome 14 at region 14q21-22. *Mamm. Genome* **1997**, *8*, 706–707.

80. Kadrofske, M. M.; Openo, K. P.; Wang, J. L. The human LGALS3 (galectin-3) gene: Determination of the gene structure and functional characterization of the promoter. *Arch. Biochem. Biophys.* **1998**, *349*, 7–20.
81. Raimond, J.; Rouleux, F.; Monsigny, M.; Legrand, A. The second intron of the human galectin-3 gene has a strong promoter activity down-regulated by p53. *FEBS Lett.* **1995**, *363*, 165–169.
82. Ahmed, H.; Cappello, F.; Rodolico, V.; Vasta, G. R. Evidence of heavy methylation in the galectin 3 promoter in early stages of prostate adenocarcinoma: Development and validation of a methylated marker for early diagnosis of prostate cancer. *Transl. Oncol.* **2009**, *2*, 146–156.
83. Saraswati, S.; Block, A. S.; Davidson, M. K.; Rank, R. G.; Mahadevan, M.; Diekman, A. B. Galectin-3 is a substrate for prostate specific antigen (PSA) in human seminal plasma. *Prostate* **2010**, *71*, 197–208.
84. Yang, R. Y.; Hill, P. N.; Hsu, D. K.; Liu, F. T. Role of the carboxyl-terminal lectin domain in self-association of galectin-3. *Biochemistry* **1998**, *37*, 4086–4092.
85. Kuklinski, S.; Probstmeier, R. Homophilic binding properties of galectin-3: Involvement of the carbohydrate recognition domain. *J. Neurochem.* **1998**, *70*, 814–823.
86. Lepur, A.; Salomonsson, E.; Nilsson, U. J.; Leffler, H. Ligand induced galectin-3 self-association. *J. Biol. Chem.* **2012**, *287*, 21751–21756.
87. Hughes, R. C. Secretion of the galectin family of mammalian carbohydrate-binding proteins. *Biochim. Biophys. Acta* **1999**, *1473*, 172–185.
88. Menon, R. P.; Hughes, R. C. Determinants in the N-terminal domains of galectin-3 for secretion by a novel pathway circumventing the endoplasmic reticulum-Golgi complex. *Eur. J. Biochem.* **1999**, *264*, 569–576.
89. Mehul, B.; Hughes, R. C. Plasma membrane targetting, vesicular budding and release of galectin 3 from the cytoplasm of mammalian cells during secretion. *J. Cell. Sci.* **1997**, *110*, 1169–178.
90. Sato, S.; Hughes, R. C. Regulation of secretion and surface expression of Mac-2, a galactoside-binding protein of macrophages. *J. Biol. Chem.* **1994**, *269*, 4424–4430.
91. Gaudin, J. C.; Mehul, B.; Hughes, R. C. Nuclear localisation of wild type and mutant galectin-3 in transfected cells. *Biol. Cell.* **2000**, *92*, 49–58.
92. Davidson, P. J.; Davis, M. J.; Patterson, R. J.; Ripoche, M. A.; Poirier, F.; Wang, J. L. Shuttling of galectin-3 between the nucleus and cytoplasm. *Glycobiology* **2002**, *12*, 329–337.
93. Lindstedt, T.; Apodaca, G.; Barondes, S. H.; Mostov, K.; Leffler, H. Apical secretion nof a cytosolic protein by Madin-Darby canine kidney cells. Evidence for polarized release of an endogenous lectin by a nonclassical secretory pathway. *J. Biol. Chem.* **1993**, *268*, 11750–11757.
94. Sato, S.; Burdett, I.; Hughes, R. C. Secretion of the baby hamster kidney 30-kDa galactose-binding lectin from polarized and nonpolarized cells: A pathway independent of the endoplasmic reticulum-Golgi complex. *Exp. Cell. Res.* **1993**, *207*, 8–18.

95. Furtak, V.; Hatcher, F.; Ochieng, J. Galectin-3 mediates the endocytosis of beta-1 integrins by breast carcinoma cells. *Biochem. Biophys. Res. Commun.* **2001**, *289*, 845–850.
96. Schneider, D.; Greb, C.; Koch, A.; Straube, T.; Elli, A.; Delacour, D.; Jacob, R. Trafficking of galectin-3 through endosomal organelles of polarized and non-polarized cells. *Eur. J. Cell. Biol.* **2010**, *89*, 788–798.
97. Lepur, A.; Carlsson, M.; Novak, R.; Dumic, J.; Nilsson, U.; Leffler, H. Galectin-3 endocytosis by carbohydrate independent and dependent pathways in different macrophage like cell types. *Biochim. Biophys. Acta* **2012**, *1820*, 804–818.
98. Davidson, P. J.; Li, S. Y.; Lohse, A. G.; Vandergaast, R.; Verde, E.; Pearson, A.; Patterson, R. J.; Wang, J. L.; Arnoys, E. J. Transport of galectin-3 between the nucleus and cytoplasm. I. Conditions and signals for nuclear import. *Glycobiology* **2006**, *16*, 602–611.
99. Li, S. Y.; Davidson, P. J.; Lin, N. Y.; Patterson, R. J.; Wang, J. L.; Arnoys, E. J. Transport of galectin-3 between the nucleus and cytoplasm. II. Identification of the signal for nuclear export. *Glycobiology* **2006**, *16*, 612–622.
100. Nakahara, S.; Oka, N.; Wang, Y.; Hogan, V.; Inohara, H.; Raz, A. Characterization of the nuclear import pathways of galectin-3. *Cancer Res.* **2006**, *66*, 9995–10006.
101. Zhu, W. Q.; Ochieng, J. Rapid release of intracellular galectin-3 from breast carcinoma cells by fetuin. *Cancer Res.* **2001**, *61*, 1869–1873.
102. Baptiste, T. A.; James, A.; Saria, M.; Ochieng, J. Mechano-transduction mediated secretion and uptake of galectin-3 in breast carcinoma cells: Implications in the extracellular functions of the lectin. *Exp. Cell. Res.* **2007**, *313*, 652–664.
103. Wang, L.; Inohara, H.; Pienta, K. J.; Raz, A. Galectin-3 is a nuclear matrix protein which binds RNA. *Biochem. Biophys. Res. Commun.* **1995**, *217*, 292–303.
104. Dagher, S. F.; Wang, J. L.; Patterson, R. J. Identification of galectin-3 as a factor in pre-mRNA splicing. *Proc. Natl. Acad. Sci. U.S.A.* **1995**, *92*, 1213–1217.
105. Vyakarnam, A.; Dagher, S. F.; Wang, J. L.; Patterson, R. J. Evidence for a role for galectin-1 in pre-mRNA splicing. *Mol. Cell. Biol.* **1997**, *17*, 4740–4737.
106. Wang, W.; Park, J. W.; Wang, J. L.; Patterson, R. J. Immunoprecipitation of spliceosomal RNAs by antisera to galectin-1 and galectin-3. *Nucleic Acids Res.* **2006**, *34*, 5166–5174.
107. Park, J. W.; Voss, P. G.; Grabski, S.; Wang, J. L.; Patterson, R. J. Association of galectin-1 and galectin-3 with Gemin4 in complexes containing the SMN protein. *Nucleic Acids Res.* **2001**, *29*, 3595–3602.
108. Wang, J. L.; Gray, R. M.; Haudek, K. C.; Patterson, R. J. Nucleocytoplasmic lectins. *Biochim. Biophys. Acta* **2004**, *1673*, 75–93.
109. Paces-Fessy, M.; Boucher, D.; Petit, E.; Paute-Briand, S.; Blanchet-Tournier, M. F. The negative regulator of Gli, Suppressor of fused (Sufu), interacts with SAP18, Galectin3 and other nuclear proteins. *Biochem. J.* **2004**, *378*, 353–362.

110. Fukumori, T.; Oka, N.; Takenaka, Y.; Nangia-Makker, P.; Elsamman, E.; Kasai, T.; Shono, M.; Kanayama, H. O.; Ellerhorst, J.; Lotan, R.; Raz, A. Galectin-3 regulates mitochondrial stability and antiapoptotic function in response to anticancer drug in prostate cancer. *Cancer Res.* **2006**, *66*, 3114–3119.
111. Nangia-Makker, P.; Nakahara, S.; Hogan, V.; Raz, A. Galectin-3 in apoptosis, a novel therapeutic target. *J. Bioenerg. Biomembr.* **2007**, *39*, 79–84.
112. Song, S.; Mazurek, N.; Liu, C.; Sun, Y.; Ding, Q. Q.; Liu, K.; Hung, M. C.; Bresalier, R. S. Galectin-3 mediates nuclear beta-catenin accumulation and Wnt signaling in human colon cancer cells by regulation of glycogen synthase kinase-3beta activity. *Cancer Res.* **2009**, *69*, 1343–1349.
113. Shimura, T.; Takenaka, Y.; Tsutsumi, S.; Hogan, V.; Kikuchi, A.; Raz, A. Galectin-3, a novel binding partner of beta-catenin. *Cancer Res.* **2004**, *64*, 6363–6367.
114. Shi, Y.; He, B.; Kuchenbecker, K. M.; You, L.; Xu, Z.; Mikami, I.; Yagui-Beltran, A.; Clement, G.; Lin, Y. C.; Okamoto, J.; Bravo, D. T.; Jablons, D. M. Inhibition of Wnt-2 and galectin-3 synergistically destabilizes beta-catenin and induces apoptosis in human colorectal cancer cells. *Int. J. Cancer* **2007**, *121*, 1175–1181.
115. Weinberger, P. M.; Adam, B. L.; Gourin, C. G.; Moretz, W. H., 3rd; Bollag, R. J.; Wang, B. Y.; Liu, Z.; Lee, J. R.; Terris, D. J. Association of nuclear, cytoplasmic expression of galectin-3 with beta-catenin/Wnt-pathway activation in thyroid carcinoma. *Arch. Otolaryngol. Head Neck Surg.* **2007**, *133*, 503–510.
116. Elad-Sfadia, G.; Haklai, R.; Balan, E.; Kloog, Y. Galectin-3 augments K-Ras activation and triggers a Ras signal that attenuates ERK but not phosphoinositide 3-kinase activity. *J. Biol. Chem.* **2004**, *279*, 34922–34930.
117. Shalom-Feuerstein, R.; Levy, R.; Makovski, V.; Raz, A.; Kloog, Y. Galectin-3 regulates RasGRP4-mediated activation of N-Ras and H-Ras. *Biochim. Biophys. Acta* **2008**, *1783*, 985–993.
118. Warfield, P. R.; Makker, P. N.; Raz, A.; Ochieng, J. Adhesion of human breast carcinoma to extracellular matrix proteins is modulated by galectin-3. *Invasion Metastasis* **1997**, *17*, 101–112.
119. Ochieng, J.; Warfield, P.; Green-Jarvis, B.; Fentie, I. Galectin-3 regulates the adhesive interaction between breast carcinoma cells and elastin. *J. Cell. Biochem.* **1999**, *75*, 505–514.
120. Goetz, J. G.; Joshi, B.; Lajoie, P.; Strugnell, S. S.; Scudamore, T.; Kojic, L. D.; Nabi, I. R. Concerted regulation of focal adhesion dynamics by galectin-3 and tyrosine-phosphorylated caveolin-1. *J. Cell. Biol.* **2008**, *180*, 1261–1275.
121. Saravanan, C.; Liu, F. T.; Gipson, I. K.; Panjwani, N. Galectin-3 promotes lamellipodia formation in epithelial cells by interacting with complex N-glycans on alpha3beta1 integrin. *J. Cell. Sci.* **2009**, *122*, 3684–3693.
122. Schnitzer, J. E.; Oh, P.; Pinney, E.; Allard, J. Filipin-sensitive caveolae-mediated transport in endothelium: Reduced transcytosis, scavenger endocytosis, and capillary permeability of select macromolecules. *J. Cell. Biol.* **1994**, *127*, 1217–1232.

123. Qaddoumi, M. G.; Gukasyan, H. J.; Davda, J.; Labhasetwar, V.; Kim, K. J.; Lee, V. H. Clathrin and caveolin-1 expression in primary pigmented rabbit conjunctival epithelial cells: Role in PLGA nanoparticle endocytosis. *Mol. Vis.* **2003**, *9*, 559–568.
124. Gong, H. C.; Honjo, Y.; Nangia-Makker, P.; Hogan, V.; Mazurak, N.; Bresalier, R. S.; Raz, A. The NH2 terminus of galectin-3 governs cellular compartmentalization and functions in cancer cells. *Cancer Res.* **1999**, *59*, 6239–6245.
125. Shankar, J.; Wiseman, S. M.; Meng, F.; Kasaian, K.; Strugnell, S.; Mofid, A.; Gown, A.; Jones, S. J.; Nabi, I. R. Coordinate expression of galectin-3 and caveolin-1 in thyroid cancer. *J. Pathol.* **2012**, *228*, 56–66.
126. Iurisci, I.; Tinari, N.; Natoli, C.; Angelucci, D.; Cianchetti, E.; Iacobelli, S. Concentrations of galectin-3 in the sera of normal controls and cancer patients. *Clin. Cancer Res.* **2000**, *6*, 1389–1393.
127. Sakaki, M.; Oka, N.; Nakanishi, R.; Yamaguchi, K.; Fukumori, T.; Kanayama, H. O. Serum level of galectin-3 in human bladder cancer. *J. Med. Invest.* **2008**, *55*, 127–132.
128. Balasubramanian, K.; Vasudevamurthy, R.; Venkateshaiah, S. U.; Thomas, A.; Vishweshwara, A.; Dharmesh, S. M. Galectin-3 in urine of cancer patients: Stage and tissue specificity. *J. Cancer. Res. Clin. Oncol.* **2009**, *135*, 355–363.
129. Fukumori, T.; Kanayama, H. O.; Raz, A. The role of galectin-3 in cancer drug resistance. *Drug Resist. Update* **2007**, *10*, 101–108.
130. Nakahara, S.; Oka, N.; Raz, A. On the role of galectin-3 in cancer apoptosis. *Apoptosis* **2005**, *10*, 267–275.
131. Califice, S.; Castronovo, V.; Bracke, M.; van den Brule, F. Dual activities of galectin-3 in human prostate cancer: Tumor suppression of nuclear galectin-3 vs tumor promotion of cytoplasmic galectin-3. *Oncogene* **2004**, *23*, 7527–7536.
132. Honjo, Y.; Inohara, H.; Akahani, S.; Yoshii, T.; Takenaka, Y.; Yoshida, J.; Hattori, K.; Tomiyama, Y.; Raz, A.; Kubo, T. Expression of cytoplasmic galectin-3 as a prognostic marker in tongue carcinoma. *Clin. Cancer. Res.* **2000**, *6*, 4635–4640.
133. Buttery, R.; Monaghan, H.; Salter, D. M.; Sethi, T. Galectin-3: Differential expression between small-cell and non-small-cell lung cancer. *Histopathology* **2004**, *44*, 339–344.
134. Szoke, T.; Kayser, K.; Trojan, I.; Kayser, G.; Furak, J.; Tiszlavicz, L.; Baumhakel, J. D.; Gabius, H. J. The role of microvascularization and growth/adhesion-regulatory lectins in the prognosis of non-small cell lung cancer in stage II. *Eur. J. Cardiothorac. Surg.* **2007**, *31*, 783–87.
135. Bresalier, R. S.; Byrd, J. C.; Wang, L.; Raz, A. Colon cancer mucin: A new ligand for the beta-galactoside-binding protein galectin-3. *Cancer Res.* **1996**, *56*, 4354–4357.
136. Nakamura, M.; Inufusa, H.; Adachi, T.; Aga, M.; Kurimoto, M.; Nakatani, Y.; Wakano, T.; Nakajima, A.; Hida, J. I.; Miyake, M.; Shindo, K.; Yasutomi, M. Involvement of galectin-3 expression in colorectal cancer progression and metastasis. *Int. J. Oncol.* **1999**, *15*, 143–148.

137. Legendre, H.; Decaestecker, C.; Nagy, N.; Hendlisz, A.; Schuring, M. P.; Salmon, I.; Gabius, H. J.; Pector, J. C.; Kiss, R. Prognostic values of galectin-3 and the macrophage migration inhibitory factor (MIF) in human colorectal cancers. *Mod. Pathol.* **2003**, *16*, 491–504.
138. Gasbarri, A.; Marchetti, C.; Iervasi, G.; Bottoni, A.; Nicolini, A.; Bartolazzi, A.; Carpi, A. From the bench to the bedside. Galectin-3 immunodetection for improving the preoperative diagnosis of the follicular thyroid nodules. *Biomed. Pharmacother.* **2004**, *58*, 356–359.
139. Finley, D. J.; Arora, N.; Zhu, B.; Gallagher, L.; Fahey, T. J., 3rd Molecular profiling distinguishes papillary carcinoma from benign thyroid nodules. *J. Clin. Endocrinol. Metab.* **2004**, *89*, 3214–3223.
140. Lin, C. I.; Whang, E. E.; Abramson, M. A.; Donner, D. B.; Bertagnolli, M. M.; Moore, F. D., Jr.; Ruan, D. T. Galectin-3 regulates apoptosis and doxorubicin chemoresistance in papillary thyroid cancer cells. *Biochem. Biophys. Res. Commun.* **2009**, *379*, 626–631.
141. Turkoz, H. K.; Oksuz, H.; Yurdakul, Z.; Ozcan, D. Galectin-3 expression in tumor progression and metastasis of papillary thyroid carcinoma. *Endocr. Pathol.* **2008**, *19*, 92–96.
142. Kawachi, K.; Matsushita, Y.; Yonezawa, S.; Nakano, S.; Shirao, K.; Natsugoe, S.; Sueyoshi, K.; Aikou, T.; Sato, E. Galectin-3 expression in various thyroid neoplasms and its possible role in metastasis formation. *Hum. Pathol.* **2000**, *31*, 428–433.
143. Castronovo, V.; Van Den Brule, F. A.; Jackers, P.; Clausse, N.; Liu, F. T.; Gillet, C.; Sobel, M. E. Decreased expression of galectin-3 is associated with progression of human breast cancer. *J. Pathol.* **1996**, *179*, 43–48.
144. Shekhar, M. P.; Nangia-Makker, P.; Nangia-Makker, P.; Tait, L.; Tait, L.; Miller, F.; Miller, F.; Raz, A.; Raz, A. Alterations in galectin-3 expression and distribution correlate with breast cancer progression: Functional analysis of galectin-3 in breast epithelial-endothelial interactions. *Am. J. Pathol.* **2004**, *165*, 1931–1941.
145. Jones, C.; Mackay, A.; Grigoriadis, A.; Cossu, A.; Reis-Filho, J. S.; Fulford, L.; Dexter, T.; DaviesBulmer, S., K.; Ford, E.; Parry, S.; Budroni, M.; Palmieri, G.; Neville, A. M.; O'Hare, M. J.; Lakhani, S. R. Expression profiling of purified normal human luminal and myoepithelial breast cells: Identification of novel prognostic markers for breast cancer. *Cancer Res.* **2004**, *64*, 3037–3045.
146. Kim, M. K.; Sung, C. O.; Do, I. G.; Jeon, H. K.; Song, T. J.; Park, H. S.; Lee, Y. Y.; Kim, B. G.; Lee, J. W.; Bae, D. S. Overexpression of galectin-3 and its clinical significance in ovarian carcinoma. *Int. J. Clin. Oncol.* **2011**, *16*, 352–358.
147. Yamamoto-Sugitani, M.; Kuroda, J.; Ashihara, E.; Nagoshi, H.; Kobayashi, T.; Matsumoto, Y.; Sasaki, N.; Shimura, Y.; Kiyota, M.; Nakayama, R.; Akaji, K.; Taki, T.; Uoshima, N.; Kobayashi, Y.; Horiike, S.; Maekawa, T.; Taniwaki, M. Galectin-3 (Gal-3) induced by leukemia microenvironment promotes drug resistance and bone marrow lodgment in chronic myelogenous leukemia. *Proc. Natl. Acad. Sci. U.S.A* **2011**, *108*, 17468–17473.

148. Vereecken, P.; Zouaoui Boudjeltia, K.; Debray, C.; Awada, A.; Legssyer, I.; Sales, F.; Petein, M.; Vanhaeverbeek, M.; Ghanem, G.; Heenen, M. High serum galectin-3 in advanced melanoma: Preliminary results. *Clin. Exp. Dermatol.* **2006**, *31*, 105–109.
149. Prieto, V. G.; Mourad-Zeidan, A. A.; Melnikova, V.; Johnson, M. M.; Lopez, A.; Diwan, A. H.; Lazar, A. J.; Shen, S. S.; Zhang, P. S.; Reed, J. A.; Gershenwald, J. E.; Raz, A.; Bar-Eli, M. Galectin-3 expression is associated with tumor progression and pattern of sun exposure in melanoma. *Clin. Cancer Res.* **2006**, *12*, 6709–6715.
150. Isic, T.; Savin, S.; Cvejic, D.; Marecko, I.; Tatic, S.; Havelka, M.; Paunovic, I. Serum Cyfra 21.1 and galectin-3 protein levels in relation to immunohistochemical cytokeratin 19 and galectin-3 expression in patients with thyroid tumors. *J. Cancer Res. Clin. Oncol.* **2010**, *136*, 1805–1812.
151. Saussez, S.; Lorfevre, F.; Lequeux, T.; Laurent, G.; Chantrain, G.; Vertongen, F.; Toubeau, G.; Decaestecker, C.; Kiss, R. The determination of the levels of circulating galectin-1 and -3 in HNSCC patients could be used to monitor tumor progression and/or responses to therapy. *Oral Oncol.* **2008**, *44*, 86–93.
152. Barrow, H.; Guo, X.; Wandall, H. H.; Pedersen, J. W.; Fu, B.; Zhao, Q.; Chen, C.; Rhodes, J. M.; Yu, L. G. Serum galectin-2, -4, and -8 are greatly increased in colon and breast cancer patients and promote cancer cell adhesion to blood vascular endothelium. *Clin. Cancer. Res.*, *17*, 7035–7046.
153. Matsuda, Y.; Yamagiwa, Y.; Fukushima, K.; Ueno, Y.; Shimosegawa, T. Expression of galectin-3 involved in prognosis of patients with hepatocellular carcinoma. *Hepatol. Res.* **2008**, *38*, 1098–1111.
154. Raz, A.; Lotan, R. Lectin-like activities associated with human and murine neoplastic cells. *Cancer Res.* **1981**, *41*, 3642–3647.
155. Al-Mehdi, A. B.; Tozawa, K.; Fisher, A. B.; Shientag, L.; Lee, A.; Muschel, R. J. Intravascular origin of metastasis from the proliferation of endothelium-attached tumor cells: A new model for metastasis. *Nat. Med.* **2000**, *6*, 100–102.
156. Glinsky, V. V.; Glinsky, G. V.; Rittenhouse-Olson, K.; Huflejt, M. E.; Glinskii, O. V.; Deutscher, S. L.; Quinn, T. P. The role of Thomsen-Friedenreich antigen in adhesion of human breast and prostate cancer cells to the endothelium. *Cancer Res.* **2001**, *61*, 4851–4857.
157. Dennis, J. W.; Granovsky, M.; Warren, C. E. Glycoprotein glycosylation and cancer progression. *Biochim. Biophys. Acta* **1999**, *1473*, 21–34.
158. Granovsky, M.; Fata, J.; Pawling, J.; Muller, W. J.; Khokha, R.; Dennis, J. W. Suppression of tumor growth and metastasis in Mgat5-deficient mice. *Nat. Med.* **2000**, *6*, 306–312.
159. Couldrey, C.; Green, J. E. Metastases: The glycan connection. *Breast Cancer Res.* **2000**, *2*, 321–323.
160. Partridge, E. A.; Le Roy, C.; Le Roy, C.; Di Guglielmo, G. M.; Di Guglielmo, G. M.; Pawling, J.; Pawling, J.; Cheung, P.; Cheung, P.; Granovsky, M.; Granovsky, M.; Nabi, I. R.; Nabi, I. R.; Wrana, J. L.; Wrana, J. L.; Dennis, J. W.; Dennis, J. W. Regulation of cytokine receptors by Golgi N-glycan processing and endocytosis. *Science* **2004**, *306*, 120–124.

161. Ochieng, J.; Warfield, P. Galectin-3 binding potentials of mouse tumor EHS and human placental laminins. *Biochem. Biophys. Res. Commun.* **1995**, *217*, 402–406.
162. Kuwabara, I.; Liu, F. T. Galectin-3 promotes adhesion of human neutrophils to laminin. *J. Immunol.* **1996**, *156*, 3939–3944.
163. Ohannesian, D. W.; Lotan, D.; Thomas, P.; Jessup, J. M.; Fukuda, M.; Gabius, H. J.; Lotan, R. Carcinoembryonic antigen and other glycoconjugates act as ligands for galectin-3 in human colon carcinoma cells. *Cancer Res.* **1995**, *55*, 2191–2199.
164. Glinskii, O. V.; Huxley, V. H.; Huxley, V. H.; Glinsky, G. V.; Glinsky, G. V.; Pienta, K. J.; Pienta, K. J.; Raz, A.; Raz, A.; Glinsky, V. V.; Glinsky, V. V. Mechanical entrapment is insufficient and intercellular adhesion is essential for metastatic cell arrest in distant organs. *Neoplasia* **2005**, *7*, 522–527.
165. Kunzli, B. M.; Berberat, P. O.; Zhu, Z. W.; Martignoni, M.; Kleeff, J.; Tempia-Caliera, A. A.; Fukuda, M.; Zimmermann, A.; Friess, H.; Buchler, M. W. Influences of the lysosomal associated membrane proteins (Lamp-1, Lamp-2) and Mac-2 binding protein (Mac-2-BP) on the prognosis of pancreatic carcinoma. *Cancer* **2002**, *94*, 228–239.
166. Sarafian, V.; Jadot, M.; Foidart, J. M.; Letesson, J. J.; Van den Brule, F.; Castronovo, V.; Wattiaux, R.; Coninck, S. W. Expression of Lamp-1 and Lamp-2 and their interactions with galectin-3 in human tumor cells. *Int. J. Cancer.* **1998**, *75*, 105–111.
167. Fukushi, J.; Makagiansar, I. T.; Stallcup, W. B. NG2 proteoglycan promotes endothelial cell motility and angiogenesis via engagement of galectin-3 and alpha3beta1 integrin. *Mol. Biol. Cell.* **2004**, *15*, 3580–3590.
168. Wen, Y.; Makagiansar, I. T.; Fukushi, J.; Liu, F. T.; Fukuda, M. N.; Stallcup, W. B. Molecular basis of interaction between NG2 proteoglycan and galectin-3. *J. Cell. Biochem.* **2006**, *98*, 115–127.
169. Bafna, S.; Kaur, S.; Batra, S. K. Membrane-bound mucins: The mechanistic basis for alterations in the growth and survival of cancer cells. *Oncogene* **2010**, *29*, 2893–2904.
170. Yu, L. G.; Andrews, N.; Zhao, Q.; McKean, D.; Williams, J. F.; Connor, L. J.; Gerasimenko, O. V.; Hilkens, J.; Hirabayashi, J.; Kasai, K.; Rhodes, J. M. Galectin-3 interaction with Thomsen-Friedenreich disaccharide on cancer-associated MUC1 causes increased cancer cell endothelial adhesion. *J. Biol. Chem.* **2007**, *282*, 773–781.
171. Zhao, Q.; Guo, X.; Nash, G. B.; Stone, P. C.; Hilkens, J.; Rhodes, J. M.; Yu, L. G. Circulating galectin-3 promotes metastasis by modifying MUC1 localization on cancer cell surface. *Cancer Res.* **2009**, *69*, 6799–6806.
172. Zhao, Q.; Barclay, M.; Hilkens, J.; Guo, X.; Barrow, H.; Rhodes, J. M.; Yu, L. G. Interaction between circulating galectin-3 and cancer-associated MUC1 enhances tumour cell homotypic aggregation and prevents anoikis. *Mol. Cancer* **2010**, *9*, 154.
173. Seelenmeyer, C.; Wegehingel, S.; Lechner, J.; Nickel, W. The cancer antigen CA125 represents a novel counter receptor for galectin-1. *J. Cell. Sci.* **2003**, *116*, 1305–1318.

174. Argueso, P.; Guzman-Aranguez, A.; Mantelli, F.; Cao, Z.; Ricciuto, J.; Panjwani, N. Association of cell surface mucins with galectin-3 contributes to the ocular surface epithelial barrier. *J. Biol. Chem.* **2009**, *284*, 23037–23045.
175. de Bruijn, H. W.; van der Zee, A. G.; Aalders, J. G. The value of cancer antigen 125 (CA 125) during treatment and follow-up of patients with ovarian cancer. *Curr. Opin. Obstet. Gynecol.* **1997**, *9*, 8–13.
176. Han, L. Y.; Karavasilis, V.; Hagen, T.; Nicum, S.; Thomas, K.; Harrison, M.; Papadopoulos, P.; Blake, P.; Barton, D. P.; Gore, M.; Kaye, S. B. Doubling time of serum CA125 is an independent prognostic factor for survival in patients with ovarian cancer relapsing after first-line chemotherapy. *Eur. J. Cancer* **2010**, *46*, 1359–1364.
177. Gaetje, R.; Winnekendonk, D. W.; Ahr, A.; Kaufmann, M. Ovarian cancer antigen CA 125 influences adhesion of human and mammalian cell lines in vitro. *Clin. Exp Obstet. Gynecol.* **2002**, *29*, 34–36.
178. Inohara, H.; Raz, A. Functional evidence that cell surface galectin-3 mediates homotypic cell adhesion. *Cancer Res.* **1995**, *55*, 3267–3671.
179. Rabinovich, G. A. Galectin-1 as a potential cancer target. *Br. J. Cancer* **2005**, *92*, 1188–1192.
180. Bian, C. F.; Zhang, Y.; Sun, H.; Li, D. F.; Wang, D. C. Structural basis for distinct binding properties of the human galectins to Thomsen-Friedenreich antigen. *PLoS One* **2011**, *6*, e25007.
181. Raz, A.; Zhu, D. G.; Hogan, V.; Shah, N.; Raz, T.; Karkash, R.; Pazerini, G.; Carmi, P. Evidence for the role of 34-kDa galactoside-binding lectin in transformation and metastasis. *Int. J. Cancer* **1990**, *46*, 871–877.
182. Bresalier, R. S.; Mazurek, N.; Sternberg, L. R.; Byrd, J. C.; Yunker, C. K.; Nangia-Makker, P.; Raz, A. Metastasis of human colon cancer is altered by modifying expression of the beta-galactoside-binding protein galectin 3. *Gastroenterology* **1998**, *115*, 287–296.
183. Nangia-Makker, P.; Hogan, V.; Honjo, Y.; Baccarini, S.; Tait, L.; Bresalier, R.; Raz, A. Inhibition of human cancer cell growth and metastasis in nude mice by oral intake of modified citrus pectin. *J. Natl. Cancer Inst.* **2002**, *94*, 1854–1862.
184. Pienta, K. J.; Naik, H.; Akhtar, A.; Yamazaki, K.; Replogle, T. S.; Lehr, J.; Donat, T. L.; Tait, L.; Hogan, V.; Raz, A. Inhibition of spontaneous metastasis in a rat prostate cancer model by oral administration of modified citrus pectin [see comments]. *J. Natl. Cancer Inst.* **1995**, *87*, 348–353.
185. Hayashi, A.; Gillen, A. C.; Lott, J. R. Effects of daily oral administration of quercetin chalcone and modified citrus pectin. *Altern. Med. Rev.* **2000**, *5*, 546–552.
186. Chauhan, D.; Li, G.; Podar, K.; Hideshima, T.; Neri, P.; He, D.; Mitsiades, N.; Richardson, P.; Chang, Y.; Schindler, J.; Carver, B.; Anderson, K. C. A novel carbohydrate-based therapeutic GCS-100 overcomes bortezomib resistance and enhances dexamethasone-induced apoptosis in multiple myeloma cells. *Cancer Res.* **2005**, *65*, 8350–8358.

187. Wang, Y. G.; Kim, S. J.; Baek, J. H.; Lee, H. W.; Jeong, S. Y.; Chun, K. H. Galectin-3 increases the motility of mouse melanoma cells by regulating matrix metalloproteinase-1 expression. *Exp. Mol. Med.* **2012**, *44*, 387–393.
188. Kim, S. J.; Shin, Y. J.; Lee, K. D.; Bae, Y. K.; Choi, I. J.; Park, S. H.; Chun, K. H. Galectin-3 facilitates cell motility in gastric cancer by up-regulating proteaseactivated receptor-1 (PAR-1) and matrix metalloproteinase-1 (MMP-1). *PLoS One* **2011**, *6*, e25103.
189. Fernandez, P. L.; Merino, M. J.; Gomez, M.; Campo, E.; Medina, T.; Castronovo, V.; Sanjuan, X.; Cardesa, A.; Liu, F. T.; Sobel, M. E. Galectin-3 and laminin expression in neoplastic and non-neoplastic thyroid tissue. *J. Pathol.* **1997**, *181*, 80–86.
190. Goetz, J. G. Bidirectional control of the inner dynamics of focal adhesions promotes cell migration. *Cell. Adhes. Migr.* **2009**, *3*, 185–190.
191. Melo, F. H.; Butera, D.; Junqueira Mde, S.; Hsu, D. K.; da Silva, A. M.; Liu, F. T.; Santos, M. F.; Chammas, R. The promigratory activity of the matricellular protein galectin-3 depends on the activation of PI-3 kinase. *PLoS One* **2011**, *6*, e29313.
192. Chen, X.; Brewer, M. A.; Zou, C.; Campagnola, P. J. Adhesion and migration of ovarian cancer cells on crosslinked laminin fibers nanofabricated by multiphoton excited photochemistry. *Integr. Biol. (Cambridge)* **2009**, *1*, 469–476.
193. Delacour, D.; Koch, A.; Ackermann, W.; Eude-Le Parco, I.; Elsasser, H. P.; Poirier, F.; Jacob, R. Loss of galectin-3 impairs membrane polarisation of mouse enterocytes in vivo. *J. Cell. Sci.* **2008**, *121*, 458–465.
194. Inohara, H.; Raz, A. Effects of natural complex carbohydrate (citrus pectin) on murine melanoma cell properties related to galectin-3 functions. *Glycoconjugate J.* **1994**, *11*, 527–532.
195. Wang, Y.; Nangia-Makker, P.; Tait, L.; Balan, V.; Hogan, V.; Pienta, K. J.; Raz, A. Regulation of prostate cancer progression by galectin-3. *Am. J. Pathol.* **2009**, *174*, 1515–1523.
196. Honjo, Y.; Nangia-Makker, P.; Inohara, H.; Raz, A. Down-regulation of galectin-3 suppresses tumorigenicity of human breast carcinoma cells. *Clin. Cancer. Res.* **2001**, *7*, 661–668.
197. Eude-Le Parco, I.; Gendronneau, G.; Dang, T.; Delacour, D.; Thijssen, V. L.; Edelmann, W.; Peuchmaur, M.; Poirier, F. Genetic assessment of the importance of galectin-3 in cancer initiation, progression, and dissemination in mice. *Glycobiology* **2009**, *19*, 68–75.
198. Abdel-Aziz, H. O.; Murai, Y.; Takasaki, I.; Tabuchi, Y.; Zheng, H. C.; Nomoto, K.; Takahashi, H.; Tsuneyama, K.; Kato, I.; Hsu, D. K.; Liu, F. T.; Hiraga, K.; Takano, Y. Targeted disruption of the galectin-3 gene results in decreased susceptibility to NNK-induced lung tumorigenesis: An oligonucleotide microarray study. *J. Cancer Res. Clin. Oncol.* **2008**, *134*, 777–788.
199. Radosavljevic, G.; Jovanovic, I.; Majstorovic, I.; Mitrovic, M.; Lisnic, V. J.; Arsenijevic, N.; Jonjic, S.; Lukic, M. L. Deletion of galectin-3 in the host attenuates metastasis of murine melanoma by modulating tumor adhesion and NK cell activity. *Clin. Exp. Metastasis* **2011**, *28*, 451–462.

200. Califice, S.; Castronovo, V.; Van Den Brule, F. Galectin-3 and cancer (Review). *Int. J. Oncol.* **2004**, *25*, 983–992.
201. Liu, F. T.; Rabinovich, G. A. Galectins as modulators of tumour progression. *Nat. Rev. Cancer* **2005**, *5*, 29–41.
202. Newlaczyl, A. U.; Yu, L. G. Galectin-3: A jack-of-all-trades in cancer. *Cancer Lett.* **2011**, *313*, 123–128.
203. Takenaka, Y.; Inohara, H.; Yoshii, T.; Oshima, K.; Nakahara, S.; Akahani, S.; Honjo, Y.; Yamamoto, Y.; Raz, A.; Kubo, T. Malignant transformation of thyroid follicular cells by galectin-3. *Cancer Lett.* **2003**, *195*, 111–119.
204. Yoshii, T.; Inohara, H.; Takenaka, Y.; Honjo, Y.; Akahani, S.; Nomura, T.; Raz, A.; Kubo, T. Galectin-3 maintains the transformed phenotype of thyroid papillary carcinoma cells. *Int. J. Oncol.* **2001**, *18*, 787–792.
205. Yang, R.-Y.; Hsu, D.; Liu, F.-T. Expression of galectin-3 modulates T-cell growth and apoptosis. *Proc. Natl. Acad. Sci. U.S.A.* **1996**, *93*, 6737–6742.
206. Song, Y. K.; Billiar, T. R.; Lee, Y. J. Role of galectin-3 in breast cancer metastasis: Involvement of nitric oxide. *Am. J. Pathol.* **2002**, *160*, 1069–1075.
207. Fukumori, T.; Takenaka, Y.; Oka, N.; Yoshii, T.; Hogan, V.; Inohara, H.; Kanayama, H. O.; Kim, H. R.; Raz, A. Endogenous galectin-3 determines the routing of CD95 apoptotic signaling pathways. *Cancer Res.* **2004**, *64*, 3376–3379.
208. Moon, B. K.; Lee, Y. J.; Battle, P.; Jessup, J. M.; Raz, A.; Kim, H. R. Galectin-3 protects human breast carcinoma cells against nitric oxide-induced apoptosis: Implication of galectin-3 function during metastasis. *Am. J. Pathol.* **2001**, *159*, 1055–1060.
209. Yu, F.; Finley, R. L., Jr.; Raz, A.; Kim, H. R. Galectin-3 translocates to the perinuclear membranes and inhibits cytochrome c release from the mitochondria. A role for synexin in galectin-3 translocation. *J. Biol. Chem.* **2002**, *277*, 15819–15827.
210. Shalom-Feuerstein, R.; Cooks, T.; Raz, A.; Kloog, Y. Galectin-3 regulates a molecular switch from N-Ras to K-Ras usage in human breast carcinoma cells. *Cancer Res.* **2005**, *65*, 7292–7300.
211. Gressett, S. M.; Shah, S. R. Intricacies of bevacizumab-induced toxicities and their management. *Ann. Pharmacother.* **2009**, *43*, 490–501.
212. Colnot, C.; Ripoche, M. A.; Milon, G.; Montagutelli, X.; Crocker, P. R.; Poirier, F. Maintenance of granulocyte numbers during acute peritonitis is defective in galectin-3-null mutant mice. *Immunology* **1998**, *94*, 290–296.
213. Boileau, C.; Poirier, F.; Pelletier, J. P.; Guevremont, M.; Duval, N.; Martel-Pelletier, J.; Reboul, P. Intracellular localisation of galectin-3 has a protective role in chondrocyte survival. *Ann. Rheum. Dis.* **2008**, *67*, 175–181.
214. Doverhag, C.; Hedtjarn, M.; Poirier, F.; Mallard, C.; Hagberg, H.; Karlsson, A.; Savman, K. Galectin-3 contributes to neonatal hypoxic-ischemic brain injury. *Neurobiol. Dis.* **2010**, *38*, 36–46.
215. Iacobini, C.; Menini, S.; Ricci, C.; Fantauzzi, C. B.; Scipioni, A.; Salvi, L.; Cordone, S.; Delucchi, F.; Serino, M.; Federici, M.; Pricci, F.; Pugliese, G. Galectin-3 ablation protects mice from diet-induced NASH: A major scavenging role for galectin-3 in liver. *J. Hepatol.* **2011**, *54*, 975–983.

216. Kolatsi-Joannou, M.; Price, K. L.; Winyard, P. J.; Long, D. A. Modified citrus pectin reduces galectin-3 expression and disease severity in experimental acute kidney injury. *PLoS One* **2011**, *6*, e18683.
217. Zhou, X.; Chen, H.; Wang, Q.; Zhang, L.; Zhao, J. Knockdown of Mgat5 inhibits CD133+ human pulmonary adenocarcinoma cell growth in vitro and in vivo. *Clin. Invest. Med.* **2011**, *34*, E155–E162.
218. Oishi, T.; Itamochi, H.; Kigawa, J.; Kanamori, Y.; Shimada, M.; Takahashi, M.; Shimogai, R.; Kawaguchi, W.; Sato, S.; Terakawa, N. Galectin-3 may contribute to Cisplatin resistance in clear cell carcinoma of the ovary. *Int. J. Gynecol. Cancer* **2007**, *17*, 1040–1046.
219. Kobayashi, T.; Shimura, T.; Yajima, T.; Kubo, N.; Araki, K.; Wada, W.; Tsutsumi, S.; Suzuki, H.; Kuwano, H.; Raz, A. Transient silencing of galectin-3 expression promotes both in vitro and in vivo drug-induced apoptosis of human pancreatic carcinoma cells. *Clin. Exp. Metastasis* **2011**, *28*, 367–376.
220. Openo, K. P.; Kadrofske, M. M.; Patterson, R. J.; Wang, J. L. Galectin-3 expression and subcellular localization in senescent human fibroblasts. *Exp. Cell Res.* **2000**, *255*, 278–290.
221. Di Lella, S.; Sundblad, V.; Cerliani, J. P.; Guardia, C. M.; Estrin, D. A.; Vasta, G. R.; Rabinovich, G. A. When galectins recognize glycans: From biochemistry to physiology and back again. *Biochemistry* **2011**, *50*, 7842–7857.
222. Melo, F. H.; Butera, D.; Junqueira Mde, S.; Hsu, D. K.; da Silva, A. M.; Liu, F. T.; Santos, M. F.; Chammas, R. The promigratory activity of the matricellular protein galectin-3 depends on the activation of PI-3 kinase. *PLoS One*, *6*, e29313.
223. Chen, Y.; Wang, B. C.; Xiao, Y. PI3K: A potential therapeutic target for cancer. *J. Cell Physiol.* **2012**, *227*, 2818–2821.

Chapter 13

Angiostatic Cancer Therapy by Targeting Galectins in the Tumor Vasculature

Iris A. Schulkens,[1] Arjan W. Griffioen,[1] and Victor L. Thijssen*,[1,2]

[1]Angiogenesis Laboratory, Department of Radiation Oncology and Medical Oncology, and VU University Medical Center, De Boelelaan 1118, 1081 HV Amsterdam,The Netherlands
[2]Department of Radiation Oncology, VU University Medical Center, De Boelelaan 1118, 1081 HV Amsterdam, The Netherlands
*E-mail: v.thijssen@vumc.nl

Tumors depend on a functional blood supply to grow and to facilitate metastasis. Therefore, tumors induce the growth of novel blood vessels from pre-existing capillaries, a process known as tumor angiogenesis. Interfering with this process is considered a promising cancer therapy. Recent studies indicate that galectins are involved in tumor angiogenesis and that they might provide opportunities for angiostatic cancer therapy. Here, we review the current knowledge regarding the expression and function of galectins in the tumor vasculature and their role in tumor angiogenesis. Strategies to interfere with galectin function for anti-angiogenesis therapy are discussed and the application of galectin-targeting strategies for targeted drug delivery, diagnostic imaging, and drug-sensitization are described.

Tumor Angiogenesis

The human vasculature is the biological infrastructure that facilitates the transport of nutrients, gasses and cells throughout the body. It consists of a complex network of blood vessels with an estimated length of approximately 100000 km (60000 miles). Already early during embryonic development, the first vessels arise from endothelial precursor cells that organize into a primitive network of small capillaries (*1*). This de novo formation of blood vessels, or vasculogenesis, is followed by angiogenesis, a process by which new vessels emerge from existing capillaries. Several variants of angiogenesis are known of which sprouting angiogenesis is the most extensively studied and best understood (*2*, *3*). Sprouting angiogenesis involves a series of steps which starts with the activation of endothelial cells (EC) in capillary vessels. The EC form the inner lining of all blood vessels and their activation is induced by growth factor signaling through specific receptors on the cell surface. Upon activation, several proteases are activated that degrade both the basement membrane and the extracellular matrix surrounding the EC. In addition, the EC become proliferative and migrate into the surrounding tissue creating new tubular structures. These premature growing vessels attract pericytes and smooth muscle cells for structural support and eventually a functional mature vascular network is formed (*2*, *3*).

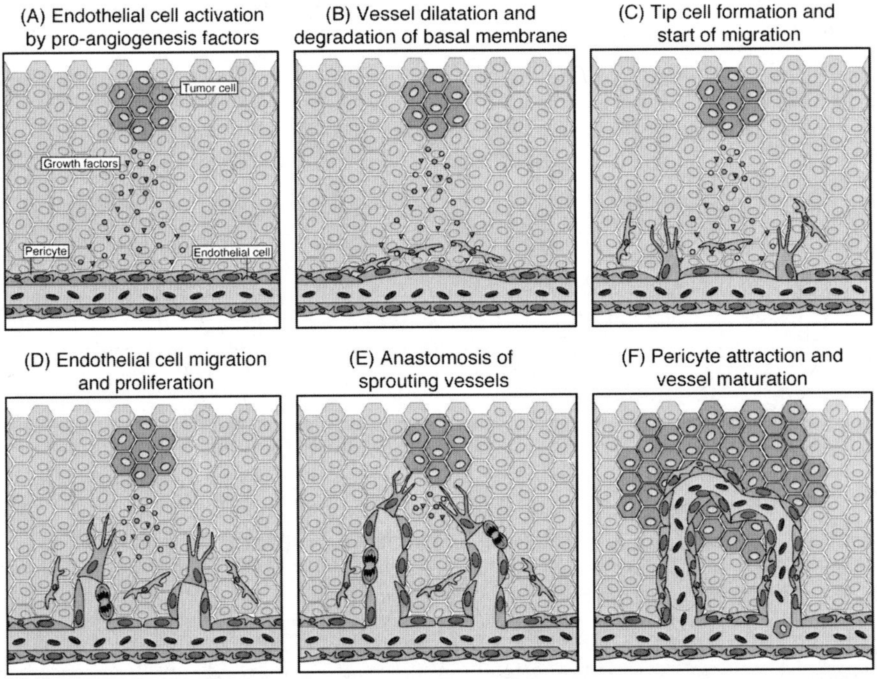

Figure 1. Tumor angiogenesis Schematic representation of the different steps of the angiogenesis cascade. First, tumor cells under metabolic stress, e.g. hypoxia, secrete growth factors that activate endothelial cells in nearby capillaries (A). The activated endothelial cells produce proteases which degrade the basal membrane, accompanied by vessel dilatation and pericyte detachment (B). Next, endothelial tip cells start to move in the direction of the growth factor gradient (C). The continuous proliferating and migrating endothelial cells form tube-like structures (D) which grow towards the tumor cells (E). Eventually the growing sprouts anastomose and a functional vessel is formed by depositing a new basal membrane and attraction of pericytes. This process will eventually allow the tumor to grow and also will facilitate tumor metastasis (F). (see color insert)

While angiogenesis is important during physiological processes like embryonic development, wound healing and inflammation, it has also been implicated in different pathologies including cancer (*4*). Tumors, like most other tissues, rely on a continuous supply of nutrients and oxygen. To grow beyond a few cubic millimeters in size tumor cells have to induce angiogenesis (*5*). Under hypoxic conditions most tumors eventually undergo the so-called angiogenic switch which results in the secretion of pro-angiogenesis growth factors. This stimulates tumor angiogenesis which in turn allows expansion of the tumor mass and facilitates tumor metastasis (Figure 1). Not surprisingly, it has been proposed that interfering with tumor angiogenesis could provide an opportunity for cancer therapy (*6*). Evidence has accumulated that galectins in the tumor endothelium might provide opportunities for targeted cancer therapy (*7*).

Galectin Expression in the Tumor Endothelium

In normal, quiescent endothelial cells the mRNA expression of galectins appears to be confined to galectin-1, -3, -8, and -9 (*8–13*) of which the latter two have been described to be subjected to alternative splicing (*12*, *14–18*). The galectin proteins can be detected at the cell surface but have also been found in the cell cytoplasm and the nucleus. This suggests a role for galectins in different cellular functions in endothelial cell biology which is supported by the observation that expression and localization of galectins changes in activated endothelial cells (*10*, *12*, *19*). For example, we observed decreased numbers of galectin-8 and -9 positive endothelial cells in the vasculature of colon tumor compared with normal colon (*12*). Additional data on the expression of these galectins in endothelial cells is limited. Most other studies assessed the endothelial expression and function of galectin-1 and/or galectin-3. We observed increased galectin-1 expression in activated EC of colon carcinoma, breast carcinoma and sarcoma as compared with EC in normal tissue (*13*). Clausse et al. demonstrated that the frequency of galectin-1 positive EC in primary prostate tissue sections increased from 7% in non-tumor associated capillaries to 64% in capillaries localized in tumor areas (*9*).

Galectin-1 expression was also found to be increased in oral squamous cell carcinoma-associated EC compared to adjacent normal tissue (*20*), and in head and neck carcinoma and lung cancer (*10*). Expression analysis of galectin-3 in tumor EC mainly concerns brain neoplasms. Endothelial galectin-3 expression was shown to change from high in low-grade astrocytomas, to intermediate in anaplastic astrocytomas, to low in glioblastomas (*21*). This was confirmed by Strik et al., who observed a reduced number of galectin-3 positive EC in glioblastoma compared with low-grade and anaplastic astrocytoma (*22*). In oligodendrogliomas, galectin-3 expression was also inversely related to malignancy (*23*). On the other hand, in a murine model of hepatocellular carcinoma, galectin-3 expression was approximately 30-fold increased in tumor-derived EC compared with normal liver-derived EC (*11*).

Endothelial galectin expression has also been studied in relation to patient survival. In 2008, D'Haene et al. evaluated the endothelial expression of galectin-1 and galectin-3 in patients with primary central nervous system lymphomas. While they did not detect any endothelial expression of galectin-1, they did find that elevated endothelial expression of galectin-3 was a prognostic factor for poor survival (*24*). In contrast, Deininger et al. found that decreased endothelial galectin-3 levels corresponded to shorter progression free and overall survival in oligodendrogliomas (*23*), suggesting that the expression levels of endothelial galectins are differently regulated depending on the tumor type or on environmental conditions.

One of the determinants that can regulate endothelial galectin expression is blood flow. Garcia-Cardena et al. showed that uneven flow dynamics, which occur in the unorganized tumor vasculature, can affect endothelial galectin-3 expression (*25*). Other factors that influence the galectin expression in tumor endothelial cells include extracellular matrix components and growth factors. For example, Baum et al. observed increased galectin-1 expression on the surface of cultured human aortic endothelial cells (HAEC) and human umbilical cord endothelial cells (HUVEC) after stimulation with minimally oxidized low density lipoprotein or with LPS and a mixture of cytokines, including IL-1β, TNFα and IFNγ (*8*). Treatment of HUVEC with the pro-inflammatory cytokine IL-1β also induced a 4-fold increased expression of galectin-3, thereby enhancing rolling of eosinophils and adhesion to EC (*26*). In addition, incubation of HUVEC and fibroblasts with conditioned media from prostate and ovary carcinoma cells significantly increases galectin-1 expression (*9*, *27*, *28*).

This suggests that the environment of a developing tumor indeed may play a role in regulating endothelial galectin-1 expression. In line with this, Glinskii et al. and others demonstrated increased mobilization of galectin-3 to the cell surface of metastasis-associated endothelium upon interaction with metastatic breast carcinoma cells (*29–31*). Also the interleukin-8-induced adhesion of neutrophils to Ea.hy926 endothelial cells markedly increased plasma membrane and cytoplasmic galectin-3 expression in the EC, while it reduced nuclear galectin-1 (*32*). In addition to growth factors and interacting cells, advanced glycation end products (AGEs) have been shown to induce galectin-3 expression in HUVEC and human micro-vascular EC (HMEC) (*33*, *34*). While data on the regulation of galectin-8 in EC is lacking, endothelial expression of galectin-9 mainly involves inflammatory and viral triggers (*35–37*). For example, galectin-9 expression was increased by stimulation of HUVEC with the pro-inflammatory cytokine IFNγ (*17*, *38*).

Altogether, these data show that multiple tumor-associated triggers can affect the expression of galectins in the tumor endothelium and that changes in endothelial galectin expression can be associated with disease outcome. Thus, analysis of galectin expression in the tumor vasculature could be of diagnostic or prognostic value.

Role of Endothelial Galectins in Tumor Angiogenesis

The previous sections show that different galectins are expressed by tumor endothelial cells and that this expression can be regulated by multiple triggers.

The functional consequence of this expression regulation has been subject to many studies. As evident from the other reviews in this issue, galectins exert a variety of activities in cell biology. They have been shown to be involved in cellular processes like proliferation (*39*, *40*), migration and adhesion (*39*, *41*), cell transformation (*42*), apoptosis (*39*, *43*) and mRNA splicing (*44*). Consequently, they are likely involved in the progression of various cancer types, as their expression is increased in e.g. melanoma, glioma, colon, prostate and head and neck cancer (reviewed by (*45*, *46*)). For example, endothelial galectin-1 might contribute to tumor progression by modifying the antitumor response, e.g. by inducing apoptosis in activated T-cells (*43*) and reducing the recruitment of lymphocytes and neutrophils to the endothelium (*47*, *48*). Additionally, endothelial galectin-1 and -3 have been shown to mediate heterotypic cancer cell adhesion, thereby potentially facilitating tumor metastasis (*9*, *30*, *31*). Here, we will only focus on the role of endothelial galectins in tumor angiogenesis.

There is ample evidence that galectins are involved in angiogenesis. We have shown that endothelial galectin-1 expression is required during the proliferation and migration of HUVEC *in vitro* (*13*). Hsieh et al. confirmed increased proliferation, migration and adhesion of HUVEC by galectin-1, which was shown to be mediated by interaction with neuropilin-1 and activation of VEGF-R2 signaling (*20*). Moreover, adding recombinant galectin-1 to EC cultures induces tube formation (*49*) as well as EC proliferation and migration (*50*). In fact, galectin-1 secreted by tumor cells can be taken up by EC, resulting in enhanced angiogenesis (*50*). A key role of galectin-1 in tumor angiogenesis *in vivo* was confirmed in galectin-1-null (gal-1$^{-/-}$) mice. Gal-1$^{-/-}$ mice that were injected with teratocarcinoma cells displayed significantly abrogated tumor growth compared to wild-type mice, which was caused by decreased vascularization of the tumor (*13*). Similar results were obtained using other tumor models (*50*).

Galectin-3 has also been shown to be involved in angiogenesis. It dose-dependently stimulates the proliferation and tube forming capacity of cultured EC (*51*, *52*). Stimulation of HUVEC with either exogenous galectin-3 or in the presence of conditioned medium from a galectin-3 secreting cell line resulted in increased tube formation (*53*). Moreover, nude mice that were injected with galectin-3 expressing cells or recombinant galectin-3 showed increased vascularization (*53*). Yang et al. demonstrated that galectin-3 significantly enhances HUVEC invasion and tube formation, which was thought to be mediated by aminopeptidase N (APN / CD13). APN is located on the endothelial cell surface and binds to galectin-3 in a carbohydrate dependent manner. Knockdown of APN reduced invasion and tube formation, and galectin-3 could no longer induce both processes (*54*). The involvement of galectin-3 in angiogenesis *in vivo* was also revealed in a mouse corneal micro-pocket assay by Markowska et al. (*55*, *56*). Stimulation with galectin-3 resulted in increased angiogenesis, which required both the C- and the N-terminal domain of the protein. Furthermore, VEGF- and bFGF-mediated angiogenesis was reduced in galectin-3-null mice.

Integrin $\alpha v\beta 3$ was thought to be involved in the angiogenic activity of galectin-3, since anti- $\alpha v\beta 3$ integrin antibodies inhibited galectin-3 mediated angiogenesis (*55*). More recently, Markowska et al. showed that galectin-3 induces phosphorylation of VEGF-R2 and retains VEGF-R2 on the plasma membrane of EC (*56*). While all these findings indicate a role in angiogenesis, Eude-Le Parco et al. did not see any difference in the occurrence or progression of spontaneous tumor models in galectin-3 deficient mice compared to normal mice (*57*). This highlights the necessity for further studies to determine the exact role of galectin-3 in tumor angiogenesis.

Angiogenic properties of galectin-8 were recently reported by Delgado et al. Bovine aortic EC (BAEC) and human micro-vascular EC cultured on matrigel supplemented with galectin-8 showed significantly increased tube formation (*16*). Exogenous galectin-8 also stimulated BAEC migration, whereas knockdown of endogenous galectin-8 hampered capillary formation and migration of BAEC (*16*). Furthermore, galectin-8 was shown to induce angiogenesis in vivo in a matrigel plug assay. The angiogenic properties of galectin-8 were mediated by CD166, as it was demonstrated that anti-CD166 antibodies hampered galectin-8 induced BAEC migration and tube formation (*16*). The potential role of galectin-9 in angiogenesis is still unresolved.

In summary, endothelial galectins appear to be involved in cell function during angiogenesis, both *in vitro* and *in vivo*. However, the exact role of all the galectins in tumor angiogenesis is not completely understood and further studies are required. Nevertheless, interfering with endothelial galectin function might provide an opportunity to perform angiostatic cancer therapy.

Targeting Endothelial Galectins for Diagnosis or Therapy

Several targeting strategies have been applied to block galectin function, including the use of antibodies, carbohydrates, and proteins. These different strategies have shown that targeting galectins can affect tumor progression at multiple levels by interfering with tumor angiogenesis, tumor immune escape and metastasis formation (*7*). Again, here we will only discuss the effects of targeting endothelial galectins on angiogenesis.

Targeting endothelial cells with galectin blocking antibodies has been shown to efficiently reduce their angiogenic capacity. For example, incubation with polyclonal anti-galectin-1 antibody was shown to inhibit migration of EC *in vitro* (*13*). In addition, this antibody reduced angiogenesis *in vivo* in a chorioallantoic membrane (CAM) assay (*13*). Blocking galectin-3 with polyclonal antibody decreased capillary tube formation by HUVEC (*53*) and was shown to hamper angiogenesis *in vivo* in the ischemic rat brain (*52*). These results suggest that targeting galectins with antibodies is a good strategy to interfere with endothelial cell function. However, Fukushi et al. demonstrated that anti-galectin-3 antibody did not affect matrigel-, laminin-, or fibronectin-induced transwell migration of EC (*58*). Apparently the effect of galectin-targeting antibodies is dependent on the context and the type of assay in which they are used. Furthermore, the effect of blocking antibodies might depend on the binding site on the galectin, e.g. near the carbohydrate binding pocket or at the site responsible for di- or oligo-merization.

Another approach used to target galectins involves blocking the carbohydrate recognition domain with competing carbohydrates. An example of a simple competing carbohydrate is lactose. This compound was shown to inhibit galectin-mediated HUVEC migration and capillary tube formation (*16*, *20*, *53*). However, lactose binds to multiple galectins with only low affinity, making it less appropriate for therapeutic applications. Another more potent disaccharide inhibitor is thiodigalactoside (TDG) which was shown to impair both galectin-1- and galectin-8-mediated tube formation (*16*, *49*). Thiodigalactoside also inhibits EC proliferation and migration *in vitro* (*16*, *49*). *In vivo*, intra-tumor treatment with TDG dose-dependently inhibited tumor growth in melanoma and mammary carcinoma mouse models (*49*).

Moreover, immunohistochemical staining of sections from TDG-treated wild-type tumors revealed that the number and diameter of the blood vessels was markedly reduced. On the other hand, tumor cells that were depleted of galectin-1 displayed hampered growth in these mice and additional treatment with TDG no longer affected the tumor growth, suggesting that TDG impairs tumor progression by inhibition of galectin-1 in tumor cells. This was supported by the observation that in galectin-1 knock out tumors no significant differences in tumor vascularization were observed after treatment with TDG (*49*). Rabinovich et al. designed three synthetic lactulose amines (SLA) derivatives that were found to differentially inhibit the binding of galectin-1 and -3 to the highly glycosylated 90K. In addition, the compounds selectively inhibited EC tube formation on matrigel (*59*). Thus far, the antitumor activity of these compounds has not been tested which is also true for two taloside compounds that bind to the carbohydrate recognition domain of galectin-1 and -3 and that might be used for inhibiting these galectins (*60*).

A more complex galectin-binding carbohydrate that has been shown to have anti-tumor activity is a modified form of citrus pectin (MCP). Galectin-3-induced endothelial tube formation was considerably reduced by MCP (*53*). In addition, MCP prevents the binding of galectin-3 to HUVEC and blocks the galectin-3-induced chemotaxis of these cells (*61*). Finally, MCP was shown to impair tumor vascularization *in vivo* resulting in hampered tumor growth (*61*).

While targeting galectins with carbohydrates show promising results, a more specific way of galectin-targeting might be achieved by peptides and proteins. In search for peptides with angiostatic properties, the synthetic 33-mer peptide anginex was found to inhibit EC migration, proliferation and sprouting *in vitro* (*62*). In addition, anginex inhibits angiogenesis *in vivo* and hampers tumor growth in mice models (*62*, *63*). Using yeast-two-hybrid analysis galectin-1 was identified as the main receptor of anginex (*13*). This was confirmed in galectin-1 deficient mice, in which tumor angiogenesis could no longer be inhibited by anginex treatment (*13*). Further studies showed that anginex also inhibits galectin-1-mediated membrane translocation of activated H-Ras in endothelial cells which could account for the inhibitory effects on cell proliferation (*50*). More recently it was suggested that binding of anginex affects the carbohydrate binding affinity and specificity of galectin-1 (*64*) which might be exploited for future therapeutic applications.

Apart from galectin-binding peptides, dominant negative isoforms of galectins have also been described to possess angiostatic activity. For example, a N-terminally truncated form of galectin-3 (galectin-3C), which retains its carbohydrate binding capacity but lacks the ability to cross-link carbohydrate-containing ligands on cell surfaces and ECM, acts as a dominant-negative inhibitor of full-length galectin-3 function by competing with its carbohydrate binding ability (*55*, *65*). Unlike full-length galectin-3, galectin-3C fails to induce HUVEC migration and network formation *in vitro* and angiogenesis *in vivo* (*55*). In tumor models, treatment with galectin-3C inhibits tumor growth although a direct link with angiogenesis was not presented (*65*, *66*). Nevertheless, the development of additional dominant negative isoforms of e.g. galectin-1 might provide novel therapeutic opportunities. Altogether, different strategies have been developed to interfere with galectin function during angiogenesis (summarized in Table 1). While pre-clinical data are promising the evidence for therapeutic efficacy in patients is still lacking. At present it is difficult to determine which strategy will be most effective and it cannot be excluded that combining different approaches might lead to the most potent therapy.

Table 1. Stimulatory effects of galectins on different steps of the angiogenic cascade and potential inhibitors

		Inhibitors[1]			
Process	*Stimulatory galectins*	*knock-down*[2]	*anti-body*	*carbohydrate*	*peptide/ protein*
Activation	gal-1, gal-3			Lac	Ax
Migration[3]	gal-1, gal-3, gal-8	gal-1, gal-8	gal-1	Lac, TDG	Ax, Gal-3C
Proliferation	gal-1, gal-3	gal-1		TDG	Ax
Sprouting	gal-1, gal-3	gal-3			
Tube formation[3]	gal-1, gal-3, gal-8	gal-8	gal-3	Lac, TDG, SLA, MCP	Ax, Gal-3C
Angiogenesis in vivo	gal-1, gal-3, gal-8	gal-1	gal-1, gal-3	MCP	Ax, Gal-3C

[1] Lac = lactose, TDG = thiodigalactoside, SLA = synthetic lactulose amines, MCP = modified citrus pectin, Ax = anginex.
[2] Either by siRNA of antisense oligo's.
[3] Inhibitory effects influenced by the type of adhesive matrix used in the assay.

Apart from direct therapeutic applications, targeting the endothelial galectins could also be used for e.g. specific delivery of anticancer drugs or for molecular imaging of tumor angiogenesis, an emerging diagnostic method (*67*). For example, fluorescently labeled anginex specifically homes to the tumor vasculature (*63*), and Brandwijk et al. showed that anginex-conjugated liposomes specifically bind to and are taken up by cultured HUVEC (*68*). Interestingly, anginex-conjugated paramagnetic liposomes showed increased contrast in MRI, indicating that anginex might be used for diagnostic imaging applications (*68*). Indeed, Kluza and colleagues recently demonstrated that conjugating paramagnetic liposomes to both anginex and RGD-peptide (targeting integrin $\alpha v\beta_3$) enhanced the uptake by HUVEC and significantly inhibited EC proliferation (*69*). This dual-targeting approach could be used for both therapeutic and diagnostic applications by loading these nanoparticles with e.g. MRI contrast agents. Moreover, treatment of melanoma MA148 tumor-bearing mice with anginex that was conjugated to the cytotoxic drug 6-hydroxypropylacylfulvene (HPAF) inhibited tumor growth significantly more than equivalent doses of either compound alone (*70*).

Microvessel density was still reduced by the conjugate, indicating that the conjugate does not affect the angiostatic properties of anginex (*70*). More importantly, the conjugate showed less toxicity compared to the unconjugated HPAF (*70*).

Another indirect application of targeting endothelial galectins appears to involve sensitization to cytotoxic therapies. For example, Mirandola et al. observed that treatment with galectin-3C enhanced the antitumor activity of bortezomib in a xenograft mouse model of human multiple myeloma (*65*). Targeting galectin-3 with MCP and Lac-*L*-Leu sensitized murine angiosarcoma cells for the cytotoxic drug doxorubicin (*71*). In addition, mice that were grafted with melanoma cells transfected with anti-galectin-1 siRNA displayed increased sensitivity for the autophagic drug temozolomide (*72*). This is in line with findings of Le Mercier et al., who demonstrated that decreasing galectin-1 expression in a xenograft mouse model of glioblastoma cells by *in vivo* siRNA delivery in the brains, enhanced the therapeutic benefits of temozolomide (*73*). Finally, anginex has also been shown to enhance the effect of different anti-cancer therapies including cytotoxic therapy and radiation therapy (*74*, *75*). Additional studies suggested that this effect might be related to a transient normalization of the tumor vasculature which temporarily enhances tumor perfusion and oxygenation (*76*). Whether this is also true for other galectin inhibitors still needs to be resolved.

Taken together, galectin-targeted angiostatic therapy can directly affect tumor progression but can also be indirectly exploited for targeted delivery of anticancer drugs, for diagnostic applications, and for sensitization of tumor cells to cancer treatment.

Summary and Future Perspectives

Here, we discussed the current knowledge regarding the expression and function of galectins in the endothelium and their role in tumor angiogenesis. Endothelial cells express at least four galectins, i.e. galectin-1, -3, -8, and -9. Interestingly, the expression is affected by different triggers and additional studies are required to unravel the underlying signaling pathways that regulate the expression. In the tumor vasculature, galectin expression is predominantly increased but the number of studies that specifically addressed galectin expression in the tumor endothelium is limited. Future studies might give more insight in the relation between vascular galectin expression and disease progression or patient survival. An important observation is that endothelial galectins have been described to facilitate key events of tumor progression, including angiogenesis. Thus, interfering with galectin expression or function could provide a powerful tool for anticancer treatment. Several compounds have been described that inhibit galectin function, including antibodies, carbohydrates, and small peptides. A major future challenge will be to further develop these compounds for clinical applications. Furthermore, preclinical studies with galectin-targeting compounds suggest that endothelial galectins can also be used for e.g. targeted drug delivery, diagnostic imaging applications, and enhancing the therapeutic benefits of cytotoxic drugs. Especially the latter, i.e. combination therapy offers new opportunities for cancer treatment and should be further explored. Eventually this will lead to novel and better therapeutic modalities for cancer patients.

References

1. Carmeliet, P. Mechanisms of angiogenesis and arteriogenesis. *Nat. Med.* **2000**, *6*, 389–395.
2. Carmeliet, P. Angiogenesis in life, disease and medicine. *Nature* **2005**, *438*, 932–936.
3. Hillen, F.; Griffioen, A. W. Tumour vascularization: Sprouting angiogenesis and beyond. *Cancer Metastasis Rev.* **2007**, *26*, 489–502.
4. Griffioen, A. W.; Molema, G. Angiogenesis: Potentials for pharmacologic intervention in the treatment of cancer, cardiovascular diseases, and chronic inflammation. *Pharmacol. Rev.* **2000**, *52*, 237–268.
5. Folkman, J.; Cole, P.; Zimmerman, S. Tumor behavior in isolated perfused organs: In vitro growth and metastases of biopsy material in rabbit thyroid and canine intestinal segment. *Ann. Surg.* **1966**, *164*, 491–502.
6. Folkman, J. Tumor angiogenesis: Therapeutic implications. *N. Engl. J. Med.* **1971**, *285*, 1182–1186.
7. Thijssen, V. L.; Poirier, F.; Baum, L. G.; Griffioen, A. W. Galectins in the tumor endothelium: Opportunities for combined cancer therapy. *Blood* **2007**, *110*, 2819–2827.
8. Baum, L. G.; Seilhamer, J. J.; Pang, M.; Levine, W. B.; Beynon, D.; Berliner, J. A. Synthesis of an endogeneous lectin, galectin-1, by human endothelial cells is up-regulated by endothelial cell activation. *Glycoconjugate J.* **1995**, *12*, 63–68.
9. Clausse, N.; van den Brule, F.; Waltregny, D.; Garnier, F.; Castronovo, V. Galectin-1 expression in prostate tumor-associated capillary endothelial cells is increased by prostate carcinoma cells and modulates heterotypic cell-cell adhesion. *Angiogenesis* **1999**, *3*, 317–325.
10. Lotan, R.; Belloni, P. N.; Tressler, R. J.; Lotan, D.; Xu, X. C.; Nicolson, G. L. Expression of galectins on microvessel endothelial cells and their involvement in tumour cell adhesion. *Glycoconjugate J.* **1994**, *11*, 462–468.
11. Ryschich, E.; Lizdenis, P.; Ittrich, C.; Benner, A.; Stahl, S.; Hamann, A.; Schmidt, J.; Knolle, P.; Arnold, B.; Hammerling, G. J.; et al. Molecular fingerprinting and autocrine growth regulation of endothelial cells in a murine model of hepatocellular carcinoma. *Cancer Res* **2006**, *66*, 198–211.
12. Thijssen, V. L.; Hulsmans, S.; Griffioen, A. W. The galectin profile of the endothelium; altered expression and localization in activated and tumor endothelial cells. *Am. J. Pathol.* **2008**, *172*, 545–553.

13. Thijssen, V. L.; Postel, R.; Brandwijk, R. J.; Dings, R. P.; Nesmelova, I.; Satijn, S.; Verhofstad, N.; Nakabeppu, Y.; Baum, L. G.; Bakkers, J.; et al. Galectin-1 is essential in tumor angiogenesis and is a target for antiangiogenesis therapy. *Proc. Natl. Acad. Sci. U.S.A* **2006**, *103*, 15975–15980.
14. Bidon-Wagner, N.; Le Pennec, J. P. Human galectin-8 isoforms and cancer. *Glycoconjugate J.* **2004**, *19*, 557–563.
15. Cueni, L. N.; Detmar, M. Galectin-8 interacts with podoplanin and modulates lymphatic endothelial cell functions. *Exp. Cell Res.* **2009**, *315*, 1715–1723.
16. Delgado, V. M.; Nugnes, L. G.; Colombo, L. L.; Troncoso, M. F.; Fernandez, M. M.; Malchiodi, E. L.; Frahm, I.; Croci, D. O.; Compagno, D.; Rabinovich, G. A.; et al. Modulation of endothelial cell migration and angiogenesis: A novel function for the "tandem-repeat" lectin galectin-8. *FASEB J.* **2011**, *25*, 242–254.
17. Imaizumi, T.; Kumagai, M.; Sasaki, N.; Kurotaki, H.; Mori, F.; Seki, M.; Nishi, N.; Fujimoto, K.; Tanji, K.; Shibata, T. Interferon-{gamma} stimulates the expression of galectin-9 in cultured human endothelial cells. *J. Leukoc. Biol.* **2002**, *72*, 486–491.
18. Spitzenberger, F.; Graessler, J.; Schroeder, H. E. Molecular and functional characterization of galectin 9 mRNA isoforms in porcine and human cells and tissues. *Biochimie* **2001**, *83*, 851–862.
19. Whitney, P.; Maxwell, S.; Ryan, U.; Massaro, D. Synthesis and binding of lactose-specific lectin by isolated lung cells. *Am. J. Physiol.* **1985**, *248*, C258–264.
20. Hsieh, S. H.; Ying, N. W.; Wu, M. H.; Chiang, W. F.; Hsu, C. L.; Wong, T. Y.; Jin, Y. T.; Hong, T. M.; Chen, Y. L. Galectin-1, a novel ligand of neuropilin-1, activates VEGFR-2 signaling and modulates the migration of vascular endothelial cells. *Oncogene* **2008**, *27*, 3746–3753.
21. Gordower, L.; Decaestecker, C.; Kacem, Y.; Lemmers, A.; Gusman, J.; Burchert, M.; Danguy, A.; Gabius, H.; Salmon, I.; Kiss, R.; et al. Galectin-3 and galectin-3-binding site expression in human adult astrocytic tumours and related angiogenesis. *Neuropathol. Appl. Neurobiol.* **1999**, *25*, 319–330.
22. Strik, H. M.; Deininger, M. H.; Frank, B.; Schluesener, H. J.; Meyermann, R. Galectin-3: Cellular distribution and correlation with WHO-grade in human gliomas. *J. Neurooncol.* **2001**, *53*, 13–20.
23. Deininger, M. H.; Trautmann, K.; Meyermann, R.; Schluesener, H. J. Galectin-3 labeling correlates positively in tumor cells and negatively in endothelial cells with malignancy and poor prognosis in oligodendroglioma patients. *Anticancer Res.* **2002**, *22*, 1585–1592.
24. D'Haene, N.; Catteau, X.; Maris, C.; Martin, B.; Salmon, I.; Decaestecker, C. Endothelial hyperplasia and endothelial galectin-3 expression are prognostic factors in primary central nervous system lymphomas. *Br. J. Haematol.* **2008**, *140*, 402–410.
25. Garcia-Cardena, G.; Comander, J.; Anderson, K. R.; Blackman, B. R.; Gimbrone, M. A., Jr. Biomechanical activation of vascular endothelium as a determinant of its functional phenotype. *Proc. Natl. Acad. Sci. U.S.A.* **2001**, *98*, 4478–4485.

26. Rao, S. P.; Wang, Z.; Zuberi, R. I.; Sikora, L.; Bahaie, N. S.; Zuraw, B. L.; Liu, F. T.; Sriramarao, P. Galectin-3 functions as an adhesion molecule to support eosinophil rolling and adhesion under conditions of flow. *J. Immunol.* **2007**, *179*, 7800–7807.
27. He, J.; Baum, L. G. Endothelial cell expression of galectin-1 induced by prostate cancer cells inhibits T-cell transendothelial migration. *Lab. Invest.* **2006**, *86*, 578–590.
28. van den Brule, F.; Califice, S.; Garnier, F.; Fernandez, P. L.; Berchuck, A.; Castronovo, V. Galectin-1 accumulation in the ovary carcinoma peritumoral stroma is induced by ovary carcinoma cells and affects both cancer cell proliferation and adhesion to laminin-1 and fibronectin. *Lab. Invest.* **2003**, *83*, 377–386.
29. Glinskii, O. V.; Turk, J. R.; Pienta, K. J.; Huxley, V. H.; Glinsky, V. V. Evidence of porcine and human endothelium activation by cancer-associated carbohydrates expressed on glycoproteins and tumour cells. *J. Physiol.* **2004**, *554*, 89–99.
30. Glinsky, V. V.; Glinsky, G. V.; Rittenhouse-Olson, K.; Huflejt, M. E.; Glinskii, O. V.; Deutscher, S. L.; Quinn, T. P. The role of Thomsen-Friedenreich antigen in adhesion of human breast and prostate cancer cells to the endothelium. *Cancer Res.* **2001**, *61*, 4851–4857.
31. Khaldoyanidi, S. K.; Glinsky, V. V.; Sikora, L.; Glinskii, A. B.; Mossine, V. V.; Quinn, T. P.; Glinsky, G. V.; Sriramarao, P. MDA-MB-435 human breast carcinoma cell homo- and heterotypic adhesion under flow conditions is mediated in part by Thomsen-Friedenreich antigen-galectin-3 interactions. *J. Biol. Chem.* **2003**, *278*, 4127–4134.
32. Gil, C. D.; La, M.; Perretti, M.; Oliani, S. M. Interaction of human neutrophils with endothelial cells regulates the expression of endogenous proteins annexin 1, galectin-1 and galectin-3. *Cell. Biol. Int.* **2006**.
33. Deo, P.; Glenn, J. V.; Powell, L. A.; Stitt, A. W.; Ames, J. M. Upregulation of oxidative stress markers in human microvascular endothelial cells by complexes of serum albumin and digestion products of glycated casein. *J. Biochem. Mol. Toxicol.* **2009**, *23*, 364–372.
34. Stitt, A. W.; He, C.; Vlassara, H. Characterization of the advanced glycation end-product receptor complex in human vascular endothelial cells. *Biochem. Biophys. Res. Commun.* **1999**, *256*, 549–556.
35. Imaizumi, T.; Yoshida, H.; Nishi, N.; Sashinami, H.; Nakamura, T.; Hirashima, M.; Ohyama, C.; Itoh, K.; Satoh, K. Double-stranded RNA induces galectin-9 in vascular endothelial cells: Involvement of TLR3, PI3K, and IRF3 pathway. *Glycobiology* **2007**, *17*, 12C–15C.
36. Ishikawa, A.; Imaizumi, T.; Yoshida, H.; Nishi, N.; Nakamura, T.; Hirashima, M.; Satoh, K. Double-stranded RNA enhances the expression of galectin-9 in vascular endothelial cells. *Immunol. Cell. Biol.* **2004**, *82*, 410–414.
37. Warke, R. V.; Xhaja, K.; Martin, K. J.; Fournier, M. F.; Shaw, S. K.; Brizuela, N.; de Bosch, N.; Lapointe, D.; Ennis, F. A.; Rothman, A. L.; et al. Dengue virus induces novel changes in gene expression of human umbilical vein endothelial cells. *J. Virol.* **2003**, *77*, 11822–11832.

38. Alam, S.; Li, H.; Margariti, A.; Martin, D.; Zampetaki, A.; Habi, O.; Cockerill, G.; Hu, Y.; Xu, Q.; Zeng, L. Galectin-9 protein expression in endothelial cells is positively regulated by histone deacetylase 3. *J. Biol. Chem.* **2011**, *286*, 44211–44217.
39. Perillo, N. L.; Marcus, M. E.; Baum, L. G. Galectins: Versatile modulators of cell adhesion, cell proliferation, and cell death. *J. Mol. Med.* **1998**, *76*, 402–412.
40. Scott, K.; Weinberg, C. Galectin-1: A bifunctional regulator of cellular proliferation. *Glycoconjugate J.* **2004**, *19*, 467–477.
41. Hughes, R. C. Galectins as modulators of cell adhesion. *Biochimie* **2001**, *83*, 667–676.
42. Paz, A.; Haklai, R.; Elad-Sfadia, G.; Ballan, E.; Kloog, Y. Galectin-1 binds oncogenic H-Ras to mediate Ras membrane anchorage and cell transformation. *Oncogene* **2001**, *20*, 7486–7493.
43. Perillo, N. L.; Pace, K. E.; Seilhamer, J. J.; Baum, L. G. Apoptosis of T cells mediated by galectin-1. *Nature* **1995**, *378*, 736–739.
44. Park, J. W.; Voss, P. G.; Grabski, S.; Wang, J. L.; Patterson, R. J. Association of galectin-1 and galectin-3 with Gemin4 in complexes containing the SMN protein. *Nucleic Acids Res.* **2001**, *29*, 3595–3602.
45. Danguy, A.; Camby, I.; Kiss, R. Galectins and cancer. *Biochim. Biophys. Acta* **2002**, *1572*, 285–293.
46. Lefranc, F.; Mathieu, V.; Kiss, R. Galectin-1-mediated biochemical controls of melanoma and glioma aggressive behavior. *World J. Biol. Chem.* **2011**, *2*, 193–201.
47. Cooper, D.; Norling, L. V.; Perretti, M. Novel insights into the inhibitory effects of galectin-1 on neutrophil recruitment under flow. *J. Leukoc. Biol.* **2008**, *83*, 1459–1466.
48. Norling, L. V.; Sampaio, A. L.; Cooper, D.; Perretti, M. Inhibitory control of endothelial galectin-1 on in vitro and in vivo lymphocyte trafficking. *FASEB J.* **2008**, *22*, 682–690.
49. Ito, K.; Scott, S. A.; Cutler, S.; Dong, L. F.; Neuzil, J.; Blanchard, H.; Ralph, S. J. Thiodigalactoside inhibits murine cancers by concurrently blocking effects of galectin-1 on immune dysregulation, angiogenesis and protection against oxidative stress. *Angiogenesis* **2011**, *14*, 293–307.
50. Thijssen, V. L.; Barkan, B.; Shoji, H.; Aries, I. M.; Mathieu, V.; Deltour, L.; Hackeng, T. M.; Kiss, R.; Kloog, Y.; Poirier, F. Tumor cells secrete galectin-1 to enhance endothelial cell activity. *Cancer Res.* **2010**, *70*, 6216–6224.
51. Wan, S. Y.; Zhang, T. F.; Ding, Y. Galectin-3 enhances proliferation and angiogenesis of endothelial cells differentiated from bone marrow mesenchymal stem cells. *Transplant Proc* **2011**, *43*, 3933–3938.
52. Yan, Y. P.; Lang, B. T.; Vemuganti, R.; Dempsey, R. J. Galectin-3 mediates post-ischemic tissue remodeling. *Brain Res.* **2009**, *1288*, 116–124.
53. Nangia-Makker, P.; Honjo, Y.; Sarvis, R.; Akahani, S.; Hogan, V.; Pienta, K. J.; Raz, A. Galectin-3 induces endothelial cell morphogenesis and angiogenesis. *Am. J. Pathol.* **2000**, *156*, 899–909.

54. Yang, E.; Shim, J. S.; Woo, H. J.; Kim, K. W.; Kwon, H. J. Aminopeptidase N/CD13 induces angiogenesis through interaction with a pro-angiogenic protein, galectin-3. *Biochem. Biophys. Res. Commun.* **2007**, *363*, 336–341.
55. Markowska, A. I.; Liu, F. T.; Panjwani, N. Galectin-3 is an important mediator of VEGF- and bFGF-mediated angiogenic response. *J. Exp. Med.* **2010**, *207*, 1981–1993.
56. Markowska, A. I.; Jefferies, K. C.; Panjwani, N Galectin-3 protein modulates cell surface expression and activation of vascular endothelial growth factor receptor 2 in human endothelial cells. *J. Biol. Chem.* **2011**, *286*, 29913–29921.
57. Eude-Le Parco, I.; Gendronneau, G.; Dang, T.; Delacour, D.; Thijssen, V. L.; Edelmann, W.; Peuchmaur, M.; Poirier, F. Genetic assessment of the importance of galectin-3 in cancer initiation, progression, and dissemination in mice. *Glycobiology* **2009**, *19*, 68–75.
58. Fukushi, J.; Makagiansar, I. T.; Stallcup, W. B. NG2 proteoglycan promotes endothelial cell motility and angiogenesis via engagement of galectin-3 and alpha3beta1 integrin. *Mol. Biol. Cell* **2004**, *15*, 3580–3590.
59. Rabinovich, G. A.; Cumashi, A.; Bianco, G. A.; Ciavardelli, D.; Iurisci, I.; D'Egidio, M.; Piccolo, E.; Tinari, N.; Nifantiev, N.; Iacobelli, S. Synthetic lactulose amines: Novel class of anticancer agents that induce tumor-cell apoptosis and inhibit galectin-mediated homotypic cell aggregation and endothelial cell morphogenesis. *Glycobiology* **2006**, *16*, 210–220.
60. Collins, P. M.; Oberg, C. T.; Leffler, H.; Nilsson, U. J.; Blanchard, H. Taloside inhibitors of galectin-1 and galectin-3. *Chem. Biol. Drug Des.* **2011**, *79*, 339–346.
61. Nangia-Makker, P.; Hogan, V.; Honjo, Y.; Baccarini, S.; Tait, L.; Bresalier, R.; Raz, A. Inhibition of human cancer cell growth and metastasis in nude mice by oral intake of modified citrus pectin. *J. Natl. Cancer Inst.* **2002**, *94*, 1854–1862.
62. Griffioen, A. W.; van der Schaft, D. W.; Barendsz-Janson, A. F.; Cox, A.; Struijker Boudier, H. A.; Hillen, H. F.; Mayo, K. H. Anginex, a designed peptide that inhibits angiogenesis. *Biochem. J.* **2001**, *354*, 233–242.
63. Steege, J. C.; Wagstaff, J.; Mayo, K. H.; Griffioen, A. W. The designer anti-angiogenic peptide anginex targets tumor endothelial cells and inhibits tumor growth in animal models. *FASEB J.* **2002**, *16*, 1991–1993.
64. Salomonsson, E.; Thijssen, V. L.; Griffioen, A. W.; Nilsson, U. J.; Leffler, H. The anti-angiogenic peptide anginex greatly enhances galectin-1 binding affinity for glycoproteins. *J. Biol. Chem.* **2011**, *286*, 13801–13804.
65. Mirandola, L.; Yu, Y.; Chui, K.; Jenkins, M. R.; Cobos, E.; John, C. M.; Chiriva-Internati, M. Galectin-3C inhibits tumor growth and increases the anticancer activity of bortezomib in a murine model of human multiple myeloma. *PLoS ONE* **2011**, *6*, e21811.
66. John, C. M.; Leffler, H.; Kahl-Knutsson, B.; Svensson, I.; Jarvis, G. A. Truncated galectin-3 inhibits tumor growth and metastasis in orthotopic nude mouse model of human breast cancer. *Clin. Cancer Re.s* **2003**, *9*, 2374–2383.

67. Schirner, M.; Menrad, A.; Stephens, A.; Frenzel, T.; Hauff, P.; Licha, K.; van der Schaft, D. W.; Dings, R. P.; de Lussanet, Q. G.; van Eijk, L. I.; Nap, A. W.; Beets-Tan, R. G.; Bouma-Ter Molecular imaging of tumor angiogenesis. *Ann. N. Y. Acad. Sci.* **2004**, *1014*, 67–75.
68. Brandwijk, R. J.; Mulder, W. J.; Nicolay, K.; Mayo, K. H.; Thijssen, V. L.; Griffioen, A. W. Anginex-conjugated liposomes for targeting of angiogenic endothelial cells. *Bioconjug. Chem.* **2007**, *18*, 785–790.
69. Kluza, E.; van der Schaft, D. W.; Hautvast, P. A.; Mulder, W. J.; Mayo, K. H.; Griffioen, A. W.; Strijkers, G. J.; Nicolay, K. Synergistic targeting of alphavbeta3 integrin and galectin-1 with heteromultivalent paramagnetic liposomes for combined MR imaging and treatment of angiogenesis. *Nano Lett.* **2011**, *10*, 52–58.
70. Dings, R. P.; Van Laar, E. S.; Loren, M.; Webber, J.; Zhang, Y.; Waters, S. J.; Macdonald, J. R.; Mayo, K. H. Inhibiting tumor growth by targeting tumor vasculature with galectin-1 antagonist anginex conjugated to the cytotoxic acylfulvene, 6-hydroxylpropylacylfulvene. *Bioconjug. Chem.* **2010**, *21*, 20–27.
71. Johnson, K. D.; Glinskii, O. V.; Mossine, V. V.; Turk, J. R.; Mawhinney, T. P.; Anthony, D. C.; Henry, C. J.; Huxley, V. H.; Glinsky, G. V.; Pienta, K. J.; et al. Galectin-3 as a potential therapeutic target in tumors arising from malignant endothelia. *Neoplasia* **2007**, *9*, 662–670.
72. Mathieu, V.; Le Mercier, M.; De Neve, N.; Sauvage, S.; Gras, T.; Roland, I.; Lefranc, F.; Kiss, R. Galectin-1 knockdown increases sensitivity to temozolomide in a B16F10 mouse metastatic melanoma model. *J. Invest. Dermatol.* **2007**, *127*, 2399–2410.
73. Le Mercier, M.; Mathieu, V.; Haibe-Kains, B.; Bontempi, G.; Mijatovic, T.; Decaestecker, C.; Kiss, R.; Lefranc, F. Knocking down galectin 1 in human hs683 glioblastoma cells impairs both angiogenesis and endoplasmic reticulum stress responses. *J. Neuropathol. Exp. Neurol.* **2008**, *67*, 456–469.
74. Dings, R. P.; Williams, B. W.; Song, C. W.; Griffioen, A. W.; Mayo, K. H.; Griffin, R. J. Anginex synergizes with radiation therapy to inhibit tumor growth by radiosensitizing endothelial cells. *Int. J. Cancer* **2005**.
75. Dings, R. P.; Yokoyama, Y.; Ramakrishnan, S.; Griffioen, A. W.; Mayo, K. H. The designed angiostatic peptide anginex synergistically improves chemotherapy and antiangiogenesis therapy with angiostatin. *Cancer Res.* **2003**, *63*, 382–385.
76. Dings, R. P.; Loren, M.; Heun, H.; McNiel, E.; Griffioen, A. W.; Mayo, K. H.; Griffin, R. J. Scheduling of radiation with angiogenesis inhibitors anginex and Avastin improves therapeutic outcome via vessel normalization. *Clin. Cancer Res.* **2007**, *13*, 3395–3402.

Chapter 14

Galectins and Pathologies: Role of Galectin-3 in the Communication between Leukemia Cells and the Microenvironment

Nora Heisterkamp,[*,1] Fei Fei,[1] and John Groffen[2]

[1]Section of Molecular Carcinogenesis, Division of Hematology/Oncology and The Saban Research Institute of Children's Hospital, 4650 Sunset Boulevard, Los Angeles, California 90027, USA
[2]Departments of Pediatrics and Pathology, Keck School of Medicine, University of Southern California, Los Angeles, California 90033, USA
[*]E-mail: heisterk@hsc.usc.edu

Our recent studies in a tissue co-culture model have shown that Galectin-3 is synthesized by both protective stromal cells and by precursor B-lineage acute lymphoblastic leukemia cells. Galectin-3 binds to the surface of these leukemia cells. Also, these studies, and those of others in chronic myeloid leukemia cell lines, show that drug treatment further increases expression of endogenous Galectin-3, and that elevated Galectin-3 levels protect leukemia cells. For therapeutic purposes, therefore, blocking Galectin-3 binding or reduction of Galectin-3 levels is an important goal. This may require the development of inhibitors with (1) a long half-life, (2) high specificity for Galectin-3 and (3) high affinity for its carbohydrate recognition domain. Alternative approaches include designing Galectin-3 inhibitors that are targeted to specific cell types, or the identification and targeting of the cell surface glycoproteins that regulate Galectin-3 biological effects. This mini-review describes literature data on interactions of extracellular Galectin-3 with glycoproteins on the cell surface and their possible connection to leukemia as well as the intracellular activity of Galectin-3, its possible regulation by interactions with glycoproteins, and its effect on leukemia cell resistance against therapeutic drugs. *In vitro* and *in vivo* experiments using Galectin blockers of a polysaccharide nature (GM-CT-01 and GR-MD-02) are also reviewed. Based on these data, it is reasonable to assume that interference with the carbohydrate-binding activity of Galectin-3 in a wide range of leukemias may be beneficial (1) as first-line treatment, in combination with other drugs, to enhance anti-leukemia activities (2) as a possible marker and contributor to the persistence of leukemia cells in protective niches, and the presence of minimal residual disease in the bone marrow (3) as a method to modulate supportive cells in the microenvironment of the leukemia cells, including bone marrow stromal cells.

Introduction

For successful utilization of a biomolecule as drug target in leukemia, the relative importance of that molecule to leukemia cell survival, compared to its functional significance for normal cells is a key consideration. In that respect, Galectin-3 is an interesting but complex target with multiple domains, locations and possibly functions. Galectin-3 is expressed in a number of different leukemias, but immune cells and stromal cells, which may profoundly alter the way leukemia cells respond to drugs, can also express Galectin-3. Thus, inhibition of Galectin-3 may have anti-leukemia effects through mechanisms other than direct effects on the leukemia cells.

Interactions of Extracellular Galectin-3

Galectin-3 is found both extracellularly and intracellularly. It was originally discovered as Mac-2, a cell surface marker on macrophages. Human Galectin-3 is a relatively small protein (30-35 kDa) that can be subdivided into N-terminal, R (-Pro-Gly-Tyr-Repeat) and Carbohydrate Recognition (CRD) domains of around 20, 100 and 130 aminoacids (*1*). High-affinity carbohydrate ligands identified for Galectin-3 include tri-and tetra antennary N-linked glycans that are N-acetyllactosamine modified on cell surface proteins. Galectin-3 only recognizes glycans containing a polyLacNAc extension (*2–4*) and sialylation of these glycans inhibits Galectin-3 binding (*5–7*). Interestingly, Galectin-3 is unique among galectins in that it can form pentamers through its N-terminal domain, which is located outside of the CRD. These Galectin-3 pentamers have the ability to interact with multivalent cell-surface glycoproteins and through this mechanism promote lattice formation and receptor clustering, crosstalk between cell surface carbohydrate-modified integrins and signaling receptors; and promote or prevent endocytosis of such molecules.

Thus, extracellular Galectin-3 is thought to mainly affect cell function through its carbohydrate-binding activity and interaction with cell surface proteins, forming lattices that can, for example, enhance residency at the cell surface. However, the precise biological outcome of this interaction differs, depending on the cell type and on the proteins with which it forms a lattice (*5*, *8*). For example,

Galectin-3 binding to the TGFβRII delays its constitutive endocytosis in murine mammary epithelial tumor cell lines, resulting in attenuation of TGFβ-generated signals (*9*). Interactions with the transferrin receptor CD71, the β1 integrin CD29 and the tyrosine phosphatase CD45 on T-cells promotes apoptosis (*10*), whereas interactions with CD98 (slc3a2) promotes macrophage M2 polarization (*11*). Thus, the signal generated by extracellular Galectin-3 depends on the presence and modification of glycoproteins it interacts with on the cell surface.

Leukemia Drug Resistance

Leukemia cells are protected against many drugs through interactions with their microenvironment, which consists of both the extracellular matrix and cellular components. Protective effects of stromal cells to leukemia cells when these are treated with drugs have been documented extensively by us in pre-B acute lymphoblastic leukemia (ALL) (*12–14*) and have also been reported in chronic myeloid leukemia (CML) (*15*), acute myeloid leukemia (AML) (*16*), and in chronic lymphocytic leukemia (CLL) (*17–20*). The resistance to drug treatment that this type of protection provides is named environmental-mediated drug resistance (EMDR) (*21–23*). Meads et al (*24*) argued that EMDR is likely to be a major source of relapse.

Leukemia cells make contact with the microenvironment through cell surface structures of which the protein components have been the easiest to approach experimentally and have therefore been the most well-studied. However, all cells are covered by a dense network of glycolipids, glycoproteins, glycophospholipid anchors and proteoglycans. The importance of these structures is illustrated by the fact that more than 1% of the genome is involved in generating the developmentally regulated and tissue-specific glycosylation characteristics of each cell type (*25*).

Extracellular Galectin-3 and Leukemia

This dense layer of carbohydrates constitutes the "face" of the cell that is presented towards the outside world and is the contact interface between leukemia cells and the cells in the microenvironment that protect them. Extracellular Galectin-3 is an important component of the microenvironment of non-transformed cells, mediating cell migration, cell adhesion, and cell-cell interactions through its carbohydrate-binding properties. Our data show that human or mouse pre-B ALL cells communicate with protective stromal cells in a tissue culture setting. These stromal cells secrete Galectin-3, which binds to structures on the surface of the ALL cells. The Galectin-3 is internalized and this appears to generate a signal in the ALL cells for the transcription, synthesis and cell surface expression of Galectin-3. Moreover, the treatment of the ALL cells with conventional (vincristine) or targeted (nilotinib) drug therapy at doses that allows EMDR results in enhanced Galectin-3 production (Fei et al., manuscript in preparation).

Induction of Galectin-3 in leukemia through contact with the microenvironment does not seem to be restricted to pre-B ALL. Recently, Yamamoto-Sugitani et al reported that the co-culture of the CML cell line MYL with the stromal cell line MS5, or adhesion to fibronectin, also significantly induced the synthesis of Galectin-3 mRNA. Upon co-culture with MS5 stromal cells, increased Galectin-3 protein was detected in three different CML cell lines, in the T-cell leukemia cell line Jurkat, and in the myeloid leukemia cell line HL60 (*26*).

In leukemias, different effects of extracellular stimulation through the addition of Galectin-3 have been reported. For example, extracellular supplementation with Galectin-3 did not affect the sensitivity of K562 or MYL cells to imatinib or doxorubicin (*26*). In contrast, Suziki and Abe reported that Galectin-3 induced cell death of the diffuse large B-cell lymphoma cell line HBL-2 (*27*).

Intracellular Galectin-3

In general, intracellular Galectin-3 is regarded as anti-apoptotic as shown in, among others, in the CML cell line K562 treated with cisplatin or LY294002 (*26*, *28*, *29*). Treatment of K652 with different drugs in the absence of stroma also induced increased Galectin-3 expression, and surviving cells contained elevated Galectin-3 compared to the original cells. Overexpression of Galectin-3 in K562 or knockdown of Galectin-3 levels increased or decreased sensitivity to apoptotic agents (*28*). Similar studies and results were reported in the CML cell line MYL (*26*).

In some cell types, Galectin-3 was shown to inhibit ROS production and prevent alteration of the mitochondrial membrane potential (*26*, *28–32*). The Galectin-3 CRD contains a Bcl2-homology domain (BH1) with the conserved N180-W181-G182-R183 motif that mediates complex formation with Bcl2 and protects cells from apoptosis. The same domain also mediates Galectin-3-Galectin-3 homodimer formation and Galectin-3/Galectin-3 and Galectin-3/Bcl2 interactions are specifically inhibitable by 25 mM lactose but not sucrose (*33*). Thus, the interesting possibility exists that some of the intracellular activities of Galectin-3 are also regulated by interactions of the CDR with glycoproteins or other carbohydrate-bearing macromolecules.

Which Galectin-3 Function Should Be Aimed at in Practical Therapy?

As briefly reviewed above, Galectin-3 has at least two locations and possibly distinct functions that are relevant in the context of leukemia cell survival: a direct anti-apoptotic effect inside the cell, which may be independent of glycan binding, and a possibly indirect extracellular effect in modulating signal transduction strength through carbohydrate-binding-dependent interactions.

Those therapeutics that interfere with the extracellular activities of Galectin-3 appear to be easier to target, and, based on our results in pre-B ALL, may be most relevant to the problem of environmental-mediated drug resistance and minimal residual disease.

How To Use Galectin-3 as Drug Target?

Exposure of some cell types to extracellular Galectin-3 may cause apoptosis, but available data for pre-B ALL and CML suggest that attenuation of the extracellular effects of the Galectin-3 in the microenvironment may have clinical benefit. As mentioned above, there are several theoretical ways to accomplish this:

a. Approaches to prevent expression or activation of defined, critical poly N-acetyllactosamine-modified cell surface glycoproteins with which Galectin-3 interacts. In pre-B ALL cells this could include CD45, CD43, integrin β1 or CD71, all of which are expressed on pre-B ALL cells. Although this approach would allow a fine-tuning of the effects of inhibition, it would require the precise identification of such glycoproteins and the intracellular effects of Galectin-3 engagement.
b. Approaches to increase sialylation of poly N-acetyllactosamine-modified cell surface glycoproteins with which Galectin-3 interacts, through inhibition of extracellular sialidases, or the stimulation of sialyltransferases. Sialydation is known to have a marked effect on the ability of Galectin-3 to interact with cell surface glycoproteins [reviewed in (*6*)]. However, currently, the targets for Galectin-3 binding that confer a survival benefit to leukemia cells and can be blocked by their sialylation are not known, nor have the sialyltransferases or sialidases that would regulate this modification been precisely defined in leukemia cells. That modulation of the sialylation can affect Galectin-3-mediated functions is illustrated by the report of Suzuki and Abe, who increased the pro-apoptotic effect of exogenously added Galectin-3 on the diffuse large B-cell lymphoma cell line HBL-2 by pre-treatment with *Vibrio Cholerae* neuraminidase (*27*).
c. Approaches to inhibit intracellular Galectin-3 protein production or prevent extracellular secretion of the protein. The detailed knowledge needed to manipulate these processes is not available.
d. Approaches to block the interaction of the CRD of Galectin-3 with accessible polyLacNAC-extended glycans. This is the only approach for which data are available.

To the best of our knowledge, the exact mechanism of action of such glycan-based Galectin-3 inhibitors, or their fate in either a tissue culture setting or in animals has not been documented. Those that bind to the CRD of Galectin-3 would be expected to sequester extracellular Galectin-3 produced by protective stromal cells as well as by the leukemia cells, perhaps followed by enzymatic degradation in the extracellular space. Alternatively, since Galectin-3 is able to form multimers, it is possible that some of the Galectin-3 molecules bind the inhibitor, others bind to their natural ligands on the cell surface, and that this as a whole is internalized as a large macromolecular complex. Finally, if glycan-based inhibitors are internalized in a Galectin-3 independent manner, they could form complexes with intracellular Galectin-3 and through this mechanisms block the anti-apoptotic activity of Galectin-3 in leukemia cells when these are treated with therapeutic drugs.

Evidence for Therapeutic Effect of Blocking the Interaction of the CRD of Galectin-3 with Accessible Polylacnac-Extended Glycans

a. In vitro

Exposure of pre-B ALL cells to chemotherapy (vincristine) or to targeted drugs (nilotinib) in the presence of GM-CT-01 (also known as Davanat) and GR-MD-02 (another polysaccharide), enhances the effect of the drugs on cell proliferation and viability (Fei et al,, manuscript in preparation). Yamamoto-Sugitani et al (*26*) reported that fractionated citrus pectin powder as a Galectin-3 inhibitor caused cell death in MYL cells, in MYL cells overexpressing Galectin-3, and in MYL cells treated with imatinib in the presence of MS5 stromal cells in tissue culture. The modified citrus pectin GCS-100 has been described as an inhibitor of Galectin-3 and was used to treat multiple myeloma cell lines and primary patient samples in the context of drug resistance (*34*, *35*).

b. In vivo

Few animal studies using anti-Galectin-3 reagents against hematological malignancies have been published. Demotte et al (*36*) used GCS-100 to activate tumor-infiltrating T-cells in a mouse transplant model of mastocytoma. The C-terminal end of Galectin-3 showed anti-cancer activity alone and combined with bortezomib in NOD/SCID mice transplanted with a human multiple myeloma cell line (*37*). Interestingly, these authors mentioned that "the primary activity of Gal-3C *in vivo* may be mediated by interactions involving the tumor microenvironment rather than by direct cytotoxicity to the multiple myeloma cells…"

Opportunities and Challenges

Based on the data described above, it is reasonable to assume that interference with the carbohydrate-binding activity of Galectin-3 in a wide range of leukemias may be beneficial 1) as first-line treatment in combination with other drugs, to enhance anti-leukemia activities 2) as a possible marker and contributor to the persistence of leukemia cells in protective niches, and the presence of minimal residual disease in the bone marrow 3) as a method to modulate supportive cells in the microenvironment of the leukemia cells including bone marrow fibroblasts.

A formidable challenge is to effectively ablate Galectin-3 activity and/or levels. As described in our *in vitro* studies, Galectin-3 is made by both protective stromal cells and by pre-B ALL cells. Moreover, our data indicate it is secreted by the stromal cells, and binds to the surface of pre-B ALL cells (Fei et al., manuscript in preparation). Finally, these studies, and those in the CML cell lines, show that drug treatment increases endogenous levels of Galectin-3 even further. The challenge will thus be to sufficiently block or diminish Galectin-3 as to achieve a biological effect *in vivo*. This may require the development of inhibitors with 1) a long half-life, 2) high specificity for Galectin-3 and 3) high affinity for its CRD. Alternative approaches could be to design Galectin-3 inhibitors that are targeted to specific cell types, or the identification of the cell surface glycoproteins that regulate Galectin-3 biological effects.

References

1. Newlaczyl, A. U.; Yu, L. G. Galectin-3: A jack-of-all-trades in cancer. *Cancer Lett.* **2011**, *313*, 123–128.
2. Song, X.; Xia, B.; Stowell, S. R.; Lasanajak, Y.; Smith, D. F.; Cummings, R. D. Novel fluorescent glycan microarray strategy reveals ligands for galectins. *Chem. Biol.* **2009**, *16*, 36–47.
3. Togayachi, A.; Kozono, Y.; Ishida, H.; Abe, S.; Suzuki, N.; Tsunoda, Y.; Hagiwara, K.; Kuno, A.; Ohkura, T.; Sato, N.; et al. Polylactosamine on glycoproteins influences basal levels of lymphocyte and macrophage activation. *Proc. Natl. Acad. Sci. U.S.A.* **2007**, *104*, 15829–15834.
4. Togayachi, A.; Kozono, Y.; Kuno, A.; Ohkura, T.; Sato, T.; Hirabayashi, J.; Ikehara, Y.; Narimatsu, H. Beta3GnT2 (B3GNT2), a major polylactosamine synthase: Analysis of B3GNT2-deficient mice. *Meth. Enzymol.* **2010**, *479*, 185–204.
5. Rabinovich, G. A.; Toscano, M. A.; Jackson, S. S.; Vasta, G. R. Functions of cell surface galectin-glycoprotein lattices. *Curr. Opin. Struct. Biol.* **2007**, *17*, 513–520.
6. Zhuo, Y.; Bellis, S. L. Emerging role of alpha2,6-sialic acid as a negative regulator of galectin binding and function. *J. Biol. Chem.* **2011**, *286*, 5935–5941.
7. Zhuo, Y.; Chammas, R.; Bellis, S. L. Sialylation of beta1 integrins blocks cell adhesion to galectin-3 and protects cells against galectin-3-induced apoptosis. *J. Biol. Chem.* **2008**, *283*, 22177–22185.
8. Rabinovich, G. A.; Toscano, M. A. Turning 'sweet' on immunity: Galectin-glycan interactions in immune tolerance and inflammation. *Nat. Rev. Immunol.* **2009**, *9*, 338–352.
9. Partridge, E. A.; Le Roy, C.; Di Guglielmo, G. M.; Pawling, J.; Cheung, P.; Granovsky, M.; Nabi, I. R.; Wrana, J. L.; Dennis, J. W. Regulation of cytokine receptors by Golgi N-glycan processing and endocytosis. *Science* **2004**, *306*, 120–124.

10. Stillman, B. N.; Hsu, D. K.; Pang, M.; Brewer, C. F.; Johnson, P.; Liu, F. T.; Baum, L. G. Galectin-3 and galectin-1 bind distinct cell surface glycoprotein receptors to induce T cell death. *J. Immunol.* **2006**, *176*, 778–789.
11. MacKinnon, A. C.; Farnworth, S. L.; Hodkinson, P. S.; Henderson, N. C.; Atkinson, K. M.; Leffler, H.; Nilsson, UJ; Haslett, C.; Forbes, S. J.; Sethi, T. Regulation of alternative macrophage activation by galectin-3. *J. Immunol.* **2008**, *180*, 2650–2658.
12. Fei, F.; Stoddart, S.; Groffen, J.; Heisterkamp, N. Activity of the Aurora kinase inhibitor VX-680 against Bcr/Abl-positive acute lymphoblastic leukemias. *Mol. Cancer Ther.* **2010a**, *9*, 1318–1327.
13. Fei, F.; Stoddart, S.; Muschen, M.; Kim, Y. M.; Groffen, J.; Heisterkamp, N. Development of resistance to dasatinib in Bcr/Abl-positive acute lymphoblastic leukemia. *Leukemia* **2010b**, *24*, 813–820.
14. Parameswaran, R.; Yu, M.; Lim, M.; Groffen, J.; Heisterkamp, N. Combination of drug therapy in acute lymphoblastic leukemia with a CXCR4 antagonist. *Leukemia* **2011**, *25*, 1314–1323.
15. Weisberg, E.; Azab, A. K.; Manley, P. W.; Kung, A. L.; Christie, A. L.; Bronson, R.; Ghobrial, I. M.; Griffin, J. D. Inhibition of CXCR4 in CML cells disrupts their interaction with the bone marrow microenvironment and sensitizes them to nilotinib. *Leukemia* **2012**, *26*, 985–990.
16. Zeng, Z.; Shi, Y. X.; Samudio, I. J.; Wang, R. Y.; Ling, X.; Frolova, O.; Levis, M.; Rubin, J. B.; Negrin, R. R.; Estey, E. H.; et al. Targeting the leukemia microenvironment by CXCR4 inhibition overcomes resistance to kinase inhibitors and chemotherapy in AML. *Blood* **2009**, *113*, 6215–6224.
17. Buchner, M.; Baer, C.; Prinz, G.; Dierks, C.; Burger, M.; Zenz, T.; Stilgenbauer, S.; Jumaa, H.; Veelken, H.; Zirlik, K. Spleen tyrosine kinase inhibition prevents chemokine- and integrin-mediated stromal protective effects in chronic lymphocytic leukemia. *Blood* **2010**, *115*, 4497–4506.
18. Buchner, M.; Brantner, P.; Stickel, N.; Prinz, G.; Burger, M.; Bar, C.; Dierks, C.; Pfeifer, D.; Ott, A.; Mertelsmann, R.; et al. The microenvironment differentially impairs passive and active immunotherapy in chronic lymphocytic leukaemia - CXCR4 antagonists as potential adjuvants for monoclonal antibodies. *Br. J. Haematol.* **2010**, *151*, 167–178.
19. Kurtova, A. V.; Balakrishnan, K.; Chen, R.; Ding, W.; Schnabl, S.; Quiroga, M. P.; Sivina, M.; Wierda, W. G.; Estrov, Z.; Keating, M. J.; et al. Diverse marrow stromal cells protect CLL cells from spontaneous and drug-induced apoptosis: Development of a reliable and reproducible system to assess stromal cell adhesion-mediated drug resistance. *Blood* **2009**, *114*, 4441–4450.
20. Plander, M.; Seegers, S.; Ugocsai, P.; Diermeier-Daucher, S.; Ivanyi, J.; Schmitz, G.; Hofstadter, F.; Schwarz, S.; Orso, E.; Knuchel, R.; et al. Different proliferative and survival capacity of CLL-cells in a newly established in vitro model for pseudofollicles. *Leukemia* **2009**, *23*, 2118–2128.
21. Meads, M. B.; Gatenby, R. A.; Dalton, W. S. Environment-mediated drug resistance: A major contributor to minimal residual disease. *Nat. Rev. Cancer* **2009b**, *9*, 665–674.

22. Meads, M. B.; Hazlehurst, L. A.; Dalton, W. S. The bone marrow microenvironment as a tumor sanctuary and contributor to drug resistance. *Clin. Cancer Res.* **2008**, *14*, 2519–2526.
23. Shain, K. H.; Dalton, W. S. Environmental-mediated drug resistance: A target for multiple myeloma therapy. *Exp. Rev. Hematol.* **2009**, *2*, 649–662.
24. Meads, M. B.; Gatenby, R. A.; Dalton, W. S. Environment-mediated drug resistance: A major contributor to minimal residual disease. *Nat. Rev. Cancer* **2009a**, *9*, 665–674.
25. Varki, N. M.; Varki, A. Diversity in cell surface sialic acid presentations: Implications for biology and disease. *Lab. Invest.* **2007**, *87*, 851–857.
26. Yamamoto-Sugitani, M.; Kuroda, J.; Ashihara, E.; Nagoshi, H.; Kobayashi, T.; Matsumoto, Y.; Sasaki, N.; Shimura, Y.; Kiyota, M.; Nakayama, R.; et al. Galectin-3 (Gal-3) induced by leukemia microenvironment promotes drug resistance and bone marrow lodgment in chronic myelogenous leukemia. *Proc. Natl. Acad. Sci. U.S.A* **2011**, *108*, 17468–17473.
27. Suzuki, O.; Abe, M. Cell surface N-glycosylation and sialylation regulate galectin-3-induced apoptosis in human diffuse large B cell lymphoma. *Oncol. Rep.* **2008**, *19*, 743–748.
28. Cheng, Y. L.; Huang, W. C.; Chen, C. L.; Tsai, C. C.; Wang, C. Y.; Chiu, W. H.; Chen, Y. L.; Lin, Y. S.; Chang, C. F.; Lin, C. F. Increased galectin-3 facilitates leukemia cell survival from apoptotic stimuli. *Biochem. Biophys. Res. Commun.* **2011**, *412*, 334–340.
29. Ochieng, J.; Green, B.; Evans, S.; James, O.; Warfield, P. Modulation of the biological functions of galectin-3 by matrix metalloproteinases. *Biochim. Biophys. Acta* **1998**, *1379*, 97–106.
30. Fukumori, T.; Oka, N.; Takenaka, Y.; Nangia-Makker, P.; Elsamman, E.; Kasai, T.; Shono, M.; Kanayama, H. O.; Ellerhorst, J.; Lotan, R.; et al. Galectin-3 regulates mitochondrial stability and antiapoptotic function in response to anticancer drug in prostate cancer. *Cancer Res.* **2006**, *66*, 3114–3119.
31. Matarrese, P.; Tinari, N.; Semeraro, M. L.; Natoli, C.; Iacobelli, S.; Malorni, W. Galectin-3 overexpression protects from cell damage and death by influencing mitochondrial homeostasis. *FEBS Lett.* **2000**, *473*, 311–315.
32. Yu, F.; Finley, R. L., Jr.; Raz, A.; Kim, H. R. Galectin-3 translocates to the perinuclear membranes and inhibits cytochrome c release from the mitochondria. A role for synexin in galectin-3 translocation. *J. Biol. Chem.* **2002**, *277*, 15819–15827.
33. Yang, R. Y.; Hsu, D. K.; Liu, F. T. Expression of galectin-3 modulates T-cell growth and apoptosis. *Proc. Natl. Acad. Sci. U.S.A.* **1996**, *93*, 6737–6742.
34. Chauhan, D.; Li, G.; Podar, K.; Hideshima, T.; Neri, P.; He, D.; Mitsiades, N.; Richardson, P.; Chang, Y.; Schindler, J.; et al. A novel carbohydrate-based therapeutic GCS-100 overcomes bortezomib resistance and enhances dexamethasone-induced apoptosis in multiple myeloma cells. *Cancer Res.* **2005**, *65*, 8350–8358.

35. Streetly, M. J.; Maharaj, L.; Joel, S.; Schey, S. A.; Gribben, J. G.; Cotter, F. E. GCS-100, a novel galectin-3 antagonist, modulates MCL-1, NOXA, and cell cycle to induce myeloma cell death. *Blood* **2010**, *115*, 3939–3948.
36. Demotte, N.; Wieers, G.; Van Der Smissen, P.; Moser, M.; Schmidt, C; Thielemans, K.; Squifflet, J. L.; Weynand, B.; Carrasco, J.; Lurquin, C.; et al. A galectin-3 ligand corrects the impaired function of human CD4 and CD8 tumor-infiltrating lymphocytes and favors tumor rejection in mice. *Cancer Res.* **2010**, *70*, 7476–7488.
37. Mirandola, L.; Yu, Y.; Chui, K.; Jenkins, M. R.; Cobos, E.; John, C. M.; Chiriva-Internati, M. Galectin-3C inhibits tumor growth and increases the anticancer activity of bortezomib in a murine model of human multiple myeloma. *PloS One* **2011**, *6*, e21811.

Chapter 15

Translational Rational for the Clinical Development of OTX-008: A Novel Drug That Inhibits Galectin-1 Expression in Human Cancer Models

Eric Raymond,* Lucile Astrorgue-Xerri, Maria Serova, Maria Eugenia Riveiro, and Sandrine Faivre

INSERM U728 and Department of Medical Oncology, Beaujon University Hospital (AP-HP – Paris 7 Diderot), Assistance Publique – Hôpitaux de Paris, 100 boulevard du Général Leclerc, 92110 Clichy, France
***E-mail: eric.raymond@bjn.aphp.fr**

OTX-008 (a.k.a. PTX-008 and calixarene 0118, see Chapter 3) is a first-in-class novel anticancer drug that binds to galectin-1 and reduces galectin-1 expression in cancer cells. Evidences suggest that OTX-008 inhibits cellular proliferation and reduces tumor angiogenesis in several human carcinoma models. Data were provided during the last 10 years that galectin-1 might play an important role in human tumors and, thus, galectin-1 inhibition with OTX-008 warranted to be evaluated in patients with advanced malignancies. Based on its safe toxicology profile, OTX-008 is currently tested in a Phase 1 clinical trial in Europe.

Relevance of Galectin-1 as a Target for the Treatment of Cancer

Galectins are carbohydrate-binding proteins related to lectins that are defined by their affinity for β-galactoside-containing glycans (*1*, *2*). Galectin-1 as a family member of this class of proteins plays multiple roles in various physiologic and pathologic processes (*3*). Within the tumor microenvironment, galectin-1 was first described as a determinant factor in cancer cell adhesion (*4*) and in cell-extracellular matrix interactions (*5*). Galectin-1 was also recognized to be a multifunctional protein involved in different aspects of cancer progression including cell proliferation (*5*), homotypic cell aggregation (*6*), migration (*7*, *8*), angiogenesis (*9*), and escape from immune surveillance (*10*, *11*). When secreted in the cellular microenvironment, galectin-1 may eventually dimerize and form extracellular lattices with lactosamine-enriched N- and O-glycans, facilitating growth factor/receptor signaling and cell/matrix interactions (*3*, *12*). For instance, interactions of extracellular galectin-1 with the neuropilin-1/semaphorin-3A system have been shown to enhance VEGFR2 signaling and tumor angiogenesis (*7–9*, *13–16*). Galectin-1 may also have other functions when not excreted but trapped into the cytoplasm and/or the nucleus of cancer cells (*15*). Studies have shown that the cytoplasmic localization of galectin-1 facilitates the binding H-Ras and increases Ras-GTP binding to the cell membrane, facilitating downstream activation of Raf-1 and ERK1/2-dependent survival pathways (*17–21*).

Galectin-1 Expression in Human Carcinomas

Immunohistochemical studies from series of biopsy and surgical specimens from patients with cancer have revealed that galectin-1 is frequently expressed in cancer cells. Up-regulation of galectin-1 has been associated with poor clinical prognosis and the presence of metastases in several malignancies (*22–31*) such as hepatocellular carcinoma (*27*, *28*), breast cancer (*24*), glioblastoma (*8*, *25*), neuroblastoma (*29*, *30*), lung adenocarcinoma (*7*, *31*), and head & neck squamous cell carcinoma (*23*). The presence of galectin-1 in the cytoplasm of cancer cells and in endothelial cells participating to tumor angiogenesis has suggested that galectin-1 may have important function for cancer cell survival and tumor growth.

Galectin-1 as a 'Drugable' Target for Anticancer Agents

Galectin-1 has been early recognized as a potential target for cancer treatments, and as such, several compounds have been designed to block its intracellular and/or extracellular effects in tumor progression. Scientists at the University of Minnesota and Maastricht University have designed a series of synthetic peptides, which have been modeled to reproduce the 3-dimensional β-sheet structure of platelet factor 4 and interleukin-8. Some of those peptides were also shown to bind galectin-1 (*8*, *32*). Anginex, a synthetic 33-amino acid peptide βpep-25, was the first peptide designed to bind galectin-1 that demonstrated cellular effects in cellular models. While the antiproliferative effects of anginex in cancer cells was limited, anginex displayed antiangiogenic effects by inhibiting proliferation, adhesion, and migration of tumor-activated endothelial cells (*33*), yielding antitumor activity in the mouse B16 melanoma model and in human ovarian carcinoma MA148 xenografts (*34*, *35*).

Mechanistically, anginex functions *in vitro* as an anti-angiogenic agent that specifically inhibits endothelial cells proliferation and angiogenesis. Anginex is cytotoxic towards angiogenically-activated endothelial cells since it inhibits their adhesion to the extracellular matrix, resulting in apoptosis and cell death. Thus, it is likely that anginex interacts with endothelial (cell-surface) adhesion molecules that are upregulated during endothelial cell proliferation. Using the mouse aortic ring assay, significant inhibition of sprout formation in *ex vivo* models were observed using anginex at relatively high concentrations (*37*). The activity of anginex in tumor models in mice was found to be dose-dependent and primarily mediated by angiogenesis inhibition, since microvessel density was significantly decreased in treated tumors (*13*, *35*, *36*). Further studies into the structure-activity relationships of anginex led to the design of a non-peptidic calixarene-based compound 0118 (*37*) that was found to target galectin-1 (*38*).

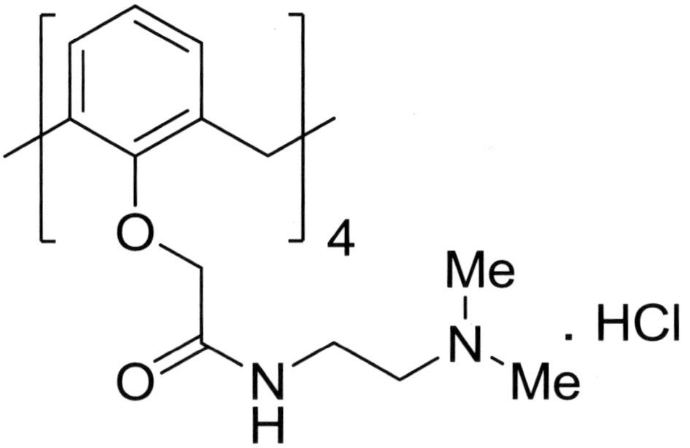

Figure 1. Chemical formula of OTX-008. It is a N-(2-dimethylamino)ethyl)acetamidyl calix[4]arene, hydrochloride salt of 937.2 molecular weight (free base).

PTX-008: A Drug That Inhibits Galectin-1 Expression in Cancer Cells

Given the promising results obtain with anginex, a new generation of compounds was specifically designed to improve specificity, increase affinity, and optimize pharmacological properties. The antiangiogenic peptide anginex was used as a model to design these non peptide compounds that approximate its molecular weight, mimic its peptide hydrophobic and positively charged amino acid composition, and its surface topology of the functionally critical β -sheet conformation (*34–37*). One of these nonpeptidic topomimetics, OTX-008 (0118, Figure 1), was shown to be a potent angiogenesis inhibitor *in vitro*, as well as *in vivo*, recapitulating most of the effects of anginex on endothelial cell proliferation and migration in in vitro experiments (*37*).

In our department, we completed the preclinical evaluation of OTX-008 to focus on its direct effects on cancer cells. We found that OTX-008 displayed potent antiproliferative effects on cancer cells in culture. Dose-dependent and duration-of-exposure-dependent decreased galectin-1 expressions were observed in cancer cells exposed to OTX-008 either in culture or in xenografts. Mechanisms by which OTX-008 reduces galectin-1 expression remain unclear. No change in galectin-1 mRNA expression was observed in cancer cells treated with OTX-008. However, a significant increase in galectin-1 oxidation was observed in cells exposed to OTX-

008, a mechanism that may facilitated proteasome degradation of galectin-1 in the cytoplasm of cancer cells.

In cancer cells, exposure to antiproliferative concentrations of OTX-008 inhibited ERK1/2 and AKT dependent cell signalling. In cultured cancer cells, the effects of OTX-008 were primarily ‘cytostatic’, OTX-008 inducing a dose-dependent accumulation of cells in late G2 phase of cell cycle without apoptosis induction. The antiproliferative effects of OTX008 were higher in cancer cells with low levels of Gal-1 mRNA and protein expression and high levels of epithelial differentiation markers such as E-cadherin, claudin-4, keratin-8, and keratin-18. Conversely, cancer cells expressing high levels of Gal-1 mRNA and protein and high levels of mesenchymal differentiation markers such as vimentin, FGFR1, N-cadherin, ZEB1, and TWIST were markedly more resistant to the antiproliferative effects of OTX008. In cultured cancer cells, OTX-008 was also shown to closely mimic inhibition of galectin-1 by shRNA, reducing migration and invasion in scratch test and matrigel assays, respectively.

Potential of OTX-008 in Combination with Other Anticancer Drugs

Combination studies showed that OTX-008 displays at least additive, often synergistic effects with several cytotoxic drugs, including cisplatin, oxaliplatin, 5-FU, gemcitabine and taxotere. PTX-008 also potentiated the antiproliferative and antitumor effects of sunitinib in human tumor models. Those preliminary evidences suggest that inhibition of galectin-1 using PTX-008 may improve the antiproliferative effects of several anticancer drugs in clinical trials and that modulation of galectin-1 may be used to enhance the activity of cytotoxic agents and sunitinib (unpublished data from our laboratory).

Antitumor Effects of OTX008 in Mouse Models

In vivo, we showed that OTX008 displays antitumor activity in human ovarian cancer models as well as human head & neck cancer xenografts and murine melanoma. OTX008 treatment reduced Gal-1 expression, delayed tumor growth, and inhibited the development of secondary tumors in SQ20B tumors that develop subcutaneous metastasis. Staining of sections from OTX008 treated tumors showed down-regulation of Galecin-1 expression, decreased tumor cell proliferation, and inhibit angiogenesis and normalize tumor blood vessels. These effects were similar to that observed in the SQ20B model using shRNA to silence Galectin-1 protein. Preliminary PK assessments showed that OTX008 can be orally absorbed rapidly (Tmax 0.25 to 0.50 hr), reaching a Cmax of 4.66 μg/mL, then rapidly distributed through the body (distribution half-life of 32 min), and cleared from plasma with an estimated elimination half-life of about 10 hr. Repeated dosing showed no drug accumulation, OTX008 being still detectable in plasma after 24 hours. Interestingly, OTX008 accumulated in tumor after repeated treatments. OTX008 levels in tumors reached Cmax at 0.5 hr, detectable drug level being still measureable in the tumor up to 24 hr after exposure. However, OTX-008 display poor oral bioavailability and other routes of drug administration have been tested. As optimal antitumor effects have been observed when cancer cells and tumor were protractedly exposed to OTX-008, the subcutaneous administration was tested in animal studies. The subcutaneous administration of OTX-008 was shown to be the most efficient to provide tumor growth inhibition. Furthermore, the subcutaneous administration of OTX-008 was well tolerated in animal. Therefore subcutaneous administration of OTX-008 was further considered for clinical trials. The adverse effects of OTX-008 were evaluated in 28-day repeated subcutaneous dose toxicity studies with 14-day recovery in rats and dogs. The highest non-severely toxic dose or maximally tolerated dose was 30 mg/kg/day in rats and 15 mg/kg/day in dogs. Few non-specific inflammatory changes and edema were observed in the skin at the injection sites, adjacent skin, and adjacent skeletal muscle on Day 28 at dose $\geq$5 mg/kg in female and 15 mg/kg in male.

Inhibition of Galectin-1 Using OTX-008 in Patients with Cancer

Based on strong preclinical evidence showing activity of OTX-008 in several human cancer models and its safe toxicity profile, a multicenter phase I clinical trial has been started in February 2012 in Europe. This trial will investigate several dose level of OTX-008 looking at pharmacokinetic and pharmacodynamic parameters in human. In this study, OTX-008 is administered subcutaneously daily until tumor progression to patients with advanced metastatic tumors that progressed under prior treatment with registered therapies. So far, few patients have been treated at the first dose levels of OTX-008 and only minor local inflammatory reaction at the site of injection were reported. Subcutaneous injections at the first dose-levels have yielded high plasma exposure, which is in the range of active concentrations for sensitive human cancer cell lines. At this time, it is too early to comment on the antitumor activity.

Conclusions and Perspectives

Galectin-1 is one of the most important lectins to date participating in the malignant tumor development since its expression is upregulated in tumors and is associated with poor prognosis. The antiangiogenic peptide anginex was used as a model to design nonpeptidic compounds that approximate the molecular dimensions of the peptide, its hydrophobic and positively charged amino acid composition, and the surface topology of the functionally critical amphipathic β-sheet conformation. OTX-008, one of these nonpeptidic topomimetics of anginex, displays antiproliferative effects in cancer cells and shows potent antiantiangiogenic effects in animal models. OTX-008 is currently investigated in clinical trial.

References

1. Barondes, S. H.; Castronovo, V.; Cooper, D. N.; et al. Galectins: A family of animal beta galactoside-binding lectins. *Cell* **1994**, *76*, 597–598.
2. Liu, F. T.; Rabinovich, G. A. Galectins as modulators of tumour progression. *Nat. Rev. Cancer* **2005**, *5*, 29–41.
3. Camby, I; Le Mercier, M.; Lefranc, F.; Kiss, R. Galectin-1: A small protein with major functions. *Glycobiology* **2006**, *16*, 137R–157R.
4. Ellerhorst, J.; Nguyen, T.; Cooper, D. N.; Lotan, D.; Lotan, R. Differential expression of endogenous galectin-1 and galectin-3 in human prostate cancer cell lines and effects of overexpressing galectin-1 on cell phenotype. *Int. J. Oncol.* **1999**, *14*, 217–224.
5. van den Brüle, F.; Califice, S.; Garnier, F.; Fernandez, P. L.; Berchuck, A.; Castronovo, V. Galectin-1 accumulation in the ovary carcinoma peritumoral stroma is induced by ovary carcinoma cells and affects both cancer cell proliferation and adhesion to laminin-1 and fibronectin. *Lab. Invest.* **2003**, *83*, 377–386.
6. Tinari, N.; Kuwabara, I.; Huflejt, M. E.; Shen, P. F.; Iacobelli, S.; Liu, F. T. Glycoprotein 90K/MAC-2BP interacts with galectin-1 and mediates galectin-1-induced cell aggregation. *Int. J. Cancer* **2001**, *91*, 167–172.
7. Wu, M. H.; Hong, T. M.; Cheng, H. W.; et al. Galectin-1-mediated tumor invasion and metastasis, up-regulated matrix metalloproteinase expression, and reorganized actin cytoskeletons. *Mol. Cancer Res.* **2009**, *7*, 311–318.
8. Camby, I.; Belot, N.; Lefranc, F.; et al. Galectin-1 modulates human glioblastoma cell migration into the brain through modifications to the actin cytoskeleton and levels of expression of small GTPases. *J. Neuropathol. Exp. Neurol.* **2002**, *61*, 585–596.
9. Thijssen, V. L.; Postel, R.; Brandwijk, R. J.; et al. Galectin-1 is essential in tumor angiogenesis and is a target for antiangiogenesis therapy. *Proc. Natl. Acad. Sci. U.S.A.* **2006**, *103*, 15975–15980.
10. Rubinstein, N.; Alvarez, M.; Zwirner, N. W.; Toscano, M. A.; Ilarregui, J. M.; Bravo, A.; Mordoh, J.; Fainboim, L.; Podhajcer, O. L.; Rabinovich, G. A. Targeted inhibition of galectin-1 gene expression in tumor cells results in heightened T cell-mediated rejection: A potential mechanism of tumor-immune privilege. *Cancer Cell* **2004**, *5*, 241–251.
11. Juszczynski, P.; Ouyang, J.; Monti, S.; Rodig, S. J.; Takeyama, K.; Abramson, J.; Chen, W.; Kutok, J. L.; Rabinovich, G. A.; Shipp, M. A. The AP1-dependent secretion of galectin-1 by Reed Sternberg cells fosters immune privilege in classical Hodgkin lymphoma. *Proc. Natl. Acad. Sci. U.S.A.* **2007**, *104*, 13134–13139.
12. Sacchettini, J. C.; Baum, L. G.; Brewer, C. F. Multivalent protein-carbohydrate interactions. A new paradigm for supermolecular assembly and signal transduction. *Biochemistry* **2001**, *40*, 3009–3015.
13. Thijssen, V. L.; Barkan, B.; Shoji, H.; et al. Tumor cells secrete galectin-1 to enhance endothelial cell activity. *Cancer Res.* **2010**, *70*, 6216–6224.

14. Hsieh, S. H.; Ying, N. W.; Wu, M. H.; et al. Galectin-1, a novel ligand of neuropilin-1, activates VEGFR-2 signaling and modulates the migration of vascular endothelial cells. *Oncogene* **2008**, *27*, 3746–3753.
15. Rabinovich, G. A. Galectin-1 as a potential cancer target. *Br. J. Cancer* **2005**, *92*, 1188–1192.
16. Thijssen, V. L.; Hulsmans, S.; Griffioen, A. W. The galectin profile of the endothelium: Altered expression and localization in activated and tumor endothelial cells. *Am. J. Pathol.* **2008**, *17*, 545–553.
17. Paz, A.; Haklai, R.; Elad-Sfadia, G.; Ballan, E.; Kloog, Y. Galectin-1 binds oncogenic H-Ras to mediate Ras membrane anchorage and cell transformation. *Oncogene* **2001**, *20*, 7486–7493.
18. Lee, M. Y.; Lee, S. H.; Park, J. H.; Han, H. J. Interaction of galectin-1 with caveolae induces mouse embryonic stem cell proliferation through the Src, ERas, Akt and mTOR signaling pathways. *Cell. Mol. Life Sci.* **2009**, *66*, 1467–1478.
19. Elad-Sfadia, G.; Haklai, R.; Ballan, E.; Gabius, H. J.; Kloog, Y. Galectin-1 augments Ras activation and diverts Ras signals to Raf-1 at the expense of phosphoinositide 3-kinase. *J. Biol. Chem.* **2002**, *277*, 37169–37175.
20. Belanis, L.; Plowman, S. J.; Rotblat, B.; Hancock, J. F.; Kloog, Y. Galectin-1 is a novel structural component and a major regulator of h-ras nanoclusters. *Mol. Biol. Cell* **2008**, *19*, 1404–1414.
21. Rotblat, B.; Belanis, L.; Liang, H.; et al. H-Ras nanocluster stability regulates the magnitude of MAPK signal output. *PLoS One* **2010**, *5*, e11991.
22. Yamaoka, K.; Mishima, K.; Nagashima, Y.; Asai, A.; Sanai, Y.; Kirino, T. Expression of galectin-1 mRNA correlates with the malignant potential of human gliomas and expression of antisense galectin-1 inhibits the growth of 9 glioma cells. *J. Neurosci. Res.* **2000**, *59*, 722–730.
23. Chiang, W. F.; Liu, S. Y.; Fang, L. Y.; et al. Overexpression of galectin-1 at the tumor invasion front is associated with poor prognosis in early-stage oral squamous cell carcinoma. *Oral Oncol.* **2008**, *44*, 325–334.
24. Jung, E. J.; Moon, H. G.; Cho, B. I.; et al. Galectin-1 expression in cancer-associated stromal cells correlates tumor invasiveness and tumor progression in breast cancer. *Int. J. Cancer* **2007**, *120*, 2331–2338.
25. Rorive, S.; Belot, N.; Decaestecker, C.; et al. Galectin-1 is highly expressed in human gliomas with relevance for modulation of invasion of tumor astrocytes into the brain parenchyma. *Glia* **2001**, *33*, 241–255.
26. Demydenko, D.; Berest, I. Expression of galectin-1 in malignant tumors. *Exp. Oncol.* **2009**, *31*, 74–9.
27. Spano, D.; Russo, R.; Di Maso, V.; et al. Galectin-1 and its involvement in hepatocellular carcinoma aggressiveness. *Mol. Med.* **2010**, *16*, 102–115.
28. Espelt, M. V.; Croci, D. O.; Bacigalupo, M. L.; Carabias, P.; Manzi, M.; Elola, M. T.; Muñoz, M. C.; Dominici, F. P.; Wolfenstein-Todel, C.; Rabinovich, G. A.; Troncoso, M. F. Novel roles of galectin-1 in hepatocellular carcinoma cell adhesion, polarization, and in vivo tumor growth. *Hepatology* **2011**, *53*, 2097–2106.

29. Cimmino, F.; Schulte, J. H.; Zollo, M.; Koster, J.; Versteeg, R.; Iolascon, A.; Eggert, A.; Schramm, A. Galectin-1 is a major effector of TrkB-mediated neuroblastoma aggressiveness. *Oncogene* **2009**, *28*, 2015–2023.
30. Soldati, R.; Berger, E.; Zenclussen, A. C.; Jorch, G.; Lode, H. N.; Salatino, M.; Rabinovich, G. A.; Fest, S. Neuroblastoma triggers an immunoevasive program involving galectin-1-dependent modulation of T cell and dendritic cell compartments. *Int. J. Cancer* **2011**, *131*, 1131–1141.
31. Banh, A.; Zhang, J.; Cao, H.; Bouley, D. M.; Kwok, S.; Kong, C.; Giaccia, A. J.; Koong, A. C.; Le, Q. T. Tumor galectin-1 mediates tumor growth and metastasis through regulation of T-cell apoptosis. *Cancer Res.* **2011**, *71*, 4423–4431.
32. Mayo, K. H.; Ilyina, E; Park, H. A recipe for designing water-soluble, beta-sheet-forming peptides. *Protein Sci.* **1996**, *5*, 1301–1315.
33. Griffioen, A. W.; van der Schaft, D. W.; Barendsz-Janson, A. F.; et al. Anginex, a designed peptide that inhibits angiogenesis. *Biochem. J.* **2001**, *354*, 233–242.
34. van der Schaft, D. W.; Dings, R. P.; de Lussanet, Q. G.; et al. The designer anti-angiogenic peptide anginex targets tumor endothelial cells and inhibits tumor growth in animal models. *FASEB J.* **2002**, *16*, 1991–1993.
35. Dings, R. P.; van der Schaft, D. W.; Hargittai, B.; Haseman, J; Griffioen, A. W.; Mayo, K. H. Anti-tumor activity of the novel angiogenesis inhibitor anginex. *Cancer Lett.* **2003**, *194*, 55–66.
36. Dings, R. P.; Arroyo, M. M.; Lockwood, N. A.; et al. Beta-sheet is the bioactive conformation of the anti-angiogenic anginex peptide. *Biochem. J.* **2003**, *373*, 281–288.
37. Dings, R. P.; Chen, X.; Hellebrekers, D. M.; et al. Design of nonpeptidic topomimetics of antiangiogenic proteins with antitumor activities. *J. Natl. Cancer Inst.* **2006**, *98*, 932–936.
38. Dings, R. P. M.; Miller, M. C.; Nesmelova, I.; Astorgues-Xerri, L.; Kumar, N.; Serova, M.; Chen, X.; Raymond, E.; Hoye, T. R.; Mayo, K. H. Anti-tumor agent calixarene 0118 targets human galectin-1 as an allosteric inhibitor of carbohydrate binding. *J. Med. Chem.* **2012**, *55*, 5121–5129.

Chapter 16

Improving the Clinical Efficacy of Cancer Vaccines by Targeting Immune Suppression in Human Tumors

Nathalie Demotte,[1] Aristotelis Antonopoulos,[2] Jean-François Baurain,[3] Grégoire Wieërs,[1,§] Nicolas Van Baren,[1] and Pierre van der Bruggen[*,1]

[1]Ludwig Institute for Cancer Research, WELBIO, and Université catholique de Louvain, de Duve Institute, 74 av. Hippocrate, P.O. Box B1-7403, B-1200 Brussels, Belgium
[2]Division of Molecular Biosciences, Imperial College London, South Kensington Campus, SW7 2AZ, United Kingdom
[3]Department of Oncology, Université catholique de Louvain, Cliniques Universitaires Saint-Luc, 10 av. Hippocrate, B-1200 Brussels, Belgium
[§]Current address: Department of Internal Medicine, Université catholique de Louvain, Cliniques Universitaires Saint-Luc, 10 av. Hippocrate, B-1200 Brussels, Belgium
[*]E-mail: pierre.vanderbruggen@bru.licr.org

The identification of tumor-specific antigens recognized by T lymphocytes on human cancer cells has elicited numerous vaccination trials of cancer patients with defined tumor antigens. These treatments have induced T cell responses but have shown a low clinical efficacy in tumor-bearing melanoma patients. Immunosuppression at the tumor sites is the most likely explanation for the poor effectiveness of cancer vaccines. Many researchers are trying to decipher the underlying immunosuppressive mechanism. Galectin-3, a lectin secreted by tumor cells and macrophages, plays a role in the dysfunction of tumor-infiltrating T lymphocytes (TIL). We have observed that human TIL, in contrast with CD8 blood cells, show impaired IFN-γ secretion and cytotoxicity. TIL dysfunction correlates with the segregation of T cell receptor (TCR) and CD8 co-receptor at the T cell surface. Treating TIL with soluble galectin ligands or an anti-galectin-3 antibody restored IFN-γ secretion, cytotoxicity and TCR/CD8 co-localization. Our working hypothesis is that TIL, having been stimulated recently by their antigen, harbor a set of glycans that contain numerous ligands for galectins, which block their proper function. In agreement with this hypothesis, we have recently observed that, compared to resting CD8 T cell clones, the N-glycans of recently activated clones contains more multi-antennary N-glycans and consists of longer LacNAc chains. We propose that therapeutic vaccines combined with soluble galectin ligands could reverse local immunosuppression at the tumor site and may induce more tumor regressions in cancer patients than vaccination alone.

Tumor Antigens Recognized by T Lymphocytes: Targets for Therapeutic Vaccination?

In the sixties, mouse experiments demonstrated that tumors can alert immune cells and that immune responses could be tumor-specific and protective (*1*, *2*). In the seventies, it was shown that antibodies and lymphocytes derived from cancer patients preferentially recognize tumor cells versus normal cells (*3*, *4*). We had to wait for the early nineties for the first molecular identifications of the antigens recognized by T lymphocytes on human and mouse tumors (*5*, *6*). Since then, various methods that combined immunological assays with genetic and biochemical approaches result in a long list of defined human tumor antigens, several of which are being tested as targets for immunotherapy (*7*).

CD8 cytolytic T lymphocytes (CTL) are important effectors in the anti-tumor response. They recognize peptides derived from intracellular proteins. Their T cell receptor (TCR) and co-receptor CD8 cooperate in the recognition of antigenic peptides (8-11 amino acids long) presented at the cell surface by human leukocyte antigen (HLA) class I molecules. We have identified antigens encoded by human melanoma antigen (MAGE) genes that seem to be good candidates for therapeutic vaccination of cancer patients. First, these antigens are strictly tumor-specific, because the only normal cells that express the peptide-encoding gene are located in testis and placenta, which do not bear HLA molecules on their surface and therefore cannot present MAGE-derived antigens to T cells (*8*). Second, MAGE genes are expressed in a significant percentage of tumors from various histological types. Several families of genes with the same pattern of expression – *i.e.* expressed in various tumors but silent in normal tissue (with the exception of testicular and placental tissue) – have been identified: genes MAGE, BAGE, GAGE, LAGE/NY-ESO-1, SSX (*9*, *10*). We refer to them as cancer-germline genes. Several of these genes have been shown to encode antigenic peptides recognized by T cells on tumors (previously reviewed in 7).

The first therapeutic vaccinations with MAGE antigens started in 1994. Various vaccines have been used in small clinical vaccination trials: peptides and proteins with or without adjuvants, viruses containing antigen-coding sequences, antigen-presenting cells loaded with antigens (*11–17*). Patients with non-small-cell lung, esophageal, bladder and head and neck carcinoma as well as melanoma have been vaccinated (*18*).

Large clinical vaccination trials with a recombinant MAGE-3 protein mixed with an adjuvant are also ongoing. Based on encouraging results in Phase II trials in patients with metastatic melanoma (NCT00086866) and in patients with completely resected non-small cell lung cancer (NCT00290355) (*19*), a randomized, double-blind Phase III trial was initiated in 2007 in patients with MAGE-A3-positive stages IB, II, and IIIA non-small cell lung cancer, and has recruited more than 2,000 patients (MAGRIT Phase III trial, NCT00480025). The objective of this trial is to investigate the efficacy of the vaccine administered after tumor resection for preventing cancer relapse. Another Phase III trial has enrolled 1,389 patients with resectable regionally advanced melanoma (DERMA Phase III trial, NCT00796445). Disease-free survival in the overall patient population is the primary endpoint.

Does Therapeutic Vaccination of Melanoma Patients Induce Tumor Regression?

Clinical Responses

Most of our small clinical vaccination trials enrolled patients with metastatic melanoma. Different immunization modalities, mostly with MAGE-A3-derived products, have already been tried (*15*, *20*, *21*). We have not observed significant toxicity. About 10 to 20% of vaccinated melanoma patients experienced regression of metastatic lesions. This frequency is far beyond the reported incidence of spontaneous regressions of melanoma metastases, estimated at 0.2-0.3%, strongly suggesting that these regressions are linked to the vaccinations. However, only 5% of the patients experience a true clinical benefit. Some of the remissions have lasted for several years.

Immune Responses

The first attempts to detect anti-vaccine T cells in the blood of vaccinated patients were disappointing, even in patients with complete responses. A sensitive approach was developed that was based on *in vitro* restimulation of blood lymphocytes, in limiting dilution conditions, with the antigenic peptide, followed two weeks afterwards by labeling of T cells with fluorescent HLA-peptide tetramers. Tetramer-positive cells were cloned and the clones were analyzed for cytotoxicity. Their diversity was analyzed by TCR (T cell receptor) sequencing (*22*, *23*). The first surprise was the low levels of anti-vaccine T cell response found in several of the patients who displayed tumor regression after the vaccinations, usually between 10^{-5} and 10^{-6} of anti-vaccine T cells among the blood CD8 T cells. Whether new vaccination modalities that induce much higher frequencies of blood anti-vaccine T cells would lead to increased tumor regression is unclear as yet. Despite the fact that these responses were often weak, in the case of the MAGE-3.A1 antigen, they were observed mostly in patients who had tumor regression (*15*, *24*, *25*).

How can we explain that such low numbers of anti-vaccine T cells in vaccinated patients can trigger tumor rejection responses? To answer that question, the immune response of a vaccinated melanoma patient who experienced complete regression of numerous skin metastases was evaluated in detail. Pierre Coulie and colleagues evaluated the frequencies not only of the "anti-vaccine" T cells, which recognized the MAGE vaccine antigen, but also of all the "anti-tumor" T cells. To this end, blood lymphocytes were restimulated *in vitro* in limiting dilution conditions with autologous tumor cells, followed 2-3 weeks afterwards by cytolysis assays using autologous tumor cells as targets. The frequency of these "anti-tumor" T cells, which recognize all possible tumor-specific antigens on the tumor, was evaluated at 3×10^{-4} of the blood T cells before vaccination and at 3×10^{-3} after vaccination. Their diversity was analyzed by TCR sequencing. The same anti-tumor T cells were found in the blood and in different metastases. For some of them, frequency at the tumor site reached 10^{-1} of the T cells present. In contrast, no anti-vaccine T cells were detectable before vaccination and, after vaccination, frequency was around 3×10^{-6} of the blood CD8 T cells. They concluded that anti-vaccine T cells showed only a modest enrichment in the tumor site as compared to the blood, while some anti-tumor T cells showed an enrichment of several hundredfold (*26–28*).

A Scenario To Explain the Low Level of Clinical Responses

Analyses of the T cell responses of melanoma patients are in favor of the following scenario. Most melanoma patients produce a spontaneous T cell response against melanoma tumor antigens at a relatively early stage of the disease, *e.g.* primary tumor or early metastatic tumor. These T cells can eliminate some tumors at an early stage, but often they do not succeed in eliminating the tumor and they become dysfunctional. Thus the tumors of the patients about to receive the vaccine already contain dysfunctional T cells directed against tumor antigens. Presumably this "anergy" is maintained by immunosuppressive factors present in the tumor. A few patients show tumor regression following vaccination because some T cells generated by the vaccine penetrate inside the tumor, attack some tumor cells and succeed in reversing the local immunosuppression, possibly by releasing cytokines or chemokines or by reactivating effective antigen-presenting cells. This reactivates the anergic T cells located inside the tumor and elicits or attracts new anti-tumor T cells. These T cells then proceed to eliminate the tumor cells. Most patients however do not show tumor regression because the immunosuppressive environment immediately overwhelms the few anti-vaccine T cells that reach the tumor.

Accordingly, the crucial difference between the responding and the non-responding patients is probably not the intensity of their direct T cell response to the vaccine but the intensity of the immunosuppression inside the tumor. It is now clear that current cancer vaccines are safe, but lead to clinical responses only in a small minority of patients (*27*, *29–31*). It is therefore important to know which immunosuppressive mechanisms operate in human tumors if we want to improve the clinical efficacy of cancer vaccines.

Immune Suppression in Tumors

Ongoing Clinical Trials Aimed at Counteracting Tumor Immunosuppression

We would like to briefly summarize several ongoing clinical efforts to neutralize immunosuppressive mechanisms potentially at work in tumors [reviewed elsewhere (*27*, *32–37*)]. Our intention is not to be exhaustive but to give a flavor of the ongoing strategies.

Tumors can recruit suppressive cells, such as regulatory T cells, which can inhibit the function of the effector tumor-infiltrating T cells. Different treatments aimed at reducing the number of $CD25^{+}$ regulatory T cells were administered to cancer patients: cyclophosphamide, anti-CD25 monoclonal antibody Daclizumab, and Denileukin diftitox (Ontak®), an engineered protein combining IL-2 and diphtheria toxin (*38–40*). There is so far no report and no documentation of a real Treg depletion, as defined by a decreased frequency of $CD4^{+}CD25^{+}$ T cells with a demethylated intron 1 of FOXP3 (*40*, *41*).

Tumor-infiltrating T cell function can be affected metabolically by limiting their access to essential amino-acid such as tryptophan and arginine [reviewed elsewhere (*33*, *42*)]. Breakdown of tryptophan inside tumor cells, expressing indoleamine-2,3-dioxygenase (*IDO*) or tryptophan 2,3-dioxygenase (TDO), results in the consumption of available tryptophan in the local tumor environment and thus in deprivation of this essential amino-acid for the T cells (*43*, *44*). A Phase I Study of an IDO inhibitor, 1-methyl-D-tryptophan (D-1MT) is ongoing in patients with solid tumors (NCT00739609).

In vitro, the active forms of TGF-β, which can be produced by tumor cells or immune cells, are classically described as immunosuppressive and are considered as attractive therapeutic targets (*45–48*). However, considering the indirect pleiotropic roles of TGF-β, it is difficult to evaluate its impact on the function of tumor-infiltrating T lymphocytes (TIL). Phase I clinical trials with neutralizing anti-TGF-β antibodies Infliximab and GC1008 are ongoing in cancer patients. High-grade glioma patients have been treated in Phase I and II clinical trials with an antisense compound (Trabedersen), which targets mRNA encoding TGF-β2 for sequence-specific degradation. A Phase III trial is ongoing (*49*).

Effector cells may become "exhausted" through inappropriate stimulation or by chronic stimulation. Several inhibitory receptors that could down-modulate TIL activation upon antigen recognition have been considered as markers of dysfunctional or exhausted T cells. CTLA-4 molecules, expressed on T cells, can compete with CD28 for the binding to CD80/86, expressed on antigen-presenting cells and, consequently, prevent recruitment of PKC-θ at the synapse and T cell activation (*50*). Anti-CTLA-4-blocking monoclonal antibodies Ipilimumab and Tremelimumab have already been tested in many clinical trials (*51–59*). The U.S. Food and Drug Administration (FDA) and the European Agency for Medicines (EMA) approved Ipilimumab in 2011 for treatment of metastatic melanoma patients. Adverse events can be severe, long-lasting, or both, but most are reversible with appropriate treatment (*51*, *60*). PD1 receptor becomes phosphorylated upon ligand binding and, consequently, recruits SHP-1 (*61*, *62*). It is generally assumed that bringing SHP-1 (a phosphatase) close to the cytosolic parts of the TCR complex alters the phosphorylation cascade that follows antigen recognition. Blockade of PD-1/PDL-1 interactions seems to prolong survival of T cells and promote their expansion rather than reverse T cell dysfunction. Anti-PD1 antibodies CT-011 and MDX-1106 were administered in two Phase I clinical studies (*63*, *64*).

As discussed below, galectins, and in particular galectin-3, can also participate in this exhaustion phenomenon by forming glycoprotein/galectin lattices, and therefore modify receptor signaling.

Galectins as Modulators of the Immune Response in Tumors

We will focus on human lymphocytes, in particular human tumor-infiltrating lymphocytes, which can be affected by extracellular galectin-1 and galectin-3. The wide variety of biological processes influenced by galectins, including different steps of tumor progression and metastasis, has been thoroughly reviewed elsewhere (*65–68*).

Galectin-3 was detected in tumors from different histological origins, *e.g.* stomach, colon, breast, prostate and thyroid cancer, and its presence was used to differentiate between benign and malignant tumors (*69–76*). Galectin-1 expression was found to correlate with an aggressive tumor phenotype (*77–79*). The sera of melanoma and adenocarcinoma patients were reported to contain at least two times more galectin-3 than the sera from healthy donors (*80*). In head and neck squamous cell carcinoma patients, elevated galectin-1 and -3 in serum were correlated with a worse survival rate (*81*). Elevated serum levels seem to correspond to a more intense cellular and stromal galectin-3 immunostaining at the tumor site (*82*). Galectin-3 staining is particularly intense in the stroma of melanoma metastasis, more specifically between the tumor islets and around the tumor mass, where inflammatory cells are located (unpublished data). Immunohistochemical staining of galectin-1 revealed that its expression is positively associated with the malignant progression of tumors of various origins, including glioma, prostate, colon, breast, cervical and oral squamous cells (*83*). Galectin-1 and galectin-3 have been reported to be secreted by tumor cells, monocyte-derived cells, activated B cells, and activated T cells (*68*, *84*).

Little is known about the role of extracellular galectin-1 and galectin-3 on TIL function. Several studies have reported that extracellular galectin-1 and galectin-3 in tumors promote immune evasion, by inducing apoptosis of CD4 or CD8 T cells in the tumors (*66*, *77*, *85*). *In vitro*, galectin-1 added at μM concentrations can directly influence T lymphocyte function by inducing IL-10 production that could inhibit T cell function (*86*), or by diminishing IFN-γ receptor surface expression on activated T lymphocytes (*87*), attenuating IFN-γ production in T cells activated *in vitro* by anti-CD3 (*88*), and suppressing IL-2 secretion (*89*). In our studies, when galectin-3 was added at 10 nM, which is the highest concentration of galectin-3 in carcinoma ascites, we did not observe apoptosis of blood T cells, T cell clones or tumor cell lines. It is nevertheless possible that galectins could accumulate in solid tumors in confined microenvironments, and reach concentrations in the μM range.

Dysfunction of T lymphocytes Can Be Corrected by Targeting Galectins

CD8 T Cell Clones

CTL clones can be maintained in culture by stimulation every 1-2 weeks with cells presenting the antigen, in the presence of growth factors and EBV-B transformed cells as feeder cells. The functional status of CTL clones can be checked regularly by testing their capacity to lyse target cells expressing the relevant antigen and to produce cytokines upon antigenic stimulation, *e.g.* IFN-γ. Fluorescent HLA-peptide complexes –multivalent complexes of HLA molecules folded in the presence of the antigenic peptide and coupled to a fluorochrome– can be used to visualize antigen-specific CTL bearing the appropriate TCR (*90*). We observed that, compared with resting CTL collected 14 days after the last stimulation, recently activated CTL collected four days after stimulation have lost their capacity to bind HLA-tetramer complexes. They also secrete lower levels of cytokines upon a further antigenic stimulation (*91*). The decreased tetramer labeling and function was not due to a reduced surface expression of either the TCR or the CD8 co-receptor, which are both essential for tetramer labeling and activation of T lymphocytes. We decided therefore to examine by confocal microscopy the surface distribution of TCR and CD8 molecules on resting and recently activated T cells. TCR and CD8 molecules appeared to be co-localized on resting CTL, whereas TCR were segregated from CD8 molecules at the surface of recently activated CTL. These results were confirmed by fluorescence resonance energy transfer (FRET), where interactions between two proteins can be estimated at a resolution of 10 nm.

Our hypothesis to explain the separation of TCR and the CD8 molecules at the cell surface of recently activated CTL is inspired by work from the group of Dennis and Demetriou (*92*, *93*): *N*-glycosylated TCR molecules are clustered by extracellular galectin-3 and form glycoprotein-galectin lattices, which decrease the lateral mobility of TCR. In agreement with this hypothesis we observed that recently activated CTL, which were treated for 2 h with mM concentrations of galectin ligand *N*-acetyllactosamine (LacNAc), secreted more IFN-γ upon antigenic stimulation. Moreover this short LacNAc treatment restored TCR-CD8 co-localization, as measured by FRET.

Tumor-Infiltrating Lymphocytes

We collected a large number of ascites samples from patients with various tumors, in particular ovarian and pancreatic carcinoma. We also collected samples of solid tumors, mostly melanoma. CD8 T lymphocytes were isolated from these samples and tested *ex vivo* without prior *in vitro* expansion– for their capacity to secrete IFN-γ upon a non-specific stimulation, using beads coated with anti-CD3 and anti-CD28 antibodies. CD8 TIL from most of the samples secreted low levels of IFN-γ, in contrast with CD8 blood lymphocytes. Secretion of other cytokines by TIL was also low, *e.g.* IL-2 and TNF-α. These results are in line with the very few studies that have demonstrated dysfunction of human TIL (*94–98*).

Treating CD8 TIL for a few hours with mM concentrations of LacNAc increased by at least three times the secretion of IFN-γ, IL-2 and TNF-α (*99*). This holds true for 80% of the samples tested so far. LacNAc-treated CD4 TIL were also able to secrete high amounts of IFN-γ upon stimulation. The cytotoxicity of CD8 TIL was tested in a redirected killing assay, where the targets were mouse cells decorated with anti-CD3 antibodies. The cytotoxicity of CD8 TIL was minimal compared to the cytotoxicity of blood CD8 T lymphocytes, but increased greatly after an overnight LacNAc treatment.

GCS-100, a modified citrus pectin, and GM-CT-01, a galactomannan extracted from guar beans, are polysaccharides that could bind to galectins and have already been injected in humans (*100–102*). A short treatment of CD8 TIL with μM concentrations of GCS-100 boosted their cytotoxicity to an efficiency level similar to LacNAc treatment. It also boosted the secretion of cytokines by either CD8 or CD4 TIL (*99*). Experiments with GM-CT-01 are ongoing and the results are very encouraging (manuscript in preparation).

LacNAc, GCS-100, and GM-CT-01 can interact with several galectins and therefore it is difficult to attribute the effect on TIL functions of these sugars to one galectin in particular. To understand which galectins were implicated, we searched for the presence of different extracellular galectins at the TIL surface. We detected both galectin-1 and galectin-3, but failed to detect galectin-8, -9 or MGL, a lectin implicated in the regulation of T-cell function (*103*). Treating TIL with anti-galectin-3 antibody B2C10 boosted IFN-γ secretion upon stimulation to levels similar to LacNAc or GCS-100 treatments (*104*). Because B2C10 was unable to detach galectin-1 while boosting TIL function, we concluded that detaching galectin-3 from TIL is sufficient to restore function, while not excluding a contribution of other galectins. We have so far failed to identify an anti-galectin-1 antibody able to detach galectin-1 from cells and are therefore unable to examine if galectin-1 also plays a role in TIL dysfunction.

How Do Galectins Influence the Distribution of T Cell Surface Molecules?

Galectin-3 is an abundant lectin in many solid tumors and carcinomatous ascites. It can thus bind to surface glycoproteins of TIL. Glycoproteins often bear multiple copies of the sugar moieties that are recognized by galectins. The multivalent nature of galectin-glycan interactions results in high avidity in the range of 10^6 M^{-1}, and allows the formation of galectin-glycoprotein lattices [reviewed elsewhere (*105*)]. Similarly, lattices on TIL, formed by glycosylated surface receptors and extracellular galectin-3, would reduce the mobility of the former molecules, a fact that could explain the impaired function of TIL. The release of galectin-3 by soluble galectin ligands would restore the mobility of glycosylated surface receptors and boost IFN-γ secretion by TIL. Anti-galectin-3 antibody B2C10 should have a similar effect: this antibody binds to the N-terminal region of the galectin-3 and its rigid structure could prevent association of galectin-3 monomers mediated by the N-terminal region, thereby affecting the oligomerization of the lectin. Antibody B2C10 was shown to inhibit erythrocyte agglutination mediated by galectin-3 oligomerization (*104*).

The presence of galectin-glycoprotein lattices is in agreement with our observations with CTL clones and TIL. TCR and CD8 molecules are not co-localized on dysfunctional T cells and treating dysfunctional T cells with either an anti-galectin-3 antibody or galectin ligands detached galectin-3 from the T cell surface and restored the TCR-CD8 co-localization estimated by FRET (*91*, *99*). Considering that HLA-peptide tetramer binding requires TCR and CD8 cooperation, the disorganization of galectin-glycoproteins lattices in the presence of galectin ligands could explain the recovery of HLA-peptide tetramer binding on dysfunctional CTL clones that were treated with LacNAc (*91*).

A number of publications suggest that several human T cell surface glycoproteins can be linked together by galectins and form lattices. Human TCR α-chain, in contrast to the β-chain, has been shown to harbor complex N-glycans, the major natural ligands for galectin-3 (*106*, *107*). The removal of an N-glycosylation site from a human TCR α-chain was reported to result in increased avidity of T cells grafted with the gene encoding the modified TCR (*108*). Galectin-3 was reported to bind to CD45, CD29, CD43, and CD71 (*109*), and galectin-1 to CD45, CD7 and CD43 (*110*). Galectin-1/CD7 ligation was shown to induce apoptosis of CD4 T lymphocytes (*111*). It has also been shown by immunoprecipitation that galectin-3 binds to CD45 and that galectin-3 influences the CD45 partition to microdomains containing the TCR (*112*). Interestingly, CD45-TCR proximity is known to negatively regulate the TCR signaling cascade (*113*).

Glycosylation Changes at the T Cell Surface

To explain that galectin-3, alone or together with galectin-1, inhibits functions of recently activated T cells, we surmised that the recently activated T cells, compared to resting T cells, harbor a set of glycans that are either more numerous or better ligands for galectin-3. We stimulated resting CTL in the presence of swainsonine that inhibits α-mannosidase II involved in the N-glycosylation pathway. Compared to untreated cells, cells stimulated in the presence of swainsonine showed on day 4 a better TCR-CD8 co-localization and a higher ability to release IFN-γ upon antigenic stimulation (*91*).

We also characterized global changes in surface N- and O-glycans on two human CTL clones that were collected either in a resting state, 14 days after antigenic stimulation, or in a recently activated state, four days after antigenic stimulation. Applying ultra-sensitive MALDI-TOF-MS, combined with various glycosidase digestions and GC-MS linkage analyses, we made two novel observations.

Firstly, the N-glycome of recently activated cells versus resting cells consists of longer LacNAc chains, of which a portion contains more than four LacNAc moieties (poly-LacNAc). Secondly, it contains more multi-antennary N-glycans (*114*). Interestingly, our results showed that the above poly-LacNAc chains appeared to be equally distributed on all available N-glycan branches and not selectively enriched on a specific branch. In contrast, murine T cells are poor in tri- and tetra-antennary poly-LacNAc glycans (*115*). This difference could potentially explain the crucial role in mice of N-acetylglucosaminyltransferase V (Mgat5), an enzyme essential for the generation of complex tetra-antennary N-glycan, as T cells from mice lacking Mgat5, compared to their wildtype counterparts, are more sensitive to activation and have reduced poly-LacNAc motives (*92*). The glycome modifications observed on human CTL clones upon activation are expected to increase the number of galectin-3 natural ligands, but also the number of galectin-1 ligands, and favor lattices that could reduce the mobility of surface glycoproteins, as the affinity of both galectins was reported to be much higher when repeated LacNAc units are present (*116*).

We also observed that recently activated CTL clones exhibited a lower abundance of terminal α2,6-linked NeuAc residues than resting CTL (*114*). Galectin-1 binds to terminal LacNAc units, even if they are decorated with α2,3-linked NeuAc. On the contrary, galectin-1 binding is blocked by the presence of terminal α2,6-linked NeuAc (*88*, *110*, *111*, *117*, *118*). Our glycome analyses suggest therefore that more galectin-1 natural ligands are presented on recently activated CTL versus resting CTL.

All together, the results of our glycome analyses of CTL clones combined with the fact that functions of both CTL clones and TIL can be boosted by galectin ligands, support our working hypothesis: TIL are in permanent contact with tumor cells and have been stimulated by antigen recently. The resulting activation of T cells modifies the expression profiles of enzymes of the N-glycosylation pathway, increasing the expression of N-glycans at the T cell surface. Considering the high abundance of extracellular galectins in tumors, secreted by tumor cells and macrophages, this could favor the formation of galectin-glycoprotein lattices and therefore the dysfunction of some TIL.

Towards a Clinical Trial Combining Vaccination and Galectin-Binding Polysaccharides

As described above, treating TIL with modified citrus pectin GCS-100 improved their ability to secrete IFN-γ upon stimulation. We decided therefore to test the therapeutic effect of GCS-100 in tumor-bearing mice. We injected 40 mice subcutaneously in the flank with $2x10^6$ P815 mastocytoma cells. On day 4, half of the animals were vaccinated with an adenovirus encoding P815 tumor antigen P1A (*5*). Therapeutic vaccination has thus far proven ineffective at inducing tumor rejection in tumor-bearing mice (Catherine Uyttenhove & Guy Warnier, personal communication). On day 10, treatments with either PBS or GCS-100 were initiated three times a week. Three weeks later, the tumor had become undetectable in six out of the ten vaccinated mice treated with GCS-100, of which five were still alive after another three months. Control mice that received only the vaccine died. In non-vaccinated mice, the polysaccharide had no visible effect by itself. These results suggest that a combination of galectin-3 ligands and therapeutic vaccination may induce more effective tumor regression in cancer patients than vaccination alone. Setting up a clinical trial combining anti-tumoral vaccination and GCS-100 was impossible because the pharmaceutical company that produced the GCS-100 declared bankruptcy.

GM-CT-01, a galactomannan derived from guar gum, has been shown to bind to galectin-1 (*119*), and to increase the anti-tumor activity of chemotherapy drug 5-fluorouracil. It was previously injected in patients with solid tumors without major side effects (*120*). We have treated TIL samples with GM-CT-01 and the first results are encouraging. We therefore will launch a Phase I/II clinical trial combining peptide vaccination associated with intravenous injections of GM-CT-01 in patients with advanced melanoma (Fig. 1). Patients will receive sequential vaccinations with one or two peptides, MAGE-3.A1 and NA17.A2, matching the tumor antigens expressed by their tumor. Their formulation and schedule of vaccination (timing, dose, route of administration) will be similar to previous trials with these peptides (*15*, *20*, *21*). GM-CT-01 will be administered systemically by repeated intravenous infusions, in order to ensure a prolonged effect on tumor-associated lymphocytes. The treatment dose matches the total cumulative dose in previous GM-CT-01 treatment schedules (*120*). For selected patients with cutaneous or subcutaneous metastases, in addition to systemic GM-CT-01, small amounts of this drug will be injected close to metastases, to increase local concentration of the drug.

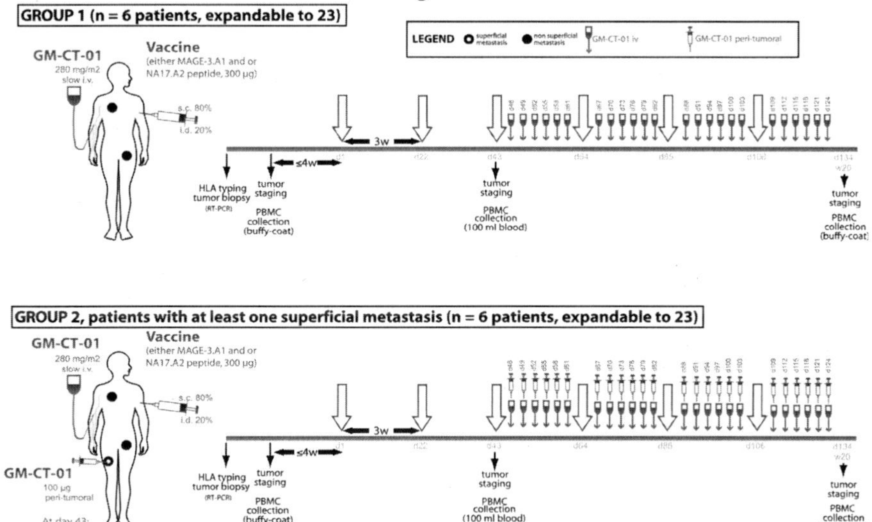

Figure 1. Treatment plan of the clinical trial involving GM-CT-01. Treatment allocation: Patients will be divided in two treatment arms. Both will run in parallel. Patients with at least one measurable lesion will be assigned to ***group 1*** *and will receive the following treatment: peptide vaccinations and systemic GM-CT-01 injections. Patients with at least one measurable and at least one superficial metastasis will be assigned in priority to* ***group 2*** *and will receive the following treatment: peptide vaccinations, systemic GM-CT-01 administrations and peri-tumoral administration of GM-CT-01 in one or two superficial metastases. (see color insert)*

Acknowledgments

We thank N. Krack for editorial assistance, and P. Coulie and N. Thrupp for critical reading. This work was supported by grants from Fondation contre le Cancer (Belgium) and Fonds de la Recherche Scientifique Médicale (Belgium). P. van der Bruggen is a "fellow du fonds Allard-Janssen pour la recherche sur le cancer". G. Wieërs was supported by a grant from the Fonds National de la Recherche Scientifique (Belgium).

References

1. Prehn, R. T.; Main, J. M. Immunity to methylcholanthrene-induced sarcomas. *J. Natl. Cancer Inst.* **1957**, *18*, 769–778.
2. Klein, G.; Sjögren, H.; Klein, E.; Hellström, K. E. Demonstration of resistance against methylcholanthrene-induced sarcomas in the primary autochthonous host. *Cancer Res.* **1960**, *20*, 1561–1572.
3. Vose, B. M.; Vanky, F.; Klein, E. Lymphocyte cytotoxicity against autologous tumour biopsy cells in humans. *Int. J. Cancer* **1977**, *20*, 512–9.
4. Hellstrom, K. E.; Brown, J. P.; Hellstrom, I Monoclonal antibodies to tumor antigens. *Contemp. Top. Immunobiol.* **1980**, *11*, 117–137.
5. Van den Eynde, B.; Lethé, B.; Van Pel, A.; De Plaen, E.; Boon, T. The gene coding for a major tumor rejection antigen of tumor P815 is identical to the normal gene of syngeneic DBA/2 mice. *J. Exp. Med.* **1991**, *173*, 1373–1384.
6. van der Bruggen, P.; Traversari, C.; Chomez, P.; Lurquin, C.; De Plaen, E.; Van den Eynde, B.; Knuth, A.; Boon, T. A gene encoding an antigen recognized by cytolytic T lymphocytes on a human melanoma. *Science* **1991**, *254*, 1643–1647.
7. van der Bruggen P.; Stroobant V.; Vigneron N.; Van den Eynde B. J. Peptide Database of T-Cell Defined Tumor Antigens. Updated January 2011. http://cancerimmunity.org/peptide/.
8. Jungbluth, A. A.; Silva, W. A., Jr.; Iversen, K.; Frosina, D.; Zaidi, B.; Coplan, K.; Eastlake-Wade, S. K.; Castelli, S. B.; Spagnoli, G. C.; Old, L. J.; Vogel, M. Expression of cancer-testis (CT) antigens in placenta. *Cancer Immun.* **2007**, *7*, 15.
9. Marsh S. G. E.; Parham P.; Barber L. D. *The HLA FactsBook*; Academic Press: London, 2000.
10. Simpson, A. J.; Caballero, O. L.; Jungbluth, A.; Chen, Y. T.; Old, L. J. Cancer/testis antigens, gametogenesis and cancer. *Nat. Rev. Cancer* **2005**, *5*, 615–625.
11. Speiser, D. E.; Lienard, D.; Rufer, N.; Rubio-Godoy, V.; Rimoldi, D.; Lejeune, F.; Krieg, A. M.; Cerottini, J. C.; Romero, P. Rapid and strong human CD8+ T cell responses to vaccination with peptide, IFA, and CpG oligodeoxynucleotide 7909. *J. Clin. Invest.* **2005**, *115*, 739–746.
12. Marchand, M.; van Baren, N.; Weynants, P.; Brichard, V.; Dréno, B.; Tessier, M.-H.; Rankin, E.; Parmiani, G.; Arienti, F.; Humblet, Y.; Bourlond, A.; Vanwijck, R.; Liénard, D.; Beauduin, M.; Dietrich, P.-Y.; Russo, V.; Kerger, J.; Masucci, G.; Jäger, E.; De Greve, J.; Atzpodien, J.;

Brasseur, F.; Coulie, P. G.; van der Bruggen, P.; Boon, T. Tumor regressions observed in patients with metastatic melanoma treated with an antigenic peptide encoded by gene *MAGE-3* and presented by HLA-A1. *Int. J. Cancer* **1999**, *80*, 219–230.

13. Slingluff, C. L., Jr.; Petroni, G. R.; Yamshchikov, G. V.; Barnd, D. L.; Eastham, S.; Galavotti, H.; Patterson, J. W.; Deacon, D. H.; Hibbitts, S.; Teates, D.; Neese, P. Y.; Grosh, W. W.; Chianese-Bullock, K. A.; Woodson, E. M.; Wiernasz, C. J.; Merrill, P.; Gibson, J.; Ross, M.; Engelhard, V. H. Clinical and immunologic results of a randomized phase II trial of vaccination using four melanoma peptides either administered in granulocyte-macrophage colony-stimulating factor in adjuvant or pulsed on dendritic cells. *J. Clin. Oncol.* **2003**, *21*, 4016–4026.
14. Kruit, W. H.; van Ojik, H. H.; Brichard, V. G.; Escudier, B.; Dorval, T.; Dréno, B.; Patel, P.; van Baren, N.; Avril, M.-F.; Piperno, S.; Khammari, A.; Stas, M.; Ritter, G.; Lethé, B.; Godelaine, D.; Brasseur, F.; Zhang, Y.; van der Bruggen, P.; Boon, T.; Eggermont, A. M.; Marchand, M. Phase 1/2 study of subcutaneous and intradermal immunization with a recombinant MAGE-3 protein in patients with detectable metastatic melanoma. *Int. J. Cancer* **2005**, *117*, 596–604.
15. van Baren, N.; Bonnet, M.-C.; Dréno, B.; Khammari, A.; Dorval, T.; Piperno-Neumann, S; Liénard, D.; Speiser, D.; Marchand, M.; Brichard, V. G.; Escudier, B.; Négrier, S.; Dietrich, P.-Y.; Maraninchi, D.; Osanto, S.; Meyer, R. G.; Ritter, G.; Moingeon, P.; Tartaglia, J.; van der Bruggen, P; Coulie, P. G.; Boon, T. Tumoral and immunologic response after vaccination of melanoma patients with an ALVAC virus encoding MAGE antigens recognized by T cells. *J. Clin. Oncol.* **2005**, *23*, 9008–9021.
16. Thurner, B.; Haendle, I.; Roder, C.; Dieckmann, D.; Keikavoussi, P.; Jonuleit, H.; Bender, A.; Maczek, C.; Schreiner, D.; von den Driesch, P.; Brocker, E. B.; Steinman, R. M.; Enk, A.; Kampgen, E.; Schuler, G. Vaccination with MAGE-3A1 peptide-pulsed mature, monocyte-derived dendritic cells expands specific cytotoxic T cells and induces regression of some metastases in advanced stage IV melanoma. *J. Exp. Med.* **1999**, *190*, 1669–1678.
17. Seremet, T.; Brasseur, F.; Coulie, P. G. Tumor-specific antigens and immunologic adjuvants in cancer immunotherapy. *Cancer J.* **2011**, *17*, 325–330.
18. Baurain, J.-F.; van der Bruggen, P.; Van den Eynde, B. J.; Coulie, P. G.; Van Baren, N. Principes généraux et premiers essais cliniques de vaccination thérapeutique contre le cancer. *Bull. Cancer* **2008**, *95*, 327–335.
19. Tyagi, P.; Mirakhur, B. MAGRIT: The largest-ever phase III lung cancer trial aims to establish a novel tumor-specific approach to therapy. *Clin. Lung Cancer* **2009**, *10*, 371–374.
20. Machiels, J. P.; van Baren, N.; Marchand, M. Peptide-based cancer vaccines. *Semin. Oncol.* **2002**, *29*, 494–502.
21. Marchand, M.; Punt, C. J. A.; Aamdal, S.; Escudier, B.; Kruit, W. H. J.; Keilholz, U.; Håkansson, L.; van Baren, N.; Humblet, Y.; Mulders, P.; Avril, M.-F.; Eggermont, A. M. M.; Scheibenbogen, C.; Uiters, J.;

Wanders, J.; Delire, M.; Boon, T.; Stoter, G. Immunization of metastatic cancer patients with MAGE-3 protein combined with adjuvant SBAS-2: Clinical report. *Eur. J. Cancer* **2003**, *39*, 70–77.
22. Coulie, P. G.; Karanikas, V.; Colau, D.; Lurquin, C.; Landry, C.; Marchand, M.; Dorval, T.; Brichard, V.; Boon, T. A monoclonal cytolytic T-lymphocyte response observed in a melanoma patient vaccinated with a tumor-specific antigenic peptide encoded by gene MAGE-3. *Proc. Natl. Acad. Sci. USA* **2001**, *98*, 10290–10295.
23. Karanikas, V.; Lurquin, C.; Colau, D.; van Baren, N.; De Smet, C.; Lethé, B.; Connerotte, T.; Corbière, V.; Demoitié, M.-A.; Liénard, D.; Dréno, B.; Velu, T.; Boon, T.; Coulie, P. G. Monoclonal anti-MAGE-3 CTL responses in melanoma patients displaying tumor regression after vaccination with a recombinant canarypox virus. *J. Immunol.* **2003**, *171*, 4898–4904.
24. Lonchay, C.; van der Bruggen, P.; Connerotte, T.; Hanagiri, T.; Coulie, P.; Colau, D.; Lucas, S.; Van Pel, A.; Thielemans, K.; van Baren, N.; Boon, T. Correlation between tumor regression and T cell responses in melanoma patients vaccinated with a MAGE antigen. *Proc. Natl. Acad. Sci. U.S.A.* **2004**, *101*, 14631–14638.
25. Carrasco, J.; Van Pel, A.; Neyns, B.; Lethé, B.; Brasseur, F.; Renkvist, N.; van der Bruggen, P.; van Baren, N.; Paulus, R.; Thielemans, K.; Boon, T.; Godelaine, D. Vaccination of a melanoma patient with mature dendritic cells pulsed with MAGE-3 peptides triggers the activity of nonvaccine anti-tumor cells. *J. Immunol.* **2008**, *180*, 3585–3593.
26. Germeau, C.; Ma, W.; Schiavetti, F.; Lurquin, C.; Henry, E.; Vigneron, N.; Brasseur, F.; Lethé, B.; De Plaen, E.; Velu, T.; Boon, T.; Coulie, P. G. High frequency of anti-tumor T cells in the blood of melanoma patients before and after vaccination with tumor antigens. *J. Exp. Med.* **2005**, *201*, 241–248.
27. Boon, T.; Coulie, P. G.; Van den Eynde, B.; van der Bruggen, P. Human T cell responses against melanoma. *Annu. Rev. Immunol.* **2006**, *24*, 175–208.
28. Lurquin, C.; Lethé, B.; Corbière, V.; Théate, I.; van Baren, N.; Coulie, P. G.; Boon, T. Contrasting frequencies of anti-tumor and anti-vaccine T cells in metastases of a melanoma patient vaccinated with a MAGE tumor antigen. *J. Exp. Med.* **2005**, *201*, 249–257.
29. Rosenberg, SA; Dudley, ME Cancer regression in patients with metastatic melanoma after the transfer of autologous antitumor lymphocytes. *Proc. Natl. Acad Sci. U.S.A.* **2004**, *101* (Suppl 2), 14639–14645.
30. Lesterhuis, W. J.; Aarntzen, E. H.; De Vries, I. J.; Schuurhuis, D. H.; Figdor, C. G.; Adema, G. J.; Punt, C. J. Dendritic cell vaccines in melanoma: From promise to proof? *Crit. Rev. Oncol. Hematol.* **2008**, *66*, 118–134.
31. Cipponi, A.; Wieers, G.; van Baren, N.; Coulie, P. G. Tumor-infiltrating lymphocytes: Apparently good for melanoma patients. But why? *Cancer Immunol. Immunother.* **2011**, *60*, 1153–1160.
32. Yaguchi, T.; Sumimoto, H.; Kudo-Saito, C.; Tsukamoto, N.; Ueda, R.; Iwata-Kajihara, T.; Nishio, H.; Kawamura, N.; Kawakami, Y. The mechanisms of cancer immunoescape and development of overcoming strategies. *Int. J. Hematol.* **2011**, *93*, 294–300.

33. Stewart, T. J.; Smyth, M. J. Improving cancer immunotherapy by targeting tumor-induced immune suppression. *Cancer Metastasis Rev.* **2011**, *30*, 125–140.
34. Lee, H.; Pal, S. K.; Reckamp, K.; Figlin, R. A.; Yu, H. STAT3: A target to enhance antitumor immune response. *Curr. Top. Microbiol. Immunol.* **2011**, *344*, 41–59.
35. de Souza, A. P.; Bonorino, C. Tumor immunosuppressive environment: Effects on tumor-specific and nontumor antigen immune responses. *Expert Rev. Anticancer Ther.* **2009**, *9*, 1317–1332.
36. Kirkwood, J. M.; Tarhini, A. A.; Panelli, M. C.; Moschos, S. J.; Zarour, H. M.; Butterfield, L. H.; Gogas, H. J. Next generation of immunotherapy for melanoma. *J. Clin. Oncol.* **2008**, *26*, 3445–3455.
37. Munn, D. H.; Mellor, A. L. Indoleamine 2,3-dioxygenase and tumor-induced tolerance. *J. Clin. Invest.* **2007**, *117*, 1147–1154.
38. Dannull, J.; Su, Z.; Rizzieri, D.; Yang, B. K.; Coleman, D.; Yancey, D.; Zhang, A.; Dahm, P.; Chao, N.; Gilboa, E; Vieweg, J. Enhancement of vaccine-mediated antitumor immunity in cancer patients after depletion of regulatory T cells. *J. Clin. Invest.* **2005**, *115*, 3623–3633.
39. Morse, M. A.; Hobeika, A. C.; Osada, T.; Serra, D.; Niedzwiecki, D.; Lyerly, H. K.; Clay, T. M. Depletion of human regulatory T cells specifically enhances antigen-specific immune responses to cancer vaccines. *Blood* **2008**, *112*, 610–618.
40. de Vries, I. J.; Castelli, C.; Huygens, C.; Jacobs, J. F.; Stockis, J.; Schuler-Thurner, B.; Adema, G. J.; Punt, C. J.; Rivoltini, L.; Schuler, G.; Coulie, P. G.; Lucas, S. Frequency of circulating Tregs with demethylated FOXP3 intron 1 in melanoma patients receiving tumor vaccines and potentially Treg-depleting agents. *Clin. Cancer Res.* **2011**, *17*, 841–848.
41. Stockis, J.; Fink, W.; François, V.; Connerotte, T.; De Smet, C.; Knoops, L.; van der Bruggen, P.; Boon, T.; Coulie, P. G.; Lucas, S. Comparison of stable human Treg and Th clones by transcriptional profiling. *Eur. J. Immunol.* **2009**, *39*, 869–882.
42. Wieërs, G.; Demotte, N.; Godelaine, D.; van der Bruggen, P. Immune suppression in tumors as a surmountable obstacle to clinical efficacy of cancer vaccines. *Cancers* **2011**, *3*, 2904–2954.
43. Uyttenhove, C.; Pilotte, L.; Theate, I.; Stroobant, V.; Colau, D.; Parmentier, N.; Boon, T.; Van den Eynde, B. J. Evidence for a tumoral immune resistance mechanism based on tryptophan degradation by indoleamine 2,3-dioxygenase. *Nat. Med.* **2003**, *9*, 1269–1274.
44. Pilotte, L.; Larrieu, P.; Stroobant, V.; Colau, D.; Dolusic, E.; Frederick, R.; De Plaen, E.; Uyttenhove, C.; Wouters, J.; Masereel, B.; Van den Eynde, B. J. Reversal of tumoral immune resistance by inhibition of tryptophan 2,3-dioxygenase. *Proc. Natl Acad. Sci. U.S.A.* **2012**, *109*, 2497–2502.
45. Letterio, J. J.; Roberts, A. B. Regulation of immune responses by TGF-beta. *Annu. Rev. Immunol.* **1998**, *16*, 137–161.
46. Li, M. O.; Wan, Y. Y.; Sanjabi, S.; Robertson, A. K.; Flavell, R. A. Transforming growth factor-beta regulation of immune responses. *Annu. Rev. Immunol.* **2006**, *24*, 99–146.

47. Taga, K.; Mostowski, H.; Tosato, G. Human interleukin-10 can directly inhibit T-cell growth. *Blood* **1993**, *81*, 2964–2971.
48. Blobe, G. C.; Schiemann, W. P.; Lodish, H. F. Role of transforming growth factor beta in human disease. *N. Engl. J. Med.* **2000**, *342*, 1350–1358.
49. Hau, P.; Jachimczak, P.; Schlingensiepen, R.; Schulmeyer, F.; Jauch, T.; Steinbrecher, A.; Brawanski, A.; Proescholdt, M.; Schlaier, J.; Buchroithner, J.; Pichler, J.; Wurm, G.; Mehdorn, M.; Strege, R.; Schuierer, G.; Villarrubia, V.; Fellner, F.; Jansen, O.; Straube, T.; Nohria, V.; Goldbrunner, M.; Kunst, M.; Schmaus, S.; Stauder, G.; Bogdahn, U.; Schlingensiepen, K. H. Inhibition of TGF-beta2 with AP 12009 in recurrent malignant gliomas: From preclinical to phase I/II studies. *Oligonucleotides* **2007**, *17*, 201–212.
50. Yokosuka, T.; Kobayashi, W.; Takamatsu, M.; Sakata-Sogawa, K.; Zeng, H.; Hashimoto-Tane, A.; Yagita, H.; Tokunaga, M.; Saito, T. Spatiotemporal basis of CTLA-4 costimulatory molecule-mediated negative regulation of T cell activation. *Immunity* **2010**, *33*, 326–339.
51. Hodi, F. S.; O'Day, S. J.; McDermott, D. F.; Weber, R. W.; Sosman, J. A.; Haanen, J. B.; Gonzalez, R.; Robert, C.; Schadendorf, D.; Hassel, J. C.; Akerley, W.; van den Eertwegh, A. J. M.; Lutzky, J.; Lorigan, P; Vaubel, J. M.; Linette, G. P.; Hogg, D.; Ottensmeier, C. H.; Lebbé, C; Peschel, C.; Quirt, I.; Clark, J. I.; Wolchok, J. D.; Weber, J. S.; Tian, J.; Yellin, M. J.; Nichol, G. M.; Hoos, A.; Urba, W. J. Improved survival with ipilimumab in patients with metastatic melanoma. *N. Engl. J. Med.* **2010**, *363*, 711–723.
52. Kirkwood, J. M.; Lorigan, P.; Hersey, P.; Hauschild, A.; Robert, C.; McDermott, D.; Marshall, M. A.; Gomez-Navarro, J.; Liang, J. Q.; Bulanhagui, C. A. Phase II trial of tremelimumab (CP-675,206) in patients with advanced refractory or relapsed melanoma. *Clin. Cancer Res.* **2010**, *16*, 1042–1048.
53. Small, E. J.; Tchekmedyian, N. S.; Rini, B. I.; Fong, L.; Lowy, I.; Allison, J. P. A pilot trial of CTLA-4 blockade with human anti-CTLA-4 in patients with hormone-refractory prostate cancer. *Clin. Cancer Res.* **2007**, *13*, 1810–1815.
54. Royal, R. E.; Levy, C.; Turner, K.; Mathur, A.; Hughes, M.; Kammula, U. S.; Sherry, R. M.; Topalian, S. L.; Yang, J. C.; Lowy, I.; Rosenberg, S. A. Phase 2 trial of single agent Ipilimumab (anti-CTLA-4) for locally advanced or metastatic pancreatic adenocarcinoma. *J. Immunother.* **2010**, *33*, 828–833.
55. Chung, K. Y.; Gore, I.; Fong, L.; Venook, A.; Beck, S. B.; Dorazio, P.; Criscitiello, P. J.; Healey, D. I.; Huang, B.; Gomez-Navarro, J.; Saltz, L. B. Phase II study of the anti-cytotoxic T-lymphocyte-associated antigen 4 monoclonal antibody, tremelimumab, in patients with refractory metastatic colorectal cancer. *J. Clin. Oncol.* **2010**, *28*, 3485–3490.
56. O'Mahony, D.; Morris, J. C.; Quinn, C.; Gao, W.; Wilson, W. H.; Gause, B.; Pittaluga, S.; Neelapu, S.; Brown, M.; Fleisher, T. A.; Gulley, J. L.; Schlom, J.; Nussenblatt, R.; Albert, P.; Davis, T. A.; Lowy, I.; Petrus, M.; Waldmann, T. A.; Janik, J. E. A pilot study of CTLA-4 blockade after cancer vaccine failure in patients with advanced malignancy. *Clin. Cancer Res.* **2007**, *13*, 958–694.

57. Vonderheide, R. H.; LoRusso, P. M.; Khalil, M.; Gartner, E. M.; Khaira, D.; Soulieres, D.; Dorazio, P.; Trosko, J. A.; Ruter, J.; Mariani, G. L.; Usari, T.; Domchek, S. M. Tremelimumab in combination with exemestane in patients with advanced breast cancer and treatment-associated modulation of inducible costimulator expression on patient T cells. *Clin. Cancer Res.* **2010**, *16*, 3485–3494.
58. Hodi, F. S.; Butler, M.; Oble, D. A.; Seiden, M. V.; Haluska, F. G.; Kruse, A.; Macrae, S.; Nelson, M.; Canning, C.; Lowy, I.; Korman, A.; Lautz, D.; Russell, S.; Jaklitsch, M. T.; Ramaiya, N.; Chen, T. C.; Neuberg, D.; Allison, J. P.; Mihm, M. C.; Dranoff, G. Immunologic and clinical effects of antibody blockade of cytotoxic T lymphocyte-associated antigen 4 in previously vaccinated cancer patients. *Proc. Natl Acad. Sci. USA* **2008**, *105*, 3005–3010.
59. Camacho, L. H.; Antonia, S.; Sosman, J.; Kirkwood, J. M.; Gajewski, T. F.; Redman, B.; Pavlov, D.; Bulanhagui, C.; Bozon, V. A.; Gomez-Navarro, J.; Ribas, A Phase I/II trial of tremelimumab in patients with metastatic melanoma. *J. Clin. Oncol.* **2009**, *27*, 1075–1081.
60. Wilgenhof, S.; Neyns, B. Anti-CTLA-4 antibody-induced Guillain-Barre syndrome in a melanoma patient. *Ann. Oncol.* **2011**, *22*, 991–993.
61. Le Drean, E.; Vely, F.; Olcese, L.; Cambiaggi, A.; Guia, S.; Krystal, G.; Gervois, N.; Moretta, A.; Jotereau, F.; Vivier, E. Inhibition of antigen-induced T cell response and antibody-induced NK cell cytotoxicity by NKG2A: Association of NKG2A with SHP-1 and SHP-2 protein-tyrosine phosphatases. *Eur. J. Immunol.* **1998**, *28*, 264–276.
62. Chemnitz, J. M.; Parry, R. V.; Nichols, K. E.; June, C. H.; Riley, J. L. SHP-1 and SHP-2 associate with immunoreceptor tyrosine-based switch motif of programmed death 1 upon primary human T cell stimulation, but only receptor ligation prevents T cell activation. *J. Immunol.* **2004**, *173*, 945–954.
63. Berger, R.; Rotem-Yehudar, R.; Slama, G.; Landes, S.; Kneller, A.; Leiba, M.; Koren-Michowitz, M.; Shimoni, A.; Nagler, A. Phase I safety and pharmacokinetic study of CT-011, a humanized antibody interacting with PD-1, in patients with advanced hematologic malignancies. *Clin. Cancer Res.* **2008**, *14*, 3044–3051.
64. Brahmer, J. R.; Drake, C. G.; Wollner, I.; Powderly, J. D.; Picus, J.; Sharfman, W. H.; Stankevich, E.; Pons, A.; Salay, T. M.; McMiller, T. L.; Gilson, M. M.; Wang, C.; Selby, M.; Taube, J. M.; Anders, R.; Chen, L.; Korman, A. J.; Pardoll, D. M.; Lowy, I.; Topalian, S. L. Phase I study of single-agent anti-programmed death-1 (MDX-1106) in refractory solid tumors: Safety, clinical activity, pharmacodynamics, and immunologic correlates. *J. Clin. Oncol.* **2010**, *28*, 3167–3175.
65. Rabinovich, G. A.; Toscano, M. A. Turning 'sweet' on immunity: Galectin−glycan interactions in immune tolerance and inflammation. *Nat. Rev. Immunol.* **2009**, *9*, 338–352.
66. Liu, F. T.; Rabinovich, G. A. Galectins as modulators of tumour progression. *Nat. Rev. Cancer* **2005**, *5*, 29–41.
67. Yang, R. Y.; Rabinovich, G. A.; Liu, F. T. Galectins: Structure, function and therapeutic potential. *Expert Rev. Mol. Med.* **2008**, *10*, e17.

68. van den Brûle, F.; Califice, S.; Castronovo, V. Expression of galectins in cancer: A critical review. *Glycoconjugate J.* **2004**, *19*, 537–542.
69. Nakamura, M.; Inufusa, H.; Adachi, T.; Aga, M.; Kurimoto, M.; Nakatani, Y.; Wakano, T.; Nakajima, A.; Hida, J. I.; Miyake, M.; Shindo, K.; Yasutomi, M. Involvement of galectin-3 expression in colorectal cancer progression and metastasis. *Int. J. Oncol.* **1999**, *15*, 143–148.
70. Baldus, S. E.; Zirbes, T. K.; Weingarten, M.; Fromm, S.; Glossmann, J.; Hanisch, F. G.; Monig, S. P.; Schroder, W.; Flucke, U.; Thiele, J.; Holscher, A. H.; Dienes, H. P. Increased galectin-3 expression in gastric cancer: Correlations with histopathological subtypes, galactosylated antigens and tumor cell proliferation. *Tumour Biol.* **2000**, *21*, 258–266.
71. Miyazaki, J.; Hokari, R.; Kato, S.; Tsuzuki, Y.; Kawaguchi, A.; Nagao, S.; Itoh, K.; Miura, S. Increased expression of galectin-3 in primary gastric cancer and the metastatic lymph nodes. *Oncol. Rep.* **2002**, *9*, 1307–1312.
72. Cindolo, L.; Benvenuto, G.; Salvatore, P.; Pero, R.; Salvatore, G.; Mirone, V.; Prezioso, D.; Altieri, V.; Bruni, C. B.; Chiariotti, L. galectin-1 and galectin-3 expression in human bladder transitional-cell carcinomas. *Int. J. Cancer* **1999**, *84*, 39–43.
73. Feilchenfeldt, J.; Totsch, M.; Sheu, S. Y.; Robert, J.; Spiliopoulos, A.; Frilling, A.; Schmid, K. W.; Meier, C. A. Expression of galectin-3 in normal and malignant thyroid tissue by quantitative PCR and immunohistochemistry. *Mod. Pathol.* **2003**, *16*, 1117–1123.
74. Bresalier, R. S.; Mazurek, N.; Sternberg, L. R.; Byrd, J. C.; Yunker, C. K.; Nangia-Makker, P.; Raz, A. Metastasis of human colon cancer is altered by modifying expression of the beta-galactoside-binding protein galectin 3. *Gastroenterology* **1998**, *115*, 287–296.
75. Than, T. H.; Swethadri, G. K.; Wong, J.; Ahmad, T.; Jamil, D.; Maganlal, R. K.; Hamdi, M. M.; Abdullah, M. S. Expression of Galectin-3 and Galectin-7 in thyroid malignancy as potential diagnostic indicators. *Singapore Med. J.* **2008**, *49*, 333–338.
76. Shen, J.; Li, C. D.; Yang, H. L.; Lu, J.; Zou, T. M.; Wang, D. L.; Deng, M. Classic chordoma coexisting with benign notochordal cell rest demonstrating different immunohistological expression patterns of brachyury and galectin-3. *J. Clin. Neurosci.* **2011**, *18*, 96–99.
77. Rubinstein, N.; Alvarez, M.; Zwirner, N. W.; Toscano, M. A.; Ilarregui, J. M.; Bravo, A.; Mordoh, J.; Fainboim, L.; Podhajcer, O. L.; Rabinovich, G. A. Targeted inhibition of galectin-1 gene expression in tumor cells results in heightened T cell-mediated rejection; A potential mechanism of tumor-immune privilege. *Cancer Cell* **2004**, *5*, 241–251.
78. Szoke, T.; Kayser, K.; Baumhakel, J. D.; Trojan, I.; Furak, J.; Tiszlavicz, L.; Horvath, . A; Szluha, K.; Gabius, H. J.; Andre, S. Prognostic significance of endogenous adhesion/growth-regulatory lectins in lung cancer. *Oncology* **2005**, *69*, 167–174.
79. Jung, E. J.; Moon, H. G.; Cho, B. I.; Jeong, C. Y.; Joo, Y. T.; Lee, Y. J.; Hong, S. C.; Choi, S. K.; Ha, W. S.; Kim, J. W.; Lee, C. W.; Lee, J. S.; Park, S. T. Galectin-1 expression in cancer-associated stromal cells correlates tumor

invasiveness and tumor progression in breast cancer. *Int. J. Cancer* **2007**, *120*, 2331–2338.
80. Iurisci, I.; Tinari, N.; Natoli, C.; Angelucci, D.; Cianchetti, E.; Iacobelli, S. Concentrations of galectin-3 in the sera of normal controls and cancer patients. *Clin. Cancer Res.* **2000**, *6*, 1389–1393.
81. Saussez, S.; Lorfevre, F.; Lequeux, T.; Laurent, G.; Chantrain, G.; Vertongen, F.; Toubeau, G.; Decaestecker, C.; Kiss, R. The determination of the levels of circulating galectin-1 and -3 in HNSCC patients could be used to monitor tumor progression and/or responses to therapy. *Oral. Oncol.* **2008**, *44*, 86–93.
82. Vereecken, P.; Zouaoui Boudjeltia, K.; Debray, C.; Awada, A.; Legssyer, I.; Sales, F.; Petein, M.; Vanhaeverbeek, M.; Ghanem, G.; Heenen, M. High serum galectin-3 in advanced melanoma: Preliminary results. *Clin. Exp. Dermatol.* **2006**, *31*, 105–109.
83. Wu, M. H.; Hong, T. M.; Cheng, H. W.; Pan, S. H.; Liang, Y. R.; Hong, H. C.; Chiang, W. F.; Wong, T. Y.; Shieh, D. B.; Shiau, A. L.; Jin, Y. T.; Chen, Y. L. Galectin-1-mediated tumor invasion and metastasis, up-regulated matrix metalloproteinase expression, and reorganized actin cytoskeletons. *Mol. Cancer Res.* **2009**, *7*, 311–318.
84. Flotte, T. J.; Springer, T. A.; Thorbecke, G. J. Dendritic cell and macrophage staining by monoclonal antibodies in tissue sections and epidermal sheets. *Am. J. Pathol.* **1983**, *111*, 112–124.
85. Perillo, N. L.; Pace, K. E.; Seilhamer, J. J.; Baum, L. G. Apoptosis of T cells mediated by galectin-1. *Nature* **1995**, *378*, 736–739.
86. van der Leij, J.; van den Berg, A.; Blokzijl, T.; Harms, G.; van Goor, H.; Zwiers, P.; van Weeghel, R.; Poppema, S.; Visser, L. Dimeric galectin-1 induces IL-10 production in T-lymphocytes: An important tool in the regulation of the immune response. *J. Pathol.* **2004**, *204*, 511–518.
87. Allione, A.; Wells, V.; Forni, G.; Mallucci, L.; Novelli, F. Beta-galactoside-binding protein (beta GBP) alters the cell cycle, up-regulates expression of the alpha- and beta-chains of the IFN-gamma receptor, and triggers IFN-gamma-mediated apoptosis of activated human T lymphocytes. *J. Immunol.* **1998**, *161*, 2114–2119.
88. Stowell, S. R.; Qian, Y.; Karmakar, S.; Koyama, N. S.; Dias-Baruffi, M.; Leffler, H.; McEver, R. P.; Cummings, R. D. Differential roles of galectin-1 and galectin-3 in regulating leukocyte viability and cytokine secretion. *J. Immunol.* **2008**, *180*, 3091–3102.
89. Rabinovich, G. A.; Ariel, A.; Hershkoviz, R.; Hirabayashi, J.; Kasai, K. I.; Lider, O. Specific inhibition of T-cell adhesion to extracellular matrix and proinflammatory cytokine secretion by human recombinant galectin-1. *Immunology* **1999**, *97*, 100–106.
90. Altman, J. D.; Moss, P. A. H.; Goulder, P. J. R.; Barouch, D. H.; McHeyzer-Williams, M. G.; Bell, J. I.; McMichael, A. J.; Davis, M. M. Phenotypic analysis of antigen-specific T lymphocytes. *Science* **1996**, *274*, 94–96.
91. Demotte, N.; Stroobant, V.; Courtoy, P. J.; Van Der Smissen, P.; Colau, D.; Luescher, I. F.; Hivroz, C.; Nicaise, J.; Squifflet, J. L.; Mourad, M.; Godelaine, D.; Boon, T.; van der Bruggen, P. Restoring the association of

the T cell receptor with CD8 reverses anergy in human tumor-infiltrating lymphocytes. *Immunity* **2008**, *28*, 414–424.

92. Demetriou, M.; Granovsky, M.; Quaggin, S.; Dennis, J. W. Negative regulation of T-cell activation and autoimmunity by Mgat5 N-glycosylation. *Nature* **2001**, *409*, 733–739.
93. Morgan, R.; Gao, G.; Pawling, J.; Dennis, J. W.; Demetriou, M.; Li, B. N-acetylglucosaminyltransferase V (Mgat5)-mediated N-glycosylation negatively regulates Th1 cytokine production by T cells. *J. Immunol.* **2004**, *173*, 7200–7208.
94. Van den Hove, L. E.; Van Gool, S. W.; Van Poppel, H.; Baert, L.; Coorevits, L.; Van Damme, B.; Ceuppens, J. L. Phenotype, cytokine production and cytolytic capacity of fresh (uncultured) tumour-infiltrating T lymphocytes in human renal cell carcinoma. *Clin. Exp. Immunol.* **1997**, *109*, 501–509.
95. Zippelius, A.; Batard, P.; Rubio-Godoy, V.; Bioley, G.; Liénard, D.; Lejeune, F.; Rimoldi, D.; Guillaume, P.; Meidenbauer, N.; Mackensen, A.; Rufer, N.; Lubenow, N.; Speiser, D.; Cerottini, J.-C.; Romero, P.; Pittet, M. J. Effector function of human tumor-specific CD8 T cells in melanoma lesions: A state of local functional tolerance. *Cancer Res.* **2004**, *64*, 2865–2873.
96. Gorgun, G.; Holderried, T. A.; Zahrieh, D.; Neuberg, D.; Gribben, J. G. Chronic lymphocytic leukemia cells induce changes in gene expression of CD4 and CD8 T cells. *J. Clin. Invest.* **2005**, *115*, 1797–1805.
97. Harlin, H.; Kuna, T. V.; Peterson, A. C.; Meng, Y.; Gajewski, T. F. Tumor progression despite massive influx of activated CD8(+) T cells in a patient with malignant melanoma ascites. *Cancer Immunol. Immunother.* **2006**, *55*, 1185–1197.
98. Luscher, U.; Filgueira, L.; Juretic, A.; Zuber, M.; Luscher, N. J.; Heberer, M.; Spagnoli, G. C. The pattern of cytokine gene expression in freshly excised human metastatic melanoma suggests a state of reversible anergy of tumor-infiltrating lymphocytes. *Int. J. Cancer* **1994**, *57*, 612–619.
99. Demotte, N.; Wieërs, G.; Van Der Smissen, P.; Moser, M.; Schmidt, C. W.; Thielemans, K.; Squifflet, J.-L.; Weynand, B.; Carrasco, J.; Lurquin, C.; Courtoy, P. J.; van der Bruggen, P. A galectin-3 ligand corrects the impaired function of human CD4 and CD8 tumor-infiltrating lymphocytes and favors tumor rejection in mice. *Cancer Res.* **2010**, *70*, 7476–7488.
100. Chauhan, D.; Li, G.; Podar, K.; Hideshima, T.; Neri, P.; He, D.; Mitsiades, N.; Richardson, P.; Chang, Y.; Schindler, J.; Carver, B.; Anderson, K. C. A novel carbohydrate-based therapeutic GCS-100 overcomes bortezomib resistance and enhances dexamethasone-induced apoptosis in multiple myeloma cells. *Cancer Res.* **2005**, *65*, 8350–8358.
101. Cotter, F.; Smith, D. A.; Boyd, T. E.; Richards, D. A.; Alemany, C.; Loesch, D.; Salogub, G; Tidmarsh, G. F.; Gammon, G. M.; Gribben, J. Single-agent activity of GCS-100, a first-in-class galectin-3 antagonist, in elderly patients with relapsed chronic lymphocytic leukemia. *J. Clin. Oncol. (Meeting Abstracts)* **2009**, *27* (Suppl.15S), Abstract 7006.

102. Grous, J. J.; Redfern, C. H.; Mahadevan, D.; Schindler, J. GCS-100, a galectin-3 antagonist, in refractory solid tumors: A phase I study. *J. Clin. Oncol. (Meeting Abstracts)* **2006**, *24* (Suppl.18S), Abstract 13023.
103. van Vliet, S. J.; Gringhuis, S. I.; Geijtenbeek, T. B.; van Kooyk, Y. Regulation of effector T cells by antigen-presenting cells via interaction of the C-type lectin MGL with CD45. *Nat. Immunol.* **2006**, *7*, 1200–1208.
104. Liu, F. T.; Hsu, D. K.; Zuberi, R. I.; Hill, P. N.; Shenhav, A.; Kuwabara, I.; Chen, S. S. Modulation of functional properties of galectin-3 by monoclonal antibodies binding to the non-lectin domains. *Biochemistry* **1996**, *35*, 6073–6079.
105. Rabinovich, G. A.; Toscano, M. A.; Jackson, S. S.; Vasta, G. R. Functions of cell surface galectin-glycoprotein lattices. *Curr. Opin. Struct. Biol.* **2007**, *17*, 513–520.
106. Clevers, H.; Alarcon, B.; Wileman, T.; Terhorst, C. The T cell receptor/CD3 complex: A dynamic protein ensemble. *Annu. Rev. Immunol.* **1988**, *6*, 629–662.
107. Patnaik, S. K.; Potvin, B.; Carlsson, S.; Sturm, D.; Leffler, H.; Stanley, P. Complex N-glycans are the major ligands for galectin-1, -3, and -8 on Chinese hamster ovary cells. *Glycobiology* **2006**, *16*, 305–317.
108. Kuball, J.; Hauptrock, B.; Malina, V.; Antunes, E.; Voss, R. H.; Wolfl, M.; Strong, R.; Theobald, M.; Greenberg, P. D. Increasing functional avidity of TCR-redirected T cells by removing defined N-glycosylation sites in the TCR constant domain. *J. Exp. Med.* **2009**, *206*, 463–475.
109. Stillman, B. N.; Hsu, D. K.; Pang, M.; Brewer, C. F.; Johnson, P.; Liu, F. T.; Baum, L. G. Galectin-3 and galectin-1 bind distinct cell surface glycoprotein receptors to induce T cell death. *J. Immunol.* **2006**, *176*, 778–789.
110. Earl, LA; Bi, S; Baum, LG N- and O-glycans modulate galectin-1 binding, CD45 signaling, and T cell death. *J. Biol. Chem.* **2010**, *285*, 2232–2344.
111. Pace, K. E.; Hahn, H. P.; Pang, M.; Nguyen, J. T.; Baum, L. G. CD7 delivers a pro-apoptotic signal during galectin-1-induced T cell death. *J. Immunol.* **2000**, *165*, 2331–2334.
112. Chen, I. J.; Chen, H. L.; Demetriou, M. Lateral compartmentalization of T cell receptor versus CD45 by galectin-N-glycan binding and microfilaments coordinate basal and activation signaling. *J. Biol. Chem.* **2007**, *282*, 35361–35372.
113. Irles, C.; Symons, A.; Michel, F; Bakker, T. R.; van der Merwe, P. A.; Acuto, O. CD45 ectodomain controls interaction with GEMs and Lck activity for optimal TCR signaling. *Nat. Immunol.* **2003**, *4*, 189–197.
114. Antonopoulos, A.; Demotte, N.; Stroobant, V.; Haslam, S. M.; van der Bruggen, P.; Dell, A. Loss of effector function of human cytolytic T lymphocytes is accompanied by major alterations in N- and O-glycosylation. *J. Biol. Chem.* **2012**, *287*, 11240–11251; epub ahead of print: Feb. 13.
115. Antonopoulos, A.; North, S. J.; Haslam, S. M.; Dell, A. Glycosylation of mouse and human immune cells: Insights emerging from N-glycomics analyses. *Biochem. Soc. Trans.* **2011**, *39*, 1334–1340.
116. Hirabayashi, J.; Hashidate, T.; Arata, Y.; Nishi, N.; Nakamura, T.; Hirashima, M.; Urashima, T.; Oka, T.; Futai, M.; Muller, W. E.; Yagi, F.;

Kasai, K. Oligosaccharide specificity of galectins: A search by frontal affinity chromatography. *Biochim. Biophys. Acta* **2002**, *1572*, 232–254.

117. Leppanen, A.; Stowell, S.; Blixt, O.; Cummings, R. D. Dimeric galectin-1 binds with high affinity to alpha2,3-sialylated and non-sialylated terminal N-acetyllactosamine units on surface-bound extended glycans. *J. Biol. Chem.* **2005**, *280*, 5549–5562.
118. Lobsanov, Y. D.; Gitt, M. A.; Leffler, H.; Barondes, S. H.; Rini, J. M. X-ray crystal structure of the human dimeric S-Lac lectin, L-14-II, in complex with lactose at 2.9-A resolution. *J. Biol. Chem.* **1993**, *268*, 27034–27038.
119. Miller, M. C.; Klyosov, A.; Mayo, K. H. The alpha-galactomannan Davanat binds galectin-1 at a site different from the conventional galectin carbohydrate binding domain. *Glycobiology* **2009**, *19*, 1034–1045.
120. Klyosov A. A.; Zomer E.; Platt D. DAVANAT® and Colon Cancer: Preclinical and Clinical (Phase I) Studies. In *Carbohydrate Drug Design*; Klyosov, A. A., Witczak, Z. J., Platt, D., Eds.; ACS Symposium Series 932; American Chemical Society: Washington, DC, 2006; pp 67−104.

Chapter 17

Targeting Galectin-3 Unveils the Complexity of Multiple Myeloma: A Sweet Context

Leonardo Mirandola,[1,2,4] Yuefei Yu,[2] Constance M. John,[3] Marjorie Jenkins,[2,4] Everardo Cobos,[2,4] and Maurizio Chiriva-Internati[*,2,4]

[1]Department of Health Sciences, Università degli Studi di Milano, Milano, Italy
[2]Department of Internal Medicine, Pharmaceutical Sciences, Surgery, Obstetrics & Gynecology at the Division of Hematology & Oncology, School of Medicine, Texas Tech University, Health Sciences Center and Southwest Cancer Treatment and Research Center, 3601 4th St., Mail Stop 9410, Lubbock, Texas 79430, USA
[3]MandalMed, 665 3rd Street, Suite 250, San Francisco, California 94107, USA
[4]Laura W. Bush Institute for Women's Health and Center for Women's Health and Gender-Based Medicine, Amarillo, Texas 79106, USA
[*]E-mail: maurizio.chiriva@ttuhsc.edu

After decades of research, multiple myeloma is still a fatal disease accounting for almost one out of five cases of all hematological malignancies. Recent evidences indicate that novel pharmacological agents, such as thalidomide, lenalidomide and bortezomib, improve the response rate and extend the overall survival. Yet, prolonged therapies are required to prevent or control recurrence, ultimately resulting in treatment-related toxicities seriously affecting the patients' quality of life. The urgent need of innovative therapeutic approaches may be answered by molecules disrupting the interactions between myeloma cells and the local microenvironment. Specifically, Galectin-3 plays key roles in the connections linking tumor cells with bone marrow stroma and the extracellular matrix. We evaluate here the multifaceted outcomes and potential applications of treatments based on Galectin-3C, a truncated dominant negative inhibitor of endogenous Galectin-3. Additionally, we hypothesize the molecular mechanism of action of Galectin-3C and present the future challenges and unique opportunities that a Galectin-3-tailored anti-myeloma therapy may offer in the near future.

Optimal Treatments for Multiple Myeloma: A Still Puzzling Clinical Problem

Multiple myeloma (MM) is a malignant tumor of the plasma cells, accounting for almost 1% of a overall neoplasia and 13% of hematological malignancies (*1*). It may be diagnosed *de novo* or evolve from a premalignant condition termed monoclonal gammopathy of undetermined significance. This can progresses to smoldering myeloma and eventually to symptomatic MM. Recently, the introduction of autologous hematopoietic stem cell (HSC) transplantation and the availability of novel drugs, such as thalidomide, lenalidomide, and bortezomib, have extended overall survival (*2*). Despite these developments, MM remains an incurable disease for the large majority of patients.

Current treatment options include a wide array of approaches basing on diagnosis, age, and co-morbidities. The different approaches are mainly dependent on the eligibility of the patient for HSC transplantation. The use of thalidomide, lenalidomide, or bortezomib for induction regimens before transplantation has increased the probability of complete response (*3*). Combined therapy with dexamethasone plus thalidomide, bortezomib, or lenalidomide has been proven very effective in raising the complete response rate (*4*, *5*). Bortezomib, in particular, significantly improved the outcome of thalidomide and dexamethasone combination, with respect to both response rate and progression-free survival (*6*). Presently, the most effective induction approach seems to be the so-called "total therapy", that relies on all available agents followed by high-dose treatment with melphalan (two cycles), then administration of autologous peripheral-blood HSC (tandem transplantation) (*7*). However, because of the serious treatment-related toxicities, single transplantation appears to be the option of choice for the majority of subjects, with thalidomide, lenalidomide, or bortezomib-based induction, followed by post-transplant consolidation (*3*).

In case transplantation cannot be performed, the combination of melphalan and prednisone plus either thalidomide or bortezomib is the standard of care (*8*). An alternative combination therapy consisting of lenalidomide plus dexamethasone increased the complete response rate and progression-free survival compared to high-dose dexamethasone alone (*9*). Consolidation and maintenance therapy are widely applied, yet no specific guidelines are available. Consolidation after autologous transplantation includes four courses of combined bortezomib, thalidomide, and dexamethasone (*10*). Maintenance therapy with thalidomide improved the rate of progression-free survival, but peripheral neuropathy hinders the long-term use of thalidomide (*11*, *12*).

Unfortunately, hematologic toxicities are relatively frequent with the use of thalidomide, lenalidomide, or bortezomib. Quite often these events require treatment suspension (*13*). In newly diagnosed subjects, the incidence of venous and arterial thrombosis is higher when either thalidomide or lenalidomide is combined with dexamethasone or other chemotherapies (*14*). Bortezomib and thalidomide are associated with peripheral neuropathy, while lenalidomide has been correlated with severe neuropathy (*5, 15, 16*). Overall, recent studies show that treatment-related adverse effects are unavoidable, and highlight the need to carefully evaluate and predict toxicities when planning treatment, especially for elderly patients. Side effects of chemotherapies are gaining increasing relevance as potentially more toxic combination regimens become the standard of care (*17*). Proper management of treatment-related morbidities is required to ensure that patients are given the best possible treatment, to maximize drug effectiveness, and extend survival (*18*). Efficient management and (whenever possible) relief from treatment side effects are expected to improve the quality of life of patients, especially in prolonged regimens, when treatment discontinuation is frequent.

Multiple Myeloma Microenvironment, Drug Resistance and Galectins: Potential Role of Galectin-3

While new drugs such as thalidomide, lenalidomide, and bortezomib have extended the survival time, MM mortality has not significantly decreased and the median survival remains at only approximately 5 years (*19–22*). Therefore, the urgent need for new and less toxic combination treatments is evident. A major challenge is identifying finding new targets for the development of tailored therapy, to achieve higher long-term response and lower treatment-related side effects, and to overall improve the quality of life of patients.

Since improved drugs and new therapeutic strategies are being developed, why is chemo-resistance still one of the main clinical issues in the treatment of MM? This question may be answered by considering the ineffectiveness of current agents in disrupting the vicious circle established by tumor cells within their neoplastic niche. However, the answer to such a central and apparently simple question presents unexpected complexities. Indeed, MM is unique among hematological malignancies in its ability to produce multiple lesions within the bone marrow (BM) that resemble solid tumors in many aspects. Notably, the pathological nature of the bone lesions strongly depends on the interaction with the microenvironment (*23*).

It has been established that MM cells are capable of profoundly altering the BM cellular and cytokine milieu, which in turns protects malignant cells from chemotherapeutics and maintains tumor growth (*24*). The cross-talk between MM and the BM niche largely relies on tumor cell adhesive properties, and accordingly extracellular matrix (ECM) adhesion-mediated drug resistance has been widely reported in MM experimental models (*25–28*). Accordingly, MM cells aberrantly express a wide array of integrin subunits, such as α4, α5, αv, β1, β2, β3, and β7 (*27, 29–32*). The most relevant in mediating adhesion-dependent migration, homing, invasion and drug resistance are integrins α4β1 (*32, 33*), α5β1 (*34*), αvβ3 (*35*), and β7 (*36*).

Angiogenesis is correlated with MM progression (*37*). The expansion of malignant plasma cells in the bone marrow causes bone remodelling typified by greater bone resorption and lower bone formation accompanied by neovascularization that is indicative of disease progression. Upon adhesive interactions, stromal and MM cells secrete angiogenic factors such as vascular endothelial growth factor (VEGF) and basic fibroblast growth factor (bFGF) (*38*, *39*). Interestingly, interaction between VEGF-R2 and αVβ3 integrin potentiate their intracellular signals (*40*).

Novel agents including thalidomide and thalidomide analogs such as lenalidomide as well as bortezomib are thought to target both the tumor cell and its BM microenvironment (*41*). Although these drugs may overcome some adhesion-mediated drug resistance, inability to achieve long-term remission or cure coupled with the serious toxicities discussed above indicate the need for novel pharmacological targets.

A promising new approach is based on the altered glycobiology of MM cells within the BM microenvironment. Indeed galectins, a class of S-type lectins which bind β-galactose-containing glycoconjugates (*42*, *43*), are aberrantly expressed by many tumors, including MM (*44–46*). Galectins are thought to have important roles in cell cycle progression (*47*), apoptosis (*48*) and metastases (*49*). Their primary ligands, β-galactoside-containing glycoproteins, are major components of the ECM (*50*) and of cell adhesion molecules (*51*). Accordingly, galectins can act as molecular bridges by linking ECM proteins with cell surface receptors, thus altering cellular interactions (*52*, *53*).

The potential of galectin targeting to reverse or block MM interactions with the BM microenvironment is a still largely unexplored field. The Gal-3 inhibitor GCS-100, a modified citrus pectin, was reported to reduce paracrine MM growth triggered by adherence to bone marrow stromal cells *in vitro* and block vascular endothelial growth-factor–induced migration of MM cells (*54*). These effects were associated with increased sensitivity to dexamethasone, melphalan, and doxorubicin, but were not accompanied by any toxic effect on normal (non-tumoral) lymphocytes (*54*). However, the molecular mechanisms accounting for the benefits of Gal-3 targeting in MM cells are still to be detailed.

Here we aim to briefly discuss our intriguing findings which suggest the great but comparatively unknown potential of Gal-3 as the target for novel, effective, and non-toxic treatment for MM. We hold that optimizing a Gal-3-tailored approach will enable a powerful opportunity to fulfill the urgent need of breakthrough therapies affording a better quality of life and possibly a cure for MM patients.

Pre-Clinical Study of Galectin-3 Inhibition in Multiple Myeloma

We have recently evaluated the biological and molecular outcomes of Gal-3 inhibition in human MM cells (*55*). Our strategy was based on the use of an *N*-terminally truncated Gal-3, termed Gal-3C (*56*). Among known galectins, Gal-3 has a unique structure consisting of an unusual, non-carbohydrate binding domain fused to its single carboxyl-terminal carbohydrate recognition domain (CRD). The amino-terminal domain of Gal-3 is required for dimerization that facilitates carbohydrate binding, because the CRD alone lacks the cooperative binding abilities of the intact protein (*53*, *57–60*). Consisting of the 143 C-terminal residues, Gal-3C retains the carbohydrate binding properties but lacks the multimerization ability of Gal-3 that increases its avidity for carbohydrates. Therefore, Gal-3C is thought to act as a competitive inhibitor of Gal-3, by preventing homophilic cross-linking of glycoconjugates (*56*).

At first, we tested the effect of Gal-3C on the proliferation of nine human MM cell lines cultured *in vitro*. Surprisingly, we noticed a limited effect on cell growth which was not of significantly greater magnitude when increasing concentrations of Gal-3C were used ranging from 0.4-20 μg/ml (*55*). Overall, the magnitude of the effects observed with any of the cell lines was slight.

Because Gal-3C had dramatically reduced metastases in a murine model of breast cancer (*56*), we tested the effect of Gal-3C on the migration and invasion of MM cells using an *in vitro* transwell insert model. Our data show that Gal-3C is a very effective inhibitor of SDF-1α-induced chemotaxis and ECM invasion by MM cells (*55*). Since migration in response to SDF-1α and ECM degradation are key steps in the progression of human MM (*27*, *61–63*), these results should be particularly relevant to the clinical disease and highlight the possible translational potential of Gal-3C-based therapies.

The effectiveness in preventing MM migration and invasion but the inability to reduce cell growth and significantly induce MM cell apoptosis are in contrast with two reports showing that the modified citrus pectin Gal-3 inhibitor, GCS-100, significantly induced apoptosis, reduced proliferation, and inhibited cell cycle in cultured human MM cell lines (*54*, *64*). It is known that Gal-3 exists as a secreted as well as an intracellular (cytoplasmatic and nuclear) protein (*65*). While extracellular galectins are able to crosslink cell-surface glycoconjugates, which in turn modulate adhesive interactions with ECM or adjacent cells, intracellular galectins play relevant roles in basic cellular functions, such as the regulation of growth, apoptosis and cell-cycle progression (*66–68*). Gal-3 can be uptaken by cells by both carbohydrate-dependent and independent mechanisms (*69*). Our data suggest that Gal-3C is similarly absorbed and secreted by cells in a carbohydrate-dependent mechanism (*70*). More data are required to establish whether there are differences between GCS-100 and Gal-3C in cellular uptake or subcellular localization that could be important in the difference in their activity.

However, it is clear that very different doses were employed in the *in vitro* studies of GCS-100 and Gal-3C (*64*, *71*, *72*). The molecular weight of both GCS-100 and Gal-3C is approximately 15kDa (*73*). At the 50% level the most effective doses for inhibition of proliferation and induction of apoptosis with GCS-100 were approximately 250-500 μg/ml with maximal response at 1.0 mg/ml. With Gal-3C, the doses tested ranged from 0.4-20 μg/ml with most maximal responses at approximately 1-2 μg/ml, more than 2 orders of magnitude lower than GCS-100 by weight and by molarity. Since GCS-100 presents more than one ligand for Gal-3, in that sense its molarity could be considered to be even higher than Gal-3C which has a single CRD per molecule.

There is growing evidence that in addition to multimerization mediated by the *N*-terminal domain (*74*, *75*), the CRD of Gal-3 can bind to itself in a manner that does not facilitate carbohydrate binding (*69*, *72*, *76*). . Therefore, at high concentrations the homophilic binding of the CRD of Gal-3C would compete with its carbohydrate binding and this could explain our inability to achieve greater inhibition of proliferation of MM cells with higher concentrations of Gal-3C. However, it may be relevant to mention that serum concentrations of Gal-3 in cancer have been found to be in most studies at the highest levels <1 μg/ml (*77–80*) and, thus, achieving levels of 2-5 μg/ml Gal-3C are likely to be sufficient to inhibit the homophilic carbohydrate binding of Gal-3 and, therefore, to be therapeutic by that mechanism.

Although GCS-100 was efficacious in reducing proliferation and inducing apoptosis in the cultured MM cells, its potency was relatively low, implying that a high concentration of GCS-100 is required to inhibit Gal-3, or that other mechanisms are important in its activity but are not understood. A potentially important issue is that there could be some issue regarding the feasibility of achieving levels of >0.5 mg/ml GCS-100 *in vivo*.

Our model predicts that Gal-3C at least partially acts to inhibit Gal-3-mediated interactions between MM cells and the bone microenvironment. This theory is supported by our recent reports evaluating the outcome of Gal-3C on MM-induced angiogenesis and on human MM cells growing *in vivo* (*55*). These data are in contrast to the very low efficacy shown by Gal-3C in reducing the proliferation of cultured MM cells alone. Gal-3C dramatically and significantly reduced MM cell growth in xenografted mice and improved the therapeutic benefits of bortezomib, without producing any evident toxic effects. When delivered intravenously using an osmotic mini-pump in NOD/SCID mice subcutaneously xenografted with the U266 MM cell line, Gal-3C was statistically significantly more effective than bortezomib as a single agent in reducing tumor burden. Overall our data support our model by which we would expect that a complex multi-cellular model may be required to adequately mimic the MM-bone microenvironment so that data obtained *in vitro* regarding the effects of inhibiting Gal-3 would reflect *in vivo* efficacy and potency.

In the view of future clinical applications, it is important to note that the combination of Gal-3C with bortezomib significantly reduced tumor growth as compared to either single agent after 14 days of treatment. The remarkable benefits observed *in vivo* are likely due to the ability of Gal-3C to function as a pan-galectin inhibitor. Indeed, other members of the galectin family, such as galectin-1 (*81*, *82*) and galectin-8, are involved in MM growth and survival (*55*). However, Gal-3C is expected to compete with galectins-1 and -8 for binding ligands important in cancer such as the polylactosaminylated *N*-glycosylated products of Mgat5 (*83*, *84*). Gal-3C had more affinity to $LacNAc_2$, $LacNAc_3$, and $LacNAc_5$, than galectin-1 and similar or more affinity than galectin-8 (*85*).

To further investigate the mechanism of action of Gal-3C, we focused on its effect on angiogenesis. This would have important implications for clinical application, because of the aforementioned role of angiogenesis in promoting MM progression (*25*, *38*, *86*, *87*). Gal-3 has been shown to mediate the signaling triggered by VEGF and bFGF, promoting angiogenesis by inducing $\alpha v\beta 3$ integrin clustering and inhibiting the constitutive endocytosis of the VEGFR-2 (*88*) (Figure 1).

Our results (*55*) show that treating U266 MM cells with Gal-3C significantly impaired their ability to produce VEGF and bFGF, resulting in a limited ability of MM-conditioned media to induce the formation of vessel-like structures in vascular endothelial cells (HUVEC) cultured *in vitro*. Additionally, media from Gal-3C-treated U266 cells was ineffective in driving HUVEC chemotaxis when compared with untreated MM cells. As expected, medium from control U266 cells induced αvβ3 integrin clustering in endothelial cells, but the medium from Gal-3C-treated MM cells did not.

Perhaps most importantly, the benefits displayed by Gal-3C in protecting xenografted mice from tumor burden were not associated with any evident toxicity. This suggests that, when translated into a clinical setting, Gal-3C-based therapies could reduce the effective dose of bortezomib or other chemotherapeutics mitigating adverse effects and allowing prolonged treatments and a better quality of life.

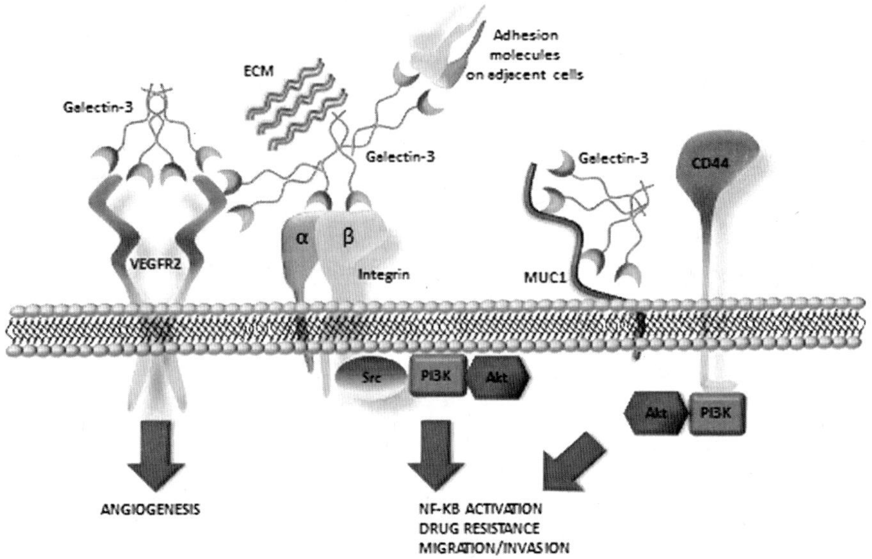

Figure 1. Main interactions between Gal-3 and molecules relevant in MM pathobiology. (see color insert)

Gal-3C Pharmacodynamic Challenges: Possible Molecular Mechanisms Altered by Gal-3c in Multiple Myeloma

The reported biological outcomes of a Gal-3C-based therapy could represent a breakthrough in the field of MM treatment. Although the pharmacodynamic mechanisms of Gal-3C are still to be detailed, there are intriguing hypotheses to be tested in the near future, particularly concerning the observed synergism with bortezomib. Figure 1 depicts the main roles of Gal-3 in MM pathobiology that could be blocked by Gal-3C.

Recent findings indicate that the effects of bortezomib on the NF-κB pathway could be more complex than just blocking the degradation of IKB. Indeed, it has been shown that bortezomib paradoxically induced the canonical NF-kB pathway by triggering IKKβ-mediated phosphorylation of IKBα (*89*). Of note, IKKβ activation is thought to limit bortezomib therapeutic efficacy (*89*). Interestingly, Gal-3 was reported to trigger integrin clustering and CD44 activation by interacting with MUC-1 (*90–92*) (Figure 1). These interactions ultimately result in NF-κB activation through the Src/PI3K/Akt pathway (*93–96*) (Figure 1). Therefore, we hypothesize that Gal-3C is able to reduce NF-κB activation by blocking Gal-3 interactions with αvβ3 integrin and MUC-1.

The dramatic inhibition of MM migration and invasive potential afforded by Gal-3C and the effectiveness in blocking MM-induced angiogenesis *in vitro* without toxicity for normal vascular endothelial cells (*55*) indicate the need to evaluate Gal-3C in animal models that most closely resemble the disease seen in humans. We present a pilot study for the evaluation of Gal-3C ability to interfere with MM-induced angiogenesis *in vivo*. A subcutaneous U266 tumor was established in NOD/SCID mice as described (*55*). 10^7 U266 MM cells and 10^6 HUVEC were dispersed in 300 μL Matrigel™. HUVEC were infected to stably express the GFP reporter as previously reported (*97*). This cell suspension was subcutaneously injected in recipient NOD/SCID mice and allowed to grow until a palpable mass was evident (two weeks). Mice were given Gal-3C or PBS (untreated controls) as recently described (*55*). After two weeks mice were sacrificed, pictures were taken, the tumor masses were disrupted and analyzed by flow-cytometry for the measurement of GFP-expressing vascular endothelial cells. Figure 2 shows that U266 MM cells induced a macroscopically evident vascularization (Figure 2A). Tumor growth was also evidently reduced in Gal-3C treated mice (Figure 2A). Flow-cytometry analysis revealed a significant ~50% reduction of GFP^+ HUVEC frequency in the tumor mass of Gal-3C-treated mice compared with untreated controls (Figure 2B).

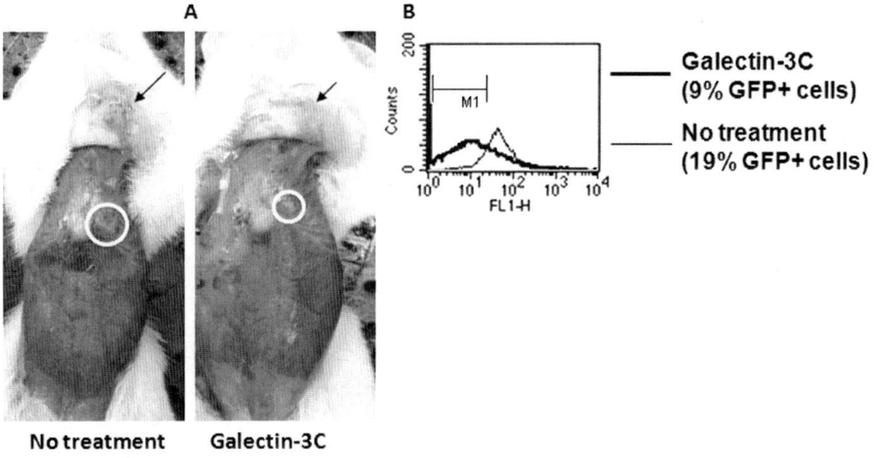

Figure 2. Representative results of Gal-3C treatment outcome on in vivo MM-induced angiogenesis. A) White circles mark the subcutaneous tumors. The arrows show the macroscopic evidence of sub-cutaneous capillaries. B) Flow-cytometry assessment of GFP-expressing HUVEC cells in tumor masses. The frequency of positive cells is shown. (see color insert)

The Pre-Clinical Challenges of Gal-3 Studies in Multiple Myeloma

The full therapeutic potential of Gal-3C is still to be tested in animal models of MM producing disseminated disease. Indeed, the presence of multiple bone lesions is characteristic of advanced MM in patients, and the BM niche protects tumor cells from therapeutic interventions (*98–101*). Such models will be critical to understand the role of Gal-3 in the interactions of MM with the BM environment and may be critical in enabling a paradigm-shifting view of MM pathophysiology. To this goal, we hold that the two of the best options for testing Gal-3 targeted therapeutics in MM animal models are the NOG and the NRG murine strains. NOG are NOD/SCID mice carrying nonfunctional IL-2 receptor gamma chain (NOD/SCID/γc^{null}): this strain is more permissive than the NOD/SCID and can be easily xenografted with human MM cell lines or even primary human MM cells, to produce a disease similar to that seen in patients, including multiple metastatic sites and bone lesions (*102–104*).

The NRG strain is a further optimization of the NOD strain, carrying double genetic disruptions of the Rag1 and the IL-2 receptor gamma chain genes (NOD-$Rag1^{null}$ $IL2rg^{null}$). The NRG has been reported to tolerate higher levels of radiation compared with NOD/SCID and NOG strains and to allow for efficient engraftment of human hematopoietic stem cells (*103*). Accordingly, we were the first to validate the NRG strain to establish an innovative model of MM, allowing for the growth and the spread of MM cell lines and primary patients' cells as well (*105*). This model would be instrumental to study the efficacy of Gal-3C *in vivo* to prevent MM cell lines and primary cells from infiltrating the bone marrow, orchestrating neo-angiogenesis, altering the microenvironment and acquiring drug resistance.

Increasing evidences highlight that a key point in the clinical management of MM is the impaired anti-tumor immune response in MM patients (*106–109*). Gal-3 has relevant activity in immune cells, including macrophages, dendritic cells, eosinophils, mast cells, NK cells and activated T and B cells (*110*). Particularly with effector T cells, Gal-3 has been shown to induce apoptosis (*111*) and to inhibit T-cell activation by forming complexes with TCR glycans, preventing the TCR clustering that is required for signal transduction (*112*). Oppositely, Gal-3 has been reported to stimulate the suppressive functions of regulatory T cells (Treg) (*113*). It is therefore notable that MM cells are very effective in evading immunosurveillance by affecting, among other mechanisms, the expansion of Treg and simultaneous reduction of T-cell cytotoxic activity (*109*). Therefore, it will be important to assess the possibility that Gal-3C can contribute to the restoration of an effective anti-myeloma response. Since this cannot be done in immunodeficient animals, the need for immune-competent models is evident.

Currently available immunocompetent murine models of MM include the 5TMM series (*114*), the LAGlambda-1 (*115*) or IL-6 transgenic strain (*116*). These models will allow for evaluation of possible effects of the therapy on the interaction between tumor cells and the immune system. However, they present three major drawbacks (*117*). They cannot recapitulate the complexity and heterogeneity of human MM, they are not suitable to study treatment outcome on patients-derived MM cells, and they could be biased by molecular and biological differences existing between murine and human MM cells.

Because Gal-3C potentially acts through multiple and complex mechanisms involving the interactions between a number of different cell types and ECM molecules, it would be advisable to perform future pre-clinical evaluations in murine models capable of closely mimicking the MM microenvironment. Such an ideal model would afford for human MM cell lines and primary cells engraftment, disseminated disease in multiple bone sites, and interaction with an active immune system. A possible answer to this need may already exist, and relies on the NRG strain, that has been shown to support the engraftment and reconstitution of a functional human hematopoietic system (*103*). Such humanized mice (*118*, *119*) could be challenged with human MM primary cells or cell lines. Finally, upon disease establishment, Gal-3C outcomes (as a single agent or in combination with standard therapies) could be fully detailed and pre-clinically validated.

Translational Challenges: Delivering Gal-3c to the Bedside

Ideally, clinical application of Gal-3C-based treatments would be in the context of an optimized delivery system. In fact, our study describes the need to administer Gal-3C intravenously at a constant rate (*55*). Indeed, although in a previous study on a CD-1 nude mouse model of metastatic human breast cancer (*56*) Gal-3C was injected intramuscularly, our recent data (*55*) suggest that sustained delivery may be preferable for maximal response to treatment. This finding is in accordance with a previous report indicating that the elimination half-life of Gal-3C in the serum of mice is approximately 3 hours (*56*). We achieved continuous intravenous administration by implanting a Gal-3C-loaded osmotic mini-pump directly connected to the jugular vein, thus creating a central venous access (*55*). It is evident that this would not be feasible to treat MM patients, and that there is the need to optimize an alternative delivery route with similar performances as the osmotic pump. Biodegradable polymer-based nanoparticles (NP) may represent a valuable option (*120*). They consist of nano-scale particles (less than 1 μm in diameter) that are synthesized from natural or synthetic polymers.

Drugs can be incorporated into the NP by a number of techniques (entrapment in the polymer matrix, coating by a shell-like polymer membrane, chemical conjugation to the polymer, or absorption to the particle's surface). Interestingly, a galectin-1/gold NP complex has been recently described for the treatment of rheumatoid arthritis (*121*). One key feature of NP polymers is the possibility to control the drug release rate, which is likely to fit the requirement of sustained drug delivery necessary for Gal-3C therapy. Several factors can be modulated to tune the release rate of the entrapped drug, such as NP dimensions (larger NP display a smaller initial release rate but a longer overall release time than smaller NP), amount of loaded drug (the greater the drug loading the greater the burst but the shorter the overall release time), or addition of different polymers (*122*, *123*). Most importantly, the addition of polymers such as polyetilenglicol to NP has been successfully used to control the drug release (*124*, *125*). We hypothesize that a similar approach could be effectively optimized for the administration of a continuous and controlled dose of Gal-3C to human subjects.

Conclusions

Our pioneering work provided the proof-of-principle for the use of Gal-3C in MM. While this novel treatment decreased tumor growth in animal models and increased the therapeutic efficacy of standard drugs such as bortezomib, it did not trigger any apparent additional toxicity. We have also show evidence indicating that the main Gal-3C mechanism of action may not be restricted to the MM tumor cell, but rather may involve alteration of the multifaceted signaling pathways linking the MM cell with the BM niche. While detailed molecular mechanisms of Gal-3 are still to be elucidated, there is strong evidence of the potential benefits that a Gal-3C-adjuvated therapy would afford in the clinical management of MM, in terms of treatment response and quality of life improvement. To achieve this goal, we still face critical challenges, covering several areas of specialization ranging from molecular biology, to pre-clinical animal models, practical clinical issues in the management of patient, and utilization of advanced drug delivery systems.

Acknowledgments

We thank Mrs. J. Avery "Janie" Rush Endowed Chair of Excellence in Women's Health and Oncology, the Billy and Ruby Power Family and Everardo Cobos, Associate Dean of the Oncology Programs at TTUHSC. We thank Teri Fields for her assistance in editing this manuscript.

Funding

This work was supported by a National Institutes of Health grant award (CA135862-01 to C.M.J. and M. C. I.

Abbreviations

MM: multiple myeloma
BM: bone marrow
ECM: extracellular matrix
HUVEC: human umbilical cord vascular endothelial cells

References

1. Palumbo, A.; Anderson, K. Multiple Myeloma. *N. Engl. J. Med.* **2011**, *364* (11), 1046–1060.
2. Mohty, B.; et al. Treatment strategies in relapsed and refractory multiple myeloma: A focus on drug sequencing and 'retreatment' approaches in the era of novel agents. *Leukemia* **2012**, *26* (1), 73–85.
3. Stewart, A. K.; Richardson, P. G.; San-Miguel, J. F. How I treat multiple myeloma in younger patients. *Blood* **2009**, *114* (27), 5436–5443.
4. Harousseau, J. L.; et al. Bortezomib plus dexamethasone is superior to vincristine plus doxorubicin plus dexamethasone as induction treatment prior to autologous stem-cell transplantation in newly diagnosed multiple myeloma: Results of the IFM 2005-01 phase III trial. *J. Clin. Oncol.* **2010**, *28* (30), 4621–4629.
5. Rajkumar, S. V.; et al. Lenalidomide plus high-dose dexamethasone versus lenalidomide plus low-dose dexamethasone as initial therapy for newly diagnosed multiple myeloma: An open-label randomised controlled trial. *Lancet Oncol.* **2010**, *11* (1), 29–37.
6. Cavo, M.; et al. International Myeloma Working Group consensus approach to the treatment of multiple myeloma patients who are candidates for autologous stem cell transplantation. *Blood* **2011**, *117* (23), 6063–6073.
7. Nair, B.; et al. Superior results of Total Therapy 3 (2003-33) in gene expression profiling-defined low-risk multiple myeloma confirmed in subsequent trial 2006-66 with VRD maintenance. *Blood* **2010**, *115* (21), 4168–4173.
8. Reeder, C. B.; et al. Cyclophosphamide, bortezomib and dexamethasone induction for newly diagnosed multiple myeloma: High response rates in a phase II clinical trial. *Leukemia* **2009**, *23* (7), 1337–1341.

9. Zonder, J. A.; et al. Lenalidomide and high-dose dexamethasone compared with dexamethasone as initial therapy for multiple myeloma: A randomized Southwest Oncology Group trial (S0232). *Blood* **2010**, *116* (26), 5838–5841.
10. Ladetto, M.; et al. Major tumor shrinking and persistent molecular remissions after consolidation with bortezomib, thalidomide, and dexamethasone in patients with autografted myeloma. *J. Clin. Oncol.* **2010**, *28* (12), 2077–2084.
11. Barlogie, B.; et al. Thalidomide and hematopoietic-cell transplantation for multiple myeloma. *N. Engl. J. Med.* **2006**, *354* (10), 1021–1030.
12. Ludwig, H.; et al. Thalidomide maintenance treatment increases progression-free but not overall survival in elderly patients with myeloma. *Haematologica* **2010**, *95* (9), 1548–1554.
13. Palumbo, A.; et al. Prevention of thalidomide- and lenalidomide-associated thrombosis in myeloma. *Leukemia* **2008**, *22* (2), 414–423.
14. Waage, A.; et al. Melphalan and prednisone plus thalidomide or placebo in elderly patients with multiple myeloma. *Blood* **2010**, *116* (9), 1405–1412.
15. Palumbo, A.; et al. Bortezomib-melphalan-prednisone-thalidomide followed by maintenance with bortezomib-thalidomide compared with bortezomib-melphalan-prednisone for initial treatment of multiple myeloma: A randomized controlled trial. *J. Clin. Oncol.* **2010**, *28* (34), 5101–5109.
16. Richardson, P. G.; et al. Bortezomib or high-dose dexamethasone for relapsed multiple myeloma. *N. Engl. J. Med.* **2005**, *352* (24), 2487–2498.
17. Richardson, P. G.; et al. A Phase 2 Study of bortezomib in relapsed, refractory myeloma. *N. Engl. J. Med.* **2003**, *348* (26), 2609–2617.
18. Palumbo, A.; et al. Practical management of adverse events in multiple myeloma: Can therapy be attenuated in older patients? *Blood Rev.* **2011**, *25* (4), 181–191.
19. Kaufman, J.; Gleason, C.; Lonial, S. Treatment of relapsed and refractory myeloma. *Curr. Hematol. Malig. Rep.* **2009**, *4* (2), 99–107.
20. Mahindra, A.; Cirstea, D.; Raje, N. Novel therapeutic targets for multiple myeloma. *Future Oncol.* **2010**, *6* (3), 407–418.
21. Palumbo, A.; Rajkumar, S. V. Multiple myeloma: Chemotherapy or transplantation in the era of new drugs. *Eur. J. Haematol.* **2010**, *84* (5), 379–390.
22. Zhou, Y.; Barlogie, B.; Shaughnessy, J. D., Jr. The molecular characterization and clinical management of multiple myeloma in the post-genome era. *Leukemia* **2009**, *23* (11), 1941–56.
23. Mirandola, L.; et al. Notching from T-cell to B-cell lymphoid malignancies. *Cancer Lett.* **2011**, *308* (1), 1–13.
24. Abildgaard, N.; et al. Comparison of five biochemical markers of bone resorption in multiple myeloma: Elevated pre-treatment levels of S-ICTP and U-Ntx are predictive for early progression of the bone disease during standard chemotherapy. *Br. J. Haematol.* **2003**, *120* (2), 235–242.
25. Abe, M. Targeting the interplay between myeloma cells and the bone marrow microenvironment in myeloma. *Int. J. Hematol.* **2011**, *94* (4), 334–343.
26. Anderson, K. C. New insights into therapeutic targets in myeloma. *Hematol. Am. Soc. Hematol. Educ. Prog.* **2011**, 184–190.

27. Katz, B. Z. Adhesion molecules: The lifelines of multiple myeloma cells. *Semin. Cancer Biol.* **2010**, *20* (3), 186–195.
28. Mahindra, A.; Hideshima, T.; Anderson, K. C. Multiple myeloma: Biology of the disease. *Blood Rev* **2010**, *24* (1), S5–S11.
29. Cook, G.; Dumbar, M.; Franklin, I. M. The role of adhesion molecules in multiple myeloma. *Acta Haematol.* **1997**, *97* (1−2), 81–89.
30. Damiano, J. S. Integrins as novel drug targets for overcoming innate drug resistance. *Curr. Cancer Drug Targets* **2002**, *2* (1), 37–43.
31. Damiano, J. S.; Dalton, W. S. Integrin-mediated drug resistance in multiple myeloma. *Leuk. Lymphoma* **2000**, *38* (1−2), 71–81.
32. Sanz-Rodriguez, F.; Teixido, J. VLA-4-dependent myeloma cell adhesion. *Leuk. Lymphoma* **2001**, *41* (3−4), 239–45.
33. Parmo-Cabanas, M.; et al. Integrin alpha4beta1 involvement in stromal cell-derived factor-1alpha-promoted myeloma cell transendothelial migration and adhesion: Role of cAMP and the actin cytoskeleton in adhesion. *Exp. Cell Res.* **2004**, *294* (2), 571–580.
34. Damiano, J. S.; et al. Cell adhesion mediated drug resistance (CAM-DR): Role of integrins and resistance to apoptosis in human myeloma cell lines. *Blood* **1999**, *93* (5), 1658–1667.
35. Ria, R.; et al. Alpha(v)beta(3) integrin engagement enhances cell invasiveness in human multiple myeloma. *Haematologica* **2002**, *87* (8), 836–845.
36. Neri, P.; et al. Integrin beta7-mediated regulation of multiple myeloma cell adhesion, migration, and invasion. *Blood* **2011**, *117* (23), 6202–6213.
37. Kumar, S.; et al. Bone marrow angiogenic ability and expression of angiogenic cytokines in myeloma: Evidence favoring loss of marrow angiogenesis inhibitory activity with disease progression. *Blood* **2004**, *104* (4), 1159–1165.
38. Jakob, C.; et al. Angiogenesis in multiple myeloma. *Eur. J. Cancer* **2006**, *42* (11), 1581–1590.
39. Corre, J.; et al. Bone marrow mesenchymal stem cells are abnormal in multiple myeloma. *Leukemia* **2007**, *21* (5), 1079–1088.
40. Tanaka, Y.; et al. Myeloma cell-osteoclast interaction enhances angiogenesis together with bone resorption: A role for vascular endothelial cell growth factor and osteopontin. *Clin. Cancer Res.* **2007**, *13* (3), 816–823.
41. Mahindra, A.; Hideshima, T.; Anderson, K. C. Multiple myeloma: Biology of the disease. *Blood Rev.* **2010**, *24* (Supplement 1) (0), S5–S11.
42. Di Lella, S.; et al. When galectins recognize glycans: From biochemistry to physiology and back again. *Biochemistry* **2011**, *50* (37), 7842–7857.
43. Laderach, D. J.; et al. Dissecting the signal transduction pathways triggered by galectin-glycan interactions in physiological and pathological settings. *IUBMB Life* **2010**, *62* (1), 1–13.
44. Newlaczyl, A. U.; Yu, L. G. Galectin-3: A jack-of-all-trades in cancer. *Cancer Lett.* **2011**, *313* (2), 123–128.
45. van den Brule, F.; Califice, S.; Castronovo, V. Expression of galectins in cancer: A critical review. *Glycoconjugate J.* **2004**, *19* (7−9), 537–542.

46. Lahm, H.; et al. Tumor galectinology: Insights into the complex network of a family of endogenous lectins. *Glycoconjugate J.* **2004**, *20* (4), 227–238.
47. Yang, R. Y.; et al. Cell cycle regulation by galectin-12, a new member of the galectin superfamily. *J Biol Chem* **2001**, *276* (23), 20252–20260.
48. Takenaka, Y.; et al. Nuclear export of phosphorylated galectin-3 regulates its antiapoptotic activity in response to chemotherapeutic drugs. *Mol. Cell Biol.* **2004**, *24* (10), 4395–4406.
49. Kuwabara, I.; Sano, H.; Liu, F. T. Functions of galectins in cell adhesion and chemotaxis. *Methods Enzymol.* **2003**, *363*, 532–552.
50. He, J.; Baum, L. G. Galectin interactions with extracellular matrix and effects on cellular function. *Methods Enzymol5* **2006**, *417*, 247–256.
51. Fred Brewer, C. Binding and cross-linking properties of galectins. *Biochim. Biophys. Acta* **2002**, *19*, 2–3.
52. Bornstein, P.; Sage, E. H. Matricellular proteins: Extracellular modulators of cell function. *Curr. Opin. Cell Biol.* **2002**, *14* (5), 608–616.
53. Ochieng, J.; Leite-Browning, M. L.; Warfield, P. Regulation of cellular adhesion to extracellular matrix proteins by galectin-3. *Biochem. Biophys. Res. Commun.* **1998**, *246* (3), 788–791.
54. Chauhan, D.; et al. A novel carbohydrate-based therapeutic GCS-100 overcomes bortezomib resistance and enhances dexamethasone-induced apoptosis in multiple myeloma cells. *Cancer Res.* **2005**, *65* (18), 8350–8358.
55. Mirandola, L.; et al. Galectin-3C inhibits tumor growth and increases the anticancer activity of bortezomib in a murine model of human multiple myeloma. *PLoS One* **2011**, *6* (7), 13.
56. John, C. M.; et al. Truncated galectin-3 inhibits tumor growth and metastasis in orthotopic nude mouse model of human breast cancer. *Clin. Cancer Res.* **2003**, *9* (6), 2374–2383.
57. Massa, S. M.; et al. L-29, an endogenous lectin, binds to glycoconjugate ligands with positive cooperativity. *Biochemistry* **1993**, *32* (1), 260–267.
58. Hsu, D. K.; Zuberi, R. I.; Liu, F. T. Biochemical and biophysical characterization of human recombinant IgE-binding protein, an S-type animal lectin. *J. Biol. Chem.* **1992**, *267* (20), 14167–14174.
59. Ochieng, J.; et al. Structure-function relationship of a recombinant human galactoside-binding protein. *Biochemistry* **1993**, *32* (16), 4455–4460.
60. Seetharaman, J.; et al. X-ray crystal structure of the human galectin-3 carbohydrate recognition domain at 2.1-A resolution. *J Biol Chem* **1998**, *273* (21), 13047–13052.
61. Alsayed, Y.; et al. Mechanisms of regulation of CXCR4/SDF-1 (CXCL12)-dependent migration and homing in multiple myeloma. *Blood* **2007**, *109* (7), 2708–2717.
62. Kim, S. W.; et al. Dexamethasone and hypoxia upregulate CXCR4 expression in myeloma cells. *Leuk. Lymphoma* **2009**, *50* (7), 1163–1173.
63. Vande Broek, I.; et al. Extravasation and homing mechanisms in multiple myeloma. *Clin. Exp. Metastasis* **2008**, *25* (4), 325–334.
64. Streetly, M. J.; et al. GCS-100, a novel galectin-3 antagonist, modulates MCL-1, NOXA, and cell cycle to induce myeloma cell death. *Blood* **2010**, *115* (19), 3939–3948.

65. Liu, F. T.; Rabinovich, G. A. Galectins as modulators of tumour progression. *Nat. Rev. Cancer* **2005**, *5* (1), 29–41.
66. Hsu, D. K.; Yang, R. Y.; Liu, F. T. Galectins in apoptosis. *Methods Enzymol.* **2006**, *417*, 256–273.
67. Davidson, P. J.; et al. Shuttling of galectin-3 between the nucleus and cytoplasm. *Glycobiology* **2002**, *12* (5), 329–337.
68. Nakahara, S.; et al. Characterization of the nuclear import pathways of galectin-3. *Cancer Res.* **2006**, *66* (20), 9995–10006.
69. Lepur, A.; et al. Galectin-3 endocytosis by carbohydrate independent and dependent pathways in different macrophage like cell types. *Biochim. Biophys. Acta* **2012**, *1820*, 804–818.
70. Jarvis, G. A.; et al.Galectin-3C, Human Lectin for Treatment of Cancer. In *The Galectins*, Volume 2, 2013.
71. Chauhan, D.; et al. A novel carbohydrate-based therapeutic GCS-100 overcomes bortezomib resistance and enhances dexamethasone-induced apoptosis in multiple myeloma cells. *Cancer Res.* **2005**, *65* (18), 8350–8358.
72. Mirandola, L.; et al. Galectin-3C inhibits tumor growth and increases the anticancer activity of bortezomib in a murine model of human multiple myeloma. *PLoS One* **2011**, *6* (7), e21811.
73. Eliaz, I.; et al. The effect of modified citrus pectin on urinary excretion of toxic elements. *Phytother. Res.* **2006**, *20* (10), 859–864.
74. Liu, F. T.; et al. Modulation of functional properties of galectin-3 by monoclonal antibodies binding to the non-lectin domains. *Biochemistry* **1996**, *35* (19), 6073–6079.
75. Ahmad, N.; et al. Galectin-3 precipitates as a pentamer with synthetic multivalent carbohydrates and forms heterogeneous cross-linked complexes. *J. Biol. Chem.* **2004**, *279* (12), 10841–10847.
76. Yang, R. Y.; et al. Role of the carboxyl-terminal lectin domain in self-association of galectin-3. *Biochemistry* **1998**, *37* (12), 4086–4092.
77. Sakaki, M.; et al. Serum level of galectin-3 in human bladder cancer. *J. Med. Invest.* **2008**, *55* (1−2), 127–132.
78. Vereecken, P.; et al. Evaluation of the prognostic significance of serum galectin-3 in American Joint Committee on Cancer stage III and stage IV melanoma patients. *Melanoma Res.* **2009**, *19* (5), 316–320.
79. Iurisci, I.; et al. Concentrations of galectin-3 in the sera of normal controls and cancer patients. *Clin Cancer Res* **2000**, *6* (4), 1389–1393.
80. Vereecken, P.; et al. High serum galectin-3 in advanced melanoma: Preliminary results. *Clin. Exp. Dermatol* **2006**, *31* (1), 105–109.
81. Abroun, S.; et al. Galectin-1 supports the survival of CD45RA(-) primary myeloma cells in vitro. *Br J Haematol* **2008**, *142* (5), 754–765.
82. Zlei, M.; et al. Characterization of in vitro growth of multiple myeloma cells. *Exp. Hematol.* **2007**, *35* (10), 1550–1561.
83. Granovsky, M.; et al. Suppression of tumor growth and metastasis in Mgat5-deficient mice. *Nat. Med.* **2000**, *6* (3), 306–312.
84. Lagana, A.; et al. Galectin binding to Mgat5-modified N-glycans regulates fibronectin matrix remodeling in tumor cells. *Mol. Cell Biol.* **2006**, *26* (8), 3181–3193.

85. Hirabayashi, C.; Imai, Y. Studies on MMA-tBB resin. I. Comparison of TBB and other initiators in the polymerization of PMMA/MMA resin. *Dent. Mater. J.* **2002**, *21* (4), 314–321.
86. Anargyrou, K.; et al. Novel anti-myeloma agents and angiogenesis. *Leuk. Lymphoma* **2008**, *49* (4), 677–689.
87. Cibeira, M. T.; et al. Bone marrow angiogenesis and angiogenic factors in multiple myeloma treated with novel agents. *Cytokine* **2008**, *41* (3), 244–253.
88. Markowska, A. I.; Liu, F. T.; Panjwani, N. Galectin-3 is an important mediator of VEGF- and bFGF-mediated angiogenic response. *J. Exp. Med.* **2010**, *207* (9), 1981–1993.
89. Hideshima, T.; et al. Bortezomib induces canonical nuclear factor-kappaB activation in multiple myeloma cells. *Blood* **2009**, *114* (5), 1046–1052.
90. Schmidmaier, R.; et al. Inhibition of lymphocyte function associated antigen 1 by LFA878 induces apoptosis in multiple myeloma cells and is associated with downregulation of the focal adhesion kinase/phosphatidylinositol 3 kinase/Akt pathway. *Int. J. Oncol.* **2007**, *31* (4), 969–976.
91. Segarra, M.; et al. Thalidomide decreases gelatinase production by malignant B lymphoid cell lines through disruption of multiple integrin-mediated signaling pathways. *Haematologica* **2010**, *95* (3), 456–463.
92. Zhao, Q.; et al. Circulating galectin-3 promotes metastasis by modifying MUC1 localization on cancer cell surface. *Cancer Res.* **2009**, *69* (17), 6799–6806.
93. Antonov, A. S.; et al. AlphaVbeta3 integrin regulates macrophage inflammatory responses via PI3 kinase/Akt-dependent NF-kappaB activation. *J. Cell. Physiol.* **2011**, *226* (2), 469–476.
94. Ju, J. H.; et al. CD24 enhances DNA damage-induced apoptosis by modulating NF-kappaB signaling in CD44-expressing breast cancer cells. *Carcinogenesis* **2011**, *32* (10), 1474–1483.
95. Yasuda, T. Activation of Akt leading to NF-kappaB up-regulation in chondrocytes stimulated with fibronectin fragment. *Biomed. Res.* **2011**, *32* (3), 209–215.
96. Noble, P. W.; et al. Hyaluronan fragments activate an NF-kappa B/I-kappa B alpha autoregulatory loop in murine macrophages. *J. Exp. Med.* **1996**, *183* (5), 2373–2378.
97. Yu, Y.; et al. Protective CD8+ T-cell responses to cytomegalovirus driven by rAAV/GFP/IE1 loading of dendritic cells. *J. Transl. Med.* **2008**, *6*, 56.
98. Fowler, J. A.; et al. Bone marrow stromal cells create a permissive microenvironment for myeloma development: A new stromal role for wnt inhibitor dkk1. *Cancer Res.* **2012**, *72* (9), 2183–2189.
99. Longo, V.; et al. Therapeutic approaches to myeloma bone disease: An evolving story. *Cancer Treat. Rev.* **2012**, *9*, 9.
100. Morgan, G. J.; Wu, P. Targeting bone in myeloma. *Recent Results Cancer Res.* **2012**, *192*, 127–143.
101. Zangari, M.; et al. Impact of bortezomib on bone health in myeloma: A review of current evidence. *Cancer Treat. Rev.* **2012**, *6*, 6.

102. Dewan, M. Z.; et al. Prompt tumor formation and maintenance of constitutive NF-kappaB activity of multiple myeloma cells in NOD/SCID/gammacnull mice. *Cancer Sci.* **2004**, *95* (7), 564–568.
103. Pearson, T.; et al. Non-obese diabetic-recombination activating gene-1 (NOD-Rag1 null) interleukin (IL)-2 receptor common gamma chain (IL2r gamma null) null mice: A radioresistant model for human lymphohaematopoietic engraftment. *Clin. Exp. Immunol.* **2008**, *154* (2), 270–284.
104. Ito, M.; Kobayashi, K.; Nakahata, T. NOD/Shi-scid IL2rgamma(null) (NOG) mice more appropriate for humanized mouse models. *Curr. Top. Microbiol. Immunol.* **2008**, *324*, 53–76.
105. Mirandola, L.; et al. Tracking human multiple myeloma xenografts in NOD-Rag-1/IL-2 receptor gamma chain-null mice with the novel biomarker AKAP-4. *BMC Cancer* **2011**, *11*, 394.
106. Auer, R. L.; et al. T-cell replete fludarabine/cyclophosphamide reduced intensity allogeneic stem cell transplantation for lymphoid malignancies. *Br. J. Haematol.* **2012**, *157* (5), 580–585.
107. Broen, K.; et al. Induction of multiple myeloma-reactive T cells during post-transplantation immunotherapy with donor lymphocytes and recipient DCs. *Bone Marrow Transplant.* **2012**, *16* (10), 258.
108. Moeller, I.; et al. Uptake routes of tumor-antigen MAGE-A3 by dendritic cells determine priming of naive T-cell subtypes. *Cancer Immunol. Immunother.* **2012**, *6*, 6.
109. Rutella, S.; Locatelli, F. Targeting multiple-myeloma-induced immune dysfunction to improve immunotherapy outcomes. *Clin. Dev. Immunol.* **2012**, *196063*, 11.
110. Dumic, J.; Dabelic, S.; Flogel, M. Galectin-3: An open-ended story. *Biochim. Biophys. Acta* **2006**, *4*, 616–635.
111. Fukumori, T.; et al. CD29 and CD7 mediate galectin-3-induced type II T-cell apoptosis. *Cancer Res.* **2003**, *63* (23), 8302–8311.
112. Demetriou, M.; et al. Negative regulation of T-cell activation and autoimmunity by Mgat5 N-glycosylation. *Nature* **2001**, *409* (6821), 733–739.
113. Radosavljevic, G.; et al. The roles of Galectin-3 in autoimmunity and tumor progression. *Immunol. Res.* **2012**, *52* (1–2), 100–110.
114. Vanderkerken, K.; et al. Organ involvement and phenotypic adhesion profile of 5T2 and 5T33 myeloma cells in the C57BL/KaLwRij mouse. *Br. J. Cancer* **1997**, *76* (4), 451–460.
115. Campbell, R. A.; et al. LAGlambda-1: A clinically relevant drug resistant human multiple myeloma tumor murine model that enables rapid evaluation of treatments for multiple myeloma. *Int. J. Oncol.* **2006**, *28* (6), 1409–1417.
116. Kovalchuk, A. L.; et al. IL-6 transgenic mouse model for extraosseous plasmacytoma. *Proc. Natl. Acad. Sci. U.S.A.* **2002**, *99* (3), 1509–1514.
117. Mitsiades, C. S.; Anderson, K. C.; Carrasco, D. R. Mouse models of human myeloma. *Hematol. Oncol. Clin. North Am.* **2007**, *21* (6), 1051–1069.
118. Garcia, S.; Freitas, A. A. Humanized mice: Current states and perspectives. *Immunol. Lett.* **2012**, *9*, 9.

119. Su, L. Studying human immunology and immunopathology in humanized mice transplanted with human lymphoid tissues and immune cells. *Cell. Mol. Immunol.* **2012**, *9* (3), 191–192.
120. Hans, M. L.; Lowman, A. M. Biodegradable nanoparticles for drug delivery and targeting. *Curr. Opin. Solid State Mater. Sci.* **2002**, *6* (4), 319–327.
121. Huang, Y. J.; et al. Multivalent structure of galectin-1-nanogold complex serves as potential therapeutics for rheumatoid arthritis by enhancing receptor clustering. *Eur. Cells Mater.* **2012**, *23*, 170–81.
122. Leroux, J.-C.; et al. Biodegradable nanoparticles: From sustained release formulations to improved site specific drug delivery. *J. Controlled Release* **1996**, *39* (2–3), 339–350.
123. Nicoli, S.; et al. Design of triptorelin loaded nanospheres for transdermal iontophoretic administration. *Int. J. Pharm.* **2001**, *214* (1–2), 31–35.
124. Matsumoto, J.; et al. Preparation of nanoparticles consisted of poly(l-lactide)–poly(ethylene glycol)–poly(l-lactide) and their evaluation in vitro. *Int. J. Pharm.* **1999**, *185* (1), 93–101.
125. Avgoustakis, K.; et al. PLGA–mPEG nanoparticles of cisplatin: In vitro nanoparticle degradation, in vitro drug release and in vivo drug residence in blood properties. *J. Controlled Release* **2002**, *79* (1–3), 123–135.

Chapter 18

Galectins in the Blood Circulation: Potential Therapeutic Targets of Cancer Metastasis

Carrie A. Duckworth and Lu-Gang Yu*

Department of Gastroenterology, Institute of Translational Medicine and Centre for Glycobiology, University of Liverpool, Nuffield Building, Ashton Street, Liverpool L69 3GE, United Kingdom
***E-mail: lgyu@liverpool.ac.uk**

Elevated concentrations of several galectin members (e.g. galectin-2, -3, -4 and -8) occur in the bloodstream of patients with many types of cancers including colorectal, breast, bladder, head and neck, lung, pancreatic and melanoma. Patients with metastatic disease are also seen to have even higher levels of circulating galectins than those with only localized tumours. Recent investigations have demonstrated that the increased circulation of these galectins actively promotes tumour cell haematogenous dissemination in metastasis. Targeting the actions of circulating galectins in the bloodstream of cancer patients therefore represents a very promising therapeutic strategy for preventing metastasis. Such a strategy may include natural or synthetic inhibitors to target the galectin molecule directly or indirectly by targeting the galectin binding ligands in the circulation. More effective inhibitors are also likely to be those that can simultaneously target the actions of multiple galectin members.

Alteration of Circulating Galectins in Cancer Patients

Increased circulation of several galectin members including galectin-2, -3, -4 and -8 have been reported to occur in a range of cancers including colorectal (*1–3*), lung (*1*), head and neck (*4*), melanoma (*5*, *6*), breast (*1*), bladder (*7*) and pancreas (*8*). The concentrations of these galectins are often seen to be further elevated in many patients with distant metastasis (*1*, *2*) and correlate with poorer prognosis in several cancer types including ovarian, thyroid and colorectal (*1*, *2*). The source of the increased circulation of these galectins in cancer patients still remains unclear but is believed to come from not only the tumour cells but also from the peri-tumoural inflammatory and stromal cells (*2*). The expressions of galectin-4 and -8 are lower in the tissues of primary colorectal cancers in comparison to those found in normal colonic epithelial cells (*9*, *10*) but are higher in the blood circulation of cancer patients (*2*, *3*).

The expressions of galectin-1 and -3 have shown to be greater in peri-tumoural tissues compared with tumour cells themselves (*11*). Serum levels of galectins -1, -3 and -4 were significantly reduced following surgical removal of the primary tumour in patients with colorectal cancer (*1*, *3*). Galectin secretion by inflammatory cells such as monocytes, macrophages and lymphocytes (*12*) has been reported to be influenced by pro-inflammatory cytokines such as GM-CSF, TNF-α, IL-1 and IL-8 that are upregulated in cancer patients (*13*). Decreased levels of circulating galectin-1 are seen in colorectal (*14*) and breast (*2*) cancer. This has been suggested to result from circulating galectin-1 being recruited from the circulation into the tumour stromal compartment (*14*), or potentially by being bound into complexes with cancer-associated serum glycoproteins (*15*). Circulating galectin-1 shows to bind almost double the amount of serum glycoprotein in patients with metastatic breast cancer compared with healthy control patients.

Galectins Modulate Cancer Cell Adhesion

Interactions between cancer cell surface associated-galectins and cell surface- or basement membrane-glycans have been shown to enhance tumour cell adhesion, invasion and intravasation of many types of tumour cell, such as melanoma, thyroid, colon and neuroendocrine (*16*). Cancer -associated galectin-1 and -3 can bind to basement membrane glycans such as fibronectin, collagen IV, elastin and laminin or to basement membrane receptors such as members of the integrin family and increases cancer cell adhesion (*17*). Galectin-8 shows high binding affinity to several integrin members and also to a splice variant of the adhesion molecule CD44 (*18*). Substrate-bound galectin-8 enhances cell adhesion by promoting β1-integrin clustering whilst soluble galectin-8 has been shown to prevent cell adhesion as a competitive binding inhibitor to the cell surface adhesion molecules (*19*, *20*). Extracellular galectin-3 is able to cross-link β1,6-acetyl-glucosaminyltransferase V (Mgat5)-modified N-glycans to cause fibronectin matrix remodelling via PI3K and FAK signalling (*21*) and also prevent endocytosis of epidermal growth factor receptor (EGFR) and transforming growth factor-β receptor (TGF-βR) by forming lattice structures and preventing interaction with negative regulator caveolin 1 (*22*, *23*).

Recent studies in our laboratory have revealed an interaction of cancer-associcated galectin-3 with the oncofetal Thomsen-Friedenreich (Galactose β1,3N-acetylgalactosamine α; TF) antigen (*24*) on cancer-associated transmembrane mucin protein MUC1 (*25–28*). MUC1 is a large and highly glycosylated transmembrane mucin protein that is expressed on only the apical surface of normal secretory epithelia but becomes over expressed and redistributed over the entire surface of ~90% epithelial cancer cells (*24*). Redistribution of the cell surface MUC1 in cancer cells has been shown to prevent intercellular interaction of much smaller adhesion molecules, thus weakening E-cadherin-mediated cell-cell or integrin-mediated cell-matrix adhesion, and enabling cancer cell invasion at primary tumour sites (*27*, *29–31*).

Circulating Galectins Enhance Cancer Cell Heterotypic Adhesion

Circulating galectin-3 levels have been shown to be increased up to ~30 fold in the blood stream of patients with several types of cancers compared to that of healthy people (*1*, *2*, *6–8*, *32*). We have shown that circulating galectin-3 interacts with the TF glycan on cancer-associated MUC1 which causes MUC1 cell surface polarization and exposure of the smaller cell surface adhesion molecules such as CD44 and E-selectin ligands, which are otherwise concealed by the large and extensively glycosylated MUC1 (Figure 1). This results in increased adhesion of cancer cells to the blood vascular endothelium (*28*).

Cancer cell adhesion to the blood vascular endothelium is an essential step in cancer cell haematogenous dissemination and is arbitrated by several adhesion molecules, such as integrins, selectins and their ligands on the surface of both cancer and endothelial cells. It is likely that tight adhesion of circulating tumour cells to the vascular endothelium may occur only after MUC1 cell-surface polarisation as the contact point between the two cell types is devoid of MUC1 (*25*). We have demonstrated that the interaction of cancer-associated MUC1 with galectin-3 increases cancer cell adhesion to, and migration through blood vascular endothelial cells and reduces metastasis-associated survival of athymic nude mice in an experimental metastasis model (*28*) (Figure 2).

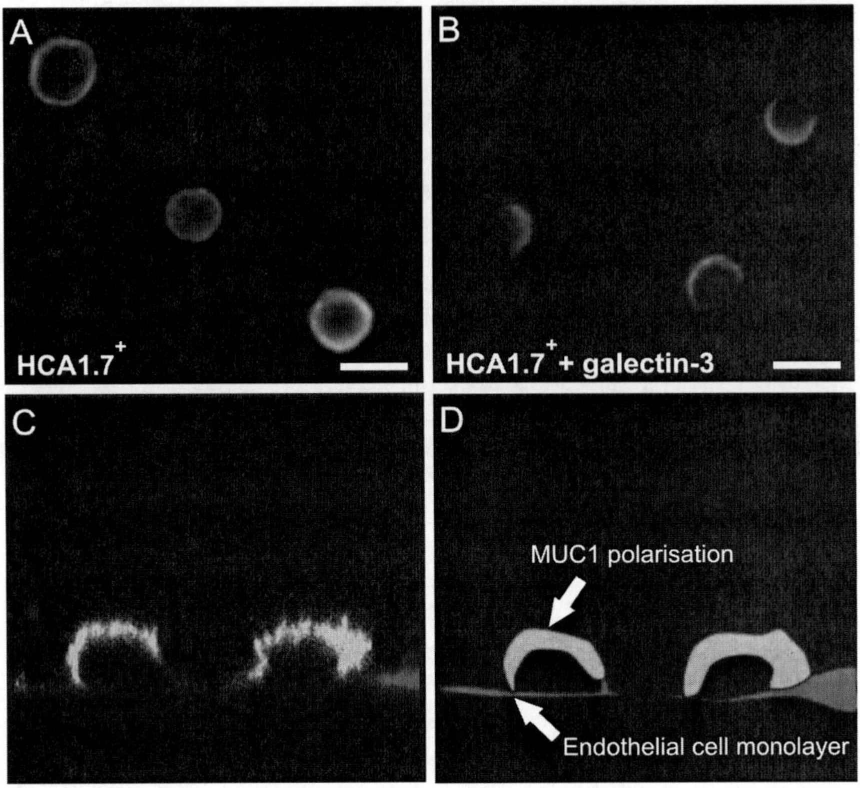

Figure 1. Galectin-3-MUC1 interaction induces MUC1 cell surface localisation. MUC1 immunohistochemistry shows homogenous MUC1 cell surface localization (A) but polarization (B) in response to galectin-3 binding (B) in the MUC1 positively-transfected HCA1.7⁺, a derivative of human breast epithelial HBL-100 cells. Confocal images (C) of galectin-3-treated HCA1.7⁺ cells in the xz plane showing absence of MUC1 (green) at the HCA1.7+ and HUVEC (red) contact points. A schematic representation of this heterotypic epithelial-endothelial adhesion illustrates the absence of MUC1 at the cell-cell junction (D). (see color insert)

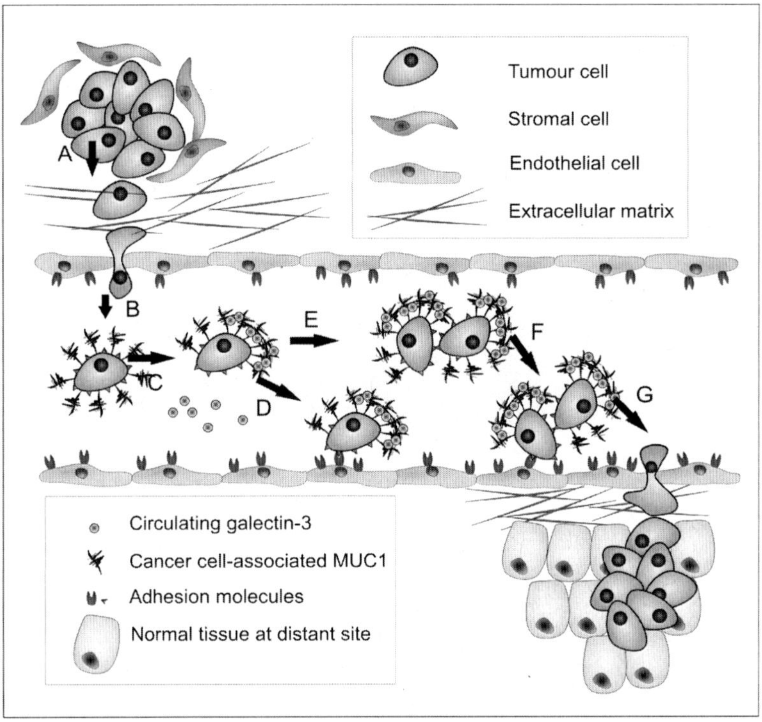

Figure 2. A schematic diagram shows how the galectin-3-MUC1 interaction in the circulation promotes cancer cell-cell and cancer cell-endothelial adhesion and metastasis. Alteration in the adhesion properties of the cancer cells with peri-tumoural stromal cells and the extracellular matrix (partly contributed by the cell-surface galectin-3) enable invasion of epithelial cancer cells through the extracellular basement matrix (A) and intravasation (B) at primary tumour sites. MUC1 over-expression on the cell surface prevents adhesion of the invaded cells with adjacent cells. MUC1 polarisation in response to binding of circulating galectin-3 induces the exposure of smaller cell surface adhesion molecules/or ligands and the cells become "sticky" (C). The "sticky" cancer cells adhere to the blood vascular endothelium (D) and they can also stick together to form micro-tumour embolic (E) (which may also subsequently bind to the endothelial cells), both of which increase cancer cell haematogenous metastasis to distant organs. (see color insert)

Circulating Galectins Promote the Formation of Tumour Micro-Emboli in the Circulation

Binding of galectin-3 (either cancer cell surface-associated galectin-3, or galectin-3 in the circulation) to cancer-associated TF glycan promotes homotypic aggregation of cancer cells in the circulation that results in the formation of micro-tumour emboli (*33–37*) and prolongs the survival of circulating tumour cells in the circulation by preventing tumour cell anoikis (*37*). Prolonged survival of the tumour cells in the circulation is known to directly increase metastasis (*38*, *39*). The formation of micro-tumour emboli in the circulation also helps mechanical trappment of the circulating tumour cells in micro-vasculature, contributing to their haematogenous dissemination (*40–42*). There is evidence that mechanical entrapment alone may not be sufficient for malignant cell arrest in target organs (*33*) and cancer cell adhesion to the endothelium is essential for cancer cell metastatic dissemination (*33*). Nethertheless, enhanced survival of tumour cells in the circulation increases the chances of their subsequent adhesion to the endothelium and extravasation into distant organs.

Recent studies have shown that circulating galectins -2, -4 and -8, levels of which are also increased in cancer patients, behave similarly to galectin-3 and may also be involved in promoting cancer cell adhesion to vascular endothelial cells by binding to cancer-associated TF antigen on MUC1 (*2*). It should be mentioned that the ultimate effects of these circulating galectins on metastasis promotion in cancer patients are likely to be influenced also by the presence of other galectin binding ligands in the circulation (*2*, *43*). This is supported by the discovery that the increased mortality-associated with higher circulating galectin-2 levels in colon cancer patients is significantly reduced when auto-anti-MUC1 antibodies with specificity for the TF epitope of MUC1 are also present in the circulation (*2*).

Targeting Galectins in the Circulation

Thus, increased circulation of galectins promotes several important steps of the cancer metastatic cascade including cancer cell heterotypic adhesion to blood vascular endothelium, cancer cell homotypic aggregation for the formation of micro-tumour emboli and angiogenesis. Targeting the actions of circulating galectins therefore represents a promising therapeutic strategy for preventing metastasis and improving patient survival. The minimal phenotypic abnormalities in mice deficient in several of the galectin family, shown in several studies (*44–46*), certainly point to such a clinically viable strategy. Effective approaches of such a strategy can include natural or synthetic inhibitors that target either the galectin molecules directly or the galectin binding ligands indirectly.

D-galactose has been shown to reduce liver metastasis when it was administered via intraperitoneal injections in experimental animal models (*47*). Monovalent carbohydrates such as galactose however tend to have weak millimolar affinity for galectins (*48*). Linking the sugars together in a multivalent fashion has been shown to greatly increase their affinity and specificity for galectin binding (*48*, *49*). The context of interaction, such as galectin-1 binding immobilised LacNAc (K_d 2-10μM) compared to LacNAc in solution (K_d 20-70μM) dramatically alters their binding affinity (*50*), suggesting that binding affinities of galectins to therapeutic inhibitors may be substantially reduced in the circulation.

The tailored synthesis of methyl β-lactoside derivatives by homology based modelling may enable the targeting of specific galectins (*51*). Potential galectin inhibitors have been created by targeting the C-3′ atom in 3′-amino-N-acetyllactosamine and the compounds with greatest affinity and specificity for galectin-3 contained an aromatic amide at C-3′ of the galactose moiety (*52*). Aromatic lactose 2-O-esters have been shown to inhibit the bindings of galectins -1, -3 and -9 (N-terminus) by interaction with arginine residues (*53*). Galectin-3 binding was selectively inhibited by tri-valent clusters of 2-propynyl-lactoside (*54*). Multi-valent enhancement in affinity has been shown specifically for galectins -1, -3, -4 (N-terminus), -5 and -9 (N-terminus) (*50*, *55–59*). However, carbohydrate-galectin inhibition may have high affinity and specificity without multivalency as is the case for galectin-8 (N-terminal CRD) bound by NeuAcα2,3Lac (*60*), small monosaccharide units of 3C triazol-1-yl-O-galactopyranosyl aldoximes bound to galectin-3 (*61*) and β-thiogalactoside modifications for the selective inhibition of galectin-7 (*62*). Short peptides have also demonstrated the ability to specifically inhibit galectin -3 (*63*).

Identification of galectin inhibitors from natural sources is another attractive approach. Pectic polysaccharides from dietary sources have been used to modify the actions of galectins, showing anti-cancer and anti-metastatic properties *in vitro* and *in vivo* (*64–68*). Modified citrus pectin, an indigestible polysaccharide from the pulp and peel of citrus fruits that are subjected to high pH and temperature treatment to yield galactose-rich forms (*67–70*) has been shown to inhibit galectin-3-associated tumour cell proliferation and angiogenesis *in vitro,* and metastasis of colon, breast (*69*), and prostate cancer *in vivo* when administered orally (*70*). Galectin-3 inhibitory activity has also been observed by treatment of breast carcinoma cell line MDA-MB-231 and buccal mucosal primary cultures from cancer patients and normal control patients with other pectic polysaccharides such as *Decalepis hamiltonii* (swallow root) (*65*). An increasing number of natural polysaccharides are now being tested for prevention of cancer initiation, promotion and metastasis. Recently, modified apple polysaccharide administered in the diet has been shown to prevent colitis-associated colon cancer, possibly by binding to galectin-3 in outbred ICR mice (*71*).

A truncated form of galectins-3 (galectin-3C), which contains only the galectin-3 C-terminal CRD so it is unable to form multimers through its N-terminal, has been shown to reduce tumour size in a multiple myeloma tumour model in NOD/SCID mice when administered into the animals via intravenous osmotic mini pump (*72*). Galectin-3C also reduced tumour size and metastasis of orthotopically implanted breast cancer cell line MDA-MD-435 when administered intramuscularly (*73*).

Antibodies raised against different regions of the galectin-3 molecule have been tested and shown to be able to modulate the ability of galectin-3 to form multimers (*74*). Portal vein injection of anti-galectin-3 antibody decreased liver metastasis of the adenocarcinoma cell lines XK4-A3 and RPMI 4788 by up to 90% (*75*).

Another promising approach, although much less well explored so far, for preventing galectin-mediated metastasis is to target the galectin ligands on cancer or endothelial cells. These galectin ligands include the cancer-associated TF (Gal β1-3 GalNAcα) disaccharide, MUC1 and endothelial-associated integrins (*76*, *77*). Administration of anti-TF antibody (clone JAA-F11) (*78*) in a murine model of breast cancer is able to inhibit lung metastasis and improve prognosis (*78*, *79*). Administration of a synthetic TF-mimic peptide, lactulose-L-leucine has been shown to prevent bone metastasis in prostate (*34*), and breast (*80*) cancer murine models (*35*). These TF-mimic peptides, which have the advantage of being much smaller single chain entities rather than multivalent IgM antibodies, have been conjugated to radionuclides to detect breast cancer in nude mice for PET imaging (*81*). Conjugation of such peptides with cytotoxic agents may provide a targeted approach to tumour-specific killing.

Concluding Remarks

Increased circulation of several members of the galectin family is now known to be significantly elevated in the bloodstream of many types of human cancers. Recent investigations have demonstrated that the increased circulation of these galactoside-binding proteins promote tumour cell haematogenous dissemination and metastasis. Targeting the actions of circulating galectins therefore represents a very promising strategy for the development of novel therapeutic agents to prevent metastasis and improve patient survival. Such a strategy could include natural or synthetic inhibitors to galectins or galectin binding ligands in the circulation. As several galectin members are often seen to be increased in the blood circulation of cancer patients, and many of them seem to have common binding ligands and produce similar biological influences on metastasis, a more effective approach of targeting circulating galectin-mediated metastasis will be the identification or design of effective inhibitors that can simultaneously target multiple galectin members, either the galectin carbohydrate binding domains or their common binding ligands.

References

1. Iurisci, I.; Tinari, N.; Natoli, C.; et al. Concentrations of galectin-3 in the sera of normal controls and cancer patients. *Clin. Cancer Res.* **2000**, *6* (4), 1389–1393.
2. Barrow, H.; Guo, X.; Wandall, H. H.; et al. Serum galectin-2, -4, and -8 are greatly increased in colon and breast cancer patients and promote cancer cell

adhesion to blood vascular endothelium. *Clin. Cancer Res.* **2011**, *17* (22), 7035–7046.

3. Watanabe, M.; Takemasa, I.; Kaneko, N.; et al. Clinical significance of circulating galectins as colorectal cancer markers. *Oncol. Rep.* **2011**, *25* (5), 1217–1226.
4. Saussez, S.; Lorfevre, F.; Lequeux, T.; et al. The determination of the levels of circulating galectin-1 and -3 in HNSCC patients could be used to monitor tumor progression and/or responses to therapy. *Oral Oncol.* **2008**, *44* (1), 86–93.
5. Vereecken, P.; Debray, C.; Petein, M.; et al. Expression of galectin-3 in primary and metastatic melanoma: Immunohistochemical studies on human lesions and nude mice xenograft tumors. *Arch. Dermatol. Res.* **2005**, *296* (8), 353–358.
6. Vereecken, P.; Heenen, M. Serum galectin-3 in advanced melanoma patients: A hypothesis on a possible role in melanoma progression and inflammation. *J Int. Med. Res.* **2006**, *34* (1), 119–120.
7. Sakaki, M.; Oka, N.; Nakanishi, R.; et al. Serum level of galectin-3 in human bladder cancer. *J. Med. Invest.* **2008**, *55* (1-2), 127–132.
8. Xie, L.; Ni, W. K.; Chen, X. D.; et al. The expressions and clinical significances of tissue and serum galectin-3 in pancreatic carcinoma. *J. Cancer Res. Clin. Oncol.* **2012**, *138*, 1035–1043.
9. Nagy, N.; Bronckart, Y.; Camby, I.; et al. Galectin-8 expression decreases in cancer compared with normal and dysplastic human colon tissue and acts significantly on human colon cancer cell migration as a suppressor. *Gut* **2002**, *50* (3), 392–401.
10. Rechreche, H; Mallo, G. V.; Montalto, G; et al. Cloning and expression of the mRNA of human galectin-4, an S-type lectin down-regulated in colorectal cancer. *Eur. J. Biochem.* **1997**, *248* (1), 225–230.
11. Sanjuan, X.; Fernandez, P. L.; Castells, A; et al. Differential expression of galectin 3 and galectin 1 in colorectal cancer progression. *Gastroenterology* **1997**, *113* (6), 1906–1915.
12. Rabinovich, G. A.; Vidal, M. Galectins and microenvironmental niches during hematopoiesis. *Curr. Opin. Hematol.* **2011**, *18* (6), 443–451.
13. Miles, F. L.; Pruitt, F. L.; van Golen, K. L.; et al. Stepping out of the flow: Capillary extravasation in cancer metastasis. *Clin. Exp. Metastasis* **2008**, *25* (4), 305–324.
14. Sheng, T. H.; Rong, L. X.; Li, Z. Y.; et al. Tissue and serum galectin-1 expression in patients with colorectal carcinoma. *Hepatogastroenterology* **2012**, *59* (114), 389–394.
15. Carlsson, M. C.; Balog, C. I.; Kilsgard, O.; et al. Different fractions of human serum glycoproteins bind galectin-1 or galectin-8, and their ratio may provide a refined biomarker for pathophysiological conditions in cancer and inflammatory disease. *Biochim. Biophys. Acta* **2012**, *1820*, 1366–1372.
16. Liu, F. T.; Rabinovich, G. A. Galectins as modulators of tumour progression. *Nat. Rev. Cancer* **2005**, *5* (1), 29–41.
17. Dumic, J.; Dabelic, S.; Flogel, M. Galectin-3: An open-ended story. *Biochim. Biophys. Acta* **2006**, *1760* (4), 616–635.

18. Cummings, R. D.; Liu, F. T. *Galectins* **2009**.
19. Levy, Y.; Arbel-Goren, R.; Hadari, Y. R.; et al. Galectin-8 functions as a matricellular modulator of cell adhesion. *J. Biol. Chem.* **2001**, *276* (33), 31285–31295.
20. Hadari, Y. R.; Arbel-Goren, R.; Levy, Y; et al. Galectin-8 binding to integrins inhibits cell adhesion and induces apoptosis. *J. Cell Sci.* **2000**, *113* (Pt 13), 2385–2397.
21. Lagana, A.; Goetz, J. G.; Cheung, P.; et al. Galectin binding to Mgat5-modified N-glycans regulates fibronectin matrix remodeling in tumor cells. *Mol. Cell Biol.* **2006**, *26* (8), 3181–3193.
22. Partridge, E. A.; Le, R. C.; Di Guglielmo, G. M.; et al. Regulation of cytokine receptors by Golgi N-glycan processing and endocytosis. *Science* **2004**, *306* (5693), 120–124.
23. Lajoie, P.; Partridge, E. A.; Guay, G.; et al. Plasma membrane domain organization regulates EGFR signaling in tumor cells. *J. Cell Biol.* **2007**, *179* (2), 341–356.
24. Yu, L. G. The oncofetal Thomsen-Friedenreich carbohydrate antigen in cancer progression. *Glycoconjugate J.* **2007**, *24* (8), 411–420.
25. Yu, L. G.; Andrews, N.; Zhao, Q.; et al. Galectin-3 interaction with Thomsen-Friedenreich disaccharide on cancer-associated MUC1 causes increased cancer cell endothelial adhesion. *J Biol. Chem.* **2007**, *282* (1), 773–781.
26. Campbell, B. J.; Finnie, I. A.; Hounsell, E. F.; et al. Direct demonstration of increased expression of Thomsen-Friedenreich (TF) antigen in colonic adenocarcinoma and ulcerative colitis mucin and its concealment in normal mucin. *J. Clin. Invest.* **1995**, *95* (2), 571–576.
27. Ligtenberg, M. J.; Buijs, F.; Vos, H. L.; et al. Suppression of cellular aggregation by high levels of episialin. *Cancer Res.* **1992**, *52* (8), 2318–2324.
28. Zhao, Q.; Guo, X.; Nash, G. B.; et al. Circulating galectin-3 promotes metastasis by modifying MUC1 localization on cancer cell surface. *Cancer Res.* **2009**, *69* (17), 6799–6806.
29. Hilkens, J.; Buijs, F.; Hilgers, J.; et al. Monoclonal antibodies against human milk-fat globule membranes detecting differentiation antigens of the mammary gland and its tumors. *Int. J. Cancer* **1984**, *34* (2), 197–206.
30. Wesseling, J.; van der Valk, S. W.; Vos, H. L.; et al. Episialin (MUC1) overexpression inhibits integrin-mediated cell adhesion to extracellular matrix components. *J. Cell Biol.* **1995**, *129* (1), 255–265.
31. Wesseling, J.; van der Valk, S. W.; Hilkens, J. A mechanism for inhibition of E-cadherin-mediated cell-cell adhesion by the membrane-associated mucin episialin/MUC1. *Mol. Biol. Cell* **1996**, *7* (4), 565–577.
32. Saussez, S.; Glinoer, D.; Chantrain, G.; et al. Serum galectin-1 and galectin-3 levels in benign and malignant nodular thyroid disease. *Thyroid* **2008**, *18* (7), 705–712.
33. Glinskii, O. V.; Huxley, V. H.; Glinsky, G. V.; et al. Mechanical entrapment is insufficient and intercellular adhesion is essential for metastatic cell arrest in distant organs. *Neoplasia* **2005**, *7* (5), 522–527.

34. Glinskii, O. V.; Sud, S.; Mossine, V. V.; et al. Inhibition of prostate cancer bone metastasis by synthetic TF antigen mimic/galectin-3 inhibitor lactulose-L-leucine. *Neoplasia* **2012**, *14* (1), 65–73.
35. Glinsky, V. V.; Glinsky, G. V.; Rittenhouse-Olson, K.; et al. The role of Thomsen-Friedenreich antigen in adhesion of human breast and prostate cancer cells to the endothelium. *Cancer Res.* **2001**, *61* (12), 4851–4857.
36. Glinsky, V. V.; Glinsky, G. V.; Glinskii, O. V.; et al. Intravascular metastatic cancer cell homotypic aggregation at the sites of primary attachment to the endothelium. *Cancer Res.* **2003**, *63* (13), 3805–3811.
37. Zhao, Q.; Barclay, M.; Hilkens, J.; et al. Interaction between circulating galectin-3 and cancer-associated MUC1 enhances tumour cell homotypic aggregation and prevents anoikis. *Mol. Cancer* **2010**, *9*, 154.
38. Takaoka, A.; Adachi, M.; Okuda, H.; et al. Anti-cell death activity promotes pulmonary metastasis of melanoma cells. *Oncogene* **1997**, *14* (24), 2971–2977.
39. Yawata, A.; Adachi, M.; Okuda, H.; et al. Prolonged cell survival enhances peritoneal dissemination of gastric cancer cells. *Oncogene* **1998**, *16* (20), 2681–2686.
40. Al-Mehdi, A. B.; Tozawa, K; Fisher, A. B.; et al. Intravascular origin of metastasis from the proliferation of endothelium-attached tumor cells: A new model for metastasis. *Nat. Med.* **2000**, *6* (1), 100–102.
41. Fidler, I. J. The pathogenesis of cancer metastasis: The 'seed and soil' hypothesis revisited. *Nat. Rev. Cancer* **2003**, *3* (6), 453–458.
42. Pantel, K.; Brakenhoff, R. H. Dissecting the metastatic cascade. *Nat. Rev. Cancer* **2004**, *4* (6), 448–456.
43. Cederfur, C.; Salomonsson, E.; Nilsson, J.; et al. Different affinity of galectins for human serum glycoproteins: Galectin-3 binds many protease inhibitors and acute phase proteins. *Glycobiology* **2008**, *18* (5), 384–394.
44. Hsu, D. K.; Yang, R. Y.; Pan, Z.; et al. Targeted disruption of the galectin-3 gene results in attenuated peritoneal inflammatory responses. *Am. J. Pathol.* **2000**, *156* (3), 1073–1083.
45. Poirier, F.; Robertson, E. J. Normal development of mice carrying a null mutation in the gene encoding the L14 S-type lectin. *Development* **1993**, *119* (4), 1229–1236.
46. Tsuboi, Y.; Abe, H.; Nakagawa, R.; et al. Galectin-9 protects mice from the Shwartzman reaction by attracting prostaglandin E2-producing polymorphonuclear leukocytes. *Clin. Immunol.* **2007**, *124* (2), 221–233.
47. Beuth, J; Ko, H. L.; Oette, K.; et al. Inhibition of liver metastasis in mice by blocking hepatocyte lectins with arabinogalactan infusions and D-galactose. *J. Cancer Res. Clin. Oncol.* **1987**, *113* (1), 51–55.
48. Vrasidas, I.; Andre, S.; Valentini, P.; et al. Rigidified multivalent lactose molecules and their interactions with mammalian galectins: A route to selective inhibitors. *Org. Biomol. Chem.* **2003**, *1* (5), 803–810.
49. Andre, S.; Pieters, R. J.; Vrasidas, I.; et al. Wedgelike glycodendrimers as inhibitors of binding of mammalian galectins to glycoproteins, lactose maxiclusters, and cell surface glycoconjugates. *ChemBioChem* **2001**, *2* (11), 822–830.

50. Leppanen, A.; Stowell, S.; Blixt, O.; et al. Dimeric galectin-1 binds with high affinity to alpha2,3-sialylated and non-sialylated terminal N-acetyllactosamine units on surface-bound extended glycans. *J. Biol. Chem.* **2005**, *280* (7), 5549–5562.
51. Solis, D.; Romero, A.; Kaltner, H.; et al. Different architecture of the combining site of the two chicken galectins revealed by chemical mapping studies with synthetic ligand derivatives. *J. Biol. Chem.* **1996**, *271* (22), 12744–12748.
52. Sorme, P.; Qian, Y.; Nyholm, P. G.; et al. Low micromolar inhibitors of galectin-3 based on 3′-derivatization of N-acetyllactosamine. *ChemBioChem* **2002**, *3* (2–3), 183–189.
53. Cumpstey, I.; Salomonsson, E.; Sundin, A.; et al. Studies of arginine-arene interactions through synthesis and evaluation of a series of galectin-binding aromatic lactose esters. *ChemBioChem* **2007**, *8* (12), 1389–1398.
54. Andre, S.; Liu, B.; Gabius, H. J.; et al. First demonstration of differential inhibition of lectin binding by synthetic tri- and tetravalent glycoclusters from cross-coupling of rigidified 2-propynyl lactoside. *Org. Biomol. Chem.* **2003**, *1* (22), 3909–3916.
55. Aplander, K.; Tejler, J.; Toftered, J.; et al. Synthesis of a 3′-naphthamido-LacNAc fluorescein conjugate with high selectivity and affinity for galectin-3. *Carbohydr. Res.* **2006**, *341* (10), 1363–1369.
56. Tejler, J; Leffler, H.; Nilsson, U. J. Synthesis of O-galactosyl aldoximes as potent LacNAc-mimetic galectin-3 inhibitors. *Bioorg. Med. Chem. Lett.* **2005**, *15* (9), 2343–2345.
57. Tejler, J.; Tullberg, E.; Frejd, T.; et al. Synthesis of multivalent lactose derivatives by 1,3-dipolar cycloadditions: Selective galectin-1 inhibition. *Carbohydr. Res.* **2006**, *341* (10), 1353–1362.
58. Tejler, J; Skogman, F.; Leffler, H.; et al. Synthesis of galactose-mimicking 1H-(1,2,3-triazol-1-yl)-mannosides as selective galectin-3 and 9N inhibitors. *Carbohydr. Res.* **2007**, *342* (12–13), 1869–1875.
59. Andre, S.; Sansone, F.; Kaltner, H.; et al. Calix[n]arene-based glycoclusters: Bioactivity of thiourea-linked galactose/lactose moieties as inhibitors of binding of medically relevant lectins to a glycoprotein and cell-surface glycoconjugates and selectivity among human adhesion/growth-regulatory galectins. *ChemBioChem* **2008**, *9* (10), 1649–1661.
60. Carlsson, S.; Oberg, C. T.; Carlsson, M. C.; et al. Affinity of galectin-8 and its carbohydrate recognition domains for ligands in solution and at the cell surface. *Glycobiology* **2007**, *17* (6), 663–676.
61. Tejler, J.; Salameh, B.; Leffler, H.; et al. Fragment-based development of triazole-substituted O-galactosyl aldoximes with fragment-induced affinity and selectivity for galectin-3. *Org. Biomol. Chem.* **2009**, *7* (19), 3982–3990.
62. Cumpstey, I.; Carlsson, S.; Leffler, H.; et al. Synthesis of a phenyl thio-beta-D-galactopyranoside library from 1,5-difluoro-2,4-dinitrobenzene: Discovery of efficient and selective monosaccharide inhibitors of galectin-7. *Org. Biomol. Chem.* **2005**, *3* (10), 1922–1932.

63. Zou, J.; Glinsky, V. V.; Landon, L. A.; et al. Peptides specific to the galectin-3 carbohydrate recognition domain inhibit metastasis-associated cancer cell adhesion. *Carcinogenesis* **2005**, *26* (2), 309–318.
64. Olano-Martin, E.; Rimbach, G. H.; Gibson, G. R.; et al. Pectin and pectic-oligosaccharides induce apoptosis in in vitro human colonic adenocarcinoma cells. *Anticancer Res.* **2003**, *23* (1A), 341–346.
65. Sathisha, U. V.; Jayaram, S.; Harish Nayaka, M. A.; et al. Inhibition of galectin-3 mediated cellular interactions by pectic polysaccharides from dietary sources. *Glycoconjugate J.* **2007**, *24* (8), 497–507.
66. Inohara, H.; Raz, A. Effects of natural complex carbohydrate (citrus pectin) on murine melanoma cell properties related to galectin-3 functions. *Glycoconjugate J.* **1994**, *11* (6), 527–532.
67. Platt, D.; Raz, A. Modulation of the lung colonization of B16-F1 melanoma cells by citrus pectin. *J. Natl. Cancer Inst.* **1992**, *84* (6), 438–42.
68. Glinsky, V. V.; Raz, A. Modified citrus pectin anti-metastatic properties: One bullet, multiple targets. *Carbohydr. Res.* **2009**, *344* (14), 1788–1791.
69. Nangia-Makker, P.; Hogan, V.; Honjo, Y.; et al. Inhibition of human cancer cell growth and metastasis in nude mice by oral intake of modified citrus pectin. *J. Natl. Cancer Inst.* **2002**, *94* (24), 1854–1862.
70. Pienta, K. J.; Naik, H.; Akhtar, A.; et al. Inhibition of spontaneous metastasis in a rat prostate cancer model by oral administration of modified citrus pectin. *J. Natl. Cancer Inst.* **1995**, *87* (5), 348–353.
71. Li, Y.; Liu, L.; Niu, Y.; et al. Modified apple polysaccharide prevents against tumorigenesis in a mouse model of colitis-associated colon cancer: Role of galectin-3 and apoptosis in cancer prevention. *Eur. J. Nutr.* **2012**, *51* (1), 107–117.
72. Mirandola, L.; Yu, Y.; Chui, K.; et al. Galectin-3C inhibits tumor growth and increases the anticancer activity of bortezomib in a murine model of human multiple myeloma. *PLoS One* **2011**, *6* (7), e21811.
73. John, C. M.; Leffler, H.; Kahl-Knutsson, B.; et al. Truncated galectin-3 inhibits tumor growth and metastasis in orthotopic nude mouse model of human breast cancer. *Clin. Cancer Res.* **2003**, *9* (6), 2374–2383.
74. Liu, F. T.; Hsu, D. K.; Zuberi, R. I.; et al. Modulation of functional properties of galectin-3 by monoclonal antibodies binding to the non-lectin domains. *Biochemistry* **1996**, *35* (19), 6073–6079.
75. Inufusa, H.; Nakamura, M.; Adachi, T.; et al. Role of galectin-3 in adenocarcinoma liver metastasis. *Int. J. Oncol.* **2001**, *19* (5), 913–919.
76. Broxterman, H. J.; Georgopapadakou, N. H. Anticancer therapeutics: A surge of new developments increasingly target tumor and stroma. *Drug Resist. Updates* **2007**, *10* (4–5), 182–193.
77. Zhao, Y.; Bachelier, R.; Treilleux, I.; et al. Tumor alphavbeta3 integrin is a therapeutic target for breast cancer bone metastases. *Cancer Res.* **2007**, *67* (12), 5821–5830.
78. Almogren, A.; Abdullah, J.; Ghapure, K.; et al. Anti-Thomsen-Friedenreich-Ag (anti-TF-Ag) potential for cancer therapy. *Front. Biosci, Scholar Ed.* **2012**, *4*, 840–863.

79. Heimburg, J.; Yan, J.; Morey, S.; et al. Inhibition of spontaneous breast cancer metastasis by anti-Thomsen-Friedenreich antigen monoclonal antibody JAA-F11. *Neoplasia* **2006**, *8* (11), 939–948.
80. Glinsky, G. V.; Price, J. E.; Glinsky, V. V.; et al. Inhibition of human breast cancer metastasis in nude mice by synthetic glycoamines. *Cancer Res.* **1996**, *56* (23), 5319–5324.
81. Kumar, S. R.; Gallazzi, F. A.; Quinn, T. P.; et al. (64)Cu-labeled peptide for PET of breast carcinomas expressing the Thomsen-Friedenreich carbohydrate antigen. *J. Nucl. Med.* **2011**, *52* (11), 1819–1826.

Galectin Mechanisms and Therapeutic Approaches in Inflammation and Fibrosis

Chapter 19

A Therapeutic Role for Galectins in Acute Inflammation?

Dianne Cooper*

William Harvey Research Institute, Barts and The London School of Medicine and Dentistry, Queen Mary University of London, Charterhouse Square, London, EC1M 6BQ, United Kingdom
***E-mail: d.cooper@qmul.ac.uk**

The inflammatory response has evolved as a protective mechanism against invading pathogens and tissue damage. However, if the inflammatory response is not contained both spatially and temporally, damage to host tissue or development of chronic pathologies can ensue. Current anti-inflammatory therapies have largely focused on the inhibition of the plethora of pro-inflammatory mediators that drive the inflammatory response and although effective many of these agents are not without side-effects. The search for novel anti-inflammatory agents is therefore still the focus of intense research. Recent studies have indicated that galectins may represent a class of endogenous proteins whose biology can be harnessed for therapeutic gain in inflammatory pathologies. This review will focus on what is known to date about the role of galectins in acute inflammation and which of these lectins represent potential novel therapeutic agents.

Introduction

Inflammation occurs as a result of tissue injury or infection in a bid, by the host, to limit damage, remove the offending agent and restore tissue homeostasis. It is a process that is crucial to host survival as evidenced by genetic diseases such as leukocyte adhesion deficiency, a class of conditions in which neutrophil trafficking is compromised; patients suffer recurrent bacterial infections and have a poor survival prognosis (*1*). Uncontrolled inflammation however, is associated with many disease states including atherosclerosis, cancer, rheumatoid arthritis and Alzheimer's disease. Although these are chronic inflammatory conditions we can, throughdeciphering what drives and then shuts off an acute inflammatory response, increase our understanding of what causes inflammation to persist.A better understanding of the molecular and cellular mechanisms that promote inflammation is therefore pertinent to the design of better anti-inflammatory therapeutics.

The distinct phases of an acute inflammatory response as depicted in Figure 1 are active phenomenons driven by pro-inflammatory and pro-resolution mediators, with both pathways required for an effective response and a subsequent return to tissue homeostasis (*2*). Initiated either by infection or tissue damage, inflammation is evident macroscopically by the cardinal signs of heat, redness, pain and swelling. These signs are the result of microscopic processes that include increased vascular permeability and edema formation and the subsequent recruitment of polymorphonuclear leukocytes (PMNs) to the inflammatory foci. This is followed by a wave of monocyte recruitment, which serves, along with macrophages to clear the inflammatory site through the non-phlogisitic process of efferocytosis of apoptotic PMNpromotinga return to normal tissue homeostasis.

Although the hallmark of an inflammatory response, excessive leukocyte recruitment can result in damage to host tissue through the release of powerful proteases and reactive oxygen species, whilst failure to clear apoptotic cells can result in the exposure of novel epitopes resulting in auto-immune conditions such as lupus (*3*). Anti-inflammatory therapies may either be directed towards inhibition of the pro-inflammatory cascade or to harnessing the effects of pro-resolution factors such asresolvins, lipoxins andAnnexinA1 (*4*, *5*). Current anti-inflammatory therapies are generally targeted towards specific enzymes or mediators that drive the inflammatory response, for example COX-2 inhibitors or anti-TNF-α biologics. Whilst these therapies are potent they are not without their risks and side-effects. COX-2 inhibition has been associated with increased risk of thrombotic events (*6*) whilst TNF-α blockade has been linked to reactivation of latent *Tuberculosis* infection (*7*). It is therefore likely that future therapies will not target enzymes such as COX-2 that are central to the production of a host of inflammatory mediators. Such limitations to current therapies have led to a revision of thinking and recent evidence suggests that targeting of the pro-resolution pathway may offer a safer alternative for future therapeutics. This review will address our current understanding of those galectins shown to have a role in the process of acute inflammation and whether these galectins fall within the class of pro-inflammatory, anti-inflammatory or pro-resolving mediators.

Understanding of the actions on cell types pertinent to inflammation will further our understanding of how galectin biology might be exploited for therapeutic gain.

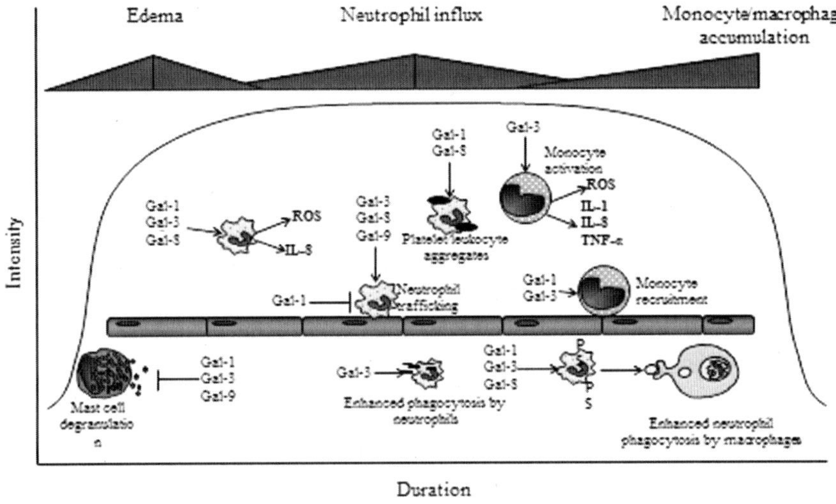

Figure 1. Schematic representing the profile of an acute inflammatory response and the major cell types involved. The acute inflammatory response is characterized by edema formation and neutrophil infiltration followed by the subsequent accumulation of monocytes and macrophages which promote resolution through the non-phlogistic phagocytosis of phosphatidylserine (PS) expressing and/or apoptotic PMN. Positive and negative effects of galectins on the various aspects of the response are indicated. (see color insert)

Galectins

Galectins are a family of evolutionary conserved carbohydrate-binding animal lectins expressed in a wide variety of tissues across species that share close sequence homology in their carbohydrate recognition domain (CRD) but exhibit distinct affinities for different saccharide ligands. The majority of galectins bind to *N*-acetyllactosamine (Galβ1,3GlcNAc or Galβ1,4GlcNAc), a common disaccharide found on many N- or O-linked glycans (*8*) with Gal-10 being an exception through its affinity for mannose-containing saccharides (*9*). Galectins can be classified based on their structure into three distinct groups: 1) proto-type galectins which have one CRD and are capable of homodimerisation (Gal-1, -2, -5, -7, -10, -13, -14, and -15), 2) chimera-type, the only member being Gal-3, which contains a single CRD with an extended N-terminus and 3) tandem repeat type which have two distinct CRDs joined by a short linker peptide (Gal-4, -6, -8, -9, and -12) (*10–12*). In terms of their ligand-binding activity galectins can be bi- or multivalent which accounts for their ability to cross-link cell surface glycoproteins. The biological response to galectins varies quite significantly between family members, which may be a result of subtle variations in their carbohydrate-binding specificities (*13*).

An ever-expanding body of literature supports a role for galectins in inflammation and autoimmune pathologies [see (*14*) and (*15*) for recent reviews]. Actions of galectinshave been identified at key stages of the inflammatory response and include: mast cell degranulation and initiation of inflammation, modulation of leukocyte trafficking, platelet activation and finally clearance of the inflammatory infiltrate and resolution of inflammation. Indicated in Figure 1 are key points of the inflammatory response where galectins have been shown to act.

Galectin Expression during Inflammation

Expression of galectins during an inflammatory response may give an insight into their actions. This is clear if one compares the early expression of cytokines such as TNF-α that drive the inflammatory response with the generation of pro-resolving mediators such as resolvins that were originally identified in murine exudates in the resolution phase of a self-limiting inflammatory response (*16*).Expression of galectins has been detected in chronic inflammatory pathologies in humans with Gal-3 present in macrophages within atherosclerotic plaques (*17*) and Gal-1, -3 and -9 detectable in synovial fluid and tissue from rheumatoid arthritis patients (*18*, *19*).

In animal models increased expression of Gal-1 and -3 can be observed in peritoneal exudates in a murine model of zymosan peritonitis (Cooper, D., Wright, R., unpublished observation) and Gal-3 levels are significantly increased in the bronchoalveolar lavage fluid of *Streptococcus pneumonia*-infected lungs (*20*, *21*). Gal-1 expression has been shown to correlate with the peak of inflammation or the onset of resolution in models of carrageenan-induced paw edema and experimental autoimmune encephalomyelitis (*22*, *23*). Interestingly, in Gal-1 null mice, Gal-9 expression increases significantly at the onset of resolution in a model of carageenan paw edema, which may suggest that in the absence of one pro-resolving galectin, another may compensate (*23*). Lidocaine, an agent shown to delay and block key events in the resolution process reduces Gal-1 expression by over 50% at the 24h time-point in a model of zymosan-induced peritonitis (*24*) further suggesting that Gal-1 may fall into the category of pro-resolving mediators.

When considering cell types pertinent to inflammation, galectins are expressed in the majority of cells, the exception being peripheral blood lymphocytes and neutrophils, which express low levels of Gal-1 and -9. In contrast vascular endothelial cells (ECs) express Gal-1, Gal-3, Gal-8 and Gal-9 under basal conditions *in vitro* (*25*, *26*) and expression is up-regulated by endothelial activation with different agents. For example, Gal-1 is increased in human umbilical vein EC (HUVEC) in response to pro-inflammatory cytokines (*25*, *26*), Gal-9 in response to IFN-γ and double-stranded RNA (*27*, *28*) and Gal-3 in response to IL-1β (*29*–*31*).

The increased vascular expression in activated endothelium along with the propensity of galectins to bind to the surface of leukocytes suggests that a loop may be in existence whereby endothelial-derived galectins act on leukocytes to either limit, in the case of Gal-1, or promote, in the case of Gal-3, -8 and -9, leukocyte recruitment. Detection of galectins within serum of type 2 diabetics (*32*) suggests that a soluble pool exists whilst studies have shown that presentation of galectins on the cell surface or extracellular matrix enhances or modifies activity (*33*). This is evident for Gal-1 expressed on the surface of HUVEC (*34*) and for immobilized galectin-8 (*35*).

Galectins in Acute Inflammation

The majority of galectin research has focused on models of auto-immunity such as experimental autoimmune encephalomyelitis and collagen induced arthritis as a result of the extensive literature reporting numerous modulatory effects on T cell biology. Studies focusing on acute inflammation are relatively scarce in comparison. *In vitro* studies have addressed the effects of galectins on the biology of mast cells, neutrophils and macrophages, all of which are key components of an acute inflammatory response whilst galectin null mice have been used in models of peritonitis, sepsis and paw edema to address the role of endogenous galectins. These findings are summarized below.

Galectin-1

Data acquired from both *in vitro*studies using recombinant Gal-1 and *in vivo* studies in Gal-1 null mice suggest that Gal-1 is a genuine therapeutic target for inflammatory conditions. Gal-1 null mice are healthy and viable but once challenged exhibit distinct phenotypes.

The first evidence of a role for Gal-1 in acute inflammation came from the Rabinovich laboratory and assessed the effects of recombinant Gal-1 administration in a model of phospholipase A2 induced paw edema (*36*). In-line with its proposed anti-inflammatory properties, significantly fewer degranulated mast cells were observed in the paws of rats treated with Gal-1 and this correlated with a reduction in edema and neutrophil infiltration, furthermore Gal-1 suppressed arachidonic acid release and PGE_2 production from LPS stimulated peritoneal macrophages (*36*). Edema formation in response to carageenan administration in the murine paw is also reduced, as is neutrophil infiltration, following administration of recombinant Gal-1, although a direct effect on mast cells was not shown (*23*). Unexpectedly, edema formation in the Gal-1 knockout mice was also reduced in comparison to wild-type animals, an effect that may have been a consequence of increased Gal-9 expression.

These findings underscore the importance of assessing the function of both the exogenous and endogenous galectin as administration of the recombinant protein can clearly function in a different manner to the endogenous protein. This may indicate differential actins of the extracellular protein versus intracellular, although this remains to be confirmed. In this respect, conditional galectin knockout mice would be advantageous and may give a more accurate reflection of galectin function in particular cell types. It also emphasizes the need for further studies in which the recombinant protein is given back to knockout animals to determine whether the null phenotype is reversed, or alternatively neutralizing antibodies or small molecule inhibitors are given to wild-type animals. Again, this will give further insight into the mechanism of action of Gal-1 in these models.

The initial study of Rabinovich hinted at a role for Gal-1 in suppressing neutrophil infiltration to the site of inflammation, a role that has since been confirmed. Neutrophils have been identified as a target for Gal-1, with increased binding upon neutrophil activation or post-transmigration reported (*37*, *38*). Intra-vital microscopy studies coupled with *in vitro* flow chamber assays have shown direct effects of recombinant Gal-1 on neutrophil trafficking (*39*, *40*) whilst Gal-1 administration also reduced neutrophil recruitment to the peritoneum in a model of zymosan induced peritonitis (*41*).

A role for the endogenous protein is supported by data reporting that knockdown of endothelial Gal-1 results in increased numbers of neutrophils being captured and subsequently rolling on TNF-α stimulated HUVEC under flow whilst significantly increased numbers of leukocytes emigrate from the microcirculation in IL-βand PAF inflamed cremasters of Gal-1 knockout mice (*39*). A direct mechanism for these inhibitory effects of Gal-1 on neutrophil trafficking has still to be elucidated but may be partly due to a distinct modulation of adhesion molecule expression on the neutrophil (*39*, *41*).

The inhibitory properties of Gal-1 on neutrophil recruitment have been observed using low (nM) concentrations of recombinant Gal-1 or through knockdown/knockout of the endogenous protein. The actions of galectins are however complex and at higher (μM) concentrations Gal-1 activates NADPH oxidase resulting in superoxide generation by primed neutrophils (*37*). This dichotomy of responses at different concentrations of Gal-1 indicates the need for further investigation of the function of Gal-1 during acute inflammation. In particular, Gal-1 receptors on neutrophils need to be identified such that the mechanism of action can be fully delineated. The effects mediated by high Gal-1 concentrations are likely to be mediated through a different receptor than those observed at low concentrations as indicated by the requirement for neutrophil priming for elicitation of superoxide generation. Although it is unlikely that μM concentrations of Gal-1 would be achieved *in vivo* these findings indicate the need for careful titration of active therapeutic doses.

Monocytes and macrophages are both a source of and a target for Gal-1 (*42*, *43*). Consistent with its largely anti-inflammatory properties, Gal-1 inhibits LPS-induced iNOS expression and consequently nitric oxide generation (*44*) as well as TNF-α and IFN-γ release from macrophages (*45*). These effects, combined with down-regulation of FcγRI and MHC-II expression suggest Gal-1 promotes alternative activation and deactivation of inflammatory macrophages (*46*).

One area of Gal-1 biology that requires further investigation if Gal-1 is to be considered an anti-inflammatory therapeutic is that of its effects on platelet biology. Platelets, in addition to their role in hemostasis, play an important role in the propagation of inflammation (*47*). This occurs through their interactions with endothelial cells and leukocytes, as well as the generation of cytokines and chemokines within the vasculature, with circulating platelet-leukocyte aggregates serving as a marker of inflammation in numerous inflammatory pathologies such as cardiovascular disease (*48*) and rheumatoid arthritis (*49*).

Recent studies have identified a role for galectins in modulating platelet behaviour; Gal-1 triggers platelet activation and the formation of platelet-leukocyte aggregates likely due to its ability to strongly induce p-selectin expression by platelets enabling their interaction with PSGL-1 on the surface of leukocytes, an interaction that results in reciprocal activation of both cell types (*50*). Gal-1 is also able to promote release of vWF from platelet alpha granules further supporting a role in platelet adhesion and thrombus formation (*51*, *52*). Use of a Gal-1 blocking antibody and studies on Gal-1 null mice also indicate a role for endogenous Gal-1 in promoting thrombus formation with prolonged bleeding times in Gal-1 null mice and decreased time to initial thrombus formation in a model of ferric chloride-induced injury (*50*, *53*). The pro-adhesive, pro-aggregatory effects of Gal-1 on platelets clearly suggest the need for further basic science studies *in vivo* to identify its effects on this important aspect of inflammation.

For an acute inflammatory response to resolve the influx of neutrophils has to be terminated and cleared. Clearance of neutrophils from the inflammatory foci is carried out by tissue resident macrophages, which ingest neutrophils that have undergone apoptosis. This process is awry in conditions such as atherosclerosis where apoptotic cells persist within plaques (*54*). Whilst galectins do not appear to induce neutrophil apoptosis they have been found to induce phosphatidylserine (PS) exposure on the surface of activated neutrophils, which serves as an "eat-me" signal and promotes subsequent phagocytosis (*38*). This process has been termed "preaparesis" and is suggested as an alternative anti-inflammatory mechanism of neutrophil clearance (*55*).

The induction of PS exposure on the surface of neutrophils by galectins is a reversible phenomenom indicating that this process is not always indicative of a commitment to apoptosis. The ability of Gal-1 to promote neutrophil clearance combined with its inhibitory effects on neutrophil trafficking suggest a pro-resolutory role for this protein. One caveat with regards to induction of PS exposure by Gal-1 was that relatively high (10μM) concentrations of were required. Even if these concentrations are achievable *in vivo*, evidence suggests that high concentrations of Gal-1 may tip the balance in favour of pro-inflammatory actions of this protein, both with regards to neutrophil activation and promotion of platelet adhesion and thrombus formation.

In-line with the potential pro-resolving effects of Gal-1 recent *in vitro* evidence has implicated a role as a chemotactic factor for monocytes but not macrophages via a pertussis toxin-sensitive pathway (*56*), a role that has also been confirmed *in vivo* in a model of zymosan induced peritonitis (*41*).Enhanced recruitment of monocytes to the inflammatory site is in-line with the potential pro-resolving effects of Gal-1 as monocyte recruitment and differentiation into macrophages is a crucial component of resolution and clearance of the inflammatory infiltrate (*57*).

On balance, the evidence to date suggests that Gal-1 is a valid therapeutic target for inflammatory conditions, The development of stable dimeric forms of Gal-1 that retain activity at low concentrations and in the absence of reducing agents as recently described (*58*) is likely to facilitate the research effort in this direction.

Galectin-3

In contrast to Gal-1, the actions of Gal-3 are suggestive of a pre-dominantly pro-inflammatory role. This however also renders Gal-3 a viable therapeutic target and the advent of specific Gal-3 inhibitors and their potential success in the cancer field and models of fibrosis is evidence of this (*59*, *60*). In-line with its pro-inflammatory actions Gal-3 induces degranulation of both IgE-sensitised and non-sensitised mast cells (*61*) and also induces mast cell apoptosis in a caspase-3 dependent manner (*62*). A role for intracellular Gal-3 is also apparent; mast cells isolated from Gal-3 null mice exhibit impaired degranulation and reduced generation of cytokines upon cross-linking of FcepsilonRI (*63*).

In contrast to Gal-1, Gal-3 is one of a small number of molecules that have been proposed to act as a soluble adhesion protein (*64*). Recombinant Gal-3 enhances adherence of human neutrophils to endothelial cell monolayers as well as the matrix proteins laminin and fibronectin*in vitro* (*15*, *21*, *65*) although it is not directly chemotactic for neutrophils (*66*). Studies investigating the putative Gal-3 receptor on neutrophils, CD66b, found that cross-linking of antibodies binding to this protein resulted in increased adhesion of the neutrophils to endothelial cells as well as release of IL-8 (*67–69*).

In vivo, Gal-3 appears to mediate neutrophil recruitment in β2 integrin-independent models such as *S. pneumoniae infection* (*70*) with significant levels of Gal-3 (>50μg/ml) detectable in BAL fluid of mice following *S. pneumoniae* infection (*20*). The reduced neutrophil recruitment observed in Gal-3 null mice correlated with increased severity of pneumonia and increased bacterial load when compared to wild-type mice (*70*). Adding back recombinant Gal-3 to null mice restored protection against pneumonia (*20*).

A role for Gal-3 in β2 integrin-dependent models of neutrophil recruitment has also been reported with Colnot*et al* (*71*) reporting decreased numbers of neutrophils in the peritoneum of Gal-3 knockout mice 4 days post thioglycollate administration, an observation that was not due to increased apoptosis or phagocytosis. The lack of maintenance of neutrophil number was not however, reproduced in a study by Hsu *et al* (*72*) with a slight but significant reduction in neutrophil recruitment at day 1 but no difference at day 4.

In addition to its effects on neutrophil trafficking, Gal-3 activates both naive and primed neutrophils as evidenced by increased superoxide generation, L-selectin shedding, CD11b upregulation and IL-8 secretion (*20*, *64*, *73*, *74*). The pro-recruitment, pro-activation effect of Gal-3 on neutrophils suggests that inhibition of Gal-3 may be beneficial in inflammatory disorders. However, given the protective effects of Gal-3 in models of pneumonia, inhibition of Gal-3 may lead to increased risk of infection.

Like Gal-1, Gal-3 is a chemoattractant for human monocytes however, more unusually it is also a macrophagechemoattractant (*75*). Expression is upregulated when monocytes differentiate into macrophages (*76*) with active secretion of Gal-3 by inflammatory macrophages observed (*77*). In-line with its largely pro-inflammatory role, exogenous Gal-3 acts on freshly isolated human monocytes to induce IL-1 and superoxide release as well as potentiating LPS-induced production (*76*, *78*) and induces TNF-α and IL-8 production in a human monocytic cell line (*79*). With regards to macrophage biology, Gal-3 is an important regulator of alternative activation; classical activation results in comparable cytokine profiles to WT cells whilst Gal-3 null macrophages exhibit significantly reduced arginase activity in response to IL-4/IL-13 (*80*). These findings combined with the increased expression and secretion of Gal-3 by alternatively activated macrophages suggests Gal-3 sustains and mediates downstream effects of this phenotype. Regulation of alternative activation of macrophages is suggestive of roles in dampening the inflammatory response and promotion of wound repair (*81*) although the need to tightly regulate such systems is emphasised by the reduced renal fibrosis observed in Gal-3 null mice (*82*, *83*).

In conjunction to its effects on neutrophils, Gal-3 also functions as an opsonin and increases the uptake of apoptotic neutrophils by human monocyte-derived macrophages (*83*) whilst mice deficient in Gal-3 exhibit reduced phagocytic clearance of apoptotic thymocytes by peritoneal macrophages (*84*). More recently, extracellular Gal-3 was identified as a ligand of the phagocytic receptor Mer receptor tyrosine kinase (MerTK); activation of this receptor through Gal-3 binding facilitated phagocytosis of apoptotic Jurkat cells by macrophages (*85*). These actions suggest that inhibition of Gal-3 may result in persistence of inflammatory infiltrates although this is not borne out by studies in Gal-3 knockout mice, which may once again be indicative of a disparity between the actions of the endogenous versus exogenous protein.

Although numerous studies have confirmed pro-inflammatory actions for Gal-3 and therefore suggest that inhibition of Gal-3 would be a viable therapeutic option for inflammatory pathologies, more evidence is required to identify specific conditions that would benefit from Gal-3 inhibition.

Galectin-8

Gal-8 has been shown to enhance neutrophil adhesion to tissue culture plates and HUVEC *in vitro* in a carbohydrate and α_M integrin (CD11b) dependent manner although evidence for a role *in vivo* is lacking (*33*, *86*). It has also been shown to induce superoxide production to levels comparable to fMLP (*33*).

As is the case for Gal-1, Gal-8 has also been shown to be a potent platelet activatorpromoting release of thromboxane A2 and ADP, alpha granule release and aggregation (*52*).

Although a limited number of studies have been performed investigating the role of Gal-8 in inflammation, initial evidence suggests its inhibition may be beneficial in some conditions, particularly those with increased risk of thrombosis.

Galectin-9

Gal-9 has numerous roles and is an exciting therapeutic target for chronic auto-immune pathologies such as rheumatoid arthritis through its ability to induce apoptosis of T cells (*87*). Its role in acute neutrophil driven pathologies however is not evident and further investigations are clearly warranted.

Gal-9 has been proposed as an autocrinestabiliser of mast cell degranulation in IgEsensitised cells (*88*), these data in conjunction with a recent study linking Gal-9 to mast cell stabilisation in a murine skin allergy model implicate a role in mast cell function downstream of IgE, however a link to mast cell function induced during acute inflammation in response to agents such as complement and bacterial products has yet to be established.

There is some evidence to support a role for Gal-9 as a chemoattractant of murine neutrophils both *in vitro* and *in vivo*in a model of the Schwartzman reaction (*89*). PMN recruited by Gal-9 into the peritoneal cavity had an anti-inflammatory phenotype that was linked to PGE_2-production suggesting Gal-9 may modulate neutrophil phenotype (*89*). The anti-inflammatory properties of Gal-9-recruited PMN were further emphasised by an enhanced inflammatory response when these mice were rendered neutropenic.

Studies using human leukocytes suggest that Gal-9 is not chemoattractive for neutrophils, at least *in vitro* (*90*) and scant evidence exists to suggest a direct role for Gal-9 in neutrophil trafficking with a single study demonstrating a pro-adhesive effect for Gal-9 in static adhesion assays using HUVEC (*86*). Such limited evidence on the role of Gal-9 in neutrophil trafficking cannot be predicative of its therapeutic potential in neutrophil driven pathologies, however it is an area that warrants further investigation. Although it seems likely that Gal-9, like Gal-8 another tandem-repeat galectin, will support leukocyte trafficking due to its ability to cross link receptors on opposing cells, the suggestion that it may alter the phenotype of the neutrophils it recruits is attractive.

Further Avenues of Study

Perhaps the area of galectin biology that still requires significant attention with regards to acute inflammation is the identification of the receptors through which galectins are acting, this along with understanding how glycosylation profiles of these receptors are altered during inflammation would allow a greater level of specificity for galectin based therapeutics. The Gal-9 receptor Tim-3 is a case in point with opposing roles in the innate and adaptive immune systems; expression of Tim-3 on monocytes and dendritic cells is linked with enhanced production of TNF-α and promotion of innate immunity, whilst its enhanced expression on TH1 cells is linked to increased apoptosis and termination of TH1 driven pathologies (*91*), effects that are both mediated through Gal-9.

The recent advent of stable forms of Gal-1 and -9 and specific inhibitors of Gal-3 is likely to advance our knowledge of galectin biology rapidly and might in the case of Gal-1 lead us to re-evaluate some of the previous findings, for example induction of apoptosis in the presence of reducing agents which have proven controversial. Forms of Gal-9 that are resistant to proteolysis are also likely to prove useful in the harsh proteolytic environment of an inflammatory lesion.

Conclusion

Anti-inflammatory therapeutics have traditionally been aimed at reducing the plethora of pro-inflammatory mediators that drive the inflammatory process. However, as our understanding of the inflammatory process increases, the mediators and pathways available as therapeutic targets increases. The wide-ranging effects of galectins on the numerous cell types that co-operate to drive and ultimately resolve an acute inflammatory response makes exploitation of their biology for therapeutic gain a challenge. Much of the research dedicated to the biology of galectins in inflammation is still at the stage of investigating the response of cells to recombinant galectins *in vitro*andclearlymore proof-of-concept studies with transgenic mice are required to detail the complex role of galectins in inflammation. However studies to date suggest that Gal-1 is a viable therapeutic proposition that warrants further investigation, whilst inhibition of Gal-3 may also prove beneficial. The role of Gal-9 in auto-immune diseases suggests it is a viable candidate for therapy however more research needs to be performed to elucidate its effects in acute inflammation.We should not be discouraged by the need for further research into this fascinating family of immune-modulators but rather seek to further our understanding of those mentioned above, with established roles in inflammation, the biology of which could then be harnessed for the development of novel therapeutics.

Funding

Funding to the Authors' laboratory for the study of galectin biology in inflammation comes from Arthritis Research UK (Non-clinical Career Development Fellowship 18103), British Heart Foundation (PhD studentship FS/10/009/28166) and the William Harvey Research Foundation.

References

1. Hanna, S.; Etzioni, A. Leukocyte adhesion deficiencies. *Ann. N. Y. Acad. Sci.* **2012**, *1250*, 50–55.
2. Gilroy, D. W.; Lawrence, T.; Perretti, M.; Rossi, A. G. Inflammatory resolution: New opportunities for drug discovery. *Nat. Rev. Drug Discovery* **2004**, *3*, 401–416.
3. Lawrence, T.; Gilroy, D. W. Chronic inflammation: A failure of resolution? *Int. J. Exp. Pathol.* **2007**, *88*, 85–94.
4. Perretti, M.; D'Acquisto, F. Annexin A1 and glucocorticoids as effectors of the resolution of inflammation. *Nat. Rev. Immunol.* **2009**, *9*, 62–70.
5. Serhan, C. N. The resolution of inflammation: The devil in the flask and in the details. *FASEB J.* **2011**, *25*, 1441–1448.

6. Mukherjee, D. Selective cyclooxygenase-2 (COX-2) inhibitors and potential risk of cardiovascular events. *Biochem. Pharmacol.* **2002**, *63*, 817–821.
7. Solovic, I.; Sester, M.; Gomez-Reino, J. J.; Rieder, H. L.; Ehlers, S.; Milburn, H. J.; Kampmann, B.; Hellmich, B.; Groves, R.; Schreiber, S.; et al. The risk of tuberculosis related to tumour necrosis factor antagonist therapies: A TBNET consensus statement. *Eur. Respir. J.* **2010**, *36*, 1185–1206.
8. Elola, M. T.; Chiesa, M. E.; Alberti, A. F.; Mordoh, J.; Fink, N. E. Galectin-1 receptors in different cell types. *J. Biomed. Sci.* **2005**, *12*, 13–29.
9. Swaminathan, G. J.; Leonidas, D. D.; Savage, M. P.; Ackerman, S. J.; Acharya, K. R. Selective recognition of mannose by the human eosinophil Charcot-Leyden crystal protein (galectin-10): A crystallographic study at 1.8 A resolution. *Biochemistry* **1999**, *38*, 13837–13843.
10. Cooper, D. N.; Barondes, S. H. God must love galectins; he made so many of them. *Glycobiology* **1999**, *9*, 979–984.
11. Leffler, H.; Carlsson, S.; Hedlund, M.; Qian, Y.; Poirier, F. Introduction to galectins. *Glycoconjugate J.* **2004**, *19*, 433–440.
12. Liu, F. T. Galectins: A new family of regulators of inflammation. *Clin. Immunol.* **2000**, *97*, 79–88.
13. Brewer, C. F.; Miceli, M. C.; Baum, L. G. Clusters, bundles, arrays and lattices: Novel mechanisms for lectin-saccharide-mediated cellular interactions. *Curr. Opin. Struct. Biol.* **2002**, *12*, 616–623.
14. Liu, F. T.; Yang, R. Y.; Hsu, D. K. Galectins in acute and chronic inflammation. *Ann. N. Y. Acad. Sci.* **2012**, *1253*, 80–91.
15. Liu, F. T.; Rabinovich, G. A. Galectins: Regulators of acute and chronic inflammation. *Ann. N. Y. Acad. Sci.* **2010**, *1183*, 158–182.
16. Norling, L. V.; Serhan, C. N. Profiling in resolving inflammatory exudates identifies novel anti-inflammatory and pro-resolving mediators and signals for termination. *J. Intern. Med.* **2010**, *268*, 15–24.
17. Nachtigal, M.; Al-Assaad, Z.; Mayer, E. P.; Kim, K.; Monsigny, M. Galectin-3 expression in human atherosclerotic lesions. *Am. J. Pathol.* **1998**, *152*, 1199–1208.
18. Ohshima, S.; Kuchen, S.; Seemayer, C. A.; Kyburz, D.; Hirt, A.; Klinzing, S.; Michel, B. A.; Gay, R. E.; Liu, F. T.; Gay, S; et al. Galectin 3 and its binding protein in rheumatoid arthritis. *Arthritis Rheum.* **2003**, *48*, 2788–2795.
19. Seki, M.; Sakata, K. M.; Oomizu, S.; Arikawa, T.; Sakata, A.; Ueno, M.; Nobumoto, A.; Niki, T.; Saita, N.; Ito, K.; et al. Beneficial effect of galectin 9 on rheumatoid arthritis by induction of apoptosis of synovial fibroblasts. *Arthritis Rheum.* **2007**, *56*, 3968–3976.
20. Farnworth, S. L.; Henderson, N. C.; Mackinnon, A. C.; Atkinson, K. M.; Wilkinson, T.; Dhaliwal, K.; Hayashi, K.; Simpson, A. J.; Rossi, A. G.; Haslett, C.; et al. Galectin-3 reduces the severity of pneumococcal pneumonia by augmenting neutrophil function. *Am. J. Pathol.* **2008**, *172*, 395–405.
21. Sato, S.; Ouellet, N.; Pelletier, I.; Simard, M.; Rancourt, A; Bergeron, M. G. Role of galectin-3 as an adhesion molecule for neutrophil extravasation during streptococcal pneumonia. *J. Immunol.* **2002**, *168*, 1813–1822.

22. Ilarregui, J. M.; Croci, D. O.; Bianco, G. A.; Toscano, M. A.; Salatino, M.; Vermeulen, M. E.; Geffner, J. R.; Rabinovich, G. A. Tolerogenic signals delivered by dendritic cells to T cells through a galectin-1-driven immunoregulatory circuit involving interleukin 27 and interleukin 10. *Nat. Immunol.* **2009**, *10*, 981–991.
23. Iqbal, A. J.; Sampaio, A. L.; Maione, F.; Greco, K. V.; Niki, T.; Hirashima, M.; Perretti, M.; Cooper, D. Endogenous galectin-1 and acute inflammation: Emerging notion of a galectin-9 pro-resolving effect. *Am. J. Pathol.* **2011**, *178*, 1201–1209.
24. Chiang, N.; Schwab, J. M.; Fredman, G.; Kasuga, K.; Gelman, S.; Serhan, C. N. Anesthetics impact the resolution of inflammation. *PLoS One* **2008**, *3*, e1879.
25. Baum, L. G.; Seilhamer, J. J.; Pang, M.; Levine, W. B.; Beynon, D.; Berliner, J. A. Synthesis of an endogeneous lectin, galectin-1, by human endothelial cells is up-regulated by endothelial cell activation. *Glycoconjugate J.* **1995**, *12*, 63–68.
26. Thijssen, V. L.; Hulsmans, S.; Griffioen, A. W. The galectin profile of the endothelium: Altered expression and localization in activated and tumor endothelial cells. *Am. J. Pathol.* **2008**, *172*, 545–553.
27. Imaizumi, T.; Kumagai, M.; Sasaki, N.; Kurotaki, H.; Mori, F.; Seki, M.; Nishi, N.; Fujimoto, K.; Tanji, K.; Shibata, T; et al. Interferon-gamma stimulates the expression of galectin-9 in cultured human endothelial cells. *J. Leukoc. Biol.* **2002**, *72*, 486–491.
28. Ishikawa, A.; Imaizumi, T.; Yoshida, H.; Nishi, N.; Nakamura, T.; Hirashima, M.; Satoh, K Double-stranded RNA enhances the expression of galectin-9 in vascular endothelial cells. *Immunol. Cell Biol.* **2004**, *82*, 410–414.
29. Darrow, A. L.; Shohet, R. V.; Maresh, J. G. Transcriptional analysis of the endothelial response to diabetes reveals a role for galectin-3. *Physiol. Genomics* **2011**, *43*, 1144–1152.
30. Deo, P.; Glenn, J. V.; Powell, L. A.; Stitt, A. W.; Ames, J. M. Upregulation of oxidative stress markers in human microvascular endothelial cells by complexes of serum albumin and digestion products of glycated casein. *J. Biochem. Mol. Toxicol.* **2009**, *23*, 364–372.
31. Rao, S. P.; Wang, Z.; Zuberi, R. I.; Sikora, L.; Bahaie, N. S.; Zuraw, B. L.; Liu, F. T.; Sriramarao, P. Galectin-3 functions as an adhesion molecule to support eosinophil rolling and adhesion under conditions of flow. *J. Immunol.* **2007**, *179*, 7800–7807.
32. Weigert, J.; Neumeier, M.; Wanninger, J.; Bauer, S.; Farkas, S.; Scherer, MN; Schnitzbauer, A.; Schaffler, A.; Aslanidis, C.; Scholmerich, J; et al. Serum galectin-3 is elevated in obesity and negatively correlates with glycosylated hemoglobin in type 2 diabetes. *J. Clin. Endocrinol. Metab.* **2010**, *95*, 1404–1411.
33. Nishi, N.; Shoji, H.; Seki, M.; Itoh, A.; Miyanaka, H.; Yuube, K.; Hirashima, M.; Nakamura, T. Galectin-8 modulates neutrophil function via interaction with integrin alphaM. *Glycobiology* **2003**, *13*, 755–763.

34. He, J.; Baum, L. G. Endothelial cell expression of galectin-1 induced by prostate cancer cells inhibits T-cell transendothelial migration. *Lab. Invest.* **2006**, *86*, 578–590.
35. Carcamo, C.; Pardo, E.; Oyanadel, C.; Bravo-Zehnder, M.; Bull, P.; Caceres, M.; Martinez, J.; Massardo, L.; Jacobelli, S.; Gonzalez, A.; et al. Galectin-8 binds specific beta1 integrins and induces polarized spreading highlighted by asymmetric lamellipodia in Jurkat T cells. *Exp. Cell Res.* **2006**, *312*, 374–386.
36. Rabinovich, G. A.; Sotomayor, C. E.; Riera, C. M.; Bianco, I.; Correa, S. G. Evidence of a role for galectin-1 in acute inflammation. *Eur. J. Immunol.* **2000**, *30*, 1331–1339.
37. Almkvist, J.; Dahlgren, C.; Leffler, H.; Karlsson, A. Activation of the neutrophil nicotinamide adenine dinucleotide phosphate oxidase by galectin-1. *J. Immunol.* **2002**, *168*, 4034–4041.
38. Dias-Baruffi, M.; Zhu, H.; Cho, M.; Karmakar, S.; McEver, R. P.; Cummings, R. D. Dimeric galectin-1 induces surface exposure of phosphatidylserine and phagocytic recognition of leukocytes without inducing apoptosis. *J. Biol. Chem.* **2003**, *278*, 41282–41293.
39. Cooper, D.; Norling, L. V.; Perretti, M. Novel insights into the inhibitory effects of Galectin-1 on neutrophil recruitment under flow. *J. Leukoc. Biol.* **2008**, *83*, 1459–1466.
40. La, M.; Cao, T. V.; Cerchiaro, G.; Chilton, K.; Hirabayashi, J.; Kasai, K.; Oliani, S. M.; Chernajovsky, Y.; Perretti, M. A novel biological activity for galectin-1: Inhibition of leukocyte-endothelial cell interactions in experimental inflammation. *Am. J. Pathol.* **2003**, *163*, 1505–1515.
41. Gil, C. D.; Gullo, C. E.; Oliani, S. M. Effect of exogenous galectin-1 on leukocyte migration: Modulation of cytokine levels and adhesion molecules. *Int. J. Clin. Exp. Pathol.* **2010**, *4*, 74–84.
42. Rabinovich, G.; Castagna, L.; Landa, C.; Riera, C. M.; Sotomayor, C. Regulated expression of a 16-kd galectin-like protein in activated rat macrophages. *J. Leukoc. Biol.* **1996**, *59*, 363–370.
43. Rabinovich, G. A.; Iglesias, M. M.; Modesti, N. M.; Castagna, L. F.; Wolfenstein-Todel, C.; Riera, C. M.; Sotomayor, C. E. Activated rat macrophages produce a galectin-1-like protein that induces apoptosis of T cells: Biochemical and functional characterization. *J. Immunol.* **1998**, *160*, 4831–4840.
44. Correa, S. G.; Sotomayor, C. E.; Aoki, M. P.; Maldonado, C. A.; Rabinovich, G. A. Opposite effects of galectin-1 on alternative metabolic pathways of L-arginine in resident, inflammatory, and activated macrophages. *Glycobiology* **2003**, *13*, 119–128.
45. Santucci, L.; Fiorucci, S.; Cammilleri, F.; Servillo, G.; Federici, B.; Morelli, A. Galectin-1 exerts immunomodulatory and protective effects on concanavalin A-induced hepatitis in mice. *Hepatology* **2000**, *31*, 399–406.
46. Barrionuevo, P.; Beigier-Bompadre, M.; Ilarregui, J. M.; Toscano, MA; Bianco, GA; Isturiz, M. A.; Rabinovich, G. A. A novel function for galectin-1 at the crossroad of innate and adaptive immunity: Galectin-1 regulates

monocyte/macrophage physiology through a nonapoptotic ERK-dependent pathway. *J. Immunol.* **2007**, *178*, 436–445.

47. Tailor, A.; Cooper, D.; Granger, D. N. Platelet-vessel wall interactions in the microcirculation. *Microcirculation* **2005**, *12*, 275–285.
48. Michelson, A. D.; Barnard, M. R.; Krueger, L. A.; Valeri, C. R.; Furman, M. I. Circulating monocyte-platelet aggregates are a more sensitive marker of in vivo platelet activation than platelet surface P-selectin: Studies in baboons, human coronary intervention, and human acute myocardial infarction. *Circulation* **2001**, *104*, 1533–1537.
49. Joseph, J. E.; Harrison, P.; Mackie, I. J.; Isenberg, D. A.; Machin, S. J. Increased circulating platelet-leucocyte complexes and platelet activation in patients with antiphospholipid syndrome, systemic lupus erythematosus and rheumatoid arthritis. *Br. J. Haematol.* **2001**, *115*, 451–459.
50. Pacienza, N.; Pozner, R. G.; Bianco, G. A.; D'Atri, L. P.; Croci, D. O.; Negrotto, S.; Malaver, E.; Gomez, R. M.; Rabinovich, G. A.; Schattner, M. The immunoregulatory glycan-binding protein galectin-1 triggers human platelet activation. *FASEB J.* **2008**, *22*, 1113–1123.
51. Romaniuk, M. A.; Negrotto, S.; Campetella, O.; Rabinovich, G. A.; Schattner, M. Identification of galectins as novel regulators of platelet signaling and function. *IUBMB Life* **2011**, *63*, 521–527.
52. Romaniuk, M. A.; Tribulatti, M. V.; Cattaneo, V.; Lapponi, M. J.; Molinas, F. C.; Campetella, O.; Schattner, M Human platelets express and are activated by galectin-8. *Biochem. J.* **2010**, *432*, 535–547.
53. Saint-Lu, N.; Oortwijn, B. D.; Pegon, J. N.; Odouard, S.; Christophe, O. D.; de Groot, PG; Denis, C. V.; Lenting, P. J. Identification of galectin-1 and galectin-3 as novel partners for von Willebrand factor. *Arterioscler. Thromb. Vasc. Biol.* **2012**, *32*, 894–901.
54. Thorp, E.; Subramanian, M.; Tabas, I The role of macrophages and dendritic cells in the clearance of apoptotic cells in advanced atherosclerosis. *Eur. J. Immunol.* **2011**, *41*, 2515–2518.
55. Stowell, S. R.; Qian, Y.; Karmakar, S.; Koyama, N. S.; Dias-Baruffi, M.; Leffler, H.; McEver, R. P.; Cummings, R. D. Differential roles of galectin-1 and galectin-3 in regulating leukocyte viability and cytokine secretion. *J. Immunol.* **2008**, *180*, 3091–3102.
56. Malik, R. K.; Ghurye, R. R.; Lawrence-Watt, D. J.; Stewart, H. J. Galectin-1 stimulates monocyte chemotaxis via the p44/42 MAP kinase pathway and a pertussis toxin-sensitive pathway. *Glycobiology* **2009**, *19*, 1402–1407.
57. Gordon, S.; Taylor, P. R. Monocyte and macrophage heterogeneity. *Nat. Rev. Immunol.* **2005**, *5*, 953–964.
58. Cedeno-Laurent, F.; Dimitroff, C. J. Galectin-1 research in T cell immunity: Past, present and future. *Clin. Immunol.* **2012**, *142*, 107–116.
59. Mackinnon, A. C.; Gibbons, M. A.; Farnworth, S. L.; Leffler, H.; Nilsson, U. J.; Delaine, T.; Simpson, A. J.; Forbes, S. J.; Hirani, N.; Gauldie, J.; et al. Regulation of transforming growth factor-beta1-driven lung fibrosis by galectin-3. *Am. J. Respir. Crit. Care Med.* **2012**, *185*, 537–546.

60. Streetly, M. J.; Maharaj, L.; Joel, S.; Schey, S. A.; Gribben, J. G.; Cotter, F. E. GCS-100, a novel galectin-3 antagonist, modulates MCL-1, NOXA, and cell cycle to induce myeloma cell death. *Blood* **2010**, *115*, 3939–3948.
61. Frigeri, L. G.; Zuberi, R. I.; Liu, F. T. Epsilon BP, a beta-galactoside-binding animal lectin, recognizes IgE receptor (Fc epsilon RI) and activates mast cells. *Biochemistry* **1993**, *32*, 7644–7649.
62. Suzuki, Y.; Inoue, T.; Yoshimaru, T.; Ra, C. Galectin-3 but not galectin-1 induces mast cell death by oxidative stress and mitochondrial permeability transition. *Biochim. Biophys. Acta* **2008**, *1783*, 924–934.
63. Chen, H. Y.; Sharma, B. B.; Yu, L.; Zuberi, R.; Weng, I. C.; Kawakami, Y.; Kawakami, T.; Hsu, D. K.; Liu, F. T. Role of galectin-3 in mast cell functions: Galectin-3-deficient mast cells exhibit impaired mediator release and defective JNK expression. *J. Immunol.* **2006**, *177*, 4991–4997.
64. Nieminen, J.; St-Pierre, C.; Sato, S. Galectin-3 interacts with naive and primed neutrophils, inducing innate immune responses. *J. Leukoc. Biol.* **2005**, *78*, 1127–1135.
65. Kuwabara, I.; Liu, F. T. Galectin-3 promotes adhesion of human neutrophils to laminin. *J. Immunol.* **1996**, *156*, 3939–3944.
66. Baseras, B.; Gaida, M. M.; Kahle, N.; Schuppel, A. K.; Kathrey, D.; Prior, B.; Wente, M.; Hansch, G. M. Galectin-3 inhibits the chemotaxis of human polymorphonuclear neutrophils in vitro. *Immunobiology* **2012**, *217*, 83–90.
67. Feuk-Lagerstedt, E.; Jordan, E. T.; Leffler, H.; Dahlgren, C.; Karlsson, A. Identification of CD66a and CD66b as the major galectin-3 receptor candidates in human neutrophils. *J. Immunol.* **1999**, *163*, 5592–5598.
68. Schroder, A. K.; Uciechowski, P.; Fleischer, D.; Rink, L. Crosslinking of CD66B on peripheral blood neutrophils mediates the release of interleukin-8 from intracellular storage. *Hum. Immunol.* **2006**, *67*, 676–682.
69. Skubitz, K. M.; Campbell, K. D.; Skubitz, A. P. CD66a, CD66b, CD66c, and CD66d each independently stimulate neutrophils. *J. Leukoc. Biol.* **1996**, *60*, 106–117.
70. Nieminen, J.; St-Pierre, C.; Bhaumik, P.; Poirier, F.; Sato, S. Role of galectin-3 in leukocyte recruitment in a murine model of lung infection by Streptococcus pneumoniae. *J. Immunol.* **2008**, *180*, 2466–2473.
71. Colnot, C.; Ripoche, M. A.; Milon, G.; Montagutelli, X.; Crocker, P. R.; Poirier, F. Maintenance of granulocyte numbers during acute peritonitis is defective in galectin-3-null mutant mice. *Immunology* **1998**, *94*, 290–296.
72. Hsu, D. K.; Yang, R. Y.; Pan, Z.; Yu, L.; Salomon, D. R.; Fung-Leung, W. P.; Liu, F. T. Targeted disruption of the galectin-3 gene results in attenuated peritoneal inflammatory responses. *Am. J. Pathol.* **2000**, *156*, 1073–1083.
73. Karlsson, A.; Follin, P.; Leffler, H.; Dahlgren, C. Galectin-3 activates the NADPH-oxidase in exudated but not peripheral blood neutrophils. *Blood* **1998**, *91*, 3430–3438.
74. Yamaoka, A.; Kuwabara, I.; Frigeri, L. G.; Liu, F. T. A human lectin, galectin-3 (epsilon bp/Mac-2), stimulates superoxide production by neutrophils. *J. Immunol.* **1995**, *154*, 3479–3487.

75. Sano, H.; Hsu, D. K.; Yu, L.; Apgar, J. R.; Kuwabara, I.; Yamanaka, T.; Hirashima, M.; Liu, F. T. Human galectin-3 is a novel chemoattractant for monocytes and macrophages. *J. Immunol.* **2000**, *165*, 2156–2164.
76. Liu, F. T.; Hsu, D. K.; Zuberi, R. I.; Kuwabara, I.; Chi, E. Y.; Henderson, W. R., Jr. Expression and function of galectin-3, a beta-galactoside-binding lectin, in human monocytes and macrophages. *Am J Pathol* **1995**, *147*, 1016–1028.
77. Sato, S.; Hughes, R. C. Regulation of secretion and surface expression of Mac-2, a galactoside-binding protein of macrophages. *J. Biol. Chem.* **1994**, *269*, 4424–4430.
78. Jeng, K. C.; Frigeri, L. G.; Liu, F. T. An endogenous lectin, galectin-3 (epsilon BP/Mac-2), potentiates IL-1 production by human monocytes. *Immunol. Lett.* **1994**, *42*, 113–116.
79. Nishi, Y.; Sano, H.; Kawashima, T.; Okada, T.; Kuroda, T.; Kikkawa, K.; Kawashima, S.; Tanabe, M.; Goto, T.; Matsuzawa, Y.; et al. Role of galectin-3 in human pulmonary fibrosis. *Allergol. Int.* **2007**, *56*, 57–65.
80. MacKinnon, A. C.; Farnworth, S. L.; Hodkinson, PS; Henderson, N. C.; Atkinson, K. M.; Leffler, H.; Nilsson, U. J.; Haslett, C.; Forbes, S. J.; Sethi, T. Regulation of alternative macrophage activation by galectin-3. *J. Immunol.* **2008**, *180*, 2650–2658.
81. Varin, A.; Gordon, S. Alternative activation of macrophages: Immune function and cellular biology. *Immunobiology* **2009**, *214*, 630–641.
82. Henderson, N. C.; Mackinnon, A. C.; Farnworth, S. L.; Kipari, T.; Haslett, C.; Iredale, J. P.; Liu, F. T.; Hughes, J.; Sethi, T. Galectin-3 expression and secretion links macrophages to the promotion of renal fibrosis. *Am. J. Pathol.* **2008**, *172*, 288–298.
83. Karlsson, A.; Christenson, K.; Matlak, M.; Bjorstad, A.; Brown, K. L.; Telemo, E.; Salomonsson, E.; Leffler, H.; Bylund, J. Galectin-3 functions as an opsonin and enhances the macrophage clearance of apoptotic neutrophils. *Glycobiology* **2009**, *19*, 16–20.
84. Sano, H.; Hsu, D. K.; Apgar, J. R.; Yu, L.; Sharma, B. B.; Kuwabara, I.; Izui, S.; Liu, F. T. Critical role of galectin-3 in phagocytosis by macrophages. *J. Clin. Invest.* **2003**, *112*, 389–397.
85. Caberoy, N. B.; Alvarado, G.; Bigcas, J. L.; Li, W. Galectin-3 is a new MerTK-specific eat-me signal. *J. Cell. Physiol.* **2012**, *227*, 401–407.
86. Yamamoto, H.; Nishi, N.; Shoji, H.; Itoh, A.; Lu, L. H.; Hirashima, M.; Nakamura, T. Induction of cell adhesion by galectin-8 and its target molecules in Jurkat T-cells. *J. Biochem.* **2008**, *143*, 311–324.
87. Zhu, C.; Anderson, A. C.; Schubart, A.; Xiong, H.; Imitola, J.; Khoury, S. J.; Zheng, X. X.; Strom, T. B.; Kuchroo, V. K. The Tim-3 ligand galectin-9 negatively regulates T helper type 1 immunity. *Nat. Immunol.* **2005**, *6*, 1245–1252.
88. Niki, T.; Tsutsui, S.; Hirose, S.; Aradono, S.; Sugimoto, Y.; Takeshita, K.; Nishi, N.; Hirashima, M. Galectin-9 is a high affinity IgE-binding lectin with anti-allergic effect by blocking IgE-antigen complex formation. *J. Biol. Chem.* **2009**, *284*, 32344–32352.

89. Tsuboi, Y.; Abe, H.; Nakagawa, R.; Oomizu, S.; Watanabe, K.; Nishi, N.; Nakamura, T.; Yamauchi, A.; Hirashima, M. Galectin-9 protects mice from the Shwartzman reaction by attracting prostaglandin E2-producing polymorphonuclear leukocytes. *Clin. Immunol.* **2007**, *124*, 221–233.
90. Matsumoto, R.; Matsumoto, H.; Seki, M.; Hata, M.; Asano, Y.; Kanegasaki, S.; Stevens, R. L.; Hirashima, M. Human ecalectin, a variant of human galectin-9, is a novel eosinophil chemoattractant produced by T lymphocytes. *J. Biol. Chem.* **1998**, *273*, 16976–16984.
91. Anderson, A. C.; Anderson, D. E.; Bregoli, L.; Hastings, W. D.; Kassam, N.; Lei, C.; Chandwaskar, R.; Karman, J.; Su, E. W.; Hirashima, M.; et al. Promotion of tissue inflammation by the immune receptor Tim-3 expressed on innate immune cells. *Science* **2007**, *318*, 1141–1143.

Chapter 20

Galectins in Immune and Inflammatory Diseases: Insights from Experiments with Galectin Deficient Mice

Daniel K. Hsu,[1,2] Ri-Yao Yang,[2] Agnes Fermin,[2] and Fu-Tong Liu*,[1,2]

[1]Institute of Biomedical Sciences, Academia Sinica, Taipei, Taiwan
[2]Department of Dermatology, University of California-Davis, Sacramento, California
***E-mail: fliu@ucdavis.edu**

Defining the properties of the multifunctional galectin family are particularly challenging, but has been facilitated by the creation of transgenic animals. In these respects, functions of broadly studied galectin-1, -3, and -9, have advanced considerably as a result of close examinations of knockout mice. While the pro-apoptotic properties of extracellular galectin-1 and -9 were determined in vitro, the spectrum of their regulatory functions in T helper cell influence was revealed by studies in galectin-1 and galectin-9 knockout (ko) mice. Both galectins were found to suppress Th1 and Th17 function by killing of these Th cells. Thus, they are both potential therapeutic agents for immune and inflammatory diseases. The functions of galectin-3 in several disease models have been explored and this protein appears to serve a pro-inflammatory role, predominantly by promoting cytokine production and infiltration of inflammatory cells, as well as prolonging inflammatory cell survival. The properties of galectin-3 as a promoter of fibrosis were confirmed as well in multiple disease models mediated by inflammatory changes. These studies support selection of galectin-3 as a therapeutic target of immune and inflammatory diseases.

Introduction

A large number of functions have been demonstrated for galectins *in vitro*. The majority of these were accomplished by adding recombinant proteins to cultured cells. Some were achieved by transfecting cells with galectins or by suppressing expression of a given galectin by siRNA or antisense oligonucleotides. An increasing number of functions have been demonstrated *in vivo*. Most of these were performed by injecting recombinant proteins either locally or systemically in experimental animals. A small number of studies were achieved by administration of plasmids coding for galectins. The roles of galectins in various diseases have been suggested through these experiments. However, additional investigations were required to establish whether they represent the functions of the endogenous proteins and reflect the roles of these proteins in the diseases in question. For some galectins, especially galectin-3, the use of their inhibitors in *in vitro* experiments has also shed light on their functions and, furthermore, some of these inhibitors were shown to be effective *in vivo*. When used in disease models, the results highlighted selective galectins as potential therapeutic targets and, moreover, they suggested the therapeutic use of these inhibitors in humans. However, the specificity of these inhibitors has not been firmly established *in vivo* and whether their effects indeed result from specifically targeting the given galectins has yet to be definitively established.

An increasing number of studies have demonstrated the roles of galectins in models of human diseases by using genetically engineered mice deficient in a given galectin (referred to as knock out (ko) mice herein). This review focuses on those diseases in which immune and inflammatory responses play an important role in their pathogenesis.

Allergic Disease

The role of galectin-3 in human asthma was addressed by the use of a mouse model in which animals were sensitized systemically with ovalbumin (OVA) and then challenged in the airways. OVA-sensitized gal3 ko mice developed lower degrees of eosinophilia and goblet cell metaplasia in the airways, after OVA challenge compared to similarly treated wild-type mice. In addition, OVA-sensitized gal3 ko mice developed significantly lower airway hyperresponsiveness after the challenge compared to wild-type mice (*1*). The role of galectin-3 in chronic asthma was subsequently studied by comparing wild-type and gal3 ko mice subjected to repetitive airway allergen challenge with OVA up to 12 wk. Gal3 ko mice contained significantly lower numbers of eosinophils in the airways compared to wild-type mice; this was correlated with lower levels of chemokines associated with eosinophil recruitment. Importantly, gal3 ko mice exhibited substantially lower degrees of airway remodeling, compared to wild-type mice, manifested as subepithelial fibrosis, smooth muscle thickness, and peribronchial angiogenesis (*2*).

In inflamed airways, galectin-3 is expressed by both epithelial cells and inflammatory cells; bronchoalveolar lavage fluid from OVA-challenged mice contained significantly higher levels of galectin-3 compared to control mice

(*1*), suggesting that galectin-3 is released by the cells under the experimental conditions. How and whether secreted galectin-3 contributes to the airway inflammatory response and which cell type(s) are influenced by galectin-3 are uncertain. The possibility also exists that galectin-3 functions intracellularly through airway epithelial cells and inflammatory cells. In both of the above models, gal3 ko mice developed a lower Th2 response, but a higher Th1 response, suggesting that galectin-3 is required for an optimal Th2 response.

The role of galectin-3 in the development of allergic skin inflammation was investigated by comparing wild-type and gal3 ko mice after repeated epicutaneous sensitization with OVA (*3*). Epidermal thickening was attenuated and dermal eosinophil infiltrations were lower in gal3 ko mice relative to wild-type. Similar to airway inflammation, gal3 ko mice exhibited Th1 polarization associated with lower levels of IgE in the serum and lower expression of interleukin-4 mRNA, but higher expression of IFNγ mRNA at OVA-treated skin sites. Finally, when exposed to OVA, recipients engrafted with T cells from gal3 ko OVA-specific T cell receptor transgenic mice developed significantly attenuated dermatitis and a markedly lower Th2 response compared with recipients of comparable wild-type T cells. These results suggest galectin-3 promotes the Th2 response through T cells. However, there is evidence that the protein functions also through dendritic cells (DCs) (*3*).

In a model of contact dermatitis, which is a manifestation of delayed-type hypersensitivity, gal3 ko mice developed lower responses relative to wild-type mice as measured by skin thickness (*4*). DCs derived from gal3 ko bone marrow exhibited defective chemotaxis toward chemokines compared to wild-type cells, and cutaneous DCs in gal3 ko mice displayed reduced migration to draining lymph nodes upon hapten stimulation, a process that is critical in the development of contact dermatitis. From the perspective of Th1-Th2 polarization, gal3 ko mice would be expected to mount a higher response, if contact sensitivity is Th1 driven through either DCs or T cells, because galectin-3 promotes the Th2 response as explained above. Thus, in this system, the positive effect of galectin-3 on DC migration may be dominating over its other effects through DCs or T cells.

The *in vivo* general inflammatory role of galectin-3 was first observed in a model of chemical peritonitis. Gal3 ko mice developed attenuated inflammatory cell infiltrations compared to wild-type mice, associated with lower numbers of neutrophils in one study (*5*), but also lower numbers of macrophages in another (*6*). Thus, galectin-3 promotes inflammatory responses in general and Th2-mediated allergic responses, in particular. These results suggest that galectin-3 may be a target for the treatment these inflammatory disorders. It is to be mentioned, however, that other investigators observed reduction of eosinophil infiltrations in rats and mice treated by intranasal delivery of cDNA encoding galectin-3 following airway antigen challenge (*7*, *8*). It thus appears that transgenic galectin-3 may not represent the functions of endogenous galectin-3 and this could be due to differences in the tissues and cells in which the transgenic protein was expressed relative to the endogenous protein. Nevertheless, these additional studies suggest that administration of galectin-3 plasmids may be suitable for treatment of allergic inflammation.

Autoimmune Disease

A number of studies demonstrated that administration of recombinant galectin-1 and -9 decreased autoimmune disease in experimental models. Data from experiments employing galectin-deficient mice are consistent with the immunosuppressive functions of these two galectins. The role of galectin-3 in mouse models of autoimmune disease has also been revealed in gal3 ko mice.

a. Systemic Lupus Erythematosus (SLE) and Experimental Autoimmune Encephalomyelitis (EAE)

Studies of aged gal1 ko mice revealed the presence of higher levels of serum anti-dsDNA antibodies compared to aged wild-type mice, suggesting that endogenous galectin-1 may suppress autoimmune responses. This is consistent with the effect of recombinant galectin-1. Specifically, SLE-prone (BWF1) mice treated with recombinant galectin-1 experienced increased rates of survival, decreased levels of serum anti-dsDNA antibodies, lower T and B cell activation, and an enhanced frequency of Tregs relative to untreated mice (*9*).

Gal1 ko mice also developed greater disease severity in mouse experimental autoimmune encephalomyelitis (EAE), an autoimmune disease of the central nervous system (CNS) driven by autoreactive Th1 and Th17 cells (*10*). Splenocytes from gal1 ko mice exhibited enhanced proliferation after restimulation with $(MOG)_{35\text{-}55}$ peptide antigen, and secreted higher levels of IFNγ and IL-17 compared to wild-type T cells. Moreover, gal1 ko CD4+ T cells produced higher levels of IFNγ and IL-2 compared to their wild-type counterparts, indicating a role for galectin-1 in the negative regulation of Th1 responses.

A vast amount of literature exists on the immunosuppressive role of galectin-1, through its effects on T cells (reviewed in (*11–13*). Galectin-1 induces apoptosis by binding to galactose-β1-4-*N*-acetylglucosamine (LacNAc) units on N- or O-linked glycans expressed on activated Th1 and Th17, but not Th2 cells (*10*). Differential cell recognition is associated with α2-6 and α2-3 sialylation on the surface of Th2 cells that masks galectin-1 ligands. Thus, galectin-1 may regulate the immune and inflammatory responses associated with autoimmune diseases by inducing T cell apoptosis or by suppressing the proliferation of self-reactive T cells [reviewed in (*14*)].

Endogenous galectin-3 has been shown to be a positive regulator of inflammatory responses in autoimmunity. Gal3 ko mice developed delayed onset of EAE, exhibited reduced leukocytic infiltrations to the CNS, and had more apoptotic cells in the CNS compared to wild-type mice (*15*). Moreover, draining lymph node cells from immunized gal3 ko mice produced lower levels of IFNγ and IL-17 and higher levels of IL-5 and IL-13 after *ex vivo* stimulation with $MOG_{35\text{-}55}$ peptide, suggesting that galectin-3 promotes pathogenic Th1 and Th17 cells and inhibits Th2 polarization. Moreover, DCs from immunized gal3 ko mice produced higher levels of IL-10, a cytokine that drives the production of inducible Tregs and is associated with immunosuppression. Whether galectin-3 exacerbates the inflammatory response in EAE indeed by promoting the production of the pathogenic cytokines IL-17 and IFNγ, while inhibiting immunosuppressive mediators, such as Treg and Th2 cells, remains to be clarified. As mentioned above, galectin-3 actually promotes Th2 responses in a number of other models. Recent work in the authors' laboratory also suggests that expression of galectin-3 in DCs negatively regulates Th17 responses to fungal pathogens (unpublished findings).

In a mouse model of arthritis induced by antigen, galectin-3 expression was reported to be correlated with disease progression and severity (*16*). Gal3 ko mice displayed less synovial joint inflammation and expressed fewer antigen-specific antibodies and lower IL-17 production compared to wild-type mice. This effect was reversed after treatment with recombinant galectin-3, which increased TNFα and IL-6 expression at early stages of the disease and enhanced the frequency of IL-17-producing T cells in gal3 ko mice. The use of gal3 ko mice supports a pathogenic role for endogenous galectin-3 in the development of rheumatoid arthritis, while the use of recombinant galectin-3 suggests that extracellular galectin-3 may partially contribute to the pro-inflammatory response.

On the other hand, galectin-3 was reported to subdue susceptibility to autoimmune disease by forming complexes with glycoproteins modified by mannosyl α1,6-glycoprotein β1,6-N-acetylglucosaminyltransferase (Mgat5). Galectin-3 was described to restrict antigen-dependent T cell receptor clustering and raising the threshold needed for T cell activation (*17*). Mgat5 ko mice (lacking cell ligands for galectin-3) exhibited increased susceptibility to EAE, delayed-type hypersensitivity, and kidney autoimmune disease, which were attributed to enhanced TCR clustering and hyperactive T cells. It is to be noted, however, the phenotypes demonstrated in mice deficient in Mgat5 may not be strictly restricted to galectin-3, because Mgat5 also regulates formation of ligands recognized by other endogenous lectins (including galectin-1) and may also contribute to functions unrelated to endogenous lectins.

Galectin-3 may function through both intracellular and extracellular mechanisms to regulate inflammatory responses and mediate cellular homeostasis, as suggested by in vitro experiments [reviewed in (*18*, *19*)]. For example, extracellular galectin-3 promotes apoptosis in activated T cells and acts as a chemoattractant for monocytes and macrophages (*20*), while intracellular galectin-3 confers the resistance of T cells to apoptosis and promotes cell proliferation (*21*). Whether the protein functions through both pathways, or predominates through either intra- or extra-cellular action is yet to be determined.

The role of galectin-9 in autoimmune responses has been studied in a mouse model of arthritis. Specifically, gal9 ko mice have been shown to develop exacerbated arthritis in a model of collagen-induced arthritis. In this model, the administration of recombinant galectin-9 after disease induction suppressed clinical symptoms and decreased proinflammatory cytokine expression, indicating a protective function for galectin-9 (*22*). Downregulation of IFNγ and IL-17 was also accompanied by increased apoptosis of Tim3-expressing Th1 and Th17 cells. Furthermore, galectin-9 therapy promoted T cell differentiation to Tregs (*22*). This is consistent with a large number of studies demonstrating the suppressive role of recombinant galectin-9 in immune and inflammatory responses [reviewed in (*23*, *24*)].

However, endogenous galectin-9 has been shown to upregulate cytokine production in a monocyte cell line by an intracellular action (*25*). Accordingly, additional studies are needed to determine whether the intracellular functions of galectin-9 are manifested in vivo. Nevertheless, the current information suggests that recombinant galectin-9 may be used therapeutically to suppress autoimmune and inflammatory responses [reviewed in (*26*)].

b. Diabetes (Nephropathy and Retinopathy)

Hyperglycemia in diabetic patients causes non-enzymatic glycosylation (glycation) of proteins and lipids, producing elevated levels of advanced glycation end products (AGEs). AGEs have been implicated in the pathogenesis of long-term diabetic complications, such as nephropathy. Galectin-3 was identified as an AGE receptor (AGE-R3) (*27*) important for the endocytosis of AGEs (*28*). A number of studies implicated galectin-3 in diabetic complications through its AGE-binding activity, while others suggested its involvement in pathogenesis of autoimmune (type 1) diabetes as a regulator of the immune response.

Exposure of C57BL/6 mice to multiple low-doses of streptozotocin induces infiltration of mononuclear cells, including macrophages, in the islets of these mice, leading to islet inflammation (insulitis), which precedes the destruction of insulin-producing beta cells. It was shown by quantitative histology of islet tissue that galectin-3 ablation significantly attenuates insulitis and beta cell loss (*29*). By this model, other investigators confirmed that gal3 ko mice were more resistant to diabetogenesis compared with wild-type counterparts. This is associated with lower levels of the inflammatory cytokines IFNγ, TNFα, and IL-17 in pancreatic draining lymph nodes. These results suggest the involvement of galectin-3 in immune-mediated beta-cell damage and diabetogenesis. Gal3 ko macrophages produced less TNFα and nitric oxide as well. Thus, it might be through this cell type that galectin-3 contributes to diabetogenesis. Whether galectin-3 functions in this model through other cell types that are also involved in the pathogenesis of diabetes remains to be determined (*30*).

By a similar model, other investigators found that gal3 ko mice developed more severe glomerulopathy, despite a similar degree of metabolic derangement, compared to wild-type counterparts (*31*). The former exhibited higher levels of renal/glomerular AGE associated with altered expression of AGE receptors. The receptors implicated in removal of AGE (macrophage scavenger receptor A and AGE-R1) were downregulated, while those mediating cell activation (RAGE and AGE-R2) were upregulated. These results suggest that galectin-3 regulates the AGE receptor pathway *in vivo* to protect animals from AGE-induced tissue injury. In another study, glomerulopathy was induced by injection of N(epsilon)-carboxymethyllysine (CML)-modified serum albumin (an AGE). Gal3 ko mice developed higher circulating and renal AGE levels and exhibited exacerbated renal function (*32*). The results are again consistent with the role of galectin-3 as an AGE receptor in vivo that confers protection against AGE-mediated tissue injury by aiding AGE disposal (*33*).

Both aging and diabetes are characterized by renal functional and structural abnormalities related to the progressive accumulation of AGEs, and cumulative oxidative stress. Iacobini et al (*34*) correlated the development of glomerular lesions with AGE levels and oxidative stress in aging gal3 ko and wild-type mice. They found that aged gal3 ko mice developed more severe glomerulopathy and higher renal extracellular matrix gene protein expression than their age-matched wild-type counterparts. AGE levels correlated significantly with renal functional and structural parameters in these mice. These data suggest that galectin-3 is involved in the AGE/AGE receptor pathway underlying age-related renal disease.

Consistent with the resistance of gal3 ko mice to diabetogenesis despite the deteriorating effects of galectin-3 deficiency on long-term diabetic complications discussed above, there are reports that galectin-3 ablation actually prevents acute pathology of diabetes. These include breakdown of the inner blood-retinal barrier (iBRB), which is central to the development of sight-threatening diabetic macular edema. When rendered diabetic with a single intraperitoneal injection of streptozotocin, gal3 ko mice exhibited significantly less diabetes-mediated iBRB dysfunction than their untreated wild-type counterparts (*35*).

In a model of oxygen-induced proliferative retinopathy, wild-type and gal3 ko mice were tested for retinal ischemia and neovascularization after perfusion of preformed AGEs. Mice treated with AGE exhibited elevated inner retinal ischemia and reduced angiogenesis. Ablation of galectin-3 abolished these effects of AGEs. The data implicate galectin-3 in mediating AGE-induced retinopathies (*36*).

While galectin-3 is well recognized as an AGE-binding protein, it is not known to what extent galectin-3's AGE-binding activity contributes to diabetic complications compared to its regulation of immune responses, gene expression, and apoptosis. Whether these effects can be reproduced in other mouse models, such as the spontaneous non-obese diabetic (NOD) mice, is an interesting topic.

Liver Disease

Several models of liver injury were studied in gal3 ko mice and the results indicated that galectin-3 is a key regulatory factor in the fibrotic response induced by injury. In chemically-induced liver fibrosis and recovery, galectin-3 functions through multiple pathways and contributes to the severity of fibrosis. Indeed, myofibroblast activation and procollagen formation *in vitro* and *in vivo* were markedly reduced in gal3 ko mice, leading to attenuated liver fibrosis in comparison with wild type animals. The reduction in hepatic fibrosis observed in gal3 ko mice occurred despite equivalent liver injury and inflammation and similar tissue expression of TGFβ, in comparison with wild type mice (*37*).

Furthermore, TGFβ failed to transactivate gal3 ko hepatic stellate cells, in contrast to wild type stellate cells; however, TGFβ-stimulated Smad-2 and -3 activation were equivalent. This study indicates that galectin-3 participates in TGF-beta-mediated myofibroblast activation and matrix production. These *in vivo* studies were recapitulated *in vitro* by effecting galectin-3 knockdown through siRNA treatment. The authors suggest prospects in providing an alternative therapeutic approach to prevention and treatment of liver fibrosis by interfering with galectin-3 expression (*37*).

Development of nonalcoholic steatohepatitis (NASH) has also been investigated in gal3 ko mice maintained on atherogenic diets. NASH was invariably present in wild type mice, but occurred at lower prevalence in a small subset of gal3 ko mice. Gal3 ko mice also displayed reduced inflammatory, degenerative and fibrotic changes compared to wild type animals, and exhibited diminished levels of disease progression, consisting of lower levels of circulating advanced lipoxidation end-products (ALE) and lower tissue ALE accumulation. In liver endothelial cells treated for galectin-3 knockdown by siRNA, a similar phenotype of reduced N(ε)-carboxymethyllysine-modified albumin uptake and ALE-receptor expression was achieved. Thus, reduction of galectin-3 levels is beneficial to repair following hepatocyte injury (*38*).

The role of galectin-3 in liver inflammation and injury were also examined using an acetaminophen (APAP) toxicity model. High dose APAP causes centrilobular hepatic necrosis and elevates serum transaminases, which is associated with increased hepatic expression of galectin-3 mRNA and protein. Immunohistochemical analysis revealed that galectin-3 was predominantly expressed by infiltrating mononuclear cells in necrotic areas. Reduced hepatotoxicity was observed in gal3 ko mice relative to wild type mice. Changes in gal3 ko mice were not due to differences in APAP metabolism or hepatic glutathione levels but correlated with reduction in APAP-induced expression of 24p3, a marker of inflammation and oxidative stress. In comparison with wild type mice, proinflammatory mediators iNOS, IL-1β, MIP-2, MMP-9, MIP-3α, as well as galectin-3-binding protein, CD98, and TNFR1 were downregulated in gal3 ko mice (*39*).

Promotion of inflammatory damage caused by expression of galectin-3 was also revealed in a model of concanavalin A-mediated hepatic toxicity. Gal3 ko mice exhibited lower numbers of activated lymphoid and DCs in the liver compared to wild type, and substantially reduced hepatitis. This was accompanied by reduced serum TNFα, IFNγ, IL-17 and IL-4, and fewer TNFα-, IFNγ-, IL-17- and IL-4-producing CD4+ cells. The numbers of IL-12-producing CD11c+ DCs were lower, while those of IL-10-producing CD4+ T cells and F4/80+ macrophages were significantly higher in livers of gal3 ko mice, relative to wild type. Increased numbers of apoptotic leukocytes in liver and splenocytes were present in gal3 ko mice. However, whether these dying cells mainly constitute the population of inflammatory cells is unknown. Pre-treatment of wild type C57BL/6 mice with galectin-3 inhibitor TD139 led to attenuation of liver injury and reduced infiltration of IFNγ-, IL-17- and IL-4-producing CD4+ T cells, increase in total number of IL-10-producing CD4+ T cells and F4/80+ CD206+ alternatively activated macrophages. Apoptosis of liver-infiltrating mononuclear cells was also prevented with this inhibitor, suggesting its utility in controlling hepatic inflammation (*40*).

Kidney Disease

As observed in hepatic repair, promotion of fibrotic injury by galectin-3 during allograft rejection due to MHC Class II mismatch was noted. In comparison with syngeneic transplants, allograft rejection is accompanied by elevated galectin-3 expression (*41*). Relative to wild type mice, allografts in gal3 ko mice exhibited attenuated interstitial fibrosis, decreased myofibroblast activation and collagen I expression, accompanied by reduced expression of YM1, a marker of alternatively activated macrophages. In addition, gal3 ko mice exhibited reduced numbers of circulating CD4-positive T cells and IL4-expressing cells, relative to wild type mice (*41*).

Consistent with prior observations associating galectin-3 and inflammation, tissue injury caused by inflammatory responses during renal ischemic-reperfusion injury was described to track with expression of galectin-3. When examined in gal3 ko mice, reduced tissue expression of MCP-1, IL-6 and IL-1β were observed relative to wild type animals, accompanied by lower macrophage infiltration and production of reactive oxygen species. Gal3 ko animals exhibited significantly lower levels of blood urea and improved tubular regeneration relative to wild type animals (*42*).

Galectin-3 is highly induced in the kidneys in a mouse model of ureteral obstruction (UUO). Gal3 ko mice exhibited increased numbers of apoptotic cells, consistent with the described anti-apoptotic property of galectin-3 (*43*), lower levels of cell proliferation and decreased levels of Endo180, an intracellular receptor for intracellular collagen degradation, but elevated levels of fibrosis compared to wild type mice. This was accompanied by lower numbers of myofibroblasts in gal3 ko mice during early stages of disease. Gal3 ko mice also exhibited lower levels of extracellular matrix synthesis than wild type mice (*44*).

These studies demonstrate that, while galectin-3 promotes inflammation during tissue injury, the protein can provide beneficial properties by limiting cell death, which is an intracellular function. When secreted, galectin-3 activates leukocytes, is a macrophage chemotactic factor, and is able to kill T cells (*11, 45*). These properties of galectin-3 are likely maintained at certain levels of equilibrium during disease processes. Future studies are required to establish which of the pathways engaged by pleiotropic galectin-3 dominates during disease.

An additional model of renal injury resulting from lipid-induced disease due to atherogenic high-fat diet caused the accumulation of oxidation products. Diseased gal3 ko mice under these conditions were observed to exhibit higher levels of oxidation products and elevated levels of fibrosis and inflammation, compared to wild type animals. The authors concluded that galectin-3 serves to protect tissue damage resulting from accumulation of oxidation products by contributing to their clearance as an AGE receptor (*46*).

Heart/Lung Disease

Consistent with its proinflammatory functions, galectin-3 participates in exacerbating vascular disease in mouse models of atherosclerosis. The ApoE ko mouse strain, an established model of spontaneously-occurring atherosclerosis, was crossed to produce ApoE ko/gal3 ko animals. In comparison to ApoE ko mice, which developed aortic atheromatous plaques and periaortic vascular channels in an age-dependent manner, ApoE ko/gal3 ko animals did not display age-dependent disease progression. Following longer periods of disease induction, ApoE ko/gal3 ko mice exhibited lower numbers of atherosclerotic lesions and fewer atheromatous plaques, concomitant with lower numbers of perivascular inflammatory infiltrates (*47*).

In contrast to the ApoE ko model, gal3 ko mice on atherogenic diets displayed larger aortic lesions than wild type and lesions with greater complexity as evident by the presence of increased inflammatory changes. In accordance with prior observations associating galectin-3 with promotion of the Th2 response, aortic lesions of gal3 ko animals contained Th1-polarized T cells. Increased levels of macrophage infiltration and inflammatory mediators were also present in gal3 ko animals, compared to wild type, as well as. oxidized LDLs and lipoxidation products, and their receptors (*48*). Apparently contradicting observations between this model and the ApoE ko model described above may be due to in part to the degree of intensity of disease induction, which is greater in the diet-induced model. Analyses for the presence or absence of Th polarization in the ApoE ko model may shed light on these contrasting results.

Like galectin-3, galectin-1 exhibits pleiotropic properties and is highly expressed in pulmonary mesenchymal cells derived from a model of chronic hypoxic pulmonary hypertension. Severity of disease was less pronounced in gal1 ko animals than wild type animals, as measured by right ventricular pressure (RVP), and this was not caused by differences in the extents of muscularization in microvessels. To examine the role of vasoreactivity, acute hypoxic stress was induced and peak RVP was found to be lower in wild type compared to gal1 ko animals. The results suggest that differences between wild type and gal1 ko mice occur because of the smooth muscle cell contractile responses to hypoxia as opposed to vascular tone in these mice before exposure to chronic hypoxia. This is supported by the observation that smooth muscle cell vasoreactivity in gal1 ko mice was significantly greater than wild type mice under induction with vasoconstrictive agents during acute hypoxia, and not in the absence of hypoxia. Consistent with early observations in myoblast studies (*49*, *50*), these results suggest that galectin-1 regulates smooth muscle cell interactions with the extracellular matrix in response to hypoxia, but not vascular tone (*51*).

Conclusions

Generation of galectin ko mice have provided essential tools to delineate functions of galectins. Animal models have been crucial in many instances where functions observed *in vitro* were confirmed in ko mice. In particular, the immunosuppressive functions of galectin-1 and -9 suggested by in vitro studies were demonstrated with the use of gal1 ko and gal 9 ko mice, respectively. Likewise, the pro-inflammatory and antiapoptotic functions of galectin-3 suggested by *in vitro* studies were described in a number of experiments of the galectin-3 ko strain in multiple diseases and tissue systems (Figure 1). Additional experiments are still needed to link the *in vitro* and *in vivo* observations mechanistically and these knock out mice will continue to serve as valuable tools in dissecting the pleiotropic functions of these galectins. In particular, both intra- and extra-cellular functions *in vivo* could be addressed by engrafting either ko or wild-type cells into the opposing genotype.

Additional challenges remain in dissecting gene function with respect to extrapolation of mouse studies to human disease. Advances in gene manipulation by genetic and transcriptional disruptions and availability of mouse strains capable of adopting human cells and tissues will permit examination of more humanized organ systems. Nevertheless, results from knock out mice now suggest that galectin-3 may be a therapeutic target for a number of immune and inflammatory diseases, and contributed to validation of recombinant galectin-1 and -9 as potential biologics for some diseases.

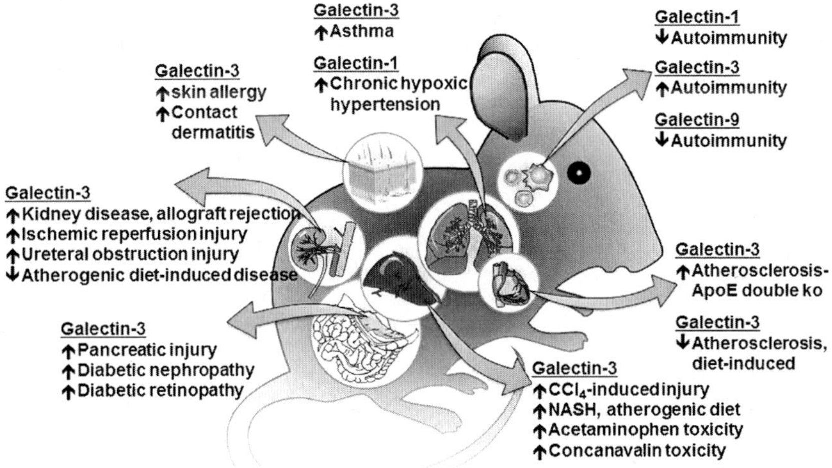

Figure 1. Disease involvement by tissues and organs in galectin-1-, galectin-3- and galectin-9-deficient mice. Arrows indicate upregulation and downregulation, observed experimentally. (see color insert)

Diabetes
Galectin-3: ↑ immune-β-cell damage, diabetogenesis, IFNγ, IL-17, TNFα, NO, insulinitis, β-cell loss
Nephropathy: ↑ beneficial AGE receptor expression, renal function
Retinopathy: ↑ loss of inner blood-retinal barrier, AGE-induced suppression of angiogenesis

Kidney disease
Galectin-3:
Allograft rejection:↑myofibroblast activation, interstitial fibrosis; ↓ IL-4 producing T cells
Ischemic reperfusion injury: ↑inflammatory cytokines, macrophage infiltration, tubular destruction
Ureteral obstruction:↓ cell apoptosis; ↑fibrosis, Endo180 (intracellular collagen degradation)
Atherogenic disease:↓ oxidation products, fibrosis, inflammation

Skin allergy
Galectin-3: ↑ eosinophilia, skin thickness, serum IgE, IL-4, Th2-polarized T cells, Th2 DC antigen presentation
Contact dermatitis: ↑ skin thickness, DC chemotaxis, LN trafficking

Asthma
Galectin-3: ↑ eosinophilia, goblet cell metaplasia, airway remodeling, eotaxin-1, IL-5, IL-13 (Th2), fibrosis, smooth muscle hypertrophy, peribronchial angiogenesis
Galectin-1:
Chronic hypoxic hypertension: ↑ severity right ventricular pressure; ↓ smooth muscle vasoreactivity (acute hypoxia only)

Atherosclerosis-ApoE ko
Galectin-3: ↑ atheromatous plaques, periaortic vascular channels, age-dependent disease progression
Atherosclerosis, diet-induced: ↓ aortic lesion size and complexity, macrophage invasion, inflammatory mediators, apoptosis, lipoxidation products; ↑ Th2 response

Autoimmunity
Galectin-1: ↓ T, B cell activation, autoantibodies, IFNγ, IL-1, IL-17; ↑Treg, patient survival
Galectin-3: ↓ IFNγ, IL-6, IL-17, TNFα, activated T, B cell, Treg, IL-10;↑IL-5, IL-13, inflammation, autoantibodies
Galectin-9: ↓ IFNγ, IL-17, disease severity; ↑Th1, Th17 cell apoptosis, Treg, TGFβ-induced FoxP3

Liver injury
Galectin-3
CCl_4-induced: ↑ myofibroblast activation, collagen deposition & fibrosis, ↑ Stellate cell activation by TGFβ
NASH-atherogenic diet: ↑ inflammation, degenerative/fibrotic change, ALE accumulation, inflammatory cytokines, ER stress, hepatocyte apoptosis
Acetaminophen toxicity: ↑ 24p3 expression, hepatotoxicity, proinflammatory mediators, CD98, TNFR1
Concanavalin toxicity: ↑ activated lymphocytes, DC, inflammatory cytokines; ↓ IL-10 secreting T cells, F4/80+ macrophages

References

1. Zuberi, R. I.; Hsu, D. K.; Kalayci, O.; Chen, H. Y.; Sheldon, H. K.; Yu, L.; Apgar, J. R.; Kawakami, T.; Lilly, C. M.; Liu, F. T. Critical role for galectin-3 in airway inflammation and bronchial hyperresponsiveness in a murine model of asthma. *Am. J. Pathol.* **2004**, *165*, 2045–2053.
2. Ge, X. N.; Bahaie, N. S.; Kang, B. N.; Hosseinkhani, M. R.; Ha, S. G.; Frenzel, E. M.; Liu, F. T.; Rao, S. P.; Sriramarao, P. Allergen-induced airway remodeling is impaired in galectin-3-deficient mice. *J. Immunol.* **2010**, *185*, 1205–1214.
3. Saegusa, J.; Hsu, D. K.; Chen, H. Y.; Yu, L.; Fermin, A.; Fung, M. A.; et al. Galectin-3 is critical for the development of the allergic inflammatory response in a mouse model of atopic dermatitis. *Am. J. Pathol.* **2009**, *174*, 922–931.
4. Hsu, D. K.; Chernyavsky, A. I.; Chen, H. Y.; Yu, L.; Grando, S. A.; Liu, F. T. Endogenous galectin-3 is localized in membrane lipid rafts and regulates migration of dendritic cells. *J. Invest. Dermatol.* **2009b**, *129*, 573–583.
5. Colnot, C.; Ripoche, M. A.; Milon, G.; Montagutelli, X.; Crocker, P. R.; Poirier, F. Maintenance of granulocyte numbers during acute peritonitis is defective in galectin-3-null mutant mice. *Immunology* **1998**, *94*, 290–296.
6. Hsu, D. K.; Yang, R. Y.; Yu, L.; Pan, Z.; Salomon, D. R.; Fung-Leung, W. P.; Liu, F. T. Targeted disruption of the galectin-3 gene results in attenuated peritoneal inflammatory responses. *Am. J. Pathol.* **2000**, *156*, 1073–1083.
7. del Pozo, V.; Rojo, M.; Rubio, M. L.; Cortegano, I.; Cardaba, B.; Gallardo, S.; Ortega, M.; Civantos, E.; Lopez, E.; C. Martin-Mosquero, C.; Peces-Barba, G.; Palomino, P.; Gonzalez-Mangado, N.; Lahoz, C. Gene therapy with galectin-3 inhibits bronchial obstruction and inflammation in antigen-challenged rats through interleukin-5 gene downregulation. *Am. J. Respir. Crit. Care Med.* **2002**, *166*, 732–737.
8. Lopez, E.; Del Pozo, V.; Miguel, T.; Sastre, B.; Seoane, C.; Civantos, E.; Llanes, E.; Baeze, M. L.; Palomino, P.; Cardaba, B.; Gallardo, S.; Manzarbeitia, F.; Zubeldia, J. M.; Lahoz, C. Inhibition of chronic airway inflammation and remodeling by galectin-3 gene therapy in a murine model. *J. Immunol.* **2006**, *176*, 1943–1950.
9. Liu, S. D.; Lee, S.; Cava, A. L.; Motran, C. C.; Hahn, B. H.; Miceli, M. C. Galectin-1-induced down-regulation of T lymphocyte activation protects (NZB x NZW) F1 mice from lupus-like disease. *Lupus* **2011**, *20*, 473–484.
10. Toscano, M. A.; Bianco, G. A.; Ilarregui, J. M.; Croci, D. O.; Correale, J.; Hernandez, J. D.; Zwirner, N. W.; Poirier, F.; Riley, E. M.; Baum, L. G.; Rabinovich, G. A. Differential glycosylation of T(H)1, T(H)2 and T(H)-17 effector cells selectively regulates susceptibility to cell death. *Nat. Immunol.* **2007**, *8*, 825–834.
11. Dhirapong, A.; Lleo, A.; Leung, P.; Gershwin, M. E.; Liu, F. T. The immunological potential of galectin-1 and -3. *Autoimmun. Rev.* **2009**, *8*, 360–363.
12. He, J.; Baum, L. G. Galectin interactions with extracellular matrix and effects on cellular function. *Methods Enzymol.* **2006**, *417*, 247–256.

13. Rabinovich, G. A.; Toscano, M. A. Turning 'sweet' on immunity: Galectin-glycan interactions in immune tolerance and inflammation. *Nat. Rev. Immunol.* **2009**, *9*, 338–352.
14. Ilarregui, J. M.; Rabinovich, G. A. Tolerogenic dendritic cells in the control of autoimmune neuroinflammation: An emerging role of protein-glycan interactions. *Neuroimmunomodulation* **2010**, *17*, 157–160.
15. Jiang, H.-R.; Al Rasebi, Z.; Mensah-Brown, E.; Shahin, A.; Xu, D.; Goodyear, C. S.; Fukada, S. Y.; Liu, F.-T.; Liew, F. Y.; Lukic, M. L. Galectin-3 deficiency reduces the severity of experimental autoimmune encephalomyelitis. *J. Immunol.* **2009**, *182*, 1167–1173.
16. Forsman, H.; Islander, U.; Andréasson, E.; Andersson, A.; Önnheim, K.; Karlström, A.; Sävman, K.; Magnusson, M.; Brown, K. L.; Karlsson, A. Galectin 3 aggravates joint inflammation and destruction in antigen-induced arthritis. *Arthritis Rheum.* **2011**, *63*, 445–454.
17. Demetriou, M.; Granovsky, M.; Quaggin, S.; Dennis, J. W. Negative regulation of T-cell activation and autoimmunity by Mgat5N-glycosylation. *Nature* **2001**, *409*, 733–739.
18. Chen, H. Y.; Liu, F. T.; Yang, R. Y. Roles of galectin-3 in immune responses. *Arch. Immunol. Ther. Exp* . **2005**, *53*, 497–504.
19. Hsu, D. K.; Chen, H. Y.; Liu, F. T. Galectin-3 regulates T-cell functions. *Immunol. Rev.* **2009a**, *230*, 114–127.
20. Sano, H.; Hsu, D. K.; Yu, L.; Apgar, J. R.; Kuwabara, I.; Yamanaka, T.; Hirashima, M.; Liu, F.-T. Human galectin-3 is a novel chemoattractant for monocytes and macrophages. *J. Immunol.* **2000**, *165*, 2156–2164.
21. Yang, R.-Y.; Hsu, D. K.; Liu, F.-T. Expression of galectin-3 modulates T-cell growth and apoptosis. *Proc. Natl. Acad. Sci. U.S.A.* **1996**, *93*, 6737–6742.
22. Seki, M.; Oomizu, S.; Sakata, K.-M.; Sakata, A.; Arikawa, T.; Watanabe, K.; Ito, K.; Takeshita, K.; Niki, T.; Saita, N.; Nishi, N.; Yamauchi, A.; Katoh, S.; Matsukawa, A.; Kuchroo, V.; Hirashima, M Galectin-9 suppresses the generation of Th17, promotes the induction of regulatory T cells, and regulates experimental autoimmune arthritis. *Clin. Immunol.* **2008**, *127*, 78–88.
23. Hirashima, M.; Kashio, Y.; Nishi, N.; Yamauchi, A.; Imaizumi, T. A.; Kageshita, T.; Saita, N.; Nakamura, T. Galectin-9 in physiological and pathological conditions. *Glycoconjugate J.* **2004**, *19*, 593–600.
24. Sakuishi, K.; Jayaraman, P.; Behar, S. M.; Anderson, A. C.; Kuchroo, V. K. Emerging Tim-3 functions in antimicrobial and tumor immunity. *Trends Immunol.* **2011**, *32*, 345–349.
25. Matsuura, A.; Tsukada, J.; Mizobe, T.; Higashi, T.; Mouri, F.; Tanikawa, R.; Yamauchi, A.; Hirashima, M.; Tanaka, Y. Intracellular galectin-9 activates inflammatory cytokines in monocytes. *Genes Cells* **2009**, *14*, 511–521.
26. Sakuishi, K.; Jayaraman, P.; Behar, S. M.; Anderson, A. C.; Kuchroo, V. K. Emerging Tim-3 functions in antimicrobial and tumor immunity. *Trends Immunol.* **2011**, *32*, 345–349.
27. Vlassara, H.; Li, Y. M.; Imani, F.; Wojciechowicz, D.; Yang, Z.; Liu, F. T.; Cerami, A. Identification of galectin-3 as a high-affinity binding protein

for advanced glycation end products (AGE): A new member of the AGE-receptor complex. *Mol. Med.* **1995**, *1*, 634–646.

28. Zhu, W.; Sano, H.; Nagai, R.; Fukuhara, K.; Miyazaki, A.; Horiuchi, S. The role of galectin-3 in endocytosis of advanced glycation end products and modified low density lipoproteins. *Biochem. Biophys. Res. Commun.* **2001**, *280*, 1183–1188.
29. Mensah-Brown, E.; Shahin, A.; Parekh, K.; Hakim, A. A.; Shamisi, M. A.; Hsu, D. K.; Lukic, M. L. Functional capacity of macrophages determines the induction of type 1 diabetes. *Ann. N. Y. Acad. Sci.* **2006**, *1084*, 49–57.
30. Mensah-Brown, E. P.; Al Rabesi, Z.; Shahin, A.; Al Shamsi, M.; Arsenijevic, N.; Hsu, D. K.; Liu, F.-T.; Lukic, M. L. Targeted disruption of the galectin-3 gene results in decreased susceptibility to multiple low dose streptozotocin-induced diabetes in mice. *Clin. Immunol.* **2009**, *130*, 83–88.
31. Pugliese, G.; Pricci, F.; Iacobini, C.; Leto, G.; Amadio, L.; Barsotti, P.; Frigeri, L.; Hsu, D. K.; Vlassara, H.; Liu, F.-T.; Di Mario, U. Accelerated diabetic glomerulopathy in galectin-3/AGE receptor 3 knockout mice. *FASEB J.* **2001**, *15*, 2471–2479.
32. Iacobini, C.; Amadio, L.; Oddi, G.; Ricci, C.; Barsotti, P.; Missori, S.; Sorchini, M.; Di Mario, U.; Pricci, F.; Pugliese, G. Role of galectin-3 in diabetic nephropathy. *J. Am. Soc. Nephrol.* **2003**, *14*, S264–S270.
33. Iacobini, C.; Menini, S.; Oddi, G.; Ricci, C.; Amadio, L.; Pricci, F.; Olivieri, A.; Sorcini, M.; Di Mario, U.; Pesce, C.; Pugliese, G. Galectin-3/AGE-receptor 3 knockout mice show accelerated AGE-induced glomerular injury: Evidence for a protective role of galectin-3 as an AGE receptor. *FASEB J.* **2004**, *18*, 1773–1775.
34. Iacobini, C.; Oddi, G.; Menini, S.; Amadio, L.; Ricci, C.; Di Pippo, C.; Sorcini, M.; Pricci, F.; Pugliese, F.; Pugliese, G. Development of age-dependent glomerular lesions in galectin-3/AGE-receptor-3 knockout mice. *Am. J. Physiol.: Renal Physiol.* **2005**, *289*, F611–F621.
35. Canning, P.; Glenn, J. V.; Hsu, D. K.; Liu, F. T.; Gardiner, T. A.; Stitt, A. W. Inhibition of advanced glycation and absence of galectin-3 prevent blood-retinal barrier dysfunction during short-term diabetes. *Exp. Diabetes Res.* **2007**, *2007*, 51837.
36. Stitt, A. W.; McGoldrick, C.; Rice-McCaldin, A.; McCance, D. R.; Glenn, J. V.; Hsu, D. K.; Liu, F.-T.; Thorpe, S. R.; Gardiner, T. A. Impaired retinal angiogenesis in diabetes: Role of advanced glycation end products and galectin-3. *Diabetes* **2005**, *54*, 785–794.
37. Henderson, N. C.; Mackinnon, A. C.; Farnworth, S. L.; Poirier, F.; Russo, F. P.; Iredale, J. P.; Haslett, C.; Simpson, K. J.; Sethi, T. Galectin-3 regulates myofibroblast activation and hepatic fibrosis. *Proc. Natl. Acad. Sci. U.S.A.* **2006**, *103*, 5060–5065.
38. Iacobini, C.; Menini, S.; Ricci, C.; Fantauzzi, C. B.; Scipioni, A.; Salvi, L.; Cordone, S.; Delucci, F.; Serino, M.; Federici, M.; Pricci, F.; Pugliese, G. Galectin-3 ablation protects mice from diet-induced NASH: A major scavenging role for galectin-3 in liver. *J. Hepatol.* **2011**, *54*, 975–983.

39. Dragomir, A. C.; Sun, R.; Mishin, V.; Hall, L. B.; Laskin, J. D.; Laskin, D. L. Role of galectin-3 in acetaminophen-induced hepatotoxicity and inflammatory mediator production. *Toxicol. Sci.* **2012**, *127*, 609–619.
40. Volarevic, V.; Milovanovic, M.; Ljujic, B.; Pejnovic, N.; Arsenijevic, N.; Nilsson, U.; Leffler, H.; Lujic, M. L. Galectin-3 deficiency prevents concanavalin A-induced hepatitis in mice. *Hepatology* **2012**, *55*, 1954–1964.
41. Dang, Z.; MacKinnon, A.; Marson, L. P.; Sethi, T. Tubular atrophy and interstitial fibrosis after renal transplantation is dependent on galectin-3. *Transplantation* **2012**, *93*, 477–484.
42. Fernandes Bertocchi, A. P.; Campanhole, G.; Wang, P. H.; Goncalves, G. M.; Damiao, M. J.; Cenedeze, M. A.; Beraldo, F. C.; de Paula Antunes Teixeira, V.; Dos Reis, M. A.; Mazzali, M.; Pacheco-Silva, A.; Camara, N. O. A role for galectin-3 in renal tissue damage triggered by ischemia and reperfusion injury. *Transplant Int.* **2008**, *21*, 999–1007.
43. Liu, F.-T.; Rabinovich, G. A. Galectins as modulators of tumour progression. *Nat. Rev. Cancer* **2005**, *5*, 29–41.
44. Okamura, D. M.; Pasichnyk, K.; Lopez-Guisa, J. M.; Collins, S.; Hsu, D. K.; Liu, F.-T.; Eddy, A. A. Galectin-3 preserves renal tubules and modulates extracellular matrix remodeling in progressive fibrosis. *Am. J. Physiol.: Renal Physiol.* **2011**, *300*, F245–F253.
45. Henderson, N. C.; Sethi, T. The regulation of inflammation by galectin-3. *Immunol. Rev.* **2009**, *230*, 160–171.
46. Iacobini, C.; Menini, S.; Ricci, C.; Scipioni, A.; Sansoni, V.; Mazzitelli, G.; Cordone, S.; Pesce, C.; Pugliese, F.; Pricci, F.; Pugliese, G. Advanced lipoxidation end-products mediate lipid-induced glomerular injury: Role of receptor-mediated mechanisms. *J. Pathol.* **2009b**, *218*, 360–369.
47. Nachtigal, M.; Ghaffar, A.; Mayer, E. P. Galectin-3 gene inactivation reduces atherosclerotic lesions and adventitial inflammation in ApoE-deficient mice. *Am. J. Pathol.* **2008**, *172*, 247–255.
48. Iacobini, C.; Menini, S.; Ricci, C.; Scipioni, A.; Sansoni, V.; Cordone, S.; Taurino, M.; Serino, M.; Marano, G.; Federici, M.; Pricci, F.; Pugliese, G. Accelerated lipid-induced atherogenesis in galectin-3-deficient mice: Role of lipoxidation via receptor-mediated mechanisms. *Arterioscler., Thromb., Vasc. Biol.* **2009a**, *29*, 831–836.
49. Cooper, D. N. W.; Barondes, S. H. Evidence for export of a muscle lectin from cytosol to extracellular matrix and for a novel secretory mechanism. *J. Cell. Biol.* **1990**, *110*, 1681–1691.
50. Gu, M.; Wang, W.; Song, W. K.; Cooper, D. N. W.; Kaufman, S. J. Selective modulation of the interaction of a7b1 integrin with fibronectin and laminin by L-14 lectin during skeletal muscle differentiation. *J. Cell Sci.* **1994**, *107*, 175–181.
51. Case, D.; Irwin, D.; Ivester, C.; Harral, J.; Morris, K.; Imamura, M.; Roedersheimer, M.; Patterson, A.; Carr, M.; Hagen, M.; Savedra, M.; Crossno, J.; Young, K. A.; Dempsey, E. C.; Poirier, F.; West, J.; Majka, S. Mice deficient in galectin-1 exhibit attenuated physiological responses to chronic hypoxia-induced pulmonary hypertension. *Am. J. Physiol.: Lung Cell. Mol. Physiol.* **2007**, *292*, L154–L164.

Chapter 21

Autoimmune Disorders in Galectin-3 Deficient Mice

Vladislav Volarevic and Miodrag L. Lukic*

Centre for Molecular Medicine and Stem Cell Research, Faculty of Medical Sciences, University of Kragujevac, 69 Svetozara Markovica Street, 34000 Kragujevac, Serbia
***E-mail: miodrag.lukic@medf.kg.ac.rs**

Despite the fact that all galectins have a galactose-defined specificity, galectin-3 has important pro-inflammatory role while other members of the galectin family, including galectin-1, galectin-2, galectin-4, galectin-9, mainly have anti-inflammatory effects in autoimmune disorders. The basis for such a completely opposite effect of galectin-3 in immune regulation remains unclear and merits further in-depth investigation. It is important that galectin-3 has pro-inflammatory role in T-cell mediated diseases: Con A induced hepatitis, MLD-STZ diabetes, EAE and antigen induced arthritis. Targeting galectin-3 as endogenous inflammatory mediator should serve as a platform for designing novel drugs with aim to prevent or resolve the inflammatory response in T cell mediated autoimmune pathology.

Introduction

A family of beta-galactosides-binding proteins, galectins, has recently emerged as novel molecules with immunoregulatory functions. Among them, galectin-3 is the most ubiquitously expressed by immunocompetent and inflammatory cells, either constitutively or in an inducible fashion (*1*). It is expressed by macrophages, dendritic cells (DCs), eosinophils, mast cells, natural killer (NK) cells and activated T and B lymphocytes giving a broad spectrum of involvement in the immune response (*1*).

Depending on the type and status of immune cells, galectin-3 can be found within the nucleus, in the cytoplasm, on the cell surface and in the extracellular compartment (*2*). Galectin-3 is usually present in the cytoplasm, but it is translocated to the nucleus in proliferating cells, and is present in perinuclear regions in tumor cells following apoptotic stimuli, in cytoplasmic vesicles during glycoprotein sorting and in membrane ruffles of activated DCs (*2*).

Galectin-3 binds and interacts with numerous ligands in the intra- and extra-cellular environment (*3, 4*). Intracellularly, galectin-3 is engaged in processes that are pivotal for basic cellular functions, such as pre-mRNA splicing (*5, 6*) regulation of cell growth, cell cycle progression and apoptosis (*4*).

In the presence of carbohydrate ligands, galectin-3 is able to form pentamer through its NH2-terminal domain, can cross-link cell surface glycoconjugates forming lattice-like structures and modulates a signaling cascade in the cells (*7*). It is well known that extracellular galectin-3 acts as an adhesion molecule by cross-linking adjacent cells, and cells and extracellular matrix (*3, 4*). It is able to oligomerize and participates in multivalent interactions with cell surface and extracellular matrix glycans, through lectin-carbohydrate interactions, affecting migration of immune cells (*3, 4*).

Galectin 3 in Immune Response

Galectin-3 serves as a chemoattractant for monocytes and macrophages (*8*). Galectin-3 knockout mice (gal-$3^{-/-}$) exhibit reduced inflammatory responses measured by decreased numbers of leukocyte infiltrates, while the addition of recombinant galectin-3 significantly increased the presence of monocytes at the site of infection leading to exacerbation of immune response (*3*).

Galectin-3 is important for alternative activation of macrophages (*9*). It binds to Cluster of differentiation (CD)98 receptor, promotes phosphoinositide 3-kinase (PI3K) activation that leads to alternative activation of macrophages. Knockdown of the galectin-3 gene in 129sv mice specifically restrains IL-4/IL-13-induced alternative macrophage activation in bone marrow-derived macrophages *in vitro* and in resident lung and recruited peritoneal macrophages *in vivo* without affecting IFN-γ/ lipopolysaccharide (LPS)-induced classical activation or IL-10-induced deactivation (*9*). IL-4-mediated alternative macrophage activation is inhibited by deletion of galectin-3 and is blocked by bis-(3-deoxy-3-(3-methoxybenzamido)-beta-D-galactopyranosyl) sulfane, a specific inhibitor of extracellular galectin-3 carbohydrate binding. In addition, an increased expression and secretion of galectin-3 correlates with other phenotypic markers of alternative macrophage activation, while LPS-induced classical macrophage activation results with inhibition of galectin-3 expression and release (*9*).

Galectin-3 plays an important role in phagocytosis (*10*). It acts as an opsonin and enhances macrophage clearance of apoptotic neutrophils (*10*). Macrophages of gal-$3^{-/-}$ mice had a delayed phagocytic response and ingested fewer cells than the wild type (WT) mice. Endogenous galectin-3 translocates to the phagosomes in cells that have engulfed erythrocytes contributing to FcgR-mediated phagocytosis (*11*).

It was shown that galectin-3 increases phagocytic activity of neutrophils in CD66a and CD66b-dependent manner (*12*). In addition, galectin-3 is important both for migration and activation of neutrophils (*3*). Recombinant galectin-3 promotes the adhesion of human neutrophils to laminin (*13*) and endothelial cells (*14*), potentiates LPS-induced production of interleukin (IL)-1 (*15*), triggers the production of superoxide anion and induces a respiratory burst in LPS-stimulated neutrophils (*3*).

Galectin-3 is important for migration and cytokine production of DCs (*16*). In comparison with WT mice, bone marrow derived DCs of gal-$3^{-/-}$ mice have a defective migratory response to chemokines *in vitro* and reduced migration to lymph nodes *in vivo* (*17*). Intracellular galectin-3 was found to have a suppressive effect on the production of IL-12 by DCs attenuating Th1 immune response (*18*, *19*). It was recently shown that galectin-3 silencing in DCs enhances T cell activation and interferon-γ (IFN-γ) production (*20*). Knockdown of galectin-3 in DCs enhanced allogeneic T cell responses: allogeneic CD4+ T cells incubated with galectin-3 knockdown DCs produced more IFN-γ and less IL-10 compared with control cells (*20*). The percentage of apoptotic T cells was significantly higher in cultures with control DCs than that with galectin-3 knockdown DCs indicating that DC-expressed galectin-3 is regulatory molecule that favors the inhibition of T cell activation (*20*).

Galectin-3 induces mediator release by mast cells, through the cross-linking of FcεRI and/or FcεRI–IgE complex, since both FcεRI and IgE were shown to be galectin-3 binding-partners (*3*, *21*). It also acts as a mediator of IgE production in B lymphocytes (*3*).

Galectin-3 is significantly expressed on the cell surface of eosinophils isolated from patients with allergic diseases and has an important role in eosinophil rolling (*22*). It functions as a cell surface adhesion molecule that acts either independently or in cooperation with selectins and integrins augmenting the multistep cascade resulting with eosinophil recruitment to the sites of allergic inflammation (*22*). An endogenous galectin-3 promotes inflammatory response in murine model of astma: significantly fewer eosinophils and less airway hyperresponsiveness was noticed in ovalbumin-sensitized galectin-$3^{-/-}$ mice compared to similarly treated WT mice (*3*). Opposite, pharmacological application of galectin-3 suppresses inflammation in rat model of astma: intratracheal instillation of galectin-3-expression plasmid inhibits bronchial obstruction and inflammation through IL-5 gene down-regulation (*3*). In accordance, the exposure of human eosinophils to galectin-3 results in a selective inhibition of IL-5 expression, on both protein and mRNA level due to signal transduction from galectin-3 stimulated FcγRII (*3*).

Galectin 3 is important for NK cell-mediated cytotoxicity (*23*, *24*). Galectin-$3^{-/-}$ mice constitutively have a significantly higher percentage of effective cytotoxic CD27(high)CD11b(high) NK cells as well as the percentage of immature CD27(high)CD11b(low) NK cells (*23*). In contrast, CD27(low)CD11b(high) less functionally exhausted NK cells and NK cells bearing inhibitory KLRG1 receptor are numerous in WT mice (*23*). Galectin-3 reduces the affinity of major histocompatibility complex class I-related chain A (MICA) for NK-activating receptor NKG2D, thereby severely impairing NK cell activation and silencing the NK cells (*24*). This galectin-3 dependent mode of NK cell silencing could be important for evasion of NK cell immunity by tumor cells.

Galectin-3 is not expressed in resting primary T cells (*25*). However, the expression of galectin-3 is noticed both in activated and memory T cells suggesting that galectin-3 expression is upregulated upon differentiation of naive T cells (*2*). In mouse CD4+ and CD8+ T cells, galectin-3 expression is inducible upon activation with CD3 antibody, the plant lectin concanavalin A (Con A) plus IL-2, and calcium ionophores (*26*). Interestingly, galectin-3 expression levels are low following induction by CD3 antibody, Con A, or IL-2 alone, suggesting that a combination of receptor cross-linking and proliferative stimulus is required for galectin-3 expression in T cells (*26*).

Galectin-3 is expressed in human immunodeficiency virus type I (HIV-I) and human lymphotropic virus type I (HTLV-I) infected T lymphocytes (*2*). Galectin-3 expression was also described in biopsies of patients with T-cell lymphoma (*2*). These virus infected and tumor cells may be considered to be in a permanent state of activation and dysregulated pathways in these cells likely contribute to galectin-3 induction (*2*).

Galectin-3 is expressed in CD4+CD25+Foxp3+ T regulatory (Tregs) cells. Both galectin-3 mRNA and protein expression were observed in circulating Tregs, and were also found to be induced following Foxp3 transfection into CD4+ effector cells (*27*).

The effect of galectin-3 in the regulation of T cell function depends on its localization. Extracellular galectin-3 promotes migration and interferes with adhesion of thymocytes with stromal cells, induces T cell activation, apoptosis and suppresses IL-5 production in primary T cells and cell lines. When delivered extracellularly, galectin-3 is capable to activate T cells. In Jurkat E6-1 T cells, galectin-3 induces secretion of IL-2 in a manner that is similar to action of the plant lectin from Phaseolus vulgaris (PHA). As it was previously described in eosinophils, recombinant galectin-3 inhibits IL-5 but not IL-4 expression in activated T lymphocytes (*2*).

Extracellular galectin-3 has been shown to induce apoptosis in T cells, including human T leukemia cell lines and activated mouse T cells (*28*, *29*). Secreted galectin-3 binds mainly to CD45, CD71 or CD7 and CD29 molecules resulting in the activation of the mitochondrial pathway including cytochrome-c release and caspase-3 activation leading to apoptosis of T cells (*29*).

Intracellular galectin-3 promotes cell growth, inhibits apoptosis and attenuates TCR signaling in primary T cells and cell lines (*2*).

Galectin-3 is the only member of the galectin family, known by now, that acts as anti-apoptotic molecule. It is interesting to notice that there is 28% identity and 48% similarity between protein sequences of galectin-3 and anti-apoptotic molecule Bcl-2 (*2*). Complementarity determining region (CRD) of galectin-3 contains the NWGR motif (residues 180–183), highly conserved in Bcl-2 family members, essential for anti-apoptotic activity of galectin-3. The anti-apoptotic effect of the intracellular galectin-3 is well documented (*1–4*). In the response to a variety of apoptotic stimuli, galectin-3 translocates from the cytosol or the nucleus to the perinuclear mitochondrial membrane in synexin-mediated manner, prevents mitochondrial damage and inhibits cytochrome c release, downregulating caspase activation (*3*). The anti-apoptotic effects of galectin-3 in T-cell are also mediated through its interaction with CD95 (APO-1/Fas) receptor. Intracellular galectin-3 associates with CD95 and stimulates caspase-8 activation, interferes with apoptotic signaling pathway from caspase-8 to mitochondria and inhibits C2-ceramide-induced apoptosis (*2*).

Naive gal-$3^{-/-}$ CD4+ T cells secreted more IFN-γ and IL-4 than naive gal-$3^{+/+}$ CD4+ T cells after TCR engagement indicating that intracellular galectin-3 principally acts as an inhibitory regulator of T-cell activation (*30*). Galectin-3 is able to form complexes with TCR glycans, therefore limiting TCR clustering necessary for initiation of TCR-mediated signaling (*31*). In addition, in activated T cells galectin-3 is recruited to the cytoplasmic side of the immunological synapse where it promotes TCR down-regulation through modulating function of Alix, a component of the endosomal sorting complex required for transport (ESCRT) (*30*).

The role of galectin-3 in Th1/Th2 polarization is controversial, probably because the effect of galectin-3 in T cell differentiation is disease and model-dependent. Gal- $3^{-/-}$ mice were reported to be Th2 defective in an ovalbumin-induced asthma model, but had a normal Th2 response following intestinal nematode and schistosome infection (*2*). In addition, as previously described, galectin-3 was shown to down-regulate IL-5 gene expression both in T cells and eosinophils (*3*).

Galectin-3 is constitutively expressed and secreted by human bone marrow-derived and umbilical cord blood-derived mesenchymal stem cells (MSCs) (*32*), self-renewable cells with immunomodulatory characteristics (*33*). MSCs can inhibit T-cell proliferation by engagement of the inhibitory molecules (such as programmed death 1 or interleukin 1 receptor antagonist) (*34*), by producing soluble factors that suppress T-cell proliferation (such as TGF-β or IL-10), through interacting with DCs and by increasing the number of Tregs (*35, 36*). In accordance with these mechanisms, it was recently showed that human MSCs also use secreted galectins to suppress T-cell mediated immune response (*32*).

Inhibition of galectin-1 and galectin-3 gene expression with small interfering RNAs abrogated the suppressive effect of MSC on allogeneic T cells (*32*). Specific gene silencing of galectin-3 reduced the expression of galectin-1 in MSCs, suggesting a possible interaction between these two galectins in MSC-mediated suppression of immune response. In addition, suppression of T-cell proliferation by MSCs could be abrogated by exogenous addition of β lactose, a competitive inhibitor for galectin-3 binding to cell surface glycoproteins (*32*). The restoration of T-cell proliferation in the presence of β lactose clearly indicates that the carbohydrate-recognition domain of galectin-3 is responsible for the immunosuppression of T cells and supports an extracellular mechanism of action of MSC-secreted galectin-3.

In summing up, galectin-3 can be positive and negative regulator of inflammatory response, depending on specific inflammatory conditions, galectin-3 expression and the type of targeted cell. In general, galectin-3 is a powerful pro-inflammatory molecule. It is secreted as a response to various inflammatory stimuli. Secreted galectin-3 affects virtually all inflammatory cells by an autocrine or paracrine mechanism: it is chemo attractant for neutrophils, monocytes, macrophages, it triggers respiratory burst in phagocytes and induces mediator and cytokine release by mast cells and T lymphocytes. Additionally, intracellular galectin-3 could contribute to the persistence of the inflammation by acting as an anti-apoptotic factor in promoting the survival of inflammatory cells, particularly T lymphocytes in T cell mediated pathology.

In the following we describe the role of galectin-3 in experimental, T-cell mediated inflammatory and autoimmune disorders.

Experimentally Induced Disorders in Galectin 3 Deficient Mice T Cell Mediated Hepatitis

Galectin-3 is involved in the pathogenesis of inflammatory and malignant liver diseases (*37*, *38*). It plays a major role in the removal of circulating advanced lipoxidation endproducts (ALEs) by the liver, and the deletion of galectin-3 accelerates nonalcoholic steatohepatitis (NASH) or prevents the development of ALE-induced liver injury (*37*). Galectin-3 is involved in the progression of hepatocellular carcinoma where a higher expression rate of nuclear galectin-3 shows a markedly worse prognosis in malignant and chronic inflammatory liver diseases, suggesting different roles of Gal-3 in tumors and autoimmunity (*37*, *38*).

Con A-induced liver injury is a well established experimental model of T cell mediated hepatitis (*39–43*). In this model, intravenous injection of Con A induces acute liver injury and systemic immune activation in mice that resembles the pathology of immune-mediated hepatitis in humans (*42*). Intravenously injected Con A is mainly phagocyted by liver macrophages and presented to CD4+ T lymphocytes, leading to their activation (*42*). CD4+ T lymphocytes infiltrate the liver tissue and secrete large amounts of cytokines, such as tumor necrosis factor alpha (TNF-α), IFN-γ, IL-2, IL-6, and granulocyte macrophage colony stimulating factor (*42–47*). Apart from CD4+ T cells, CD8+ T cells, as well as NK, NKT cells and macrophages could also induce hepatocyte cell death by cell to cell contact, through secretion of pro inflammatory cytokines or reactive oxygen species (*42–47*).

In Con A-induced liver injury, galectin-3 plays an important pro-inflammatory role by promoting the activation of T lymphocytes and NKT cells, maturation of DCs, secretion of pro-inflammatory cytokines, down-regulation of alternative (M2) macrophage polarization and apoptosis of mononuclear cells (MNCs) in the liver (*48*).

Gal-3$^{-/-}$ mice are less sensitive to Con A–induced hepatic injury. After Con A injection, liver tissue sections in gal-3$^{-/-}$ mice showed several solitary areas of necrotic tissue while the majority of hepatocytes were not damaged. On contrary, liver tissue sections in Con A-treated WT mice showed widespread areas of necrosis with extensive infiltration of MNCs within liver lobules and around the central veins and portal tracts, indicating the ongoing inflammatory process (*48*).

Targeted disruption of galectin-3 gene attenuated liver injury by reducing the number of effector cells, including T lymphocytes (both CD4+ and CD8+),

B lymphocytes, DCs, and NK and NKT cells, and increasing the number of IL-10-producing CD4+ T cells and alternatively activated (M2-polarized) macrophages. In addition, knockdown of galectin-3 gene, because of the lack of intracellular, anti-apoptotic galectin-3, enhanced the apoptosis of liver-infiltrating MNCs contributing to the lower number of mononuclear cells in the livers of Con A treated gal-3$^{-/-}$ mice (*48*).

The level of TNF-α, IFN-γ, IL-17 and IL-4 in the sera and total number of TNF-α-, IFN-γ-, IL-17- and IL-4-producing CD4+ cells and IL-12-producing DCs were lower in the livers of Con A treated gal-3$^{-/-}$ mice. In contrast, total number of IL-10-producing CD4+ T cells and alternatively activated macrophages were significantly higher in the livers of gal-3$^{-/-}$ mice. Additionally, the ratio between the total number of IL-10- and IFN-γ producing CD4+ T cells was significantly higher in the liver of Con A–treated gal-3$^{-/-}$ mice compared to WT mice, suggesting that, in Con A hepatitis, galectin-3 affects production of hepatoprotective IL-10 in CD4+ T cells (*48–50*).

Although there were significantly lower levels of both Th1 and Th2 cytokines in the sera of Con A treated gal-3$^{-/-}$ mice, there was no significant difference in the levels of TNF-α, IFN-γ, IL-17, IL-4 and IL-10 in supernatants of *in vitro* Con A–stimulated splenocytes isolated from healthy WT and gal-3$^{-/-}$ mice (*48*) suggesting that the inflammatory milieu of the Con A–damaged liver is most likely responsible for the difference in cytokine production of liver-infiltrating MNCs of WT and gal-3$^{-/-}$ mice.

As it is previously discussed, galectin-3 is important for the migration, adhesion, and maturation of DCs (*16–20*). IL-12, mainly produced by DCs and macrophages, is essential for the onset of Con A–induced hepatitis, because IL-12 interacts directly with NKT cells, contributes to their recruitment to the liver, and enhances immune response through increased IL-4 (*51*). Accordingly, attenuated liver injury noticed in Con A treated gal-3$^{-/-}$ mice correlates with a significantly reduced number of IL-12-producing DCs, activated NK, NKT cells and IL-4-producing CD4+ T cells that was accompanied by a decreased serum level of IL-4 (*48*). Furthermore, a decreased number of IL-12-producing DCs in livers of Con A treated gal-3$^{-/-}$ mice indicates that galectin-3 plays an important role in the antigen presentation and activation of T lymphocytes in Con A hepatitis.

Pretreatment of WT mice with selective galectin-3 inhibitor (TD139) (*52*) attenuated Con A–induced liver injury (*48*). Intraperitoneal injection of TD139 in WT mice 2 hours before and immediately after Con A injection suppressed the infiltration of IFN-γ-, IL-17- and IL-4-producing CD4+ and IFN-γ-producing CD8+ lymphocytes, increased the total number of IL-10-producing CD4+ T cells, attenuated serum levels of IFN-γ, IL-17 and IL-4, elevated the serum level of IL-10 and increased the number of alternatively activated (M2-polarized) macrophages (*48*). Knowing that galectin-3 has an important role in the phagocytic function of macrophages (*11*), it seems that pretreatment with TD139 inhibited the expression of galectin-3 on macrophages, impaired phagocytosis of Con A, and reduced the activation of CD4+ T cells, manifested by the lower number of IFN-γ-, IL-17- and IL-4-producing CD4+T cells and the higher number of CD4+IL-10- producing T lymphocytes in livers of Con A–treated mice that received TD139.

Reduced inflammation noticed in the livers of Con A treated gal-$3^{-/-}$ mice and TD139 pre-treated WT mice could be the result of both macrophage and T-cell attenuation. Consistent with recently published results in animal models of diet-induced NASH (*38*), galectin-3 deletion attenuates both Th1 and Th2 inflammatory responses in the liver and down-regulates the gene expression level of both Th1/M1 and Th2/M2 cells.

In accordance with data obtained in Con A hepatitis, it was shown that galectin-3 is highly expressed in the livers of patients suffering from acute liver disease (*48*). Compared to healthy controls, galectin-3 was strongly expressed in lining cells of hepatic sinuses both in patients with isoniazid-induced and hepatitis B virus-induced fulminant hepatitis (*48*), indicating an important role of galectin-3 in liver inflammation.

In conclusion, galectin-3 is highly expressed in inflamed liver, has an important pro-inflammatory role in fulminant hepatitis and therefore could be a potential target for therapeutic intervention in acute liver failure.

Multiple Low-Dose Streptozotocin-Induced Diabetes

Multiple low-dose streptozotocin-induced diabetes (MLD-STZ diabetes) is an experimental model of type 1 diabetes characterized by delayed and sustained hyperglycemia (*53*). The initial destruction of some β cells due to MLD-STZ, similarly to viral infection, induces the activation of autoreactive T cells to multiple diabetogenic epitopes. This "epitope spreading" leads to chronic immunopathology and β-cell loss until biochemical and histological evidence of disease is present (*53*, *54*).

The lack of galectin-3 led to resistance to the induction of MLD-STZ diabetes in susceptible C57BL/6 mice (*55*), which was associated with the lack of significant MNC infiltration in the pancreatic islets and with retention of higher insulin content when compared with WT mice. It seems that the effect of galectin-3 deficiency on immune and accessory effector cells is responsible for the attenuation of diabetogenesis. Gal-3 is required for the optimal production of IL-1 and TNF-α (*56*). In accordance, macrophages of MLD-STZ treated gal-$3^{-/-}$ mice produce lower levels of inflammatory mediators, particularly TNF-α and nitric oxide (NO). More importantly, immune cells in the draining lymph node of gal-$3^{-/-}$ mice exhibit lower expression of IFN-γ and inducible nitric oxide synthases (iNOS) and do not express TNF-alpha and IL-17 after MLD-STZ treatment. The roles of TNF-alpha and IFN-γ in β-cell damage are well established (*57*), and it could be assumed that the attenuation of their production affects diabetogenesis *in vivo*. Apart from IFN-γ, there is evidence that IL-17 can contribute to the pathogenesis of autoimmune inflammation and that IL-23/IL-17 axis also plays a role in diabetogenesis (*53*).

It is important to note that conditional and specific NF-κB blockade protects pancreatic β cells from the diabetogenic effect of MLD-STZ (*58*). As galectin-3 is able to induce NF-κB activation (*30*), it is possible that the lack of galectin-3 attenuates β cell specific activation of NF-κB and prevents the progressive loss of β cells.

Thus, it seems that in MLD-STZ diabetes model, galectin-3 acts as a pro-diabetogenic rather than a protective factor by enhancing inflammation and autoimmune response within the pancreatic islets.

Opposite to MLD-STZ diabetes, animal studies provide evidence for protective function of galectin-3 in type 2 diabetes (T2D) and its associated secondary complications (*59*, *60*). Obesity-induced insulin resistance and dysfunction of islet β cells are characteristic of the disease (*59*, *60*). Additionally, accumulation of amyloid peptide in the islets stimulates inflammasome NLRP-3-dependent cleavage of caspase-1 and production of IL-1β in resident DCs and invading macrophages (*61*). This leads to β-cell loss and immune mediated accumulation of pro-inflammatory T cells.

Late glycation products accumulate on long-lived proteins and cause tissue damage correlating with the severity of diabetic complications. Galectin-3 binds to advanced glycation end-products (AGE) and stimulates their degradation (*60*) indicating protective role of galectin-3 in obesity and T2D. Accordingly, gal-3$^{-/-}$ mice reveal elevated AGE levels and signaling and show accelerated diabetic glomerulopathy (*60*).

It can be concluded that, in contrast to the β-cell loss in type 1 diabetes, in obesity induced type 2 diabetes, galectin-3 may exert protective effect. In line with these observations are results obtained from recently published clinical study showing that systemic galectin-3 is elevated in obesity and negatively correlates with glycated hemoglobin in T2D patients (*59*) suggesting that function of galectin-3 in human metabolic diseases may be not primarily associated with inflammation.

Experimental Autoimmune Encephalomyelitis

Multiple sclerosis is the inflammatory disease of the central nervous system (CNS), characterized by inflammatory lesions, demyelination and axonal loss (*62*). Experimental autoimmune encephalomyelitis (EAE) is an animal model of CNS inflammatory demyelination, commonly used as a model of multiple sclerosis in humans (*63*). Multiple sclerosis and EAE are supposed to be T cell-mediated autoimmune diseases. EAE is induced in susceptible animals by active immunization with myelin antigens mixed with adjuvants. T lymphocytes activated by encephalytogen in the periphery differentiate in inflammatory helper T cells which are able to pass blood-brain barrier where they recognize their cognate target antigen and initiate an inflammatory cascade leading to tissue damage (*63*). EAE can also be induced by passive transfer of myelin reactive population of CD4+ T helper cells (*63*). Both Th1 and Th17 cells are thought to be responsible for the inflammatory demyelination in CNS (*62*, *63*). In EAE, Th2 lymphocytes, Tregs and related cytokines such as IL-5 and IL-10 are important in the resolution stages of the disease (*62*, *63*). T helper cell differentiation toward inflammatory phenotype depends on the function of antigen presenting cells (*64*, *65*).

Galectin-3 appears to play a role in promoting EAE. This pathogenic role is associated with the ability of galectin-3 to preferentially limit IL-10 synthesis by DCs, which in turn biases the production of IL-17 and IFN-γ and inhibits the development of Th2 and Treg cells (*66*). Galectin-3-deficient mice immunized with myelin oligodendrocyte glycoprotein (MOG35–55) peptide developed markedly attenuated EAE compared with similarly immunized WT mice (*66*). The disease attenuation was accompanied by reduced cellular infiltration of monocytes and macrophages in the CNS supporting a key role of galectin-3 in promoting inflammation via local recruitment of leukocytes (*8*). Consistent with the previously discussed anti-apoptotic role of galectin-3 (*2*, *3*), CNS of gal-3$^{-/-}$ mice consisted of markedly elevated TUNEL-positive apoptotic cells which may further explain the significantly reduced number of infiltrating leukocytes in the CNS of gal-3$^{-/-}$ mice compared with WT animals (*66*).

Gal-3$^{-/-}$ mice developed enhanced Th2 response during EAE: IL-4, IL-5, IL-10, and Treg cells were all elevated in gal-3$^{-/-}$ mice, consistent with the protective role of Th2 and Treg cells in this disease. In addition, Th1 and Th17 lymphocytes of gal-3$^{-/-}$ mice produced less IFN-γ and IL-17 that was consistent with the reduced severity of EAE in these animals (*66*).

The effect of galectin-3 on Th1, Th2, Th17, and Treg polarization may be secondary to its effect on DC functions. As it is previously discussed, DCs express a high density of galectin-3 (*17*). Bone marrow derived DCs of naive gal-3$^{-/-}$ mice and splenic DCs of immunized gal-3$^{-/-}$ mice produced markedly elevated IL-10 (but not IL-12) in response to LPS compared with WT DCs (*66*). Moreover, galectin-3-deficient DCs induced antigen specific T cells to produce more IL-4, IL-5 and IL-10, but less IL-17 (*66*), suggesting an association of galectin-3 with the promotion of Th1 cells and limiting the differentiation of Th2 cells and Treg cells during EAE.

More evidences confirmed that galectin-3 affects inflammation in the CNS during EAE. Extracellular galectin-3 is able to exert cytokine-like regulatory action, activates immune and inflammatory signaling events through phosphorylation of STAT1, STAT3, STAT5 and JAK2 amplifying the inflammatory cascade in the brain (*67*).

In apparent contrast to these data, inflammatory demyelization and neurodegeneration were enhanced in mice, which display natural deficiencies in multiple N-glycosylation pathway enzymes (*68*). These differences may be related to the fact that other related galectins (galectin-1 and galectin-9) are able to suppress Th1 and Th17 immune response (*69–71*).

Earlier report (*31*) has shown that reduction in galectin-3 functions through the deletion of Mgat5 (β1, 6N-acetylglucosaminyltransferase V) in mice and leads to heightened susceptibility to EAE. The glycosylation deficiency in Mgat5$^{-/-}$ mice affects other pathways and cell types that may also contribute to the observed autoimmunity. Mgat5- modified glycans also reduce clusters of fibronectin receptors, therefore causing accelerated focal adhesion turnover in fibroblasts and tumor cells, a functionality that may affect leukocyte motility (*31*).

In summing up, galectin-3 plays an important pathogenic role in EAE and may therefore be a potential target for therapeutic intervention in autoimmune neurological diseases.

Methylated Bovine Serum Albumin Induced Arthritis

Rheumatoid arthritis (RA) is an autoimmune disease characterized by a massive infiltration of mononuclear and polymorphonuclear cells into the joints and the development of inflammation that results in destruction of articular cartilage and adjacent bone (*72*). Although the precise mechanism that gives rise to RA is still unknown, RA is thought to be T-cell mediated autoimmune disease. Activated CD4+ T helper cells and macrophages comprise a large proportion of the inflammatory cells that invade the synovial tissue (*73*) and represent the most important effector cells in RA. Pro-inflammatory cytokines: TNF-α, IL-6, and IL-17 produced by activated CD4+ T cells and macrophages are implicated in the establishment and progression of inflammatory joint destruction in RA (*72*, *73*).

Galectin-3 plays a pathogenic role in the development and progression of methylated bovine serum albumin induced artritis (antigen induced arthritis (AIA)), a well established experimental model of RA (*74*).

Significantly reduced synovitis and joint erosion was noticed in gal-3$^{-/-}$ mice compared with WT mice (*74*). This effect was partially restored by the addition of exogenous galectin 3 to gal-3$^{-/-}$ mice. The joints from gal-3$^{-/-}$ mice receiving recombinant galectin 3 had increased synovitis compared with gal-3$^{-/-}$ mice that received vehicle, and the level of synovitis was comparable with that in the WT group, clearly indicating pathogenic role of galectin-3 in AIA (*74*).

Reduced arthritis in gal-3$^{-/-}$ mice was accompanied by a significant decrease in circulating antigen specific IgG antibodies, decreased systemic production of pro-inflammatory cytokines TNF-alpha and IL-6 and the frequency of IL-17-producing T cells (*74*). Interestingly, the significant difference in serum levels of TNF-α and IL-6 between WT and gal-3$^{-/-}$ mice was noticed only on day 10, prior to the induction of joint arthritis, suggesting that galectin 3 modulates production of TNF-α and IL-6 only at early stages of AIA (*74*).

Gal-3$^{-/-}$ mice, which were protected from AIA, displayed significantly lower infiltration of inflammatory cells in the joints and significantly lower frequency of IL-17–producing CD3+ splenocytes (*74*). IL-17 has a direct role in joint destruction and plays an essential role in mediating neutrophil migration during inflammation through chemokine release (*75*).

Sinovial fibroblasts and neutrophils are important cells involved in amplifying the local inflammation and joint damage in RA (*72–74*). Once accumulated at the site of inflammation, neutrophils are potentially responsible for damage to surrounding tissues by producing reactive oxygen species (ROS) and hydrolytic enzymes. Another hypothetical mechanism for mediating the pro-inflammatory activity of galectin-3 in AIA and RA is the direct targeting by galectin 3 of synovial fibroblasts and neutrophils locally in the joints (*74*). Galectin-3 can induce massive production of ROS from neutrophils and splenocytes (*76*, *77*) and has an important role in promoting mononuclear cell infiltration in the joints (*78*).

In line with data obtained in experimental model of RA (*74*), galectin-3 was highly expressed in the inflamed synovium and the level of galectin-3 was elevated in synovial fluid of RA patients compared to healthy controls and to patients with osteoarthritis (*79*). Upon galectin-3 stimulation, isolated synovial fibroblasts from RA patients are able to secrete significant amounts of pro-inflammatory and mononuclear cell– recruiting chemokines. It can be concluded that the elevated levels of galectin 3 in the joint stimulate fibroblasts and locally infiltrated neutrophils to produce chemokines, cytokines and ROS, involved in amplifying the immune responses and causing bone destruction.

Taken together, galectin-3 plays a pathogenic role in the development and progression of AIA and may be new molecular target for therapeutic treatment of RA.

Concluding Remarks and Future Directions

Despite the fact that all galectins have similar carbohydrate specificity, galectin-3 has important pro-inflammatory role while other members of the galectin family, including galectin-1 (*71*, *80*), galectin-2 (*81*), galectin-4 (*82*), galectin-9 (*69*, *70*), mainly have anti-inflammatory effects in autoimmune disorders. The question as to how subtle structural differences in galectin-3 with regard to other members of the family could lead to a completely opposite effect in immune regulation remains unclear and merits further in-depth investigation.

Finally, it should be concluded that galectin-3 has pro-inflammatory role in T-cell mediated diseases: Con A induced hepatitis, MLD-STZ diabetes, EAE and antigen induced arthritis. Targeting galectin-3, as endogenous inflammatory mediator, should serve as a platform for designing novel drugs with aim to prevent or resolve the inflammatory response in T cell mediated autoimmune pathology.

References

1. Radosavljevic, G.; Volarevic, V.; Jovanovic, I.; Milovanovic, M.; Pejnovic, N.; Arsenijevic, N.; Hsu, D. K.; Lukic, M. L. The roles of Galectin-3 in autoimmunity and tumor progression. *Immunol. Res.* **2012**, *52*, 100–110.
2. Hsu, D. K.; Chen, H. Y.; Liu, F. T. Galectin-3 regulates T-cell functions. *Immunol. Rev.* **2009**, *230*, 114–127.
3. Dumic, J.; Dabelic, S.; Flogel, M. Galectin-3: An open-ended story. *Biochim. Biophys. Acta* **2006**, *1760*, 616–635.
4. Liu, F. T.; Rabinovich, G. A. Galectins as modulators of tumour progression. *Nat. Rev. Cancer* **2005**, *5*, 29–41.
5. Dagher, S. F.; Wang, J. L.; Patterson, R. J. Identification of galectin-3 as a factor in pre-mRNA splicing. *Proc. Natl. Acad. Sci. U.S.A.* **1995**, *92*, 1213–1217.
6. Wang, J. L.; Gray, R. M.; Haudek, K. C.; Patterson, R. J. Nucleocytoplasmic lectins. *Biochim. Biophys. Acta* **2004**, *1673*, 75–93.
7. Ahmad, N.; Gabius, H. J.; Andre′, S.; Kaltner, H.; Sabesan, S.; Roy, R.; Liu, B.; Macaluso, F.; Brewer, C. F. Galectin-3 precipitates as a pentamer with synthetic multivalent carbohydrates and forms heterogeneous cross-linked complexes. *J. Biol. Chem.* **2004**, *279*, 10841–10847.

8. Sano, H.; Hsu, D. K.; Yu, L.; Apgar, J. R.; Kuwabara, I.; Yamanaka, T.; Hirashima, M.; Liu, F. T. Human galectin-3 is a novel chemoattractant for monocytes and macrophages. *J. Immunol.* **2000**, *165*, 2156–2164.
9. MacKinnon, A. C.; Farnworth, S. L.; Hodkinson, P. S.; Henderson, N. C.; Atkinson, K. M.; Leffler, H.; Nilsson, U. J.; Haslett, C.; Forbes, S. J.; Sethi, T. Regulation of alternative macrophage activation by galectin-3. *J. Immunol.* **2008**, *180*, 2650–2658.
10. Liu, F. T.; Hsu, D. K.; Zuberi, R. I.; Kuwabara, I.; Chi, E. Y.; Henderson, W. R., Jr Expression and function of galectin-3, a b-galactosidebinding lectin, in human monocytes and macrophages. *Am. J. Pathol.* **1995**, *147*, 1016–2109.
11. Sano, H.; Hsu, D. K.; Apgar, J. R.; Yu, L.; Sharma, B. B.; Kuwabara, I.; Izui, S.; Liu, F. T. Critical role of galectin-3 in phagocytosis by macrophages. *J. Clin. Invest.* **2003**, *112*, 389–397.
12. Feuk-Lagerstedt, E.; Jordan, E.; Leffler, H.; Dahlgren, C.; Karlsson, A. Identification of CD66a and CD66b as the major galectin-3 receptor candidates in human neutrophils. *J. Immunol.* **1999**, *163*, 5592–5598.
13. Kuwabara, I.; Liu, F. T. Galectin-3 promotes adhesion of human neutrophils to laminin. *J. Immunol.* **1996**, *156*, 3939–3944.
14. Sato, S.; Ouellet, N.; Pelletier, I.; Simard, M.; Rancourt, A.; Bergeron, M. G. Role of galectin-3 as an adhesion molecule for neutrophil extravasation during streptococcal pneumonia. *J. Immunol.* **2002**, *168*, 1813–1822.
15. Jeng, K.; Frigeri, L.; Liu, F. T. An endogenous lectin, galectin-3 (epsilon BP/Mac-2), potentiates IL-1 production by human monocytes. *Immunol. Lett.* **1994**, *42*, 113–116.
16. Larsen, L.; Chen, H. Y.; Saegusa, J.; Liu, F. T. Galectin-3 and the skin. *J. Dermatol. Sci.* **2011**, *64*, 85–91.
17. Hsu, D. K.; Chernyavsky, A. I.; Chen, H. Y.; Yu, L.; Grando, S. A.; Liu, F. T. Endogenous galectin-3 is localized in membrane lipid rafts and regulates migration of dendritic cells. *J. Invest. Dermatol.* **2009**, *129*, 573–583.
18. Bernardes, E. S.; Silva, N. M.; Ruas, L. P.; Mineo, J. R.; Loyola, A. M.; Hsu, D. K.; Liu, F. T.; Chammas, R.; Roque-Barreira, M. C. *Toxoplasma gondii* infection reveals a novel regulatory role for galectin-3 in the interface of innate and adaptive immunity. *Am. J. Pathol.* **2006**, *168*, 1910–1920.
19. Breuilh, L.; Vanhoutte, F.; Fontaine, J.; van Stijn, C. M.; Tillie-Leblond, I.; Capron, M.; Faveeuw, C.; Jouault, T.; van Die, I.; Gosset, P.; Trottein, F. Galectin-3 modulates immune and inflammatory responses during helminthic infection: Impact of galectin-3 deficiency on the functions of dendritic cells. *Infect. Immun.* **2007**, *75*, 5148–5157.
20. Mobergslien, A.; Sioud, M. Galectin-1 and -3 gene silencing in immature and mature dendritic cells enhances T cell activation and interferon-γ production. *J. Leukoc. Biol.* **2012**, *91*, 461–7.
21. Frigeri, L.; Zuberi, R.; Liu, F. T. Epsilon BP, a beta-galactoside binding animal lectin, recognizes IgE receptor (Fc epsilon RI) and activates mast cells. *Biochemistry* **1993**, *32*, 7644–7649.
22. Rao, S. P.; Wang, Z.; Zuberi, R. I.; Sikora, L.; Bahaie, N. S.; Zuraw, B. L.; Liu, F. T.; Sriramarao, P. Galectin-3 functions as an adhesion molecule to

support eosinophil rolling and adhesion under conditions of flow. *J. Immunol.* **2007**, *179*, 7800–7807.

23. Radosavljevic, G.; Jovanovic, I.; Majstorovic, I.; Mitrovic, M.; Lisnic, V. J.; Arsenijevic, N.; Jonjic, S.; Lukic, M. L. Deletion of galectin-3 in the host attenuates metastasis of murine melanoma by modulating tumor adhesion and NK cell activity. *Clin. Exp. Metastasis* **2011**, *28*, 451–462.
24. Tsuboi, S.; Sutoh, M.; Hatakeyama, S.; Hiraoka, N.; Habuchi, T.; Horikawa, Y.; Hashimoto, Y.; Yoneyama, T.; Mori, K.; Koie, T.; Nakamura, T.; Saitoh, H; Yamaya, K.; Funyu, T.; Fukuda, M.; Ohyama, C. A novel strategy for evasion of NK cell immunity by tumours expressing core2 O-glycans. *EMBO J.* **2011**, *30*, 3173–3185.
25. Chiariotti, L.; Salvatore, P.; Frunzio, R.; Bruni, C. B. Galectin genes: Regulation of expression. *Glycoconj J* **2004**, *19*, 441–449.
26. Joo, H. G.; Goedegebuure, P. S.; Sadanaga, N.; Nagoshi, M.; von Bernstorff, W.; Eberlein, T. J. Expression and function of galectin-3, a beta-galactoside-binding protein in activated T lymphocytes. *J. Leukoc. Biol.* **2001**, *69*, 555–564.
27. Ocklenburg, F.; et al. UBD, a downstream element of FOXP3, allows the identification of LGALS3, a new marker of human regulatory T cells. *Lab. Invest.* **2006**, *86*, 724–737.
28. Stillman, B. N.; Hsu, D. K.; Pang, M.; Brewer, C. F.; Johnson, P.; Liu, F. T.; Baum, L. G. Galectin-3 and galectin-1 bind distinct cell surface glycoprotein receptors to induce T cell death. *J. Immunol.* **2006**, *176*, 778–789.
29. Fukumori, T.; Takenaka, Y.; Yoshii, T.; Kim, H. R. C.; Hogan, V.; Inohara, H.; Kagawa, S.; Raz, A. CD29 and CD7 mediate galectin-3- induced type II T-cell apoptosis. *Cancer Res.* **2003**, *63*, 8302–8311.
30. Chen, H. Y.; Fermin, A.; Vardhana, S.; Weng, I. C.; Lo, K. F.; Chang, E. Y.; Maverakis, E.; Yang, R. Y.; Hsu, D. K.; Dustin, M. L.; Liu, F. T. Galectin-3 negatively regulates TCR-mediated CD4+ T-cell activation at the immunological synapse. *Proc. Natl. Acad. Sci. U.S.A.* **2009**, *106*, 14496–14501.
31. Demetriou, M.; Granovsky, M.; Quaggin, S.; Dennis, J. W. Negative regulation of T-cell activation and autoimmunity by Mgat5 N-glycosylation. *Nature* **2001**, *409*, 733–739.
32. Sioud, M. New insights into mesenchymal stromal cell-mediated T-cell suppression through galectins. *Scand. J. Immunol.* **2011**, *73*, 79–84.
33. Volarevic, V.; Ljujic, B.; Stojkovic, P.; Lukic, A.; Arsenijevic, N.; Stojkovic, M. Human stem cell research and regenerative medicine: Present and future. *Br. Med. Bull.* **2011**, *99*, 155–168.
34. Volarevic, V.; Al-Qahtani, A.; Arsenijevic, N.; Pajovic, S.; Lukic, M. L. Interleukin-1 receptor antagonist (IL-1Ra) and IL-1Ra producing mesenchymal stem cells as modulators of diabetogenesis. *Autoimmunity* **2010**, *43*, 255–263.
35. Nauta, A. J.; Fibbe, W. E. Immunomodulatory properties of mesenchymal stromal cells. *Blood* **2007**, *110*, 3499–3506.

36. Volarevic, V.; Arsenijevic, N.; Lukic, M. L.; Stojkovic, M. Concise review: Mesenchymal stem cell treatment of the complications of diabetes mellitus. *Stem Cells* **2011**, *29*, 5–10.
37. Matsuda, Y.; Yamagiwa, Y.; Fukushima, K.; Ueno, Y.; Shimosegawa, T. Expression of galectin-3 involved in prognosis of patients with hepatocellular carcinoma. *Hepatol. Res.* **2008**, *38*, 1098–1111.
38. Iacobini, C.; Menini, S.; Ricci, C.; Fantauzzi, C. B.; Scipioni, A.; Salvi, L.; Cordone, S.; Delucchi, F.; Serino, M.; Federici, M; Pricci, F.; Pugliese, G. Galectin-3 ablation protects mice from diet-induced NASH: A major scavenging role for galectin-3 in liver. *J. Hepatol.* **2011**, *54*, 975–983.
39. Xiao, X.; Zhao, P.; Rodriguez-Pinto, D.; Qi, D.; Henegariu, O.; Alexopoulou, L.; Flavell, A.; Wong, S.; Wen, L. Inflammatory regulation by TLR3 in acute hepatitis. *J. Immunol.* **2009**, *183*, 3712–3719.
40. Itoh, A.; Isoda, K.; Kondoh, M.; Kawase, M.; Kobayashi, M.; Tamesada, M.; Yagi, K. Hepatoprotective effect of syringic acid and vanillic acid on concanavalin a-induced liver injury. *Biol. Pharm. Bull.* **2009**, *32*, 1215–1219.
41. Wolf, A. M.; Wolf, D.; Avila, M. A.; Moschen, A. R.; Berasain, C.; Enrich, B.; Rumpold, H.; Tilg, H. Up-regulation of the anti-inflammatory adipokine adiponectin in acute liver failure in mice. *J. Hepatol.* **2006**, *44*, 537–543.
42. Hanson, J. C.; Bostick, M. K.; Campe, C. B.; Kodali, P.; Lee, G.; Yan, J.; Maher, J. J. Transgenic overexpression of interleukin-8 in mouse liver protects against galactosamine/endotoxin toxicity. *J. Hepatol.* **2006**, *44*, 359–367.
43. Tiegs, G.; Hentschel, J.; Wendel, A. A T cell-dependent experimental liver injury in mice inducible by concanavalin A. *J. Clin. Invest.* **1992**, *90*, 196–203.
44. Volarevic, V.; Mitrovic, M.; Milovanovic, M.; Zelen, I.; Nikolic, I.; Mitrovic, S.; Pejnovic, N.; Arsenijevic, N.; Lukic, M. Protective role of IL-33/ST2 axis in con A-induced hepatitis. *J. Hepatol.* **2012**, *56*, 26–33.
45. Wang, J.; Sun, R.; Wei, H.; Dong, Z.; Gao, B.; Poly Tian, Z. Poly I: C prevents T cell-mediated hepatitis via an NK-dependent mechanism. *J. Hepatol.* **2006**, *44*, 446–454.
46. Takeda, K.; Hayakawa, Y.; Van Kaer, L.; Matsuda, H.; Yagita, H.; Okumura, K. Critical contribution of liver natural killer T cells to a murine model of hepatitis. *Proc. Natl. Acad. Sci. U.S.A.* **2000**, *97*, 5498–5503.
47. Gantner, F.; Leist, M.; Lohse, W.; Germann, G.; Tiegs, G. Concanavalin A-induced T-cell-mediated hepatic injury in mice: The role of tumor necrosis factor. *Hepatology* **1995**, *21*, 190–198.
48. Volarevic, V.; Milovanovic, M.; Ljujic, B.; Pejnovic, N.; Arsenijevic, N.; Nilsson, U.; Leffler, H.; Lukic, M. L. Galectin-3 deficiency prevents concanavalin A-induced hepatitis in mice. *Hepatology* **2012**, *55*, 1954–1964.
49. Louis, H.; Le Moine, O.; Peny, M. O.; Quertinmont, E.; Fokan, D.; Goldman, M.; Devière, J. Production and role of interleukin-10 in concanavalin A induced hepatitis in mice. *Hepatology* **1997**, *25*, 1382–1389.

50. Erhardt, A.; Biburger, M.; Papadopoulos, T.; Tiegs, G. IL-10, regulatory T cells, and Kupffer cells mediate tolerance in concanavalin A-induced liver injury in mice. *Hepatology* **2007**, *45*, 475–485.
51. Zhu, R.; Diem, S.; Araujo, L. M.; Aumeunier, A.; Denizeau, J.; Philadelphe, E.; Damotte, D.; Samson, M.; Gourdy, P.; Dy, M.; Schneider, E.; Herbelin, A. The Pro-Th1 cytokine IL-12 enhances IL-4 production by invariant NKT cells: Relevance for T cell-mediated hepatitis. *J. Immunol.* **2007**, *178*, 5435–5442.
52. Cumpstey, I.; Sundin, A; Leffler, H.; Nilsson, U. J. C2-symmetrical thiodigalactoside bis-benzamido derivatives as high-affinity inhibitors of galectin-3: Efficient lectin inhibition through double arginine-arene interactions. *Angew. Chem., Int. Ed. Engl.* **2005**, *44*, 5110–5112.
53. Mensah-Brown, E. P.; Shahin, A.; Al-Shamisi, M.; Wei, X.; Lukic, M. L. IL-23 leads to diabetes induction after subdiabetogenic treatment with multiple low doses of streptozotocin. *Eur. J. Immunol.* **2006**, *36*, 216–223.
54. Zdravkovic, N.; Shahin, A.; Arsenijevic, N.; Lukic, M. L.; Mensah-Brown, E. P. Regulatory T cells and ST2 signaling control diabetes induction with multiple low doses of streptozotocin. *Mol. Immunol.* **2009**, *47*, 28–36.
55. Mensah-Brown, E. P.; Al Rabesi, Z.; Shahin, A.; Al Shamsi, M.; Arsenijevic, N.; Hsu, D. K.; Liu, F. T.; Lukic, M. L. Targeted disruption of the galectin-3 gene results in decreased susceptibility to multiple low dose streptozotocin-induced diabetes in mice. *Clin. Immunol.* **2009**, *130*, 83–88.
56. Jeng, K. C.; Frigeri, L. G.; Liu, F. T. An endogenous lectin, galectin-3 (epsilon BP/Mac-2), potentiates IL-1 production by human monocyte. *Immunol. Lett.* **1994**, *42*, 113–116.
57. Cnop, M.; Welsh, N.; Jonas, J. C.; Jorns, A.; Lenzen, S.; Eizirik, D. L. Mechanisms of pancreatic beta-cell death in type 1 and type 2 diabetes: Many differences, few similarities. *Diabetes* **2005**, *54*, S97–107.
58. Eldor, R.; Yeffet, A.; Baum, K; Doviner, V; Amar, D.; Ben-Neriah, Y.; Christofori, G.; Peled, A.; Carel, J. C.; Boitard, C.; Klein, T.; Serup, P.; Eizirik, D. L.; Melloul, D. Conditional and specific NF-kappaB blockade protects pancreatic beta cells from diabetogenic agents. *Proc. Natl. Acad. Sci. U.S.A.* **2006**, *103*, 5072–5077.
59. Weigert, J.; Neumeier, M.; Wanninger, J.; Bauer, S.; Farkas, S.; Scherer, M. N.; Schnitzbauer, A.; Schäffler, A.; Aslanidis, C.; Schölmerich, J.; Buechler, C Serum galectin-3 is elevated in obesity and negatively correlates with glycosylated hemoglobin in type 2 diabetes. *J. Clin. Endocrinol. Metab.* **2010**, *95*, 1404–1411.
60. Iacobini, C.; Menini, S.; Oddi, G.; Ricci, C.; Amadio, L.; Pricci, F.; Olivieri, A.; Sorcini, M.; Di Mario, U.; Pesce, C; Pugliese, G. Galectin-3/AGE-receptor 3 knockout mice show accelerated AGE-induced glomerular injury: Evidence for a protective role of galectin-3 as an AGE receptor. *FASEB J.* **2004**, *18*, 1773–1775.
61. Masters, S. L.; Dunne, A.; Subramanian, S. L.; Hull, R. L.; Tannahill, G. M.; Sharp, F. A.; Becker, C.; Franchi, L.; Yoshihara, E.; Chen, Z.; Mullooly, N.; Mielke, L. A.; Harris, J.; Coll, R. C.; Mills, K. H.; Mok, K. H.; Newsholme, P.; Nunez, G.; Yodoi, J.; Kahn, S. E.; Lavelle, E. C.;

O'Neill, L. A. Activation of the NLRP3 inflammasome by islet amyloid polypeptide provides a mechanism for enhanced IL-1beta in type 2 diabetes. *Nat. Immunol.* **2010**, *11*, 897–904.

62. Sospedra, M.; Martin, R Immunology of multiple sclerosis. *Annu. Rev. Immunol.* **2005**, *23*, 683–747.
63. Steinman, L.; Zamvil, S. How to successfully apply animal studies in experimental allergic encephalomyelitis to research on multiple sclerosis. *Ann. Neurol.* **2006**, *60*, 12–21.
64. Jiang, H. R.; Milovanović, M.; Allan, D.; Niedbala, W.; Besnard, A. G.; Fukada, S. Y.; Alves-Filho, J. C.; Togbe, D.; Goodyear, C. S.; Linington, C.; Xu, D.; Lukic, M. L.; Liew, F. Y. IL-33 attenuates EAE by suppressing IL-17 and IFN-γ production and inducing alternatively activated macrophages. *Eur. J. Immunol.* **2012**; DOI: 10.1002/eji.201141947.
65. Milovanovic, M.; Volarevic, V.; Radosavljevic, G.; Jovanovic, I.; Pejnovic, N.; Arsenijevic, N.; Lukic, M. L. IL-33/ST2 axis in inflammation and immunopathology. *Immunol. Res.* **2012**, *52*, 89–99.
66. Jiang, H. R.; Al Rasebi, Z.; Mensah-Brown, E.; Shahin, A.; Xu, D.; Goodyear, C. S.; Fukada, S. Y.; Liu, F. T.; Liew, F. Y.; Lukic, M. L. Galectin-3 deficiency reduces the severity of experimental autoimmune encephalomyelitis. *J. Immunol.* **2009**, *182*, 1167–1173.
67. Jeon, S. B.; Yoon, H. J.; Chang, C. Y.; Koh, H. S.; Jeon, S. H.; Park, E. J. Galectin-3 exerts cytokine-like regulatory actions through the JAK-STAT pathway. *J. Immunol.* **2010**, *185*, 7037–7046.
68. Grigorian, A.; Torossian, S.; Demetriou, M. T-cell growth, cell surface organization, and the galectin-glycoprotein lattice. *Immunol. Rev.* **2009**, *230*, 232–246.
69. Zhu, C.; Anderson, A. C.; Schubart, A.; Xiong, H.; Imitola, J.; Khoury, S. J.; Zheng, X. X.; Strom, T. B.; Kuchroo, V. K. The Tim-3 ligand galectin-9 negatively regulates T helper type 1 immunity. *Nat. Immunol.* **2005**, *6*, 1245–1252.
70. Seki, M.; Oomizu, S.; Sakata, K. M.; Sakata, A.; Arikawa, T.; Watanabe, K.; Ito, K.; Takeshita, K.; Niki, T.; Saita, N; Nishi, N.; Yamauchi, A.; Katoh, S.; Matsukawa, A.; Kuchroo, V.; Hirashima, M. Galectin-9 suppresses the generation of Th17, promotes the induction of regulatory T cells, and regulates experimental autoimmune arthritis. *Clin. Immunol.* **2008**, *127*, 78–88.
71. Rabinovich, G. A.; Daly, G.; Dreja, H.; Tailor, H.; Riera, C. M.; Hirabayashi, J.; Chernajovsky, Y. Recombinant galectin-1 and its genetic delivery suppress collagen-induced arthritis via T cell apoptosis. *J. Exp. Med.* **1999**, *190*, 385–398.
72. Feldmann, M.; Brennan, F. M.; Maini, R. N. Rheumatoid arthritis. *Cell* **1996**, *85*, 307–310.
73. Firestein, G. S. The T cell cometh: Interplay between adaptive immunity and cytokine networks in rheumatoid arthritis. *J Clin. Invest.* **2004**, *114*, 471–474.
74. Forsman, H.; Islander, U.; Andréasson, E.; Andersson, A.; Onnheim, K.; Karlström, A.; Sävman, K.; Magnusson, M.; Brown, KL; Karlsson, A

Galectin 3 aggravates joint inflammation and destruction in antigen-induced arthritis. *Arthritis Rheum.* **2011**, *63*, 445–454.

75. Lubberts, E.; Joosten, L. A.; Oppers, B.; van den Bersselaar, L.; Coenen-de Roo, C. J.; Kolls, J. K.; Schwarzenberger, P.; van de Loo, F. A.; van den Berg, W. B. IL-1-independent role of IL-17 in synovial inflammation and joint destruction during collagen-induced arthritis. *J. Immunol.* **2001**, *167*, 1004–1013.
76. Almkvist, J.; Faldt, J.; Dahlgren, C.; Leffler, H.; Karlsson, A. Lipopolysaccharide- induced gelatinase granule mobilization primes neutrophils for activation by galectin-3 and formylmethionyl-Leu-Phe. *Infect. Immun.* **2001**, *69*, 832–837.
77. Nieminen, J.; St-Pierre, C; Sato, S. Galectin-3 interacts with naive and primed neutrophils, inducing innate immune responses. *J. Leukoc. Biol.* **2005**, *78*, 1127–1135.
78. Filer, A.; Bik, M.; Parsonage, G. N.; Fitton, J.; Trebilcock, E.; Howlett, K.; Cook, M.; Raza, K.; Simmons, D. L.; Thomas, A. M.; Salmon, M.; Scheel-Toellner, D.; Lord, J. M.; Rabinovich, G. A.; Buckley, C. D. Galectin 3 induces a distinctive pattern of cytokine and chemokine production in rheumatoid synovial fibroblasts via selective signaling pathways. *Arthritis Rheum.* **2009**, *60*, 1604–1614.
79. Ohshima, S.; Kuchen, S.; Seemayer, C. A.; Kyburz, D.; Hirt, A.; Klinzing, S.; Michel, B. A.; Gay, R. E.; Liu, F. T.; Gay, S.; Neidhart, M. Galectin 3 and its binding protein in rheumatoid arthritis. *Arthritis Rheum* **2003**, *48*, 2788–2795.
80. Toscano, M. A.; Commodaro, A. G.; Ilarregui, J. M.; Bianco, G. A.; Liberman, A; Serra, H. M.; Hirabayashi, J.; Rizzo, L. V.; Rabinovich, G. A. Galectin-1 suppresses autoimmune retinal disease by promoting concomitant Th2- and T regulatory-mediated anti-inflammatory responses. *J. Immunol.* **2006**, *176*, 6323–6332.
81. Paclik, D.; Berndt, U.; Guzy, C.; Dankof, A.; Danese, S.; Holzloehner, P.; Rosewicz, S.; Wiedenmann, B.; Wittig, B. M.; Dignass, A. U.; Sturm, A. Galectin-2 induces apoptosis of lamina propria T lymphocytes and ameliorates acute and chronic experimental colitis in mice. *J. Mol. Med. (Berl.)* **2008**, *86*, 1395–1406.
82. Paclik, D.; Danese, S.; Berndt, U.; Wiedenmann, B.; Dignass, A.; Sturm, A. Galectin-4 controls intestinal inflammation by selective regulation of peripheral and mucosal T cell apoptosis and cell cycle. *PLoS One* **2008**, *3*, e2629.

Chapter 22

Galectin-3: A Central Regulator of Chronic Inflammation and Tissue Fibrosis

Neil C. Henderson,[*,1] Alison C. Mackinnon,[1] Claire Rooney,[2] and Tariq Sethi[*,2]

[1]MRC Centre for Inflammation Research, The Queen's Medical Research Institute, University of Edinburgh, 47 Little France Crescent, Edinburgh, EH16 4TJ, United Kingdom
[2]Department of Respiratory Medicine and Allergy, King's College London, London, United Kingdom
[*]E-mail: Neil.Henderson@ed.ac.uk (N.C.H); tariq.sethi@kcl.ac.uk (T.S.)

Fibrosis is a major cause of morbidity and mortality worldwide. Tissue injury, with chronic inflammation and fibrogenesis, results in disruption of tissue architecture and eventually organ failure. Currently, the therapeutic options for tissue fibrosis are severely limited and organ transplantation is often the only effective treatment for end-stage fibrotic diseases. However, demand for donor organs greatly outstrips supply, and so effective anti-fibrotic treatments are urgently required. In recent years, Galectin-3 has gained prominence as a central regulator of chronic inflammation and fibrogenesis. Tissue fibrosis models in multiple organs have demonstrated that galectin-3 has profound effects on organ fibrogenesis and scarring. In this review we will examine the ways in which galectin-3 regulates these processes through both direct effects on tissue myofibroblasts and also by mediating cross talk between the innate immune system and fibroblast populations in various organs. Additionally, we will discuss how the manipulation of galectin-3 using small molecule inhibitors may have clinical utility in the treatment of patients with a broad range of fibrotic diseases.

Introduction

Fibrosis represents a massive health care burden worldwide. Chronic tissue injury and fibrogenesis results in disruption of tissue architecture, organ dysfunction and eventually organ failure. Our therapeutic repertoire for the treatment of tissue fibrosis is severely limited and organ transplantation is currently the only effective treatment in end-stage fibrotic disease. However, the disparity between donor organ availability and organ demand means that many patients die. Therefore effective anti-fibrotic treatments are urgently required.

Galectin-3 is a β-galactoside-binding lectin of ~30kDa. It is unique among galectins in that it is a chimeric protein with a C-terminal carbohydrate recognition domain (CRD) linked to a proline, glycine, and tyrosine rich additional N-terminal non-CRD with multiple homologue repeats, which are involved in higher order oligomerization (*1*). Galectin-3 is pleiotropic and it's localisation within the tissue micro-environment may be extracellular, cytoplasmic or nuclear. This imparts great flexibility on galectin-3 as a key regulator of a wide range of biological processes such as adhesion (*2–4*), proliferation (*5*, *6*) and cell survival (*7*, *8*). In recent years, there has been increasing interest in the role of galectin-3 in chronic inflammation and tissue fibrogenesis. A variety of different murine models of organ fibrosis have demonstrated that galectin-3 has profound effects on the fibrotic process, mediating it's effects on multiple different cell lineages during tissue scarring (Figure 1). In this review we will examine how galectin-3 regulates chronic inflammation and fibrosis in different organs, and highlight the progress which has been made in identifying galectin-3 as an attractive therapeutic target in the search for effective anti-fibrotic therapies.

Hepatic Fibrosis

Increased hepatic galectin-3 expression has been demonstrated in cirrhotic human liver secondary to a wide range of etiologies (*9*). Although galectin-3 was not present in normal hepatocytes, immunohistochemistry of liver biopsies from both hepatitis B induced cirrhosis of the liver and hepatocellular carcinoma complicating hepatitis B infection demonstrated increased expression of galectin-3. Galectin-3 was highly expressed in cirrhotic liver in a peripheral distribution within regenerating nodules. In a further study of galectin-3 expression in human liver cirrhosis (*10*) galectin-3 expression was found to be increased in liver cirrhosis secondary to a variety of different causes with varying mechanisms of liver injury including viral-induced liver disease (Hepatitis B and C), autoimmune, copper or iron overload, primary biliary cirrhosis and alcohol-induced liver disease. Galectin-3 expression was negligible in the normal liver and increased in the cirrhotic nodules of hepatocytes, particularly at the nodule periphery. These data suggest that galectin-3 up-regulation within human liver is a basic response to liver injury, irrespective of the initiating agent or disease process.

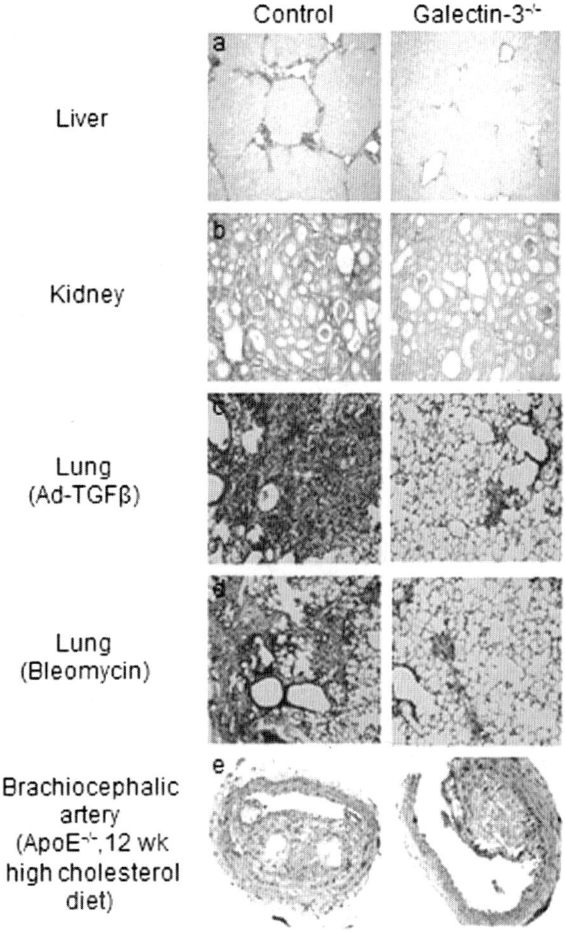

Figure 1. Galectin-3 regulates tissue fibrosis in multiple organs. a) Picrosirius red staining (collagen staining) in wild type and galectin-$3^{-/-}$ mouse liver following chronic CCl_4-induced liver fibrosis (10). b) Sirius red staining in wild type and galectin-$3^{-/-}$ mouse kidney following unilateral ureteric obstruction (UUO) induced renal fibrosis (20). c) Masson's trichrome staining (collagen staining) in wild type and galectin-$3^{-/-}$ mouse lung following adenoviral TGFβ1 (ad-TGFβ1) induced lung fibrosis (41). d) Masson's trichrome staining in wild type and galectin-$3^{-/-}$ mouse lung following bleomycin-induced lung fibrosis (41). e) Representative sections through the brachiocephalic artery of $ApoE^{-/-}$ and $ApoE^{-/-}/G\text{-}3^{-/-}$ mice (fed high cholesterol diet for 12 weeks) stained with Masson's trichrome (MacKinnon et al., unpublished data). (see color insert)

Galectin-3 expression has also been examined in murine models of hepatic fibrosis (*10*). After eight weeks of CCl_4 treatment galectin-3 expression was increased in the periportal areas and areas of bridging fibrosis in mouse liver. Dense hepatocyte galectin-3 staining was also present at the periphery of the hepatocyte nodules. Furthermore, in a rat model of reversible CCl_4 induced liver fibrosis galectin-3 expression was temporally and spatially associated with liver fibrosis, with expression minimal in normal rat liver, maximal at peak liver fibrosis, and then virtually absent again at 24 weeks (recovery from fibrosis) (*10*).

Hepatic stellate cells (Ito cells, liver specific pericytes) are the major source of extracellular matrix proteins during hepatic fibrogenesis (*11*, *12*), and therefore represent an important target in the development of anti-fibrotic therapies for liver fibrosis. Galectin-3 has been shown to stimulate the proliferation of rat and mouse hepatic stellate cells (*10*, *13*) and a number of *in vivo* studies have shown an important role for galectin-3 in the regulation of hepatic fibrosis.

Disruption of the galectin-3 gene blocked hepatic stellate cell activation and collagen expression in a CCl4-induced model of liver fibrosis (*10*). The decrease in liver fibrosis observed in the galectin-3$^{-/-}$ mouse occurred despite equivalent liver injury and inflammation, and similar tissue expression of the pro-fibrotic cytokine TGF-β. TGF-β failed to transactivate galectin-3$^{-/-}$ hepatic stellate cells, in contrast with wildtype hepatic stellate cells. However TGF-β stimulated Smad-2 and -3 phosphorylation was equivalent, suggesting that galectin-3 is required for TGF-β mediated myofibroblast activation and extracellular matrix production. Furthermore, deletion of the galectin-3 gene has also recently been shown to have anti-fibrotic effects in murine models of non-alcoholic steatohepatitis (NASH) (*14*) and biliary fibrosis (*15*) further highlighting the important role of galectin-3 in the regulation of hepatic fibrosis. These data suggest that pharmacological targeting of galectin-3 may have clinical utility in the treatment of patients with liver fibrosis.

Renal Fibrosis

Kidney fibrosis represents a major cause of morbidity and mortality worldwide. End stage renal failure secondary to renal fibrosis results in large numbers of patients becoming dialysis dependent or having to undergo kidney transplantation. At present alternative treatment options are severely limited.

The expression and subcellular distribution of galectin-3 alters with cellular differentiation. In light of this there are numerous functional roles attributed to galectin-3 in the context of the renal system. These include development, where galectin-3 plays a role in both mouse and human foetal collecting duct morphogenesis (*16*, *17*), and the addition of exogenous galectin-3 to embryonic mouse explants inhibits branching of the ureteric bud (*16*). Similarly, functional adaptation of the kidney to different physiological conditions occurs through galectin-3 dependent mechanisms. In immortalised cell lines, metabolic acidosis precipitates cellular remodelling whereby B-intercalated (bicarbonate secreting) cells are transformed into A-intercalated (acid secreting) cells, mediated by a galectin-3-hensin interaction (*18*). Mechanistically the supposition is that galectin-3 plays a role in the terminal differentiation of epithelial cells. This is also seen in examples of aberrant renal physiology: for example in acute kidney injury, a high dose folic acid nephropathy model demonstrates tubular necrosis and apoptosis with incomplete kidney healing, interstitial fibrosis, loss of peritubular capillaries and macrophage infiltration. Modified citrus pectin, which binds to and antagonises galectin-3, has been shown to be protective in this experimental model (*19*).

It has long been recognised that macrophage infiltration into the kidney is an early hallmark of many forms of renal injury. Indeed in human kidney biopsy studies there is a significant association between degree of tubulointerstitial macrophage infiltration, severity of fibrosis and progression to end stage renal failure. Recently the role of galectin-3 in renal fibrosis has been examined. Using a mouse model of renal fibrosis (unilateral ureteric obstruction, UUO) galectin-3 expression was shown to be upregulated following UUO, and deletion of galectin-3 protected against renal myofibroblast accumulation/activation and fibrogenesis (*20*). Furthermore, specific depletion of macrophages using CD11b-DTR transgenic mice reduced fibrosis severity following UUO demonstrating that macrophages are key cells in the pathogenesis of renal fibrosis. Absence of galectin-3 did not affect macrophage recruitment following UUO, or macrophage proinflammatory cytokine profiles in response to IFN-γ/LPS (*21*). Adoptive transfer of wildtype but not galectin-3$^{-/-}$macrophages did, however, restore the fibrotic phenotype in galectin-3 knockout mice.

In vitro, cross-over experiments using wildtype and galectin-3$^{-/-}$ macrophage supernatants and renal fibroblasts confirmed that secretion of galectin-3 by macrophages is a critical step in the activation of renal fibroblasts to a profibrotic phenotype (*20*). Therefore, these data demonstrate that galectin-3 expression and secretion by macrophages is a major mechanism linking macrophages to the promotion of renal fibrosis.

Recently, a second model of kidney injury has examined the role of galectin-3 in chronic allograft injury (CAI) in murine renal transplants (*22*). Chronic allograft injury (CAI) is characterized by interstitial fibrosis and tubular atrophy and results in a progressive decline in graft function, resulting in the loss of 5% of renal transplants per annum. This study used a mouse model of CAI, characterized by a single class II mismatch between BM12 donor and C57/BL6 recipient strains. Transplantation of BM12 kidneys into C57/BL6 mice was associated with interstitial fibrosis, tubular atrophy and increased galectin-3 expression compared with syngeneic controls. However, transplantation of BM12 kidneys into galectin-3$^{-/-}$ mice resulted in significant preservation of tubules and decreased interstitial fibrosis, with a reduction in myofibroblast activation and collagen I expression compared with wild type controls (*22*).

Furthermore, infiltrating leukocytes numbers were unaltered by abrogation of galectin-3, but reduced expression of YM1 (a marker of alternative macrophage activation) coupled with a reduction in the number of circulating CD4-positive T cells and reduced expression of interleukin-4 in galectin-3$^{-/-}$ mice suggest possible mechanisms by which galectin-3 may promote renal transplant fibrosis. These data suggest that galectin-3 may represent a novel therapeutic target in chronic allograft injury.

These studies highlight the importance of macrophages in two diverse models of renal fibrosis. However there remains some debate regarding the mechanism of this effect. In the UUO model, as renal fibrosis progresses, macrophage infiltration increases and galectin-3 remains upregulated. Moreover, depletion of macrophages using CD11b-DTR transgenic mice decreased fibrosis severity following UUO demonstrating that macrophages are key regulators of renal fibrosis. This is supported by other studies which show that inhibition of macrophage recruitment following UUO reduces the severity of renal fibrosis (*23–25*). However the studies in this area are not all in agreement, as adoptive transfer of macrophages at later time-points during UUO-induced renal injury have also been shown to ameliorate renal fibrosis (*26*). This may reflect the fact that macrophages play a varied and time- dependent role in both inflammatory injury and repair mechanisms, or that differentiated macrophages may fall further into as yet poorly defined sub-populations with distinct functional roles.

In the studies examining the role of galectin-3 in renal fibrosis (*20*, *22*) galectin-3 is identified as the link between macrophages, fibroblasts and the pro-fibrotic phenotype. It is known that galectin-3 mediates IL-4 induced alternative macrophage activation (*21*) and that IL-4/IL-13 activated macrophages upregulate profibrotic genes, stimulating matrix production and enhancing fibrosis (*27–29*). The concept of a galectin-3 / macrophage / fibroblast 'axis' is supported by the UUO adoptive transfer studies whereby wild type but not galectin-3$^{-/-}$ macrophages lead to myofibroblast activation and collagen deposition. Cross over supernatant experiments additionally confirmed that galectin-3 secretion by macrophages is required to activate quiescent renal fibroblasts (*20*). In keeping with this the galectin-3 knockout allograft model shows reduced levels of alternatively activated macrophages, reduced myofibroblast accumulation and fibrosis compared to controls (*22*). Therefore the results from both these models indicate a key role for galectin-3 in the pathogenesis of renal fibrosis. A better understanding of the mechanisms regulating this process and targeted strategies to inhibit galectin-3 in the kidney may allow the development of new treatments for patients with renal fibrosis.

Pulmonary Fibrosis

Galectin-3 is highly expressed on lung macrophages and to a lesser extent on bronchial epithelium and is markedly upregulated in type II alveolar epithelial cells following irradiation-induced lung injury in rats (*30*). Galectin-3 has also been shown to have an important role in the development of asthma where expression is upregulated in areas of fibroproliferation following allergen challenge (*31*, *32*). Deletion of galectin-3 results in reduced airway inflammation and interstitial fibrosis associated with reduced expression of the major pro-fibrotic cytokine TGFβ (*31*). However, overexpression of galectin-3 using adenoviral delivery itself reduced hyper-responsiveness and eosinophil accumulation in rats (*33*, *34*). This highlights that non-targeted overexpression may lead to functional effects that are quite distinct from those observed endogenously.

Galectin-3 immunostaining is also increased in the small airways of COPD patients when compared with nonsmokers and smokers (*35*) establishing an important role for this galectin in chronic lung disease. There is also convincing evidence that galectin-3 functions as an anti-apoptotic factor in lung carcinoma and is expressed within and around non-small cell lung cancer (NSCLC) but not small cell lung cancer (SCLC) in human biopsy specimens (*36*) and its presence has been shown to correlate with poor response to chemotherapy. Furthermore, genetic polymorphisms in galectin-3 have been associated with platinum-based chemotherapy response and prognosis of NSCLC (*37*).

With regard to chronic inflammatory disorders of the lung, idiopathic pulmonary fibrosis (IPF) is a chronic condition of unknown etiology with repeated acute lung injury causing progressive fibrosis and architectural distortion resulting in deterioration of lung function and ultimately respiratory failure and death. The median time to death from diagnosis of this devastating condition is 2.5 years (*38*) and the incidence of IPF continues to rise (*39*). At present no specific therapy is available. Corticosteroids alone or in combination with immunosuppressive drugs have been used with limited success (*40*) and there are no reliable prognostic factors or biomarkers to predict disease progression.

Galectin-3 is expressed in the lungs of mice exposed to the fibrotic agent bleomycin and in response to adenoviral mediated increased TGFβ, the major profibrotic cytokine in the lung (*41*). TGFβ1 induces the fibrogenic response through receptor-mediated phosphorylation of members of the Smad family of cytoplasmic transcription factors Smad2 and Smad3 (*42*) and Smad3 deficient mice are protected from TGF β1-induced fibrosis (*43*, *44*). There is also increasing evidence for a role of the wnt/β-catenin pathway in regulating TGFβ1-dependent signalling (*45*) and this pathway is aberrantly activated in IPF (*46*). Pulmonary fibrosis in two well characterized rodent models of lung fibrosis (induced by TGFβ and bleomycin), was dramatically reduced in mice deficient in galectin-3 (*41*). This was manifest by reduced TGFβ1-induced EMT and myofibroblast activation and collagen production *in vitro* and *in vivo*. Galectin-3 deletion reduced retention of TGFβ receptors at the cell surface and reduced phosphorylation and nuclear translocation of β-catenin but had no effect on Smad2/3 phosphorylation. Moreover, a novel inhibitor of galectin-3, TD139, blocked TGFβ-induced β-catenin activation *in vitro* and *in vivo* and attenuated the late stage progression of lung fibrosis following bleomycin-induced lung injury (*41*). The regulation of myofibroblast activation by galectin-3 is summarized schematically in Figure 2.

In patients with IPF there is increased lung expression of galectin-3 (*47*) and levels are elevated in bronchoalveolar lavage fluid and serum from patients with stable IPF compared to non-specific interstitial pneumonitis and controls. Moreover, serum galectin-3 rises sharply during an acute exacerbation suggesting that galectin-3 may be a marker of active fibrosis in IPF (*41*). Therefore this study identifies galectin-3 as an important regulator of lung fibrosis and provides a proof of principle for galectin-3 inhibition as a potential novel therapeutic strategy for IPF.

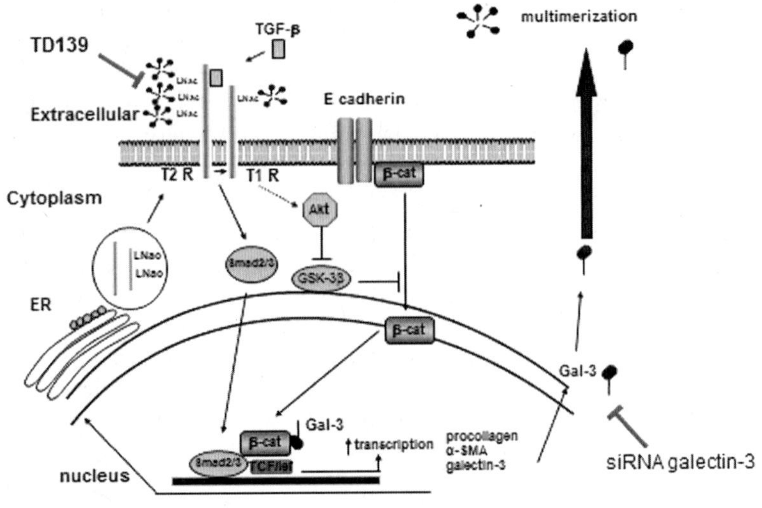

Figure 2. Schematic showing a potential mechanism for galectin-3-mediated regulation of myofibroblast activation. Galectin-3 binding to n-acetyl lactosamine residues (l-nac) on TGFβ-RII causes association with TGFβ-RI and potentiation of TGFβ signalling;- smad2/3 and Akt activation. Liberation of beta-catenin from adherens junction during myofibroblast activation is sequestered in the cytosol where its nuclear translocation is inhibited by GSK3-β. Nuclear galectin-3 complexes with beta-catenin in a transcription complex that mediates expression of mesenchymal genes and galectin-3. TD139 inhibits extracellular galectin-3 binding and function. (see color insert)

Atherosclerosis

Atherosclerosis is a major cause of cardiovascular disease (CVD) and stroke. In the U.S. it is estimated that there are around 2000 deaths from CVD each day, more each year than from cancer, respiratory disease, and accidents combined (*48*). Atherosclerosis is recognized as being a chronic inflammatory with macrophages playing a dominant role (*49*, *50*). Macrophages recruited to the vascular intima engulf lipoprotein particles and differentiate into foam cells which orchestrate lesion development by promoting inflammation, smooth muscle cell proliferation and extracellular matrix deposition (*50*).

Galectin-3 is highly expressed in human atherosclerotic plaques and in mouse models of atheroma (*51*, *52*) and is commonly used as a marker for plaque macrophages. There is currently growing interest in galectin-3 as a validated biomarker for heart failure (*53–55*) and as a predictor of response to statin therapy in heart failure (*56*) and galectin-3 undoubtedly plays an important role in atherosclerotic disease development. However, previous studies have yielded conflicting results regarding the role of galectin-3 in plaque development. The first study, using C57/Bl6 mice, showed that deletion of galectin-3 increased lesion formation in mice fed a high fat diet for 8 months (*57*). However, high fat feeding in mice without a defect in lipoprotein metabolism (e.g. $ApoE^{-/-}$ or $LDLR^{-/-}$) does not cause development of advanced lesions, and does not induce the same high levels of serum cholesterol. Therefore, this study could not address the role of galectin-3 on the later, and arguably more relevant, stages of atherosclerosis.

The second study showed that in an atherosclerosis prone model ($ApoE^{-/-}$ but on a mixed 129sv/C57/Bl6 background), galectin-3 deletion reduced plaque size in older mice (50 weeks) fed a normal diet (*58*). Differences in strain and/or serum cholesterol could be the main factor responsible for this paradox. A third study using high cholesterol feeding in $ApoE^{-/-}$C57/Bl6 mice. shows that galectin-3 deletion in atherosclerosis-prone mice fed a high cholesterol diet results in smaller and less complex plaques with reduced plaque collagen and smaller lipid core and no adverse effects on plaque vulnerability (Mackinnon et al., unpublished). The reduced plaque burden was not due to reduced serum cholesterol but was associated with reduced weight gain in galectin-$3^{-/-}$ mice. The mechanism of this reduced weight gain is unclear but it may be due to a previously described function of galectin-3 to stimulate adipocyte proliferation (*59*). Indeed, high levels of circulating galectin-3 have been associated with obesity (*60*).

Galectin-$3^{-/-}$ macrophages have a specific defect in M2 alternative macrophage activation (*21*) and there is reduced M2 marker expression in later lesions in galectin-$3^{-/-}$/$ApoE^{-/-}$mice. In humans, M2 macrophages predominate in diseased versus normal intima of carotid arteries, and patients with a predisposition towards an M2 phenotype may be more susceptible to atherosclerotic disease (*61*). Our previous work has shown that galectin-3 mediates alternative/M2 macrophage activation via activation of the dimeric transmembrane protein CD98 (*21*), a disulfide-linked 125 kDa heterodimeric type II transmembrane glycoprotein (*62*) which is highly expressed on macrophages (*63*) (summarized schematically in Figure 3). Deletion of CD98 or inhibition of CD98 function with pharmacological inhibitors prevents M2 activation (*21*). CD98 may mediate the effects of galectin-3 on M2 activation within plaques and may provide another target for therapeutic intervention.

Reduced plaque stability and rupture leading to thrombosis is the most common fatal consequence of atherosclerosis and it will be essential to address this issue in order to fully evaluate the potential of galectin-3 inhibitors as a novel therapy or as an adjunct to statin therapy. Modified citrus pectin is a naturally-occurring pectin found in the peel and pulp of citrus fruits. In the United States of America, MCP is registered as a food supplement and is generally regarded as safe (GRAS). MCP inhibits galectin-3 binding and function *in vitro* and *in vivo* (*64–66*). Administration of 1% MCP in the drinking water to $ApoE^{-/-}$ mice for 4 weeks at the end of a 10 week high cholesterol feeding regimen reduced plaque burden in the descending aorta compared to vehicle control. Therefore, strategies to inhibit galectin-3 function may reduce plaque progression and potentially represent a novel therapeutic strategy in the treatment of atherosclerotic disease.

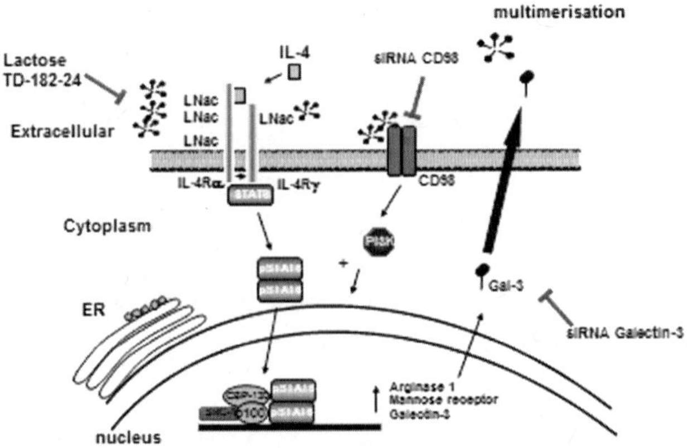

Figure 3. Schematic showing mechanism for the regulation of alternative macrophage activation by galectin-3. Galectin-3 binding to n-acetyl lactosamine residues (l-nac) on IL-4Ra and CD98 potentiates IL-4-induced STAT6 activation and CD98 mediated activation of PI3-kinase augmenting transcription of alternative activation genes arginase-1 and mannose receptor and expression of galectin-3. (see color insert)

Conclusion

In recent years it has become clear that galectin-3 has profound effects on tissue fibrosis. The majority of the *in vivo* data demonstrates a pro-fibrotic role for galectin-3, mediating myofibroblast activation and extracellular matrix deposition with disruption of tissue architecture and organ dysfunction. However, the component parts of tissue fibrogenesis are exquisitely complex and newer data has highlighted the important cross-talk between cells of the immune system and tissue myofibroblasts in the evolution and resolution of fibrosis. Galectin-3 represents an excellent example of a molecule which can exert potent effects on multiple cell types during the fibrotic process, both through direct effects on scar-secreting myofibroblasts and by altering the behaviour of innate immune cells such as macrophages. Strategies to manipulate galectin-3, such as the emerging small molecule inhibitors, will hopefully result in the development of effective anti-fibrotic therapies.

Acknowledgments

N.C.H., A.C.M. and T.S. acknowledge the support of the Wellcome Trust.

References

1. Liu, F. T. Molecular biology of IgE-binding protein, IgE-binding factors, and IgE receptors. *Crit. Rev. Immunol.* **1990**, *10*, 289–306.
2. Inohara, H.; Akahani, S.; et al. Interactions between galectin-3 and Mac-2-binding protein mediate cell-cell adhesion. *Cancer Res.* **1996**, *56*, 4530–4534.
3. Inohara, H.; Raz, A. Functional evidence that cell surface galectin-3 mediates homotypic cell adhesion. *Cancer Res.* **1995**, *55*, 3267–3271.
4. Kuwabara, I.; Liu, F. T. Galectin-3 promotes adhesion of human neutrophils to laminin. *J. Immunol.* **1996**, *156*, 3939–3944.
5. Inohara, H.; Akahani, S.; et al. Galectin-3 stimulates cell proliferation. *Exp. Cell Res.* **1998**, *245*, 294–302.
6. Moutsatsos, I. K.; Wade, M.; et al. Endogenous lectins from cultured cells: Nuclear localization of carbohydrate-binding protein 35 in proliferating 3T3 fibroblasts. *Proc. Natl. Acad. Sci. U.S.A.* **1987**, *84*, 6452–6456.
7. Akahani, S.; Nangia-Makker, P.; et al. Galectin-3: A novel antiapoptotic molecule with a functional BH1 (NWGR) domain of Bcl-2 family. *Cancer Res.* **1997**, *57*, 5272–5276.
8. Yang, R. Y.; Hsu, D. K.; et al. Expression of galectin-3 modulates T-cell growth and apoptosis. *Proc. Natl. Acad. Sci. U.S.A.* **1996**, *93*, 6737–6742.
9. Hsu, D. K.; Dowling, C. A.; et al. Galectin-3 expression is induced in cirrhotic liver and hepatocellular carcinoma. *Int. J. Cancer* **1999**, *81*, 519–526.
10. Henderson, N. C.; Mackinnon, A. C.; et al. Galectin-3 regulates myofibroblast activation and hepatic fibrosis. *Proc. Natl. Acad. Sci. U.S.A.* **2006**, *103*, 5060–5065.
11. de Leeuw, A. M.; McCarthy, S. P.; et al. Purified rat liver fat-storing cells in culture divide and contain collagen. *Hepatology* **1984**, *4*, 392–403.
12. Friedman, S. L.; Roll, F. J.; et al. Hepatic lipocytes: The principal collagen-producing cells of normal rat liver. *Proc. Natl. Acad. Sci. U.S.A.* **1985**, *82*, 8681–8685.
13. Maeda, N.; Kawada, N.; et al. Stimulation of proliferation of rat hepatic stellate cells by galectin-1 and galectin-3 through different intracellular signaling pathways. *J. Biol. Chem.* **2003**, *278*, 18938–18944.
14. Iacobini, C.; Menini, S.; et al. Galectin-3 ablation protects mice from diet-induced NASH: A major scavenging role for galectin-3 in liver. *J. Hepatol.*, *54*, 975–983.
15. Jiang, J. X.; Chen, X.; et al. Galectin-3 modulates phagocytosis-induced stellate cell activation and liver fibrosis in vivo. *Am. J. Physiol. Gastrointest. Liver Physiol.*, *302*, G439–446.
16. Bullock, S. L.; Johnson, T. M.; et al. Galectin-3 modulates ureteric bud branching in organ culture of the developing mouse kidney. *J. Am. Soc. Nephrol.* **2001**, *12*, 515–523.
17. Winyard, P. J.; Bao, Q.; et al. Epithelial galectin-3 during human nephrogenesis and childhood cystic diseases. *J. Am. Soc. Nephrol.* **1997**, *8*, 1647–1657.

18. Hikita, C.; Vijayakumar, S.; et al. Induction of terminal differentiation in epithelial cells requires polymerization of hensin by galectin 3. *J. Cell Biol.* **2000**, *151*, 1235–1246.
19. Kolatsi-Joannou, M.; Price, K. L.; et al. Modified citrus pectin reduces galectin-3 expression and disease severity in experimental acute kidney injury. *PLoS One*, *6*, e18683.
20. Henderson, N. C.; Mackinnon, A. C.; et al. Galectin-3 expression and secretion links macrophages to the promotion of renal fibrosis. *Am. J. Pathol.* **2008**, *172*, 288–298.
21. MacKinnon, A. C.; Farnworth, S. L.; et al. Regulation of alternative macrophage activation by galectin-3. *J. Immunol.* **2008**, *180*, 2650–2658.
22. Dang, Z.; MacKinnon, A.; et al. Tubular atrophy and interstitial fibrosis after renal transplantation is dependent on galectin-3. *Transplantation*, *93*, 477–484.
23. Anders, H. J.; Vielhauer, V.; et al. A chemokine receptor CCR-1 antagonist reduces renal fibrosis after unilateral ureter ligation. *J. Clin. Invest.* **2002**, *109*, 251–259.
24. Eis, V.; Luckow, B.; et al. Chemokine receptor CCR1 but not CCR5 mediates leukocyte recruitment and subsequent renal fibrosis after unilateral ureteral obstruction. *J. Am. Soc. Nephrol.* **2004**, *15*, 337–347.
25. Kitagawa, K.; Wada, T.; et al. Blockade of CCR2 ameliorates progressive fibrosis in kidney. *Am. J. Pathol.* **2004**, *165*, 237–246.
26. Nishida, M.; Okumura, Y.; et al. Adoptive transfer of macrophages ameliorates renal fibrosis in mice. *Biochem. Biophys. Res. Commun.* **2005**, *332*, 11–16.
27. Fichtner-Feigl, S.; Strober, W.; et al. IL-13 signaling through the IL-13alpha2 receptor is involved in induction of TGF-beta1 production and fibrosis. *Nat. Med.* **2006**, *12*, 99–106.
28. Liu, T.; Jin, H.; et al. Regulation of found in inflammatory zone 1 expression in bleomycin-induced lung fibrosis: Role of IL-4/IL-13 and mediation via STAT-6. *J. Immunol.* **2004**, *173*, 3425–3431.
29. Wynn, T. A. Fibrotic disease and the T(H)1/T(H)2 paradigm. *Nat. Rev. Immunol.* **2004**, *4*, 583–594.
30. Kasper, M.; Hughes, R. C. Immunocytochemical evidence for a modulation of galectin 3 (Mac-2), a carbohydrate binding protein, in pulmonary fibrosis. *J. Pathol.* **1996**, *179*, 309–316.
31. Ge, X. N.; Bahaie, N. S.; et al. Allergen-induced airway remodeling is impaired in galectin-3-deficient mice. *J. Immunol.*, *185*, 1205–1214.
32. Zuberi, R. I.; Hsu, D. K.; et al. Critical role for galectin-3 in airway inflammation and bronchial hyperresponsiveness in a murine model of asthma. *Am. J. Pathol.* **2004**, *165*, 2045–2053.
33. del Pozo, V.; Rojo, M.; et al. Gene therapy with galectin-3 inhibits bronchial obstruction and inflammation in antigen-challenged rats through interleukin-5 gene downregulation. *Am. J. Respir. Crit. Care Med.* **2002**, *166*, 732–737.
34. Lopez, E.; del Pozo, V.; et al. Inhibition of chronic airway inflammation and remodeling by galectin-3 gene therapy in a murine model. *J. Immunol.* **2006**, *176*, 1943–1950.

35. Pilette, C.; Colinet, B.; et al. Increased galectin-3 expression and intra-epithelial neutrophils in small airways in severe COPD. *Eur. Respir. J.* **2007**, *29*, 914–922.
36. Buttery, R.; Monaghan, H.; et al. Galectin-3: Differential expression between small-cell and non-small-cell lung cancer. *Histopathology* **2004**, *44*, 339–344.
37. Wu, F.; Hu, N.; et al. Galectin-3 genetic variants are associated with platinum-based chemotherapy response and prognosis in patients with NSCLC. *Cell Oncol .(Dordrecht).*
38. Gross, T. J.; Hunninghake, G. W. Idiopathic pulmonary fibrosis. *N. Engl. J. Med.* **2001**, *345*, 517–525.
39. Raghu, G.; Weycker, D.; et al. Incidence and prevalence of idiopathic pulmonary fibrosis. *Am. J. Respir. Crit. Care Med.* **2006**, *174*, 810–816.
40. Flaherty, K. R.; Toews, G. B.; et al. Steroids in idiopathic pulmonary fibrosis: A prospective assessment of adverse reactions, response to therapy, and survival. *Am. J. Med.* **2001**, *110*, 278–282.
41. Mackinnon, A. C.; Gibbons, M. A.; et al. Regulation of transforming growth factor-beta1-driven lung fibrosis by galectin-3. *Am. J. Respir. Crit. Care Med.*, *185*, 537–546.
42. Zavadil, J.; Bottinger, E. P. TGF-beta and epithelial-to-mesenchymal transitions. *Oncogene* **2005**, *24*, 5764–5774.
43. Bonniaud, P.; Kolb, M.; et al. Smad3 null mice develop airspace enlargement and are resistant to TGF-beta-mediated pulmonary fibrosis. *J. Immunol.* **2004**, *173*, 2099–2108.
44. Bonniaud, P.; Margetts, P. J.; et al. TGF-beta and Smad3 signaling link inflammation to chronic fibrogenesis. *J. Immunol.* **2005**, *175*, 5390–5395.
45. Kim, K.; Lu, Z.; et al. Direct evidence for a role of beta-catenin/LEF-1 signaling pathway in induction of EMT. *Cell Biol. Int.* **2002**, *26*, 463–476.
46. Arnold, S. A.; Rivera, L. B.; et al. Losartan slows pancreatic tumor progression and extends survival of SPARC-null mice by abrogating aberrant TGFbeta activation. *PLoS One*, *7*, e31384.
47. Nishi, Y.; Sano, H.; et al. Role of galectin-3 in human pulmonary fibrosis. *Allergol. Int* **2007**, *56*, 57–65.
48. Roger, V. L.; Go, A. S.; et al. Heart disease and stroke statistics--2011 update: A report from the American Heart Association. *Circulation*, *123*, e18–e209.
49. Swirski, F. K.; Libby, P.; et al. Ly-6Chi monocytes dominate hypercholesterolemia-associated monocytosis and give rise to macrophages in atheromata. *J. Clin. Invest.* **2007**, *117*, 195–205.
50. Swirski, F. K.; Pittet, M. J.; et al. Monocyte accumulation in mouse atherogenesis is progressive and proportional to extent of disease. *Proc. Natl. Acad. Sci. U.S.A.* **2006**, *103*, 10340–10345.
51. Arar, C.; Gaudin, J. C.; et al. Galectin-3 gene (LGALS3) expression in experimental atherosclerosis and cultured smooth muscle cells. *FEBS Lett.* **1998**, *430*, 307–311.
52. Nachtigal, M.; Al-Assaad, Z.; et al. Galectin-3 expression in human atherosclerotic lesions. *Am. J. Pathol.* **1998**, *152*, 1199–1208.

53. de Boer, R. A.; Voors, A. A.; et al. Galectin-3: A novel mediator of heart failure development and progression. *Eur. J. Heart. Fail.* **2009**, *11*, 811–817.
54. Lin, Y. H.; Lin, L. Y.; et al. The relationship between serum galectin-3 and serum markers of cardiac extracellular matrix turnover in heart failure patients. *Clin. Chim. Acta* **2009**, *409*, 96–99.
55. Lok, D. J.; Van Der Meer, P.; et al. Prognostic value of galectin-3, a novel marker of fibrosis, in patients with chronic heart failure: Data from the DEAL-HF study. *Clin. Res. Cardiol.*, *99*, 323–328.
56. Gullestad, L.; Ueland, T.; et al. Galectin-3 predicts response to statin therapy in the Controlled Rosuvastatin Multinational Trial in Heart Failure (CORONA). *Eur. Heart J.*.
57. Iacobini, C.; Menini, S.; et al. Accelerated lipid-induced atherogenesis in galectin-3-deficient mice: Role of lipoxidation via receptor-mediated mechanisms. *Arterioscler. Thromb. Vasc. Biol.* **2009**, *29*, 831–836.
58. Nachtigal, M.; Ghaffar, A.; et al. Galectin-3 gene inactivation reduces atherosclerotic lesions and adventitial inflammation in ApoE-deficient mice. *Am. J. Pathol.* **2008**, *172*, 247–255.
59. Kiwaki, K.; Novak, C. M.; et al. Galectin-3 stimulates preadipocyte proliferation and is up-regulated in growing adipose tissue. *Obesity (Silver Spring)* **2007**, *15*, 32–39.
60. Weigert, J.; Neumeier, M.; et al. Serum galectin-3 is elevated in obesity and negatively correlates with glycosylated hemoglobin in type 2 diabetes. *J Clin. Endocrinol. Metab.*, *95*, 1404–1411.
61. Waldo, S. W.; Li, Y.; et al. Heterogeneity of human macrophages in culture and in atherosclerotic plaques. *Am. J. Pathol.* **2008**, *172*, 1112–1126.
62. Verrey, F.; Closs, E. I.; et al. CATs and HATs: The SLC7 family of amino acid transporters. *Pflugers Arch.* **2004**, *447*, 532–542.
63. Dong, S.; Hughes, R. C. Macrophage surface glycoproteins binding to galectin-3 (Mac-2-antigen). *Glycoconjugate J.* **1997**, *14*, 267–274.
64. Glinsky, V. V.; Raz, A. Modified citrus pectin anti-metastatic properties: One bullet, multiple targets. *Carbohydr. Res.* **2009**, *344*, 1788–1791.
65. Nangia-Makker, P.; Hogan, V.; et al. Inhibition of human cancer cell growth and metastasis in nude mice by oral intake of modified citrus pectin. *J. Natl. Cancer Inst.* **2002**, *94*, 1854–1862.
66. Pienta, K. J.; Naik, H.; et al. Inhibition of spontaneous metastasis in a rat prostate cancer model by oral administration of modified citrus pectin. *J Natl. Cancer Inst.* **1995**, *87*, 348–353.

Chapter 23

The Role of Galectin-3 in Stellate Cell Activation and Liver Fibrosis

Joy X. Jiang,[*,1] Xiangling Chen,[1] Hiroo Fukada,[1] Dan K. Hsu,[2] Fu-tong Liu,[2] and Natalie J. Török[1]

[1]Department of Internal Medicine, Division of Gastroenterology and Hepatology, UC Davis Medical Center, 4635 2nd Avenue, Suite 1001, Sacramento, California 95817
[2]Department of Dermatology, UC Davis Medical Center, 4635 2nd Avenue, Suite 1001, Sacramento, California 95817
[*]E-mail: xiaosong.jiang@ucdmc.ucdavis.edu

Gal3 (galectin-3) has been known to be involved in the regulation of kidney, lung and liver fibrosis. We have reported a novel mechanism by which Gal3 contributes to fibrogenesis. Extracellular Gal3 is required for tethering of apoptotic bodies by HSC via cross-linking with integrin αvβ3, and consequently promoting HSC activation. On the other hand, phagocytosis induces Gal3 production by both HSC and Kupffer cells. Taken together, Gal3 may become a therapeutic target for antifibrogenic strategy.

Liver Fibrosis

Liver fibrosis is a wound-healing process that is elicited by various pathologic stimuli (*1*, *2*). In normal liver, quiescent hepatic stellate cells (HSC) exist in the Disse space between the sinusoidal endothelial cells and the parenchymal cells; and store vitamin A as fat droplets in their cytoplasm (*3*). In pathological conditions such as steatohepatitis, virus infection, and alcoholic liver injury, hepatocytes undergo apoptosis and form apoptotic bodies (AB), which can be phagocytosed by HSC (*4*, *5*). HSC become activated upon phagocytosis, which is marked with losing vitamin A droplets, proliferation and morphologically changing into myofibroblast-like cells, as well as the production of extra amount of extracellular matrix (ECM) compounds, mainly type I collagen (*5*). Accumulation of these ECM compounds leads to fibrosis and cirrhosis. Active HSC also produce fibrogenic cytokines, such as TGF-β, which is pro-apoptotic on hepatocytes and further promotes HSC activation (*4*). Therefore TGF-β perpetuates the cycle of apoptosis and phagocytosis (*6*, *7*). Thus, HSC phagocytosis is a key event in progressive liver fibrosis.

Galectin-3 in Fibrosis

Galectin-3 (Gal3), a member of β-galactoside-binding lectin family, is expressed in various types of cells and widely distributed in cell nuclei, cytoplasm and membrane and can be secreted and uptaken (*8*). Gal3, both endogenous and exogenous, is involved in the regulation of a variety of biological functions. Gal3 mediates cell proliferation (*9–11*), adhesion (*9*, *12*, *13*), trafficking (*13*, *14*) and apoptosis (*15*, *16*) in various types of cells. Gal3 also regulates phagocytosis of opsonized red blood cells (*17*) and apoptotic neutrophils by macrophages (*18*).

Accumulating evidence has shown that Gal3 is also an important regulator in fibrosis of multiple organs. Henderson et al. reported that Gal3 was upregulated in progressive fibrotic kidney in mouse and deletion of Gal3 caused improvement (*19*). High level of Gal3 was found in bronchoalveolar lavage fluid from patients with pulmonary fibrosis and it was released by alveolar macrophages (*20*). Studying different animal models, we and other groups showed that Gal3 played a role in CCl_4 (*21*) and bile duct ligation (*22*) induced liver fibrosis and non-alcoholic steatohepatitis (NASH) (*23*).

Extracellular Gal3 Facilitates Apoptotic Body Tethering by HSC

Hepatocyte apoptosis and the clearance of these apoptotic bodies by HSC are key steps during fibrogenesis (*4*, *5*). Our group has shown that HSC displayed decreased phagocytic activity when pretreated with a Gal3 competitor, β-lactose; HSC from $Gal3^{-/-}$ mice showed diminished phagocytic ability, and this could be reversed by recombinant Gal3, indicating that the extracellular Gal3 is required for HSC phagocytosis (*22*). Phagocytosis also caused upregulation of profibrogenic genes procollagen, αSMA and TGFβ in HSC (*5*, *24*); however this induction was not seen in Gal3 deficient HSC. This was also reversed by recombinant Gal3 (*22*). These data suggested that extracellular Gal3 is required for HSC phagocytosis and activation. By studying the mechanism, we found that Gal3 facilitated cross-linking the integrin αvβ3 heterodimers in HSC (*22*). In addition, blocking the β3 integrin extracellular binding sites inhibited HSC phagocytosis (*22*). These data suggested that extracellular Gal3 mediates HSC phagocytosis and activation via cross- linking to αvβ3 integrin.

Upregulation of Gal3 in Phagocytosis-Activated HSC

Gal3 was also upregulated in phagocytosis-activated HSC. A possible mechanism was an NFκB-dependent pathway, as overexpressing an IκB dominant negative mutant significantly reduced the induction of Gal3 (*22*). At protein level, our ELISA data showed that phagocytosing HSC and Kupffer cells released higher levels of Gal3 compared to the control groups (*22*). Thus Gal3 produced by active HSC contributes to fibrogenic activity by a feed-forward mechanism (Figure 1).

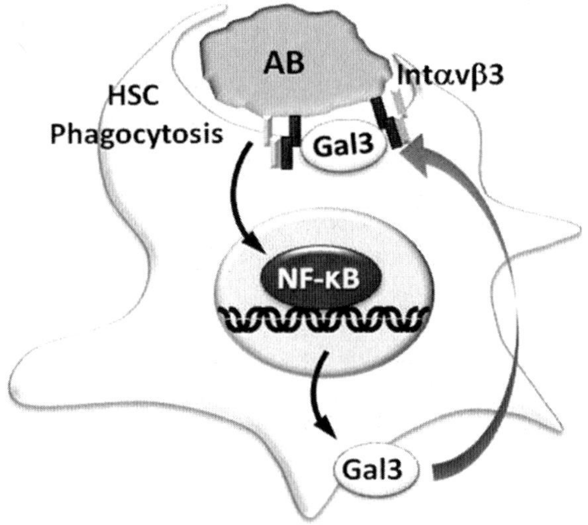

Figure 1. Graphical summary. Gal3 mediates liver fibrosis in an autocrine manner. Gal3 cross-linking with integrin αvβ3 is required for HSC phagocytosing apoptotic bodies (AB). Phagocytosis in turn induces the Gal3 expression via an NFκB-dependent pathway.

The Role of Gal3 in Liver Fibrosis: *In Vivo* Studies

Gal3 expression increased in liver from bile duct ligated (BDL) mice, mainly in myofibroblasts. Furthermore, liver fibrogenesis in Gal3$^{-/-}$ mice was attenuated (*22*).

To study the effect of Gal3 on HSC phagocytosis *in vivo*, we used a mouse model described previously (*25*). In brief, mice were injected with a lenti-viral GFP expressing vector and a TRAIL (TNF-related apoptosis-inducing ligand) adeno-viral vector sequentially, to induce hepatocyte apoptosis. As the apoptotic cells were GFP positive, it was possible to track them by the GFP and also by the active HSC marker αSMA. In this way, the *in vivo* HSC phagocytosis and activation became visible. Consistent with our *in vitro* findings, HSC in Gal3$^{-/-}$ mice showed suppressed phagocytic and fibrogenic activity (unpublished data).

Acknowledgments

This work was supported by National Institute of Diabetes and Digestive and Kidney Disease Grants 1K01DK090121-01A1, DK-069765, DK-080715 and DK-083283.

References

1. Bissell, D. M.; Roulot, D.; George, J. Transforming growth factor beta and the liver. *Hepatology* **2001**, *34* (5), 859–867.
2. Friedman, S. L. Seminars in medicine of the Beth Israel Hospital, Boston. The cellular basis of hepatic fibrosis. Mechanisms and treatment strategies. *N. Engl. J. Med.* **1993**, *328* (25), 1828–1835.
3. Geerts, A. History, heterogeneity, developmental biology, and functions of quiescent hepatic stellate cells. *Semin. Liver Dis.* **2001**, *21* (3), 311–335.
4. Oberhammer, F. A.; et al. Induction of apoptosis in cultured hepatocytes and in regressing liver by transforming growth factor beta 1. *Proc. Natl. Acad. Sci. U.S.A.* **1992**, *89* (12), 5408–5412.
5. Zhan, S. S.; et al. Phagocytosis of apoptotic bodies by hepatic stellate cells induces NADPH oxidase and is associated with liver fibrosis in vivo. *Hepatology* **2006**, *43* (3), 435–443.
6. George, J.; et al. In vivo inhibition of rat stellate cell activation by soluble transforming growth factor beta type II receptor: A potential new therapy for hepatic fibrosis. *Proc. Natl. Acad. Sci. U.S.A.* **1999**, *96* (22), 12719–12724.
7. Dooley, S.; et al. Transforming growth factor beta signal transduction in hepatic stellate cells via Smad2/3 phosphorylation, a pathway that is abrogated during in vitro progression to myofibroblasts. TGFbeta signal transduction during transdifferentiation of hepatic stellate cells. *FEBS Lett.* **2001**, *502* (1–2), 4–10.
8. Mehul, B.; Hughes, R. C. Plasma membrane targetting, vesicular budding and release of galectin 3 from the cytoplasm of mammalian cells during secretion. *J. Cell Sci.* **1997**, *110* (Pt 10), 1169–1178.
9. Lei, C. X.; et al. Interactions between galectin-3 and integrinbeta3 in regulating endometrial cell proliferation and adhesion. *Hum. Reprod.* **2009**, *24* (11), 2879–2889.
10. Inohara, H.; Akahani, S.; Raz, A. Galectin-3 stimulates cell proliferation. *Exp. Cell Res.* **1998**, *245* (2), 294–302.
11. Gustavsson, P.; et al. Galectin-3 inhibits Schwann cell proliferation in cultured sciatic nerve. *Neuroreport* **2007**, *18* (7), 669–673.
12. Kuwabara, I.; Liu, F. T. Galectin-3 promotes adhesion of human neutrophils to laminin. *J. Immunol.* **1996**, *156* (10), 3939–3944.
13. Rao, S. P.; et al. Galectin-3 functions as an adhesion molecule to support eosinophil rolling and adhesion under conditions of flow. *J. Immunol.* **2007**, *179* (11), 7800–7807.
14. Saravanan, C.; et al. Galectin-3 promotes lamellipodia formation in epithelial cells by interacting with complex N-glycans on alpha3beta1 integrin. *J. Cell Sci.* **2009**, *122* (Pt 20), 3684–3693.

15. Akahani, S.; et al. Galectin-3: A novel antiapoptotic molecule with a functional BH1 (NWGR) domain of Bcl-2 family. *Cancer Res.* **1997**, *57* (23), 5272–5276.
16. Fukumori, T.; et al. Endogenous galectin-3 determines the routing of CD95 apoptotic signaling pathways. *Cancer Res.* **2004**, *64* (10), 3376–3379.
17. Sano, H.; et al. Critical role of galectin-3 in phagocytosis by macrophages. *J. Clin. Invest.* **2003**, *112* (3), 389–397.
18. Farnworth, S. L.; et al. Galectin-3 reduces the severity of pneumococcal pneumonia by augmenting neutrophil function. *Am. J. Pathol.* **2008**, *172* (2), 395–405.
19. Henderson, N. C.; et al. Galectin-3 expression and secretion links macrophages to the promotion of renal fibrosis. *Am. J. Pathol.* **2008**, *172* (2), 288–298.
20. Nishi, Y.; et al. Role of galectin-3 in human pulmonary fibrosis. *Allergol. Int.* **2007**, *56* (1), 57–65.
21. Henderson, N. C.; et al. Galectin-3 regulates myofibroblast activation and hepatic fibrosis. *Proc. Natl. Acad. Sci. U.S.A.* **2006**, *103* (13), 5060–5065.
22. Jiang, J. X.; et al. Galectin-3 modulates phagocytosis-induced stellate cell activation and liver fibrosis in vivo. *Am. J. Physiol.: Gastrointest. Liver Physiol.* **2012**, *302* (4), G439–G446.
23. Iacobini, C.; et al. Galectin-3 ablation protects mice from diet-induced NASH: A major scavenging role for galectin-3 in liver. *J. Hepatol.* **2011**, *54* (5), 975–983.
24. Jiang, J. X.; et al. Leptin induces phagocytosis of apoptotic bodies by hepatic stellate cells via a Rho guanosine triphosphatase-dependent mechanism. *Hepatology* **2008**, *48* (5), 1497–1505.
25. Jiang, J. X.; et al. Reduced nicotinamide adenine dinucleotide phosphate oxidase 2 plays a key role in stellate cell activation and liver fibrogenesis in vivo. *Gastroenterology* **2010**, *139* (4), 1375–1384.

Chapter 24

Galectin-3 Mediated Cardiovascular Fibrogenesis: An Important Cause of Heart Failure and Cardiovascular Mortality

Wouter C. Meijers and Rudolf A. de Boer*

University Medical Center Groningen, Department of Cardiology, Groningen, The Netherlands
***E-mail: r.a.de.boer@umcg.nl**

Cardiac remodeling is the heart's primary adaptive response to injury. Remodeling is characterized by myocyte hypertrophy, but fibrosis formation in the interstitial space is also dominant. It has been established that galectin-3 plays an important role in tissue inflammation, immunity, and fibrosis. Galectin-3 is highly upregulated in adverse cardiac remodeling and heart failure (HF). Several lines of evidence suggest that galectin-3 is not only a marker (bystander) in cardiac remodeling but it may actively contribute as well. First, plasma galectin-3 is increased in human subjects prone to develop HF, and in patients with established HF galectin-3 has emerged as a useful biomarker reflecting the severity of HF. Second, galectin-3 has been shown to contribute to the formation of fibrosis (fibrogenesis) – administering exogenous galectin-3 leads to cardiac fibrosis. Reversely, disruption of galectin-3 is associated with the absence of cardiac fibrosis. The effects of galectin-3 on fibrosis have also been established in other organs, for instance kidney and liver. Since complete (genetic) disruption is not clinically feasible, pharmacological inhibition of galectin-3 is an attractive therapeutic modality to inhibit cardiac remodeling and HF development. Various food products, containing oligosaccharides such as pectins, may act as neutralizing ligands or inhibitors for galectin-3. Pectins can bind to galectin-3's carbohydrate recognition domain (CRD) and have been shown to inhibit carcinogenesis and other galectin-3-driven diseases. Recently, it has been reported that cardiac remodeling, fibrogenesis and HF development may also be amenable to inhibition of galectin-3. Circumstantial evidence for a potential role of galectin-3 comes from the observation that consumption of dietary fibers, e.g. from cereals and fruits, that are rich in pectins, has consistently been associated with a lower risk for heart disease. The search for the precise mechanism of galectin-3 in HF and better treatment aimed against galectin-3 is ongoing. Candidate anti-galectin-3 treatments will first have to be tested in animal models, and should then be further evaluated in clinical trials.

Heart Failure

Heart failure (HF) is a clinical syndrome with primary symptoms including shortness of breath and fatigue, signs including fluid retention, ánd objective evidence of abnormal structure or function of the heart. The prevalence of HF in the western world is about 1-2% (*1*) and when ≥ 75 years it is 8.4% (*2*). The life time risk for subjects from the general population to develop HF after the age of 55 is 30% (*3*). Despite optional conventional treatment (*4*) survival remains low with a medium mortality of more than 50% after 5 years (*3*). Main causes of HF are hypertension, myocardial infarction due to ischemic heart disease and cardiomyopathies.

Cardiac Remodeling and Fibrosis

The heart's general response to injury is an adaptive response that is referred to as cardiac remodeling. Hallmark events of cardiac remodeling include myocyte hypertrophy, loss of cardiomyocytes (apoptosis, necrosis), and changes in the interstitial space, predominantly fibrosis (*5*). Recently, the interest in pathways of cardiac remodeling is rising. The cardiac interstitium consists of fibroblasts, blood vessels, lymphatic vessels, adrenergic nerve endings and extra cellular matrix (ECM). The ECM comprises several proteins including collagens, fibronectin, proteoglycans and laminin, but also different proteases and growth factors, produced by cardiac fibroblasts differentiating into myofibroblasts. Besides ECM protein production, cardiac fibroblasts also facilitate mechanical, electrical and chemical signaling in the heart and influence the development and remodeling of myocardial vasculature (*6*, *7*). The function of ECM is to provide a structural network for transmitting force, generated by individual myocytes into organized systolic contraction of the heart. Furthermore, it contributes to passive stiffness in diastole and prevents overstretch, myocyte slippage, and tissue deformation during ventricular filling (*8*). As such, ECM remodeling is an essential process in cardiac remodeling (*9*).

Galectin-3

Galectin-3 is a 29-35 kDa chimaera-type galectin, which is unique because of its extended N-terminal domain linked to a single C-terminal carbohydrate-recognition domain. The galectin family consists of 3 different structures (Figure 1).

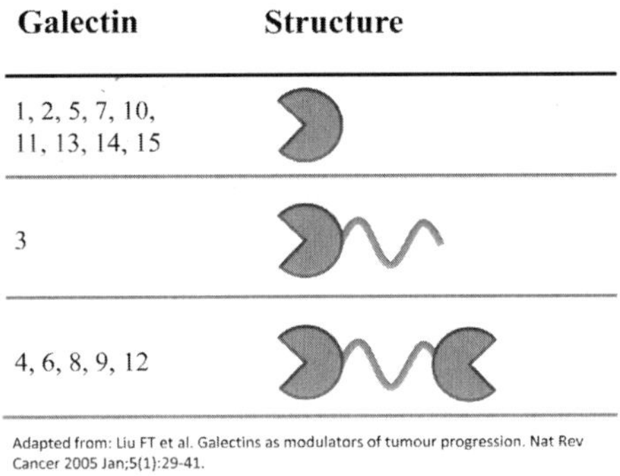

Figure 1. Galectin family and their structures.

The gene that encodes galectin-3, LGALS3, is a single gene located on chromosome 14, locus q21–q22 (*10*). Galectin-3 belongs to a family of soluble β-galactoside-binding lectins that play regulatory roles in inflammation, immunity, fibrosis, and cancer (*11*). Regulation of galectin-3 has not extensively been studied – most consistently galectins have been overexpressed in cancerous cells (*12*).

Galectin-3 and Heart Failure

In 2004, it was observed that galectin-3 is the most over-expressed gene in failing hearts from transgenic hypertensive rats, found in a microarray study (*13*).

Galectin-3 is secreted by hitherto unexplained mechanisms. An FDA-approved ELISA has been developed and allows for reliable quantitation of galectin-3 in plasma or serum. It has convincingly been shown by many groups that plasma galectin-3 levels are increased in HF, and that plasma galectin-3 levels provide strong prognostic value, independent from established predictors like age, gender and kidney function (*14*). In line with the experimental observations (vide infra) that galectin-3 is co-localized with fibrosis, it has also been observed that galectin-3 levels relate to markers of matrix turnover (*11*).

Galectin-3: Emerging Role in Adverse Cardiac Remodeling and Heart Failure

It has been described that galectin-3 interacts with a wide array of glycoproteins that are also located in het ECM in the heart, including laminin, collagen, synexin and integrins (*15*). Especially pertinent to increased galectin-3 regulation and secretion is macrophage migration. Influx of macrophages has been described in many forms of cardiac injury, including infarction, myocarditis, and also chronic LV remodeling (*16*, *17*). The chronic inflammatory state of the HF patient is supported by increased levels of CRP and high total leukocyte counts, especially in patients with increased galectin-3 (*18*).

The seminal paper from Sharma and colleagues first described galectin-3 in HF (*15*). Galectin-3 was upregulated in the left ventricular tissue of Ren2- rats, in parallel to various other ECM proteins, such as collagens, oestoactivin, fibronectin and others, supporting the paramount role galectin-3 plays in ECM homeostasis and integrity. During the compensated phase of cardiac remodeling, myocardial galectin-3 expression was increased to higher levels in rats that later progressed towards overt HF compared with rats that remained compensated. So, besides an interesting correlation, this suggested that galectin-3 would actively contribute to the progression of cardiac remodeling and HF. Further experiments showed that continuous infusion of galectin-3 for four weeks into the pericardial sac induced cardiac remodeling, myocardial fibrosis and cardiac dysfunction, with depressed LV ejection fraction, fractional shortening, and increased lung weight-to-body weight ratio compared with rats receiving placebo infusion. They also found an increase in collagen volume, especially collagen type I (*13*).

Galectin-3 colocalized to sites of extracellular matrix, fibrosis, and accumulation of ECM proteins. The observation that galectin-3 causes myocardial fibrosis and LV dysfunction has been confirmed by others (*23*).

Furthermore, independent corroborating evidence for the pivotal role of galectin-3 in tissue fibrosis was obtained studying mice deficient for the gene encoding galectin-3 (Gal3 KO mice). In a mouse model of liver fibrosis, mice with complete genetic disruption of galectin-3 had less severe fibrosis of their livers upon injection of a pro-fibrotic compound (*19*). In a subsequent study from the same group, it was shown that Gal3KO mice are also protected from renal fibrosis (*20*). In a model of unilateral uninephrectomy, Gal3KO mice showed reduced collagen deposition, less macrophage influx, although expression levels of TGF-β and Smad 2/3 phosphorylation were comparable.

Collectively, these observations clearly indicated that Galectin-3 is produced in adverse cardiac remodeling and HF, might contribute to the pathophysiology, but it remains to be resolved if targeted inhibition of galectin-3 might represent a viable target in HF treatment.

Galectin-3: Emerging Role as a Biomarker in Heart Failure

Extensive cardiac remodeling is the most important determinant of disease progression and highly correlated with poor prognosis. It is of utmost importance to recognize these patients who are at the highest risk for adverse outcome, as this allows more aggressive interventions. Circulating galectin-3 levels are an independent predictor of mortality in patients with chronic HF (*14*, *21*). Patients with chronic HF and (NYHA III/IV) with high baseline galectin-3 had worse survival independent from NT-proBNP (*14*). Furthermore, the prognostic importance of plasma galectin-3 levels appears to be stronger in patients with HF with preserved ejection fraction (HFPEF) (*21*). Additionally, patients who suffered a myocardial infarction were more prone to develop HF when their baseline galectin-3 baseline levels were increased (*22*).

In more advanced HF, the role of galectin-3 needs further study. A recent study in patients receiving cardiac resynchronization therapy (CRT) indicated that galectin/3 did not predict response to CRT (*23*).

Patients with HF who are waiting for heart transplantation (Htx) can be supported by a mechanical support device or treated with total artificial hearts (TAH) when necessary Patients who had high levels of galectin-3 before TAH implantation showed no significantly changes in galectin-3 levels 30 days after the TAH implantation. This observation suggests extracardiac production of galectin-3 in patients with end-stage HF. Higher galectin-3 levels did however still predict adverse outcome of this bridging therapy (*24*).

Besides HF, plasma galectin-3 levels predict all-cause mortality in the general population (*25*). There is evidence that highlight the importance of heart-kidney interactions in HF (*23*), but data in patients with renal disease are currently lacking. Galectin-3 is associated with kidney fibrosis in animal studies (*20*), suggesting that galectin-3 is upregulated in a cardio-renal profibrotic pathway (*23*). In patients with acute decompensated HF who have high levels of galectin-3, there is an association between high age, poor renal function, higher CRP and higher NT-proBNP (*26*).

Inhibition of Galectin-3 by Pectins

Galectin-3 may be bound by ligands, mainly carbohydrates that specifically bind to galectin-3's CRD. The CRD of galectin-3 acts as an unique on-off switch. It has been demonstrated that neutral sugar side chains, containing terminal galactose at the nonreducing end of the polysaccharide chain, bind galectin-3. The binding between the complexes seems to be a lectin-carbohydrate interaction because of the force needed to rupture the binding (*27*). Natural occurring ligands in the heart for galectin-3 are various matrix proteins and oligosaccharides. Recently, it has been acknowledged that several oligosaccharides present in various foods are also ligands to galectin-3. Pectins are typical examples of such oligosaccharides – pectins are present in fruit peels, okra, sugar beets and many more natural foods. It is believed that pectins bind to galectin-3 and render it unavailable to the endogenous ligands, thus acting as neutralizing ligands. Pectin-derived bioactive fragments bind to galectin-3's CRD with various affinity; this is subject to investigation as a pectin with strong affinity might afford protective effects in galectin-3 related disease. The potential efficacy of pectins to reduce galectin-3 bioactivity has been proven in non-cardiac disease only.

Modified citrus pectin (MCP) is the best studied pectin in this perspective. MCP is a dietary fiber that is soluble in water which is found in the peel and pulp of citrus fruits and modified by high pH and temperature (*28*, *29*).

Since galectin-3 plays an important role in cancer and metastasis development, MCP has been studied for its efficacy in preventing carcinogenesis. Fitting this hypothesis, MCP seems to be a therapeutic option in experimental and clinical colon and metastatic prostate cancer (*30*, *31*). The therapeutic pathway in controlling cancer is indeed due to blockage of galectin-3. Mice with injected melanoma cells were started on MPC treatment and showed decrease of lung colonization (*32*). MCP has shown to interfere with cell-cell interactions mediated by cell surface carbohydrate-binding galectin-3 molecules (*31*). Furthermore, in a model of unilateral ureter obstruction, MCP was shown to reduce renal fibrosis (*28*).

Inhibition of Galectin-3 in HF

The concept to inhibit galectin-3-related myocardial fibrogenesis and LV dysfunction has been explored first by Liu and colleagues (*23*).They tested N-acetyl-seryl-aspartyl-lysyl-proline (Ac-SDKP), a tetrapeptide with established anti-inflammatory and antifibrotic capacities. The potentially protective effects of Ac-SDKP have been demonstrated in HF models of hypertension and post-myocardial infarction (*33*, *34*). Ac-SDKP has inhibitory effects on the very mechanisms that are governed by galectin-3 namely, myocardial inflammation (macrophages influx), and myocardial fibrogenesis, including collagen synthesis, TGF-β1 expression, and SMAD3 phosphorylation. The authors concluded that Ac-SDKP prevented galectin-3-mediated myocardial damage via the TGF-β/SMAD3 signaling pathway (Figure 2) (*35*).

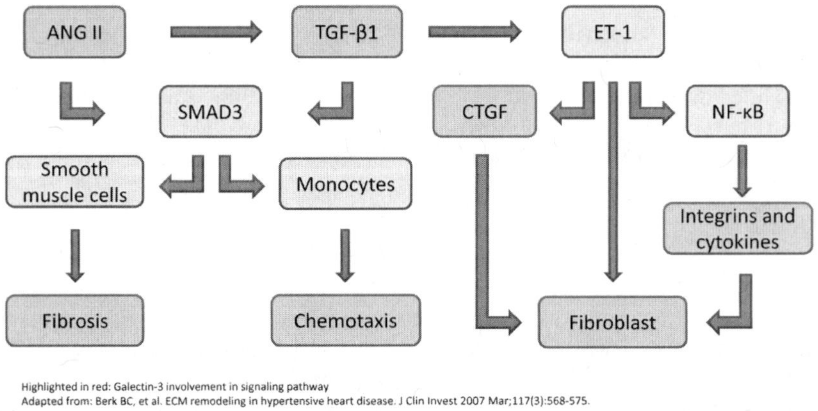

Figure 2. Common signaling pathways that contribute to myocardial fibrosis. (see color insert)

Our group has recently conducted a series of experiments to establish if galectin-3 disruption or inhibition could attenuate progressive adverse cardiac remodeling. We have studied Gal3 KO mice, and subjected the mice to two established perturbations causing LV remodeling: infusion of Angiotensin II (AngII) and transverse aortic constriction (TAC). Both perturbations led in wild type (WT) mice to progressive remodeling, characterized by LV hypertrophy, fibrosis, and associated functional abnormalities, most prominently increased LV end-diastolic pressure and impaired LV relaxation. Gal3 KO mice undergoing the same perturbations, showed identical severity of LV hypertrophy, however, myocardial fibrosis was far less prominent, and mice had less severe diastolic dysfunction (*26*).

Pharmacological inhibition of Galectin-3 was tested in a rat model of spontaneous cardiac remodeling. The galectin-3 inhibitor N-acetyl-D-Lactosamine (N-Lac) was administered to Ren-2 rats for six weeks. Ren-2 rats treated with N-Lac were protected from adverse cardiac remodeling, as indicated by better survival, better cardiac function, and less fibrosis. The improvement was associated with favorable genetic program (lower expression of genes associated with collagen synthesis and processing (*36*) (Figure 3).

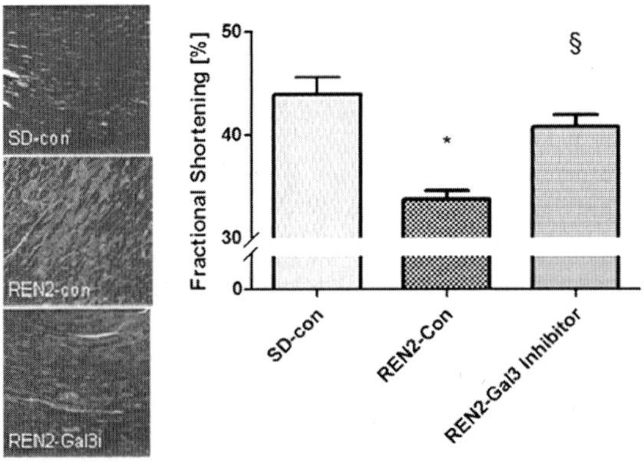

SD: Sprague-Dawley
* $p < 0.05$ vs. SD-con, § $p < 0.05$ vs. REN2-con
Adapted from: Unpublished data from the department of Experimental Cardiology, University Medical Centre Groningen

Figure 3. Fibrosis and Fractional Shortening in Ren-2 Rats (control vs. Galectin-3 inhibitor). (see color insert)

Inhibition of Galectin-3 in Heart Failure: Clinical Clues

There are no data available if galectin-3 inhibition could benefit humans suffering from HF. However, there is some circumstantial evidence to suggest this may be true. First, consumption of dietary fibers, e.g. from cereals and fruits, has consistently been associated with a lower risk for coronary artery disease (*37*). Such dietary fibers may act as galectin-3 inhibitors, although this has not formally been studied. It has been observed that diets that contain soluble fiber-rich whole grains are associated with improvement of blood-pressure control among patients treated with anti-hypertensive medication, a significant reduction in the number of anti-hypertensive medication, and improvement in serum lipids and plasma glucose. Taken these three factors into account this diet can be very effective in a reduction of cardiovascular disease risk (Table 1) (*38*). Interestingly, the intake of whole grain breakfast cereals is also associated with a lower risk of HF (*39*).

Table 1. Dietary fiber intake related to relative risk for disease based on estimates from prospective cohort studies*

Disease	*Number of patients*	*Included studies*	*Relative risk** (95% CI)*
Coronary heart disease	158.327	7	0.71 (0.47-0.95)
Stroke	134.787	4	0.74 (0.63-0.86)
Diabetes	239.485	5	0.81 (0.70-0.93)
Obesity	115.789	4	0.70 (0.62-0.78)

* Table adapted from Anderson, J.W., et al. Health benefits of dietary fiber. *Nutr. Rev.* **2009**, *67* (4), 188-205. ** Relative risks adjusted for demographic, dietary and non-dietary factors.

Future Perspectives

There is accumulating evidence that galectin-3 is important for HF development and progression. Furthermore, galectin-3 is an attractive and feasible target for therapy. What will be needed before galectin-3 inhibition becomes mainstay therapy in HF? First, we need to further dissect what precise role galectin-3 plays in the pathophysiology of HF. Second, we need to study what inhibitors may be used, study if certain types of inhibitors confer superior efficacy, and ideally, identify what sequences are involved. This will require intense interaction between biochemists, chemical, nutritional and pharmaceutical industry and academic researchers. These studies likely will be complex, given the different roles galectin-3 serves in various diseases, both cardiac and non-cardiac. Finally, we need to design elegant animal studies that proof efficacy and safety parameters. Ultimately, clinical trials should be conducted to evaluate the effect of these inhibitors, which might improve survival of patients suffering from this devastating disease.

Conflicts of Interest

BG Medicine (Waltham, MA, USA) holds certain rights with respect to the use of galectin-3 in HF. The UMCG, that employs Dr. de Boer, has received research grants from BG Medicine. Dr. de Boer received consultancy fees from BG Medicine.

References

1. Mosterd, A.; Hoes, A. W. Clinical epidemiology of heart failure. *Heart* **2007**Sep, *93* (9), 1137–1146.
2. Redfield, M. M.; Jacobsen, S. J.; Burnett, J. C., Jr; Mahoney, D. W.; Bailey, K. R.; Rodeheffer, R. J. Burden of systolic and diastolic ventricular dysfunction in the community: Appreciating the scope of the heart failure epidemic. *JAMA, J. Am. Med. Assoc.* **2003**, *289* (2), 194–202.

3. Bleumink, G. S.; Knetsch, A. M.; Sturkenboom, M. C.; Straus, S. M.; Hofman, A.; Deckers, J. W.; et al. Quantifying the heart failure epidemic: Prevalence, incidence rate, lifetime risk and prognosis of heart failure The Rotterdam Study. *Eur. Heart J.* **2004**Sep, *25* (18), 1614–1619.
4. McMurray, J.; Pfeffer, M. A. New therapeutic options in congestive heart failure: Part I. *Circulation* **2002**, *105* (17), 2099–2106.
5. Sutton, M. G.; Sharpe, N. Left ventricular remodeling after myocardial infarction: Pathophysiology and therapy. *Circulation* **2000**, *101* (25), 2981–2988.
6. Baudino, T. A.; Carver, W.; Giles, W.; Borg, T. K. Cardiac fibroblasts: Friend or foe? *Am. J. Physiol. Heart Circ. Physiol.* **2006**, *291* (3), H1015–H1026.
7. Souders, C. A.; Bowers, S. L.; Baudino, T. A. Cardiac fibroblast: The renaissance cell. *Circ Res* **2009**, *105* (12), 1164–1176.
8. Weber, K. T.; Sun, Y.; Tyagi, S. C.; Cleutjens, J. P. Collagen network of the myocardium: Function, structural remodeling and regulatory mechanisms. *J. Mol. Cell. Cardiol.* **1994**Mar, *26* (3), 279–292.
9. Zannad, F.; Rossignol, P.; Iraqi, W. Extracellular matrix fibrotic markers in heart failure. *Heart Fail Rev* **2010**, *15* (4), 319–329.
10. Raimond, J.; Zimonjic, D. B.; Mignon, C.; Mattei, M.; Popescu, N. C.; Monsigny, M.; et al. Mapping of the galectin-3 gene (LGALS3) to human chromosome 14 at region 14q21-22. *Mamm. Genome* **1997**, *8* (9), 706–707.
11. Lin, Y. H.; Lin, L. Y.; Wu, Y. W.; Chien, K. L.; Lee, C. M.; Hsu, R. B.; et al. The relationship between serum galectin-3 and serum markers of cardiac extracellular matrix turnover in heart failure patients. *Clin. Chim. Acta* **2009**, *409* (1–2), 96–99.
12. Liu, F. T.; Rabinovich, G. A. Galectins as modulators of tumour progression. *Nat. Rev. Cancer* **2005**, *5* (1), 29–41.
13. Sharma, U. C.; Pokharel, S.; van Brakel, T. J.; van Berlo, J. H.; Cleutjens, J. P.; Schroen, B.; et al. Galectin-3 marks activated macrophages in failure-prone hypertrophied hearts and contributes to cardiac dysfunction. *Circulation* **2004**Nov9, *110* (19), 3121–3128.
14. Lok, D. J.; Van Der Meer, P.; de la Porte, P. W.; Lipsic, E.; Van Wijngaarden, J.; Hillege, H. L.; et al. Prognostic value of galectin-3, a novel marker of fibrosis, in patients with chronic heart failure: Data from the DEAL-HF study. *Clin. Res. Cardiol.* **2010**, *99* (5), 323–328.
15. Ochieng, J.; Warfield, P.; Green-Jarvis, B.; Fentie, I. Galectin-3 regulates the adhesive interaction between breast carcinoma cells and elastin. *J. Cell. Biochem* **1999**, *75* (3), 505–514.
16. Neumann, F. J.; Ott, I.; Gawaz, M.; Richardt, G.; Holzapfel, H.; Jochum, M.; et al. Cardiac release of cytokines and inflammatory responses in acute myocardial infarction. *Circulation* **1995**, *92* (4), 748–755.
17. Matsumori, A.; Yamada, T.; Suzuki, H.; Matoba, Y.; Sasayama, S. Increased circulating cytokines in patients with myocarditis and cardiomyopathy. *Br. Heart. J.* **1994**, *72* (6), 561–566.
18. Ueland, T.; Aukrust, P.; Broch, K.; Aakhus, S.; Skardal, R.; Muntendam, P.; et al. Galectin-3 in heart failure: High levels are associated with all-cause mortality. *Int. J. Cardiol.* **2011**, *150* (3), 361–364.

19. Henderson, N. C.; Mackinnon, A. C.; Farnworth, S. L.; Poirier, F.; Russo, F. P.; Iredale, J. P.; et al. Galectin-3 regulates myofibroblast activation and hepatic fibrosis. *Proc. Natl. Acad. Sci. U.S.A.* **2006**, *103* (13), 5060–5065.
20. Henderson, N. C.; Mackinnon, A. C.; Farnworth, S. L.; Kipari, T.; Haslett, C.; Iredale, J. P.; et al. Galectin-3 expression and secretion links macrophages to the promotion of renal fibrosis. *Am. J. Pathol.* **2008**, *172* (2), 288–298.
21. de Boer, R. A.; Lok, D. J.; Jaarsma, T.; van der Meer, P.; Voors, A. A.; Hillege, H. L.; et al. Predictive value of plasma galectin-3 levels in heart failure with reduced and preserved ejection fraction. *Ann. Med.* **2011**, *43* (1), 60–68.
22. Grandin, E. W.; Jarolim, P.; Murphy, S. A.; Ritterova, L.; Cannon, C. P.; Braunwald, E.; et al. Galectin-3 and the development of heart failure after acute coronary syndrome: Pilot experience from PROVE IT-TIMI 22. *Clin. Chem.* **2012**, *58* (1), 267–273.
23. Lopez-Andres, N.; Rossignol, P.; Iraqi, W.; Fay, R.; Nuee, J.; Ghio, S.; et al. Association of galectin-3 and fibrosis markers with long-term cardiovascular outcomes in patients with heart failure, left ventricular dysfunction, and dyssynchrony: Insights from the CARE-HF (Cardiac Resynchronization in Heart Failure) trial. *Eur. J. Heart Fail.* **2012**, *14* (1), 74–81.
24. Milting, H.; Ellinghaus, P.; Seewald, M.; Cakar, H.; Bohms, B.; Kassner, A.; et al. Plasma biomarkers of myocardial fibrosis and remodeling in terminal heart failure patients supported by mechanical circulatory support devices. *J. Heart Lung Transplant.* **2008**, *27* (6), 589–596.
25. de Boer, R. A.; van Veldhuisen, D. J.; Gansevoort, R. T.; Muller Kobold, A. C.; van Gilst, W. H.; Hillege, H. L.; et al. The fibrosis marker galectin-3 and outcome in the general population. *J. Intern. Med.* **2012**, *272* (1), 55–64.
26. Shah, R. V.; Chen-Tournoux, A. A.; Picard, M. H.; van Kimmenade, R. R.; Januzzi, J. L. Galectin-3, cardiac structure and function, and long-term mortality in patients with acutely decompensated heart failure. *Eur. J. Heart Fail.* **2010**, *12* (8), 826–832.
27. Gunning, A. P.; Bongaerts, R. J.; Morris, V. J. Recognition of galactan components of pectin by galectin-3. *FASEB J.* **2009**, *23* (2), 415–424.
28. Kolatsi-Joannou, M.; Price, K. L.; Winyard, P. J.; Long, D. A. Modified citrus pectin reduces galectin-3 expression and disease severity in experimental acute kidney injury. *PLoS One* **2011**, *6* (4), e18683.
29. Glinsky, V. V.; Raz, A. Modified citrus pectin anti-metastatic properties: One bullet, multiple targets. *Carbohydr. Res.* **2009**, *344* (14), 1788–1791.
30. Liu, H. Y.; Huang, Z. L.; Yang, G. H.; Lu, W. Q.; Yu, N. R. Inhibitory effect of modified citrus pectin on liver metastases in a mouse colon cancer model. *World J .Gastroenterol.* **2008**, *14* (48), 7386–7391.
31. Pienta, K. J.; Naik, H.; Akhtar, A.; Yamazaki, K.; Replogle, T. S.; Lehr, J.; et al. Inhibition of spontaneous metastasis in a rat prostate cancer model by oral administration of modified citrus pectin. *J. Natl. Cancer Inst.* **1995**, *87* (5), 348–353.
32. Platt, D.; Raz, A. Modulation of the lung colonization of B16-F1 melanoma cells by citrus pectin. *J. Natl. Cancer Inst.* **1992**Mar18, *84* (6), 438–442.

33. Peng, H.; Carretero, O. A.; Liao, T. D.; Peterson, E. L.; Rhaleb, N. E. Role of N-acetyl-seryl-aspartyl-lysyl-proline in the antifibrotic and anti-inflammatory effects of the angiotensin-converting enzyme inhibitor captopril in hypertension. *Hypertension* **2007**, *49* (3), 695–703.
34. Yang, F.; Yang, X. P.; Liu, Y. H.; Xu, J.; Cingolani, O.; Rhaleb, N. E.; et al. Ac-SDKP reverses inflammation and fibrosis in rats with heart failure after myocardial infarction. *Hypertension* **2004**, *43* (2), 229–236.
35. Liu, Y. H.; D'Ambrosio, M.; Liao, T. D.; Peng, H.; Rhaleb, N. E.; Sharma, U.; et al. N-acetyl-seryl-aspartyl-lysyl-proline prevents cardiac remodeling and dysfunction induced by galectin-3, a mammalian adhesion/growth-regulatory lectin. *Am. J. Physiol. Heart Circ. Physiol.* **2009**Feb, *296* (2), H404–12.
36. Yu, L.; Ruifrok, W. P.; Sillje, H. H. W.; Bos, E.; Van Goor, H.; Van Veldhuisen, D. J.; Van Gilst, H. W.; De Boer, R. A. Pharmacological inhibition of galectin-3 attenuates adverse cardiac remodeling and heart failure. *Eur. Heart J.* **2011**.
37. Pereira, M. A.; O'Reilly, E.; Augustsson, K.; Fraser, G. E.; Goldbourt, U.; Heitmann, B. L.; et al. Dietary fiber and risk of coronary heart disease: A pooled analysis of cohort studies. *Arch. Intern. Med.* **2004**, *164* (4), 370–376.
38. Pins, J. J.; Geleva, D.; Keenan, J. M.; Frazel, C.; O'Connor, P. J.; Cherney, L. M. Do whole-grain oat cereals reduce the need for antihypertensive medications and improve blood pressure control? *J. Fam. Pract.* **2002**, *51* (4), 353–359.
39. Djousse, L.; Gaziano, J. M. Breakfast cereals and risk of heart failure in the physicians' health study I. *Arch. Intern. Med.* **2007**, *167* (19), 2080–2085.

Chapter 25

Mucins and Galectin-3 in Ocular Surface Health and Disease

Jerome Mauris and Pablo Argüeso*

Schepens Eye Research Institute and Massachusetts Eye and Ear, Department of Ophthalmology, Harvard Medical School, 20 Staniford Street, Boston, Massachusetss 02114
***E-mail: pablo.argueso@schepens.harvard.edu**

The barrier function of ocular surface epithelia is multi-level, from the stratified structure of the corneal and conjunctival epithelia, to the thick glycocalyx present on the foremost apical cell membranes. Major glycoconjugates on the epithelial glycocalyx include membrane-associated mucins, a group of heavily O-glycosylated, high molecular weight glycoproteins involved in cell protection against damage and infection. In this mini review, we summarize recent evidence indicating that mucin O-glycans associate with the carbohydrate-binding protein galectin-3 to provide barrier function at the ocular surface, and discuss the relevance of this interaction to ocular surface disease.

Anatomy of the Ocular Surface

The healthy ocular surface is composed of mucosa lining the cornea and conjunctiva, as well as the intervening transition area between them, known as the limbus (*1*). The cornea is a transparent, avascular tissue that is the primary refractive element of the visual system. The conjunctiva is a mucous membrane that covers the inner surface of the upper and lower eyelids and extends to the limbus. Both cornea and conjunctiva, as well as the limbus, are covered by a stratified, squamous, nonkeratinizing epithelium, consisting of 5 to 7 cell layers within the cornea, and 3 to 10 cell layers within the conjunctiva. The conjunctiva is unique among the nonkeratinizing squamous tissues in that secretory goblet cells are intercalated between the epithelial cells. The role of the ocular surface epithelia is to maintain optical clarity by regulating the hydration of the cornea and conjunctiva, and to protect the globe from mechanical, toxic, and infectious trauma (*2*).

Mucins and the Epithelial Glycocalyx

Traditionally, the cellular barrier function on mucosal surfaces has been ascribed to intercellular junctions that seal the paracellular space and connect individual epithelial cell membranes (*3*). It is now well accepted, however, that a second barrier is formed by dense microvilli and a complex glycocalyx containing high levels of membrane-associated mucins on the apical surface of mucosal epithelial cells (*4*).

Based on molecular characterization, cell surface mucins are defined by their unique structural characteristics, including the presence on the extracellular domain of multiple tandem repeats of amino acids rich in serine, threonine and proline residues that are densely O-glycosylated (*5*). In addition, they contain a single transmembrane domain that anchors the large ectodomain to the plasma membrane, as well as a short cytoplasmic tail with intracellular signaling capabilities (*6*). The mucin ectodomain has a long filamentous structure that can extend up to 500 nm above the plasma membrane and, therefore, provide steric hindrance (*7*). Cell surface mucins produced in the ocular surface include MUC1, MUC4 and MUC16 (*8*).

Early analyses of the chemical composition of purified ocular surface mucins revealed that approximately 55% of the mucin mass was carbohydrate, with galactose, N-acetylgalactosamine, N-acetylglucosamine and sialic acid as major constituents, and fucose, mannose, and glucose as minor components (*9*). Further structural analyses have shown that short core 1-based structures (Galβ1-3GalNAcα1-Ser/Thr, also known as the Thomsen Friedenreich or T-antigen) are prevalent at the ocular surface (*10*). This finding is supported by glycogene microarray analysis demonstrating the expression of core 1 β 1,3-galactosyltransferase (T-synthase or c1galt1), the enzyme responsible for biosynthesis of core 1 O-glycans, and Cosmc, a molecular chaperone specific for c1galt1, at the human ocular surface (*11*). Due to the presence of central tandem repeats in mucins, it is possible to speculate that hundreds of clustered core 1 O-glycans would be present on each mucin ectodomain, providing a high degree of multivalency for optimal interactions with carbohydrate-binding proteins (*12*).

Role of Galectin-3 in Barrier Function

Despite extensive molecular characterization of mucins at the ocular surface during the last 15 years, their organization at the plasma membrane and the mechanism by which they promote barrier function is not well understood. Using glycogene microarray analysis, we demonstrated that galectin-3 was one of the most highly expressed glycogenes in human conjunctival epithelium (*11*). This finding led us to evaluate the role of galectins in maintaining barrier function at the ocular surface through interaction with mucin O-glycans.

Galectins are a family of animal lectins defined by their affinity towards β-galactosides and the presence of at least one evolutionary conserved carbohydrate-binding domain (*13*). In recent years, several studies have revealed that galectin-3 exists as a monomer in solution, but that it can self-associate through intermolecular interactions involving the N-terminal domain when bound to a multivalent ligand (*14*) and, therefore, mediate crosslinking of counter-receptors (*15–18*). It has also been shown that the resulting galectin-ligand lattices on the cell surface are robust and resistant to lateral movement of membrane components (*19*).

Data from our laboratory demonstrated that galectin-3 localizes to apical membranes of apical epithelial cells in human conjunctival and corneal tissue (*20*). Moreover, galectin-3 colocalized with the membrane-associated mucins MUC1 and MUC16 on the apical surface of epithelial cells, and both mucins bound to galectin-3 affinity columns in a galactose-dependent manner, indicating that transmembrane mucins are counter-receptors for galectin-3 at the ocular surface. The relevance of this interaction to ocular surface barrier function was evaluated using the rose bengal uptake assay. Rose bengal, a derivative of fluorescein, is an organic anionic dye that has been clinically used for many decades to assess damage to the ocular surface epithelium in ocular surface disease (*21*). Stratification and differentiation of cultured immortalized corneal epithelial cells, as measured by the capacity to produce the membrane-associated mucin MUC16 and core 1 O-glycans on their apical surfaces, provide protection against rose bengal penetrance (*22*). Abrogation of the mucin-galectin interaction in this *in vitro* system, using competitive carbohydrate inhibitors of galectin binding, β-lactose and modified citrus pectin, resulted in decreased levels of galectin-3 on the cell surface with concomitant loss of barrier function, as indicated by increased permeability to rose bengal diagnostic dye (*20*). Similarly, downregulation of mucin *O*-glycosylation in corneal epithelial cells using a stable tetracycline-inducible RNA interfering system to knockdown c1galt1 also reduced cell surface galectin-3 and increased epithelial permeability. These findings indicate that galectin-3 through interactions with mucin O-glycans at the apical membrane of corneal epithelial cells forms a cell surface lattice important to barrier function.

Using cell surface biotinylation and subcellular fractionation, as well as confocal laser scanning microscopy, we recently showed that knockdown of c1galt1 in human corneal epithelial cells also stimulates the endocytosis of plasma membrane proteins and enhances the internalization of nanoparticles in a clathrin-dependent manner (*23*). Therefore, it is possible to speculate that, when bound to cell surface O-glycans, galectin-3 effectively promotes lattice formation and prevents the endocytosis of plasma membrane proteins and extracellular material.

Barrier Function in Ocular Surface Disease

Ocular surface pathology is commonly associated with loss of epithelial barrier function (*21*). Several studies have reported alterations in the biosynthesis of mucins and mucin O-glycans at the ocular surface under pathological conditions, including dry eye, allergy, pterygium, ocular rosacea, and infection [reviewed by Mantelli (*24*) and Guzman-Aranguez (*10*)]. Within these ocular surface diseases, dry eye has been extensively studied, as it affects between 6 and 43 million people in the United States alone (*25*), and the options for effective pharmacological treatment are limited.

Dry eye is a multifactorial disease of the ocular surface that is prevalent in women and that results in symptoms of discomfort, visual disturbance, and tear film instability, with potential damage to ocular surface epithelia. A number of reports have described alterations in the carbohydrate composition of the apical glycocalyx in patients with dry eye. These include a reduction in lectin and antibody binding to cell-surface carbohydrate epitopes such as sialic acid as well as core 1, and alteration in the distribution of glycosyltransferases involved in mucin-type O-glycosylation (*26–30*).

Unlike with mucins, limited research has been conducted to date on the role of galectins in ocular surface epithelial pathology. To our knowledge, only one manuscript has been published describing alterations in galectin-3 in ocular surface disease (*31*). Although the study included only a small number of patients, the authors found increased galectin-3 levels in tears of patients with ocular inflammatory disease, such as sarcoidosis and adenoviral conjunctivitis, as compared to normal individuals. This result would suggest that barrier disruption in ocular surface disease results in lack of interaction of galectin-3 with mucin O-glycans on the apical epithelial glycocalyx, followed by release of the lectin into the tear fluid.

Increased understanding of the ocular surface barrier under physiological and pathological conditions has led to interest in developing pharmaceutical agents that modulate mucin biosynthesis. Two therapeutic agents targeting the production of mucins at the ocular surface have been recently developed for dry eye and marketed in Japan as Mucosta® ophthalmic suspension (rebamipide) and DIQUAS™ ophthalmic solution (diquafosol tetrasodium). So far, however, it is not clear whether the mechanism of action of these drugs is to promote ocular surface health by restoring the mucin O-glycan and galectin-3 interaction on superficial cells at the ocular surface. Studies aimed at determining whether carbohydrate-lectin interactions on the epithelial glycocalyx can be modulated to treat patients with ocular surface barrier dysfunction are likely to prove to be rewarding.

Acknowledgments

Supported by the National Eye Institute Grant R01 EY014847 (PA).

References

1. Foster, C. S.; Azar, D. T.; Dohlman C. H.; Smolin, G. *Smolin and Thoft's, The Cornea: Scientific Foundations and Clinical Practice*, 4th ed.; Lippincott Williams & Wilkins: Philadelphia, PA, 2004.
2. Holland, E. J.; Mannis, M. J. *Ocular Surface Disease: Medical and Surgical Management*; Springer: New York, 2002.
3. Madara, J. L. Warner-Lambert/Parke-Davis Award lecture. Pathobiology of the intestinal epithelial barrier. *Am. J. Pathol.* **1990**, *137*, 1273–1281.
4. McGuckin, M. A.; Linden, S. K.; Sutton, P.; Florin, T. H. Mucin dynamics and enteric pathogens. *Nat. Rev. Microbiol.* **2011**, *9*, 265–278.
5. Gendler, S. J.; Spicer, A. P. Epithelial mucin genes. *Annu. Rev. Physiol.* **1995**, *57*, 607–634.
6. Carson, D. D. The cytoplasmic tail of MUC1: A very busy place. *Sci. Signaling* **2008**, *1*, pe35.
7. Linden, S. K.; Sheng, Y. H.; Every, A. L.; Miles, K. M.; Skoog, E. C.; Florin, T. H.; Sutton, P.; McGuckin, M. A. MUC1 limits *Helicobacter pylori* infection both by steric hindrance and by acting as a releasable decoy. *PLoS Pathog.* **2009**, *5*, e1000617.
8. Govindarajan, B.; Gipson, I. K. Membrane-tethered mucins have multiple functions on the ocular surface. *Exp. Eye Res.* **2010**, *90*, 655–663.
9. Chao, C. C.; Butala, S. M.; Herp, A. Studies on the isolation and composition of human ocular mucin. *Exp. Eye Res.* **1988**, *47*, 185–196.
10. Guzman-Aranguez, A.; Argueso, P. Structure and biological roles of mucin-type O-glycans at the ocular surface. *Ocul Surf* **2010**, *8*, 8–17.
11. Mantelli, F.; Schaffer, L.; Dana, R.; Head, S. R.; Argueso, P. Glycogene expression in conjunctiva of patients with dry eye: Downregulation of Notch signaling. *Invest. Ophthalmol. Vis. Sci.* **2009**, *50*, 2666–2672.
12. Dam, T. K.; Brewer, C. F. Effects of clustered epitopes in multivalent ligand-receptor interactions. *Biochemistry* **2008**, *47*, 8470–8476.
13. Dumic, J.; Dabelic, S.; Flogel, M. Galectin-3: An open-ended story. *Biochim. Biophys. Acta* **2006**, *1760*, 616–635.
14. Ahmad, N.; Gabius, H. J.; Andre, S.; Kaltner, H.; Sabesan, S.; Roy, R; Liu, B.; Macaluso, F.; Brewer, C. F. Galectin-3 precipitates as a pentamer with synthetic multivalent carbohydrates and forms heterogeneous cross-linked complexes. *J. Biol. Chem.* **2004**, *279*, 10841–10847.
15. Delacour, D.; Greb, C.; Koch, A.; Salomonsson, E.; Leffler, H.; Le Bivic, A.; Jacob, R. Apical sorting by galectin-3-dependent glycoprotein clustering. *Traffic* **2007**, *8*, 379–388.
16. Inohara, H.; Raz, A. Functional evidence that cell surface galectin-3 mediates homotypic cell adhesion. *Cancer Res.* **1995**, *55*, 3267–3271.
17. Lagana, A.; Goetz, J. G.; Cheung, P.; Raz, A.; Dennis, J. W.; Nabi, I. R. Galectin binding to Mgat5-modified N-glycans regulates fibronectin matrix remodeling in tumor cells. *Mol. Cell Biol.* **2006**, *26*, 3181–3193.
18. Partridge, E. A.; Le Roy, C.; Di Guglielmo, G. M.; Pawling, J.; Cheung, P.; Granovsky, M.; Nabi, I. R.; Wrana, J. L.; Dennis, J. W. Regulation of

cytokine receptors by Golgi N-glycan processing and endocytosis. *Science* **2004**, *306*, 120–124.

19. Nieminen, J; Kuno, A.; Hirabayashi, J.; Sato, S. Visualization of galectin-3 oligomerization on the surface of neutrophils and endothelial cells using fluorescence resonance energy transfer. *J. Biol. Chem.* **2007**, *282*, 1374–1383.
20. Argueso, P.; Guzman-Aranguez, A.; Mantelli, F; Cao, Z.; Ricciuto, J.; Panjwani, N. Association of cell surface mucins with galectin-3 contributes to the ocular surface epithelial barrier. *J. Biol. Chem.* **2009**, *284*, 23037–23045.
21. Kim, J. The use of vital dyes in corneal disease. *Curr. Opin. Ophthalmol.* **2000**, *11*, 241–247.
22. Argueso, P.; Tisdale, A.; Spurr-Michaud, S.; Sumiyoshi, M.; Gipson, I. K. Mucin characteristics of human corneal-limbal epithelial cells that exclude the rose bengal anionic dye. *Invest. Ophthalmol. Vis. Sci.* **2006**, *47*, 113–119.
23. Guzman-Aranguez, A.; Woodward, A. M.; Pintor, J; Argueso, P. Targeted disruption of core 1 β1,3-galactosyltransferase (C1galt1) induces apical endocytic trafficking in human corneal keratinocytes. *PLoS One*(in press).
24. Mantelli, F.; Argueso, P. Functions of ocular surface mucins in health and disease. *Curr. Opin. Allergy Clin. Immunol.* **2008**, *8*, 477–483.
25. Pflugfelder, S. C. Tear dysfunction and the cornea: LXVIII Edward Jackson Memorial Lecture. *Am. J. Ophthalmol.* **2011**, *152*, 900–909 e901.
26. Argueso, P.; Sumiyoshi, M. Characterization of a carbohydrate epitope defined by the monoclonal antibody H185: Sialic acid O-acetylation on epithelial cell-surface mucins. *Glycobiology* **2006**, *16*, 1219–1228.
27. Argueso, P.; Tisdale, A.; Mandel, U.; Letko, E.; Foster, C. S.; Gipson, I. K. The cell-layer- and cell-type-specific distribution of GalNAc-transferases in the ocular surface epithelia is altered during keratinization. *Invest. Ophthalmol. Vis. Sci.* **2003**, *44*, 86–92.
28. Danjo, Y.; Watanabe, H.; Tisdale, A. S.; George, M.; Tsumura, T.; Abelson, M. B.; Gipson, I. K. Alteration of mucin in human conjunctival epithelia in dry eye. *Invest. Ophthalmol. Vis. Sci.* **1998**, *39*, 2602–2609.
29. Versura, P.; Maltarello, M. C.; Cellini, M.; Caramazza, R.; Laschi, R. Detection of mucus glycoconjugates in human conjunctiva by using the lectin-colloidal gold technique in TEM. II. A quantitative study in dry-eye patients. *Acta Ophthalmol. (Copenhagen)* **1986**, *64*, 451–455.
30. Watanabe, H.; Maeda, N.; Kiritoshi, A.; Hamano, T.; Shimomura, Y.; Tano, Y. Expression of a mucin-like glycoprotein produced by ocular surface epithelium in normal and keratinized cells. *Am. J. Ophthalmol.* **1997**, *124*, 751–757.
31. Hrdlickova-Cela, E.; Plzak, J.; Smetana, K., Jr.; Melkova, Z.; Kaltner, H.; Filipec, M.; Liu, F. T.; Gabius, H. J. Detection of galectin-3 in tear fluid at disease states and immunohistochemical and lectin histochemical analysis in human corneal and conjunctival epithelium. *Br. J. Ophthalmol.* **2001**, *85*, 1336–1340.

Chapter 26

Role of Galectins in Wound Healing

Noorjahan Panjwani, Ph.D.*

New England Eye Center, Departments of Ophthalmology and Biochemistry, Tufts University School of Medicine, 136 Harrison Ave., Boston, Massachusetts 02111
*** E-mail: Noorjahan.panjwani@tufts.edu. Tel: 617-636-6776. Fax: 617-636-0348.**

Impaired or delayed re-epithelialization underlies serious disorders of wound healing that are painful, difficult to treat, and affect a variety of human tissues. Recent studies have provided evidence that members of the galectin class of β-galactoside-binding proteins play a crucial role in modulating re-epithelialization of wounds by novel carbohydrate-based recognition systems. Galectins constitute a family of widely distributed carbohydrate-binding proteins characterized by their affinity for β-galactoside-containing glycans found on many cell surface and extracellular matrix glycoproteins. In mammals, 15 members of the galectin family have been identified to date. Studies aimed at characterization of the role of galectins in wound healing have shown that galectin-3 promotes re-epithelialization of corneal and skin wounds, galectin-7 promotes re-epithelialization of corneal, skin and kidney wounds, and galectins-2 and-4 promote re-epithelialization of intestinal wounds. Molecular mechanisms by which galectins promote wound healing have also begun to be elucidated. Galectin-3 promotes re-epithelialization of wounds by: (i) activating α3β1-integrin–Rac1 signaling to promote formation of lamellipodia in epithelial cells, and (ii) interacting with N-glycans of laminin-332. Findings that galectins stimulate the re-epithelialization of corneal, dermal, intestinal and kidney wounds have broad implications for developing novel therapeutic strategies for the treatment of nonhealing wounds.

I. Re-Epithelialization of Wounds

Wound healing presents therapeutic challenges in a variety of clinical scenarios. Organ systems as different as cornea, skin and gastrointestinal (GI) may be the site of healing disorders that are related in their biological basis (*1–6*). These are but three of the many human organ systems in which impaired or delayed re-epithelialization may result in persistent epithelial defects which define a condition with serious medical implications.

A unified hypothesis to comprehensively explain the failure of some, and not other, wounds to heal within a normal course of time has yet to be articulated. Meanwhile, patients with debilitations caused by a range, from relatively obscure to unfortunately commonplace, disease-associated, accidental, surgical or inflicted wounds (for example of combat) rely on what we know to guide their treatment. Attempts at resolution of chronic wounds of various etiologies can be frustrating and may not have a positive outcome. Millions of individuals are affected world-wide. In the U.S. alone, combat-related and other traumatic wounds cause over 300,000 hospitalizations annually (*7*, *8*) .

In the cornea, epithelial defects may persist and threaten the integrity of the anterior stroma, causing ulceration and in the worst cases perforation of the stromal tissue resulting in significant visual loss. Chronic wounds in the elderly, decubitus ulcer, and venous statis ulcer of the skin also are attributable to delayed re-epithelialization and resultant persistent epithelial defects. Damage and impairment of the intestinal surface barrier are commonly observed in a variety of GI diseases including inflammatory bowel diseases (IBDs). The treatment goal is prompt re-epithelialization of the wound, essential for rapid resealing of the epithelial surface barrier to control inflammation and to restore intestinal homeostasis. When re-epithelialization of intestinal wounds in IBDs is delayed, uncontrolled intestinal inflammation and general immune responses become inevitable (*9*, *10*).

Failure to re-epithelialize is generally caused not by inadequate cell proliferation but is due to a reduced potential of the epithelium to migrate across the wound bed (*11–13*). Cell migration involves sequential adhesion to and release from the substrate, a complex process of cell-matrix interactions (*14–17*). Results of recent studies suggest that members of the galectin class of β-galactoside-binding proteins have a critical role in modulating cell-matrix interactions and re-epithelialization of wounds through novel carbohydrate-based recognition systems (*18–25*).

II. Galectins

Galectins constitute a family of widely distributed carbohydrate-binding proteins characterized by their affinity for β-galactoside-containing glycans found on many cell surface and extracellular matrix (ECM) glycoproteins (*26*, *27*). In mammals, there are currently 15 identified members of the galectin family. They all range in subunit size from 14- to 39-kDa. Each galectin contains a canonical carbohydrate recognition domain (CRD) of ~130 amino acids. Galectins can be expressed both intracellularly and extracellularly. Galectins do not contain a classical signal sequence or a transmembrane domain and are secreted from the cell via nonclassical pathways. Some galectins such as galectins-1, -3, -8 and -9 have wide tissue distribution, whereas others, such as galectins-4, -5 and -6, exhibit tissue specificity. There is currently intense interest in characterizing the function of galectins because so many important cellular responses such as cell adhesion (*28–30*), migration (*18*, *31*), immune response (*32*, *33*) and angiogenesis (*34–40*) are regulated by this class of lectins.

Carbohydrate-Binding Specificity of Galectins

Although all galectins specifically recognize galactose-containing glycans, each galectin has unique, fine specificity for more complex galactose-containing oligosaccharides, which occurs as a consequence of variability in the CRD sequence. Due to differences in the carbohydrate-binding specificities, each galectin associates with certain types of glycans for signaling (*41*, *42*). The differences in the sugar-binding specificity of different members of the galectin family can be profound. For example, Gal1 (Gal1) recognizes α2-3 sialylated glycans, but not α2-6 sialylated glycans; Gal2 does not bind glycans sialylated with either linkage; Gal3 binds internal N-acetyllactosamine (LacNAc) within polyLacNAc (*41*); and depending on cellular microenvironment, sialylation may also impact Gal3 binding and signaling (*43*). In summary, due to fine differences in carbohydrate-binding specificities, each galectin may interact with a discrete spectrum of glycoprotein receptors, with consequent specific downstream effects. For example, (i) the affinity of Gal1 for the blood group A tetrasaccharide is about 100-fold lower than that for Gal3 (*44*), and (ii) only Gal8, but not Gal1, Gal2, Gal3, or Gal7, interact with the glycans of a well-known lymphatic vessels glycoprotein, podoplanin (*45*).

Galectin-Glycan Lattices

All lectins are either dimers or oligomers. This multivalency allows the formation of lectin-carbohydrate lattices to cross-link and clusterize cell surface receptors including growth factor receptors and integrins. The diverse functions of galectins are thought to result from the formation of galectin–glycan lattice (*46–48*), by which the glycoprotein receptors are trapped, and thereby, precluded from undergoing endocytosis (*49*). It is by this mechanism that the interactions between galectins and N-glycans of the cell surface receptors regulate the density and distribution of cell surface receptors as well as cell responsiveness to the receptor ligand (*46–49*). For example, Gal3 interacts with the N-glycans of the epidermal growth factor (EGF) receptor in a carbohydrate-dependent manner; this delays its constitutive endocytic removal and promotes EGF signaling (*49*). Recent studies in our laboratory have revealed that Gal3 promotes cell migration and formation of lamellipodia by activating α3β1-integrin-Rac1 signaling in epithelial cells, and that carbohydrate-mediated interaction between Gal3 and complex N-glycans on the α3β1 integrin is involved in Gal3-induced lamellipodia formation and cell migration (*18*).

III. Role of Galectins in Wound Healing

A. Galectin-3

Gal3 is expressed in inflammatory cells and in epithelia and fibroblasts of various tissues (*26*). It is found on the cell surface, within ECM, and in the cytoplasm of cells, and is thought to influence cell-matrix adhesion by binding to the ECM and cell surface-glycosylated counter receptors (*e.g.* growth factor receptors, integrins, certain isoforms of laminin, fibronectin and vitronectin). In addition, this lectin is found in the nucleus of the cells and may influence cell-matrix interactions indirectly by influencing the expression of well-known cell adhesion molecules (*e.g.* $\alpha_6\beta_1$ and $\alpha_4\beta_7$integrins) and cytokines (*e.g.* IL-1).

1. Role of Gal3 in Corneal Wound Healing

In corneas, Gal3 is located in high density at sites of corneal epithelial cell-matrix adhesion (*25*), an ideal location for influencing cell-matrix interactions and cell migration. To determine whether Gal3 plays a role in re-epithelialization of corneal wounds, experiments were conducted to determine whether the rate of wound closure rate is impaired in Gal3-deficient mice. In this study, two different models of corneal wound healing were used. Corneas with excimer laser ablations or alkali-burn wounds were allowed to partially heal *in vivo* or *in vitro* for up to 22 h. At the end of the healing period, remaining wound areas were quantitated and compared among different groups. Regardless of whether the corneas were injured by excimer laser or by alkali treatment and whether the corneas were allowed to heal *in vivo* or *in vitro*, corneal epithelial wound closure rate (expressed as mm^2/h) was significantly slower in gal3$^{-/-}$mice compared with gal3$^{+/+}$ mice (Figure 1A-1E) (*25*). In contrast, no differences were found in the wound closure rates between Gal1$^{+/+}$ and Gal1$^{-/-}$groups (Figure 1F).

To determine whether delayed re-epithelialization of corneal wounds in Gal3$^{-/-}$ mice was because of a deficiency in the rate of corneal epithelial cell proliferation, normal and healing Gal3$^{+/+}$ and Gal3$^{-/-}$ corneas were labeled with BrdUrd to identify cells undergoing DNA synthesis. There was no significant difference in the number BrdUrd-labeled cells between Gal3$^{+/+}$ and Gal3$^{-/-}$ corneas (*25*), suggesting that the rate of corneal epithelial cell proliferation is not perturbed in Gal3$^{-/-}$ mice and that delayed re-epithelialization of corneal wounds in Gal3$^{-/-}$mice is most likely to be due to an impairment in the process of cell migration.

The next set of experiments was conducted to determine whether exogenous Gal3 would stimulate re-epithelialization of corneal wounds. In this study, the corneas of Gal3$^{+/+}$ mice with alkali-burn wounds were incubated in serum-free media in the presence and absence of varying amounts of recombinant Gal3. After a 20–22-h healing period, the remaining wound areas were quantified. The exogenous Gal3 stimulated the rate of wound closure in a concentration-dependent manner in Gal3$^{+/+}$ mice (Figure 2). Overall, the extent of acceleration of re-epithelialization of wounds was 43 and 71% in the presence of 10 and 20 μg/ml Gal3, respectively. It was further demonstrated that the stimulatory effect of Gal3 on the rate of corneal epithelial wound closure can be almost completely abrogated by a competing disaccharide, β-lactose, but not by an irrelevant disaccharide, sucrose. This finding suggested that the lectin CRD was directly involved in the beneficial effect of the exogenous lectin on the wound closure. In corresponding experiments, recombinant Gal1 did not stimulate the corneal epithelial wound closure rate. Subsequent studies have shown that exogenous Gal3 promotes re-epithelialization of wounds in rat corneas(Yano C, et al. IOVS2010; 51:ARVO E-Abstract 371), monkey corneas (Fujii A, et al. IOVS2012; 53:ARVO E-Abstract 3540) as well as in a rat model of dry eye(Sasaki A, et al.IOVS2012; 53:ARVO E-Abstract 2359).

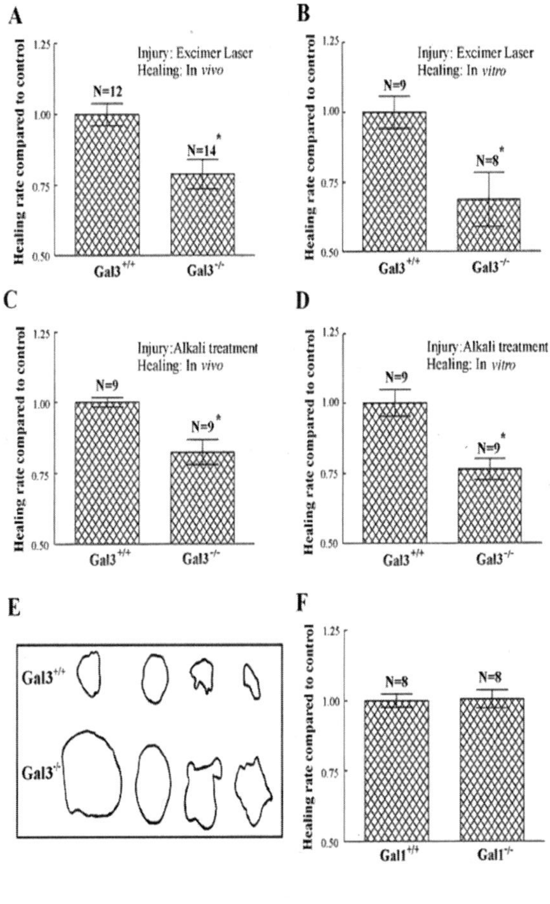

Figure 1. Corneal epithelial wound closure rate is significantly slower in gal3-/- mice. Corneas of gal3$^{+/+}$ and gal3$^{-/-}$ mice with 2-mm transepithelial excimer laser ablations or alkali-burn wounds were allowed to partially heal in vivo for 16–18 h or in vitro for 20–22 h in serum-free media. At the end of the healing period, wound areas were quantified. Regardless of injury by excimer laser (A and B) or by alkali treatment (C and D) or whether corneas were allowed to heal in vivo (A and C) or in vitro (B and D), corneal epithelial wound closure rate

*expressed in mm2/h was significantly slower in gal3$^{-/-}$ mice compared with that in the gal3$^{+/+}$ mice. A value of 1.0 was assigned to the healing rate of gal3$^{+/+}$ corneas. The values for gal3$^{-/-}$ corneas are expressed as a change in healing rate with respect to gal3$^{+/+}$ corneas. Wound closure rates expressed as mm^2/h among different groups were: (a) excimer laser in vivo: gal3$^{+/+}$, 0.076±0.003; gal3$^{-/-}$, 0.060±0.004; (b) excimer laser in vitro: gal3$^{+/+}$, 0.051±0.003; gal3$^{-/-}$, 0.035±0.005;(c) alkali injury in vivo: gal3$^{+/+}$, 0.182±0.003; gal3$^{-/-}$, 0.150±0.008; and (d) alkali injury in vitro: gal3$^{+/+}$, 0.106±0.005; gal3$^{-/-}$, 0.081±0.004. Panel E shows outlines of remaining wound areas from one of the experiments (group: alkali injury, healing in vivo). There was no difference in wound closure rate between galectin-1$^{+/+}$ and galectin-1$^{-/-}$ mice corneas (F). Mean±S.E. of two or more experiments are shown. *, $p<0.05$ compared with the respective gal3$^{+/+}$ group. (Reprinted from (25)).*

2. Role of Gal3 in Intestinal Wound Healing

In the GI tract, Gal3 is highly expressed in enterocytes and subepithelial macrophages (*50*, *51*), where it is thought to play a role in wound healing. In scratch wound-healing assays, treatment of colonic epithelial cells (T84 cells) with Gal3 for 24 hours promoted healing with a 60.4% ± 4.4 reduction in wound width (*20*). The Gal3-induced reduction in wound width was inhibited by a pan inhibitor of galectins, β-lactose, and an anti-Gal3 neutralizing antibody (−9.8% ± 24.8). It is noteworthy that the levels of Gal-3 are reduced in epithelia derived from inflammatory bowel disease (IBD) tissues (*52–54*). Whether the reduced levels of Gal3 is a causative factor in the complications related to wound healing in IBD patients remains to be determined. It is known, however, that in *in vitro* experiments, matrix metalloproteinase-7 (MMP7) which is highly expressed in IBD tissues (*52*, *53*), cleaves Gal3 and the addition of MMP7 to Gal3 abrogated the wound healing and cell migration induced by Gal3 (*20*). These findings led Puthenedam and colleagues (*20*) to propose that cleavage of Gal3 may be one mechanism by which MMP7 inhibits wound healing. This study has significance in understanding delayed wound healing in chronic intestinal diseases such as intestinal ulcers and IBD where MMP7 protein expression is elevated with a concomitant decrease in Gal3 protein expression.

B. Galectin-7

Gal7 is a prototype galectin that forms homodimers (*55*) and therefore can cross-link cell surface receptors. It is preferentially expressed in stratified epithelia, including epidermis, cornea, oral cavity, esophagus and anorectal epithelium (*56*). Major changes in Gal7 level of expression have been observed during re-epithelialization of corneal wounds and in some types of cancer such as skin tumors (*57*). Although Gal7 is considered to be a marker for stratified epithelia (*56*), it has been detected in cilia isolated from cultured human airway as well as on most cilia of multiciliated cells in human airway epithelia primary cultures (*56*, *58*, *59*). Gal7 is also expressed in primary cilia of Madin-Darby canine kidney (MDCK) cells (*60*), LLC-PK_1 (pig kidney), and mpkCCD_{c14} (mouse kidney) cells as well as on cilia in the rat renal proximal tubule (*19*). Indeed, it has been reported that Gal7 plays a role in wound healing of not only stratified epithelium such as that of cornea and skin which lack cilia, but also of simple epithelia such as that of kidney epithelium (*19*).

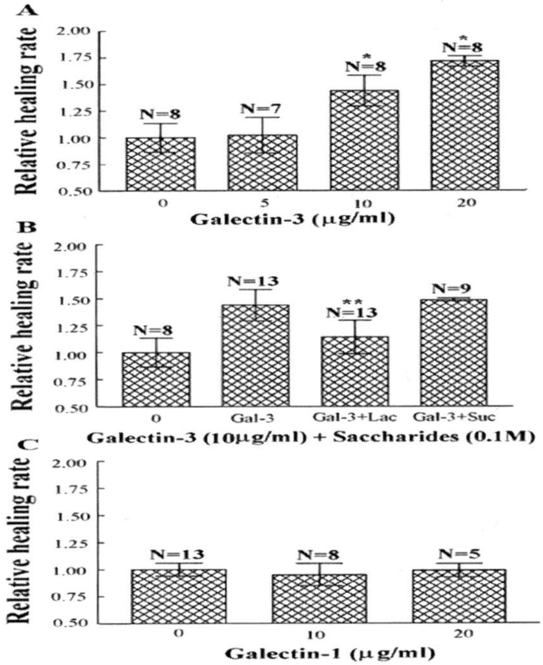

*Figure 2. Exogenous Gal3 stimulates re-epithelialization of corneal wounds. Corneas with 2-mm alkali-burn wounds were allowed to heal in organ culture in serum-free media in the presence and absence of recombinant lectins and saccharides for 20–22 h. At the end of the healing period, wound areas were quantified and compared. A, galectin-3 stimulated corneal epithelial wound closure in a dose-dependent manner.B, the stimulatory effect of exogenous galectin-3 on corneal epithelial wound closure is inhibited by β-lactose, a disaccharide that contains galactose but not by sucrose, which lacks galactose. C, unlike galectin-3, galectin-1 did not accelerate corneal epithelial wound closure in gal3$^{+/+}$ mice. A value of 1.0 was assigned to the healing rate of control corneas incubated in media alone. The value of corneas incubated in media containing galectins and saccharides is expressed as change in the healing rate with respect to the control corneas. Means ± S.E. of two or more experiments are shown. *, $p < 0.05$ compared with the other three groups in panel A; **, $p < 0.05$ compared with gal3 (10 μg/ml) and gal3 + Suc groups in panel B; Lac, β-lactose (0.1 M); Suc, sucrose (0.1 M). (Adapted from (25)).*

1. Role in Corneal Wound Healing

Studies aimed at characterization of the role of Gal7 in re-epithelialization of corneal wounds have shown that the expression level of Gal7 is markedly up-regulated in mouse corneas after injury and that exogenous Gal7 stimulates re-epithelialization of corneal wounds in organ culture specimens (*24*). The stimulatory effect of Gal7 on the rate of corneal epithelial wound closure is partially abrogated by a competing disaccharide, β-lactose, but not by an irrelevant disaccharide, sucrose; again, suggesting that the Gal7CRD is directly involved in the beneficial effect of the exogenous lectin on wound closure.

2. Role in Skin Wound Healing

Recently, Poierer et al (*23*) have produced Gal7 knockout mice and have assessed the role of this lectin in skin wound healing. To assess the extent to which Gal7 may play a role in posttraumatic skin response, superficial scratches were made along the sagittal axis of the tail of*Gal7*$^{+/+}$ and *Gal7*$^{-/-}$ adult mice. Tissue sections of injured healing tails at 24 and 48 h after injury were stained with hematoxylin and eosin and distance between the two wound margins was quantified. In these experiments, the process of wound closure was less efficient in the Gal7$^{-/-}$ mice compared to the Gal7$^{+/+}$ mice. In an ex vivo assay for wound healing, keratinocyte outgrowth from *Gal7*$^{-/-}$ skin explants was also reduced compared with the *Gal7*$^{+/+}$ controls. That Gal7 plays a role in cell migration is further supported by the findings that (i) Gal7 accumulates in podosomes, which are specialized cell–matrix adhesion complexes connecting the ECM to the microfilament network and (ii) distribution of cortactin, an actin-binding protein implicated in membrane ruffle formation, is severely affected in migrating keratinocytes lacking Gal7, suggesting that the formation and/or stabilization of actin-based lamellipodia is abnormal. In wild type animals, Gal7 specifically accumulated at the front of the leading edge keratinocytes where it colocalized with cortactin. In contrast, in the absence of Gal7, diffuse cortactin signal was observed in keratinocytes at the wound margin. In the in vivo model, the rate of wound closure rate was slower in gal7 null mice even when proliferation was blocked by mitomycin-C treatment leading the authors to conclude that as observed with Gal3, Gal7 also promotes re-epithelialization of skin wounds by influencing cell migration rather than cell proliferation.

3. Role of Gal3 in Wound Repair of Polarized Kidney Epithelial Cells

In a recent study, Rondanino et al. (*19*) have demonstrated that Gal7 modulates the length of the primary cilia and wound repair in polarized kidney epithelial cells. To characterize the role of Gal-7 in the regulating the length of the primary cilia and wound repair in kidney epithelial cells, Gal-7 expression was knocked down using shRNA and the length of cilia and wound closure rate were compared in the Gal7 shRNA- and control shRNA-expressing cells. Significantly shorter cilia were observed in Gal-7-shRNA-expressing cells compared to the control cells. In scratch wound assays, 33% reduction in wound healing was detected for Gal-7-shRNA-expressing cells compared to control cells (*19*).

C. Galectins-2 and -4

Gal-2 and Gal-4 are of special importance with respect to the GI tract. Both are expressed in GI tissues, but not in various other tissues including brain, kidney, skeletal muscle, liver, or lung tissues (*61*).

1. Role of Galectins-2 and -4 in Intestinal Epithelial Wound Healing

Exogenous Gal2 has been shown to ameliorate colitis in several models of intestinal inflammation (*62*). In an effort to characterize the role of Gal2 in wound healing, Paclik et al (*21*) assessed the effect of exogenous Gal2 on cell migration using the scratch wound assays. Confluent monolayers of Caco-2 cells were wounded with a razor blade and incubated for 24 hours in the presence or absence of 50 μg/mL Gal2. At the end of the incubation period, the wound closure rate was quantified. Gal-2 significantly enhanced epithelial cell migration over the wound edge (*21*). In these assays, exogenous Gal4 but not Gal1 also promoted wound closure. Unlike Gal3 and Gal7 which promoted cell migration but not cell proliferation of corneal and skin epithelium, both Gal2 and -4 promoted cell migration as well as proliferation of Caco-2 cells suggesting that both processes may be involved in the beneficial effect of these galectins on resealing of disrupted epithelial barrier in GI diseases (*21*).

IV. Molecular Mechanism by Which Galectins Modulate Wound Healing

A. Gal3 Promotes Wound Healing by Activating α3β1-Integrin–Rac1 Signaling

Cell migration is a complex biological process involving (i) extension of cellular protrusions such as lamellipodia or filopodia, (ii) interactions of the surface molecules of the cell protrusions with the permissive ligands in the underlying matrix to form transient cell-matrix adhesions and (iii) actomyosin-mediated cell contraction and forward movement with a concomitant detachment of adhesions at the rear end (*63*). Among the factors that regulate the process of cell migration are transmembrane integrin receptors that mediate cell-matrix adhesions as well asintracellular signaling pathways, leading to cytoskeletal reorganization and cell motility (*63*). Almost all integrins are glycosylated proteins, and, in recent years, a number of studies have revealed that integrin glycans can modulate transmembrane signaling (*64*, *65*). Specifically, it has been demonstrated that interactions between integrin glycans and carbohydrate-binding proteins, galectins, play an essential role in integrin-dependent cell adhesion and migration (*43*, *66–72*). For example, Lagana et al. (*68*) have shown that Gal3 interactions with *N*-acetylglucosaminyltransferase V (GnT-V)-modified N-glycans at the cell surface of mammary carcinoma cells promote α5β1 integrin activation and cell motility. In a recent study aimed at determining the molecular mechanism by which Gal-3 promotes epithelial cell migration during corneal wound closure, we have demonstrated that Gal-3, by interacting with GnT-V-modified complex N-glycans, activates α3β1-integrin–Rac1 signaling to promote formation of lamellipodia in epithelial cells. Based on these findings and other published studies showing that (i) α3β1-integrin-mediated Rac1 activation is essential to promote lamellipodia formation (*73*), (ii) Gal-3 cross-links cell surface receptors (e.g. EGF and TGF-β receptors) by interacting with GnT-V -modified complex N-glycans to promote their signal transduction (*49*) and (iii) clustering of integrins leads to activation of its intracellular signaling (*74–76*), we have proposed a model of Gal-3-mediated epithelial cell migration and re-epithelialization of wounds (*18*) (Figure 3). According to this model, Gal-3, by virtue of its multivalency (*77*), cross-links and clusters α3β1 integrin on the cell surface at the leading edge of the migrating epithelium. The clustering of α3β1 integrin activates FAK and Rac1 and this, in turn, promotes lamellipodia formation, cell migration, and re-epithelialization of wounds.

B. Galectin-3 Promotes Wound Healing by Interacting with N-glycans of Laminin-332

Laminin-332 (Lm332; also known as laminin-5) is a component of basement membranes in the cornea, skin and other stratified squamous epithelial tissues (*78–80*). It is overexpressed at the leading edge of wounds during healing and promotes cell migration (*81–83*) and is thought to play a critical role in re-epithelialization of wounds. A null mutation of Lm332 causes a lethal blistering disease of the skin. Although a substantial portion of laminins is constituted of N-linked glycans, the function Lm332 has been relatively under-investigated in the context of its glycosylation pattern. The glycosyltransferase, GnT-V, catalyzes addition of the β1,6-linked GlcNAc branch that serves as a substrate for polylactosamine, the high affinity ligands for Gal3. By contrast, GnT-III adds GlcNAc to the inner β-linked mannose to form bisecting GlcNAc, which suppresses both further processing by branching enzymes, such as GnT-V, and elongation of *N*-glycans (*84–86*), resulting in down-regulation of interaction with Gal3 with a concomitant reduction in cell migration and cancer metastasis (*87*). Therefore, the sugar chains may switch galectin binding on and off during wound healing as alterations in glycosylation are observed during re-epithelialization of wounds. In an elegant study, Kariya et al. (*83*) have shown that Gal3 bound to Lm332 coated wells, which greatly enhanced Lm332-dependent keratinocyte motility. However, increased cell migration on GnT-III-Lm332 substratum was not induced by exogenous Gal3, because modification of Lm332 by GnT-III reduced its ability to bind to Gal3. These results led authors to suggest that Gal3 may be a cofactor for Lm332-induced cell motility during wound healing and squamous cell carcinoma tumor progression conditions that are associated with GnT-V overexpression (*83*).

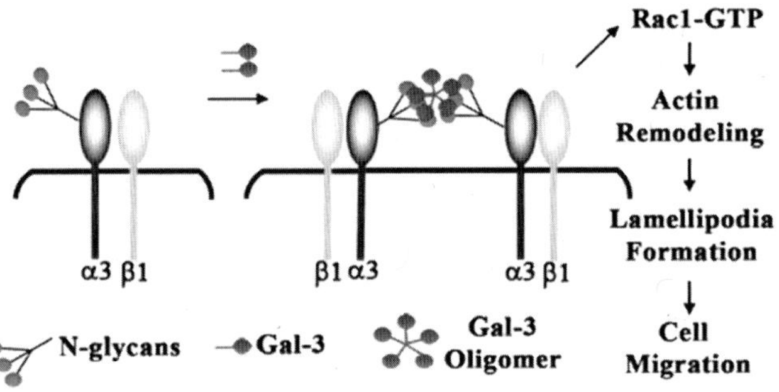

Figure 3. Proposed model of Gal-3-mediated signaling in epithelial cells leading to the formation of lamellipodial protrusions and cell migration.According to this model, Gal-3, by virtue of its multivalency, crosslinks and clusters α3β1 integrin on the cell surface at the leading edge of the migrating epithelium. The clustering of α3β1 integrin activates FAK and Rac1 and this, in turn, promotes lamellipodia formation, cell migration and reepithelialization of wounds. This model is suggested based on our findings that: (1) α3β1 integrin is a major Gal-3-binding partner and a functionblocking anti-α3 integrin mAb blocks the Gal-3-mediated lamellipodia formation, (2) Gal-3 interacts with MGAT5-modified complex N-glycans on α3β1 integrin, (3) Gal-3 activates Rac1, a member of Rho GTPases, and the published findings showing that: (i) Gal-3 cross-links cell surface receptors (e.g. EGF and TGFβ receptors) by interacting with MGAT5-modified complex N-glycans to promote their signal transduction (Partridge et al., 2004), and (ii) α3β1-integrin–Rac1 signaling is essential to promote lamellipodia formation (76). Adapted from (18). (see color insert)

V. Therapeutic Implications

There is an ongoing need for effective treatment of chronic wounds in the elderly, decubitus ulcers, and venous stasis ulcers of the skin.. At present, wound healing related complications in various GI diseases including inflammatory bowel diseases remain a major clinical challenge, as does the treatment of persistent epithelial defects of the cornea.

It has been estimated that in the United States alone in a given year nearly half a million excimer laser keratectomy procedures are performed to obviate the need for eyeglasses and contact lenses to correct myopia (*88*). If conservatively 25–30% of the adult population worldwide is myopic, the potential number of myopia surgeries is enormous. In some cases following excimer laser surgery, there is a delay in epithelial healing, which puts the pre-surgically healthy cornea at risk of developing postoperative haze, infectious keratitis, and ulceration.

Findings that galectins stimulate the re-epithelialization of corneal, dermal, intestinal and kidney wounds have broad implications for developing novel therapeutic strategies for the treatment of nonhealing wounds. The data from various independent laboratories and multiple animal species showing that Gal3 and Gal7 promote re-epithelialization of corneal, skin and/or intestinal wound provide a high level of confidence in the validity of the concept aimed at developing galectins-based drugs to promote healing of chronic wounds.

The biological role of galactins in wound healing as well as the implicit treatment potential become clearer in the context of studies of the effect of growth factors on wound healing. Epidermal growth factor, transforming growth factor-α, fibroblast growth factor, keratinocyte growth factor, and hepatocyte growth factor, all known to stimulate cell proliferation, have been tested for effectiveness in promoting corneal as well as cutaneous epithelial wound healing. Generally, the results are disappointing (*1*, *5*, *89–92*). When compared with the effects displayed with galectins, as described above, the extent of acceleration of re-epithelialization of wounds using growth factors was, according to most findings, far less (*90*, *92*). Additionally it was found that treating corneas with growth factors such as epidermal growth factor resulted in hyperplastic epithelium (*89*, *93*, *94*), a clearly undesirable condition. On the other hand, the lectins Gal3 and Gal7 were found not to induce cell mitosis in healing corneas and skin, respectively, so that galectin-based drugs may be without the drawback of causing epithelial hyperplasticity.

Confirmation of the underlying biological mechanisms of wound healing and concurrent development and trials of treatment modalities derived from these understandings will offer relief and encouragement to myriads of patients and caregivers.

Acknowledgments

I am greatly indebted to my long-time colleague and a senior Research Associate in the lab, Dr. Zhiyi Cao, who performed many of the studies described in this review and also trained all postdoctoral fellows and students who undertook studies on corneal wound healing in the author's laboratory. The work carried out in the author's laboratory was supported by a National Eye Institute (NIH) Grant EY007088, a core grant for vision research P30EY13078, New England Corneal Transplant Fund, Mass Lions Eye Research fund and an unrestricted grant from Research to Prevent Blindness.

References

1. Singer, A. J.; Clark, R. A. Cutaneous wound healing. *N. Engl. J. Med.* **1999**, *341* (10), 738–746.
2. Raja; Sivamani, K.; Garcia, M. S.; Isseroff, R. R. Wound re-epithelialization: Modulating keratinocyte migration in wound healing. *Front. Biosci.* **2007**, *12*, 2849–2868.
3. Price, R. L. *Ophthalmology Annual*; Raven Press, Ltd.: New York, 1989.
4. Fonder, M. A.; et al. Treating the chronic wound: A practical approach to the care of nonhealing wounds and wound care dressings. *J. Am. Acad. Dermatol.* **2008**, *58* (2), 185–206.
5. Eaglstein, W. H.; Falanga, V. Chronic wounds. *Surg. Clin. North Am.* **1997**, *77* (3), 689–700.

6. *Cornea*; Mosby-Year Book, Inc.: St. Louis, MO, 1997.
7. Hostetler, S. G.; Xiang, H.; Gupta, S.; Sen, C.; Gordillo, G. M. Discharge patterns of injury-related hospitalizations with an acute wound in the united states. *Wound Repair Regen* **2006**, *8* (12), 340.
8. Belmont, P. J.; Schoenfeld, A. J.; Goodman, G. Epidemiology of combat wounds in Operation Iraqi Freedom and Operation Enduring Freedom: Orthopaedic burden of disease. *J. Surg. Orthop. Adv.* **2010**, *19* (1), 2–7.
9. Dignass, A. U. Mechanisms and modulation of intestinal epithelial repair. *Inflamm. Bowel Dis.* **2001**, *7* (1), 68–77.
10. Dignass, A. U. *Epithelial Injury and Restitution*; Kluwer Academic: Dordrecht, 2002.
11. Seiler, W. O.; Stahelin, H. B.; Zolliker, R.; Kallenberger, A.; Luscher, N. J. Impaired migration of epidermal cells from decubitus ulcers in cell cultures. A cause of protracted wound healing? *Am. J. Clin. Pathol.* **1989**, *92* (4), 430–434.
12. Hanna, C Effect of IDU on DNA synthesis. During corneal wound healing. *Am. J. Ophthalmol.* **1966**, *61* (2), 279–282.
13. *The Molecular and Cellular Biology of Wound Repair*; Plenum Publishing Corp: New York, 1996.
14. Lauffenburger, D. A.; Horwitz, A. F. Cell migration: A physically integrated molecular process. *Cell* **1996**, *84* (3), 359–369.
15. Hynes, R. O. The extracellular matrix: Not just pretty fibrils. *Science* **2009**, *326* (5957), 1216–1219.
16. Gumbiner, B. M. Cell adhesion: The molecular basis of tissue architecture and morphogenesis. *Cell* **1996**, *84* (3), 345–357.
17. Bornstein, P.; Sage, E. H. Matricellular proteins: Extracellular modulators of cell function. *Curr. Opin. Cell. Biol.* **2002**, *14* (5), 608–616.
18. Saravanan, C.; Liu, F. T.; Gipson, I. K.; Panjwani, N. Galectin-3 promotes lamellipodia formation in epithelial cells by interacting with complex N-glycans on alpha3beta1 integrin. *J. Cell. Sci.* **2009**, *122* (Pt 20), 3684–3693.
19. Rondanino, C; et al. Galectin-7 modulates the length of the primary cilia and wound repair in polarized kidney epithelial cells. *Am. J. Physiol. Renal Physiol.* **2011**, *301* (3), F622–633.
20. Puthenedam, M; et al. Matrilysin-1 (MMP7) cleaves galectin-3 and inhibits wound healing in intestinal epithelial cells. *Inflamm. Bowel Dis.* **2011**, *17* (1), 260–267.
21. Paclik, D.; Lohse, K.; Wiedenmann, B.; Dignass, A. U.; Sturm, A. Galectin-2 and -4, but not galectin-1, promote intestinal epithelial wound healing in vitro through a TGF-beta-independent mechanism. *Inflamm. Bowel Dis.* **2008**, *14* (10), 1366–1372.
22. Kariya, Y.; Kawamura, C.; Tabei, T.; Gu, J. Bisecting GlcNAc residues on laminin-332 down-regulate galectin-3-dependent keratinocyte motility. *J. Biol. Chem.* **2010**, *285* (5), 3330–3340.
23. Gendronneau, G.; et al. Galectin-7 in the control of epidermal homeostasis after injury. **2008**, *19* (12), 5541–5549.
24. Cao, Z.; et al. Galectin-7 as a potential mediator of corneal epithelial cell migration. *Arch. Ophthalmol.* **2003**, *121* (1), 82–86.

25. Cao, Z.; et al. Galectins-3 and -7, but not galectin-1, play a role in re-epithelialization of wounds. *J. Biol. Chem.* **2002**, *277* (44), 42299–42305.
26. Yang, R. Y.; Rabinovich, G. A.; Liu, F. T. Galectins: Structure, function and therapeutic potential. *Expert Rev. Mol. Med.* **2008**, *10*, e17.
27. Leffler, H.; Carlsson, S.; Hedlund, M.; Qian, Y.; Poirier, F. Introduction to galectins. *Glycoconjugate J.* **2004**, *19* (7–9), 433–440.
28. Tadokoro, T.; et al. Involvement of Galectin-3 with vascular cell adhesion molecule-1 in growth regulation of mouse BALB/3T3 cells. *J. Biol. Chem.* **2009**, *284* (51), 35556–35563.
29. Friedrichs, J.; et al. Contributions of galectin-3 and -9 to epithelial cell adhesion analyzed by single cell force spectroscopy. *J. Biol. Chem.* **2007**, *282* (40), 29375–29383.
30. Diskin, S.; Cao, Z.; Leffler, H.; Panjwani, N. The role of integrin glycosylation in galectin-8-mediated trabecular meshwork cell adhesion and spreading. *Glycobiology* **2009**, *19* (1), 29–37.
31. Lagana, A.; et al. Galectin binding to Mgat5-modified N-glycans regulates fibronectin matrix remodeling in tumor cells. *Mol. Cell Biol.* **2006**, *26* (8), 3181–3193.
32. Rabinovich, G. A.; Liu, F. T.; Hirashima, M.; Anderson, A. An emerging role for galectins in tuning the immune response: Lessons from experimental models of inflammatory disease, autoimmunity and cancer. *Scand. J. Immunol.* **2007**, *66* (2–3), 143–158.
33. Liu, F. T.; Rabinovich, G. A. Galectins: Regulators of acute and chronic inflammation. *Ann. N. Y. Acad. Sci.*, *1183*, 158–182.
34. Thijssen, V. L.; et al. Galectin-1 is essential in tumor angiogenesis and is a target for antiangiogenesis therapy. *Proc. Natl. Acad. Sci. U.S.A.* **2006**, *103* (43), 15975–15980.
35. Thijssen, V. L.; Poirier, F.; Baum, L. G.; Griffioen, A. W. Galectins in the tumor endothelium: Opportunities for combined cancer therapy. *Blood* **2007**, *110* (8), 2819–2827.
36. Nangia-Makker, P.; et al. Galectin-3 induces endothelial cell morphogenesis and angiogenesis. *Am. J. Pathol.* **2000**, *156* (3), 899–909.
37. Markowska, A. I.; Liu, F. T.; Panjwani, N. Galectin-3 is an important mediator of VEGF- and bFGF-mediated angiogenic response. *J. Exp. Med.*, *207* (9), 1981–1993.
38. Markowska, A. I.; Jefferies, K. C.; Panjwani, N. Galectin-3 protein modulates cell surface expression and activation of vascular endothelial growth factor receptor 2 in human endothelial cells. *J. Biol. Chem.* **2011**, *286* (34), 29913–29921.
39. Hsieh, SH; et al. Galectin-1, a novel ligand of neuropilin-1, activates VEGFR-2 signaling and modulates the migration of vascular endothelial cells. *Oncogene* **2008**, *27* (26), 3746–3753.
40. Delgado, V. M.; et al. Modulation of endothelial cell migration and angiogenesis: A novel function for the "tandem-repeat" lectin galectin-8. *FASEB J.*, *25* (1), 242–254.

41. Stowell, S. R.; et al. Galectin-1, -2, and -3 exhibit differential recognition of sialylated glycans and blood group antigens. *J. Biol. Chem.* **2008**, *283* (15), 10109–10123.
42. Stillman, B. N.; et al. Galectin-3 and galectin-1 bind distinct cell surface glycoprotein receptors to induce T cell death. *J. Immunol.* **2006**, *176* (2), 778–789.
43. Zhuo, Y.; Chammas, R.; Bellis, S. L. Sialylation of beta1 integrins blocks cell adhesion to galectin-3 and protects cells against galectin-3-induced apoptosis. *J. Biol. Chem.* **2008**, *283* (32), 22177–22185.
44. Sparrow, C. P.; Leffler, H.; Barondes, S. H. Multiple soluble beta-galactoside-binding lectins from human lung. *J. Biol. Chem.* **1987**, *262* (15), 7383–7390.
45. Cueni, L. N.; Detmar, M. Galectin-8 interacts with podoplanin and modulates lymphatic endothelial cell functions. *Exp. Cell Res.* **2009**, *315* (10), 1715–1723.
46. Rabinovich, G. A.; Toscano, M. A.; Jackson, S. S.; Vasta, G. R. Functions of cell surface galectin-glycoprotein lattices. *Curr. Opin. Struct. Biol.* **2007**, *17* (5), 513–520.
47. Garner, O. B.; Baum, L. G. Galectin−glycan lattices regulate cell-surface glycoprotein organization and signalling. *Biochem. Soc. Trans.* **2008**, *36* (Pt 6), 1472–1477.
48. Brewer, C. F.; Miceli, M. C.; Baum, L. G. Clusters, bundles, arrays and lattices: Novel mechanisms for lectin-saccharide-mediated cellular interactions. *Curr. Opin. Struct. Biol.* **2002**, *12* (5), 616–623.
49. Partridge, E. A.; et al. Regulation of cytokine receptors by Golgi N-glycan processing and endocytosis. *Science* **2004**, *306* (5693), 120–124.
50. Lotz, M. M.; et al. Decreased expression of Mac-2 (carbohydrate binding protein 35) and loss of its nuclear localization are associated with the neoplastic progression of colon carcinoma. *Proc. Natl. Acad. Sci. U.S.A.* **1993**, *90* (8), 3466–3470.
51. Brazowski, E.; Dotan, I.; Tulchinsky, H.; Filip, I.; Eisenthal, A. Galectin-3 expression in pouchitis in patients with ulcerative colitis who underwent ileal pouch-anal anastomosis (IPAA). *Pathol. Res. Pract.* **2009**, *205* (8), 551–558.
52. Muller, S.; et al. Galectin-3 modulates T cell activity and is reduced in the inflamed intestinal epithelium in IBD. *Inflamm. Bowel Dis.* **2006**, *12* (7), 588–597.
53. Matsuno, K.; et al. The expression of matrix metalloproteinase matrilysin indicates the degree of inflammation in ulcerative colitis. *J. Gastroenterol.* **2003**, *38* (4), 348–354.
54. Jensen-Jarolim, E.; et al. The constitutive expression of galectin-3 is downregulated in the intestinal epithelia of Crohn's disease patients, and tumour necrosis factor alpha decreases the level of galectin-3-specific mRNA in HCT-8 cells. *Eur. J. Gastroenterol. Hepatol.* **2002**, *14* (2), 145–152.
55. Leonidas, D. D.; et al. Structural basis for the recognition of carbohydrates by human galectin-7. *Biochemistry* **1998**, *37* (40), 13930–13940.

56. Magnaldo, T.; Fowlis, D.; Darmon, M. Galectin-7, a marker of all types of stratified epithelia. *Differentiation* **1998**, *63* (3), 159–168.
57. Saussez, S; Kiss, R. Galectin-7. *Cell. Mol. Life Sci.* **2006**, *63* (6), 686–697.
58. Timmons, P. M.; Colnot, C.; Cail, I.; Poirier, F.; Magnaldo, T. Expression of galectin-7 during epithelial development coincides with the onset of stratification. *Int. J. Dev. Biol.* **1999**, *43* (3), 229–235.
59. Ostrowski, L. E.; et al. A proteomic analysis of human cilia: Identification of novel components. *Mol. Cell. Proteomics* **2002**, *1* (6), 451–465.
60. Poland, P. A.; et al. Identification and characterization of endogenous galectins expressed in Madin Darby canine kidney cells. *J. Biol. Chem.* **2011**, *286* (8), 6780–6790.
61. Huflejt, M. E.; Leffler, H. Galectin-4 in normal tissues and cancer. *Glycoconjugate J.* **2004**, *20* (4), 247–255.
62. Paclik, D.; et al. Galectin-2 induces apoptosis of lamina propria T lymphocytes and ameliorates acute and chronic experimental colitis in mice. *J. Mol. Med. (Berlin)* **2008**, *86* (12), 1395–1406.
63. Ridley, A. J.; et al. Cell migration: Integrating signals from front to back. *Science* **2003**, *302* (5651), 1704–1709.
64. Gu, J; Taniguchi, N. Regulation of integrin functions by N-glycans. *Glycoconjugate J.* **2004**, *21* (1-2), 9–15.
65. Bellis, S. L. Variant glycosylation: An underappreciated regulatory mechanism for beta1 integrins. *Biochim. Biophys. Acta* **2004**, *1663* (1-2), 52–60.
66. Nishi, N; et al. Galectin-8 modulates neutrophil function via interaction with integrin alphaM. *Glycobiology* **2003**, *13* (11), 755–763.
67. Levy, Y.; Ronen, D.; Bershadsky, A. D.; Zick, Y. Sustained induction of ERK, protein kinase B, and p70 S6 kinase regulates cell spreading and formation of F-actin microspikes upon ligation of integrins by galectin-8, a mammalian lectin. *J. Biol. Chem.* **2003**, *278* (16), 14533–14542.
68. Lagana, A.; et al. Galectin binding to Mgat5-modified N-glycans regulates fibronectin matrix remodeling in tumor cells. *Mol. Cell. Biol.* **2006**, *26* (8), 3181–3193.
69. Goetz, J. G.; et al. Concerted regulation of focal adhesion dynamics by galectin-3 and tyrosine-phosphorylated caveolin-1. *J. Cell. Biol.* **2008**, *180* (6), 1261–1275.
70. Friedrichs, J.; Manninen, A.; Muller, D. J.; Helenius, J. Galectin-3 regulates integrin alpha2beta1-mediated adhesion to collagen-I and -IV. *J. Biol. Chem.* **2008**, *283* (47), 32264–32272.
71. Fischer, C.; et al. Galectin-1 interacts with the {alpha}5{beta}1 fibronectin receptor to restrict carcinoma cell growth via induction of p21 and p27. *J. Biol. Chem.* **2005**, *280* (44), 37266–37277.
72. Carcamo, C.; et al. Galectin-8 binds specific beta1 integrins and induces polarized spreading highlighted by asymmetric lamellipodia in Jurkat T cells. *Exp. Cell Res.* **2006**, *312* (4), 374–386.
73. Choma, D. P.; Pumiglia, K.; DiPersio, C. M. Integrin alpha3beta1 directs the stabilization of a polarized lamellipodium in epithelial cells through activation of Rac1. *J. Cell Sci.* **2004**, *117* (Pt 17), 3947–3959.

74. Lock, J. G.; Wehrle-Haller, B.; Stromblad, S. Cell-matrix adhesion complexes: Master control machinery of cell migration. *Semin. Cancer Biol.* **2008**, *18* (1), 65–76.
75. Hynes, R. O. Integrins: Bidirectional, allosteric signaling machines. *Cell* **2002**, *110* (6), 673–687.
76. Guo, W.; Giancotti, F. G. Integrin signalling during tumour progression. *Nat. Rev. Mol. Cell Biol.* **2004**, *5* (10), 816–826.
77. Fred Brewer, C. Binding and cross-linking properties of galectins. *Biochim. Biophys. Acta* **2002**, *1572* (2–3), 255–262.
78. Rousselle, P.; Lunstrum, G. P.; Keene, D. R.; Burgeson, R. E. Kalinin: An epithelium-specific basement membrane adhesion molecule that is a component of anchoring filaments. *J. Cell Biol.* **1991**, *114* (3), 567–576.
79. Colognato, H.; Yurchenco, P. D. Form and function: The laminin family of heterotrimers. *Dev. Dyn.* **2000**, *218* (2), 213–234.
80. Carter, W. G.; Ryan, M. C.; Gahr, P. J. Epiligrin, a new cell adhesion ligand for integrin alpha 3 beta 1 in epithelial basement membranes. *Cell* **1991**, *65* (4), 599–610.
81. Ryan, M. C.; Tizard, R.; VanDevanter, D. R.; Carter, W. G. Cloning of the LamA3 gene encoding the alpha 3 chain of the adhesive ligand epiligrin. Expression in wound repair. *J. Biol. Chem.* **1994**, *269* (36), 22779–22787.
82. Nguyen, B. P.; Gil, S. G.; Carter, W. G. Deposition of laminin 5 by keratinocytes regulates integrin adhesion and signaling. *J. Biol. Chem.* **2000**, *275* (41), 31896–31907.
83. Kariya, Y.; Miyazaki, K. The basement membrane protein laminin-5 acts as a soluble cell motility factor. *Exp. Cell Res.* **2004**, *297* (2), 508–520.
84. Schachter, H. Biosynthetic controls that determine the branching and microheterogeneity of protein-bound oligosaccharides. *Biochem. Cell Biol.* **1986**, *64* (3), 163–181.
85. Gu, J.; Taniguchi, N. Potential of N-glycan in cell adhesion and migration as either a positive or negative regulator. *Cell Adhes. Migr.* **2008**, *2* (4), 243–245.
86. Gu, J.; et al. A mutual regulation between cell-cell adhesion and N-glycosylation: Implication of the bisecting GlcNAc for biological functions. *J. Proteome Res.* **2009**, *8* (2), 431–435.
87. Yoshimura, M.; Nishikawa, A.; Ihara, Y.; Taniguchi, S.; Taniguchi, N. Suppression of lung metastasis of B16 mouse melanoma by N-acetylglucosaminyltransferase III gene transfection. *Proc. Natl. Acad. Sci. U.S.A.* **1995**, *92* (19), 8754–8758.
88. *Refractive Surgery*; Thieme: New York, 1999.
89. Watanabe, K.; Nakagawa, S.; Nishida, T. Stimulatory effects of fibronectin and EGF on migration of corneal epithelial cells. *Invest. Ophthalmol. Vis. Sci.* **1987**, *28* (2), 205–211.
90. Schultz, G.; et al. Growth factors and ocular wound healing. *Eye (London)* **1994**, *8* (Pt 2), 184–187.
91. Kandarakis, A. S.; Page, C.; Kaufman, H. E. The effect of epidermal growth factor on epithelial healing after penetrating keratoplasty in human eyes. *Am. J. Ophthalmol.* **1984**, *98* (4), 411–415.

92. *Principle and Practice of Ophthalmology*; W.B. Saunders Co.: Philadelphia, 2000.
93. Singh, G.; Foster, C. S. Epidermal growth factor in alkali-burned corneal epithelial wound healing. *Am. J. Ophthalmol.* **1987**, *103* (6), 802–807.
94. Singh, G.; Foster, C. S. Gross factors in treatment of nonhealing corneal ulcers and recurrent erosions. *Cornea* **1989**, *8* (1), 45–53.

Editors' Biographies

Anatole A. Klyosov, Ph.D., D.Sc.

Anatole A. Klyosov, Ph.D., D.Sc., is Chief Scientist and founder of Galectin Therapeutics, and a co-inventor of the patented technology of the public Company based on galectin blockers, which often control angiogenesis, inflammation, immune response in humans. Before that, Dr. Klyosov was Professor of Biochemistry at Harvard Medical School for eight years, and also Vice President of Research and Development of a biotechnology and polymer engineering public company in the Boston area. Before that, he was Professor and Head of the Carbohydrates Research Laboratory at the Institute of Biochemistry, Russian Academy of Sciences. Dr. Klyosov is Fellow, the World Academy of Art and Science (since 1989), holds over 60 U.S. and international patents, has published more than 300 peer-reviewed scientific articles, written books on enzymes, carbohydrates, polymers, and biotechnology, and edited three books, *Enzyme Engineering*, *Carbohydrates in Drug Design*, and *Galectins*. Dr. Klyosov earned his Ph.D. and D.Sc. degrees in physical chemistry from Moscow University.

Peter G. Traber, MD

Peter G. Traber, M.D. is President, Chief Executive Officer, and Chief Medical Officer of Galectin Therapeutics, Inc (NASDAQ: GALT), a development stage biotechnology company that is applying its leadership in galectin science and drug development for therapies in fibrotic disease and cancer. Drug candidates based on complex carbohydrates target galectin proteins which are key mediators of biologic and pathologic function. His previous positions include President and CEO of Baylor College of Medicine, Chief Medical Officer and Senior Vice President for Clinical Development and Medical Affairs for GlaxoSmithKline, and Chief Executive Officer, Chair of Medicine and Chief of Gastroenterology at The University of Pennsylvania School of Medicine. In addition to leadership, education, and clinical medicine, Dr. Traber managed a productive molecular biology laboratory that elucidated fundamental mechanisms of intestinal cell transcription and differentiation. Dr. Traber has a B.S. degree in chemical engineering from the University of Michigan, a M.D. degree from Wayne State School of Medicine, and a certificate from the Wharton School of Business of the University of Pennsylvania. He is board certified in Internal Medicine and Gastroenterology. He previously served on the Board of the Federal Reserve Bank of Dallas, Houston Branch and Tanox, Inc. Board of Directors.

Indexes

Author Index

Subject Index

H

I

K

L